Diabetes and Hyperglycemia: A Clinician's Guide

Diabetes and Hyperglycemia: A Clinician's Guide

Edited by Jennifer Witherspoon

AMERICAN
MEDICAL PUBLISHERS
www.americanmedicalpublishers.com

American Medical Publishers,
41 Flatbush Avenue,
1st Floor, New York,
NY 11217, USA

Visit us on the World Wide Web at:
www.americanmedicalpublishers.com

ISBN: 978-1-63927-112-2

Cataloging-in-Publication Data

Diabetes and hyperglycemia : a clinician's guide / edited by Jennifer Witherspoon.
p. cm.
Includes bibliographical references and index.
ISBN 978-1-63927-112-2
1. Diabetes. 2. Hyperglycemia. 3. Diabetes--Treatment--Guidebooks.
4. Hyperglycemia--Treatment--Guidebooks. I. Witherspoon, Jennifer.
RC660 .D53 2022
616.462--dc23

Table of Contents

Preface

The main aim of this book is to educate learners and enhance their research focus by presenting diverse topics covering this vast field. This is an advanced book which compiles significant studies by distinguished experts in the area of analysis. This book addresses successive solutions to the challenges arising in the area of application, along with it; the book provides scope for future developments.

Diabetes is the condition of high blood sugar levels for a long period. It causes symptoms such as frequent urination, increased hunger and thirst, etc. Various serious complications such as cardiovascular disease, chronic kidney disease, and stroke can occur due to high blood sugar levels. One of the most complex conditions that occurs due to diabetes is hyperglycemia. It is a condition where an excessive amount of glucose circulates in the blood plasma. It is majorly caused by diabetes mellitus and acute stress such as stroke. The growth hormone, glucagon, cortisol and catecholamines may also cause hyperglycemia. Certain medications such as corticosteroids, octreotide, statins and niacin, increase the risk of hyperglycemia. It can also occur due to insulin resistance which obstructs the process of the conversion of glucose into glycogen and makes it impossible to be removed from the blood. The general symptoms of hyperglycemia include blurred vision, fatigue, restlessness, weight loss, dry and itchy skin, polyuria and polydipsia. Its treatment requires the reduction of the underlying cause like diabetes. Acute hyperglycemia is treated by giving insulin while severe hyperglycemia is treated with oral hypoglycemic therapy. This book provides comprehensive insights into hyperglycemia. The book presents researches and studies performed by experts across the globe. Those in search of information to further their knowledge will be greatly assisted by this book.

It was a great honour to edit this book, though there were challenges, as it involved a lot of communication and networking between me and the editorial team. However, the end result was this all-inclusive book covering diverse themes in the field.

Finally, it is important to acknowledge the efforts of the contributors for their excellent chapters, through which a wide variety of issues have been addressed. I would also like to thank my colleagues for their valuable feedback during the making of this book.

Editor

1

Aldose Reductase Inhibitor Protects against Hyperglycemic Stress by Activating Nrf2-Dependent Antioxidant Proteins

Kirtikar Shukla, Pabitra Bikash Pal, Himangshu Sonowal, Satish K. Srivastava, and Kota V. Ramana

Department of Biochemistry and Molecular Biology, University of Texas Medical Branch, Galveston, TX 77555, USA

Correspondence should be addressed to Kota V. Ramana; kvramana@utmb.edu

Academic Editor: Hao Wu

We have shown earlier that pretreatment of cultured cells with aldose reductase (AR) inhibitors prevents hyperglycemia-induced mitogenic and proinflammatory responses. However, the effects of AR inhibitors on Nrf2-mediated anti-inflammatory responses have not been elucidated yet. We have investigated how AR inhibitor fidarestat protects high glucose- (HG-) induced cell viability changes by increasing the expression of Nrf2 and its dependent phase II antioxidant enzymes. Fidarestat pretreatment prevents HG (25 mM)-induced Thp1 monocyte viability. Further, treatment of Thp1 monocytes with fidarestat caused a time-dependent increase in the expression as well as the DNA-binding activity of Nrf2. In addition, fidarestat augmented the HG-induced Nrf2 expression and activity and also upregulated the expression of Nrf2-dependent proteins such as hemeoxygenase-1 (HO1) and NQO1 in Thp1 cells. Similarly, treatment with AR inhibitor also induced the expression of Nrf2 and HO1 in STZ-induced diabetic mice heart and kidney tissues. Further, AR inhibition increased the HG-induced expression of antioxidant enzymes such as SOD and catalase and activation of AMPK-α1 in Thp1 cells. Our results thus suggest that pretreatment with AR inhibitor prepares the monocytes against hyperglycemic stress by overexpressing the Nrf2-dependent antioxidative proteins.

1. Introduction

Hyperglycemia is a major contributor to inflammation, apoptosis, profound vasodilation, tissue damage, and dysfunction in patients with diabetes mellitus [1]. The cytotoxicity of hyperglycemia is mediated by the increase in reactive oxygen species (ROS) which activate NF-κB and AP1 that results in the transcription of inflammatory cytokines [2]. Our recent studies indicate that inhibition of the polyol pathway enzyme aldose reductase (AR) prevents cytokine- and hyperglycemia-induced increase in inflammatory markers in macrophages, vascular cells, and diabetic mice [3, 4] by preventing the activation of NF-κB- and AP1-induced proinflammatory signals [3, 5]. We have shown that preincubation with AR inhibitor prevents hyperglycemia- and cytokine-induced proliferation of vascular cells and apoptosis of macrophages [6–8]. While these studies indicate that inhibition of AR could prevent oxidative stress-induced inflammatory response, the mechanism(s) by which inhibition of AR prepares the cells against oxidative stress is not known.

Previous studies indicate that transcription factor nuclear factor-erythroid-2-related factor 2 (Nrf2) regulates a battery of cytoprotective genes which maintain cellular redox homeostasis. Nrf2 binds to the antioxidant response element (ARE) and transcriptionally regulates the gene expression of several antioxidant and phase II detoxifying enzymes including hemeoxygenase 1 (HO1), NAD(P)H-quinone dehydrogenase 1 (NQO1), γ-glutamylcysteine synthetase (GCS), glutathione *S*-transferases (GSTs), and AR [9]. Generally, under nonstress conditions, Nrf2 complexes with an adaptor protein, Keap1, which is a regulator of the proteasomal degradation of Nrf2. However, under stress conditions, Nrf2 dissociates from Keap1 and translocates to the nucleus and transcribes the genes responsible for defense against stress. Thus, it has been well established that activation of the Nrf2 pathway in response to oxidative stress protects the cells and tissues from oxidative injury [10].

Although our previous studies indicate that AR inhibition prevents hyperglycemia-induced NF-κB-dependent inflammatory signals, it is not known how AR inhibition increases the resistance of cells to withstand oxidative stress stimuli initiated by hyperglycemia. Therefore, in this study, we examined our hypothesis that AR inhibition promotes the activation of Nrf2-mediated cytoprotective pathways that protect cells against hyperglycemic stress. Our results suggest that AR inhibitor fidarestat increases the expression as well as the DNA-binding activity of Nrf2 in Thp1 monocytes. In addition, fidarestat increased the expression of Nrf2 downstream target proteins such as HO1 and NQO1 in Thp1 cells and heart and kidney tissues of STZ-induced diabetic mice. AR inhibitor also prevented the expression of antioxidant enzymes such as SOD and catalase. Collectively, our results demonstrate that AR inhibition protects the cells against hyperglycemia-induced changes in the cell viability by activating Nrf2/HO1-mediated antioxidative pathway, which could also account for the anti-inflammatory effects of AR inhibitors in diabetes.

2. Materials and Methods

2.1. Materials. RPMI-1640, penicillin/streptomycin, and fetal bovine serum (FBS) were purchased from Invitrogen. Antibodies against Nrf2 were obtained from Santa Cruz. Antibodies against KEAP1, HO1, NQO1, phospho-AMPK-α1, AMPK-α1, GAPDH, and histone H3 were purchased from Cell Signal Inc. Fidarestat was obtained from Livwel Therapeutics Inc., USA. 3-(4,5-dimethylthiazol-2-yl)-2,5-diphenyltetrazolium-bromide (MTT) and other reagents used in Western blot analysis were obtained from Sigma. HO1 assay kit was purchased from Abcam. Nrf2 transcription factor binding assay and superoxide dismutase activity assay kits were purchased from Cayman Chemicals. Catalase activity was determined spectrophotometrically using hydrogen peroxide (30%) (Sigma-Aldrich).

2.2. Cell Culture and Treatment. Human Thp1 monocytic cells were obtained from the American Type Culture Collection (ATCC) and cultured in RPMI-1640 medium supplemented with 10% FBS and penicillin/streptomycin at 37°C in a humidified atmosphere of 5% CO_2. Prior to treatment, cells were serum starved in the respective medium containing 0.1% FBS ± fidarestat (10 μM) for 14 h and further stimulated with high glucose (25 mM; 19.5 mM glucose was added to 5.5 mM glucose containing media) for different time intervals.

2.3. Cell Viability. Cell viability was determined using a standard MTT assay [11]. Briefly, Thp1 cells were growth arrested in 0.1% FBS containing RPMI medium. Cells were preincubated with fidarestat (10 μM) for overnight (14 h) at37°C followed by incubation with HG (25 mM) for another 48 h. At the end of incubation period, cells were incubated with 10 μl MTT reagent (5 mg/ml) for 4 h at 37°C. The formazan crystals formed by the viable cells were solubilized by the addition of 100 μl DMSO. Absorbance was measured at 570 nm using a microplate reader. Cell viability was also examined by counting the live and dead cells using a hemocytometer [6]. AR activity (mU/mg protein) was measured spectrophotometrically using glyceraldehyde as a substrate [6]. Nrf2 DNA binding activity was determined by Nrf2 transcription factor assay kit as per the manufacturer's instructions (Cayman Chemical).

2.4. Immunoblot Analysis. Nuclear and cytoplasmic proteins from the treated cells were isolated using a nuclear extraction kit (Cayman Chemicals). Protein concentration in the extracts was measured with Bradford reagent (Bio-Rad). Equal amount of proteins were subjected to 12% SDS-PAGE electrophoresis followed by Western blot analysis using specific antibodies against Nrf2, Keap1, HO1, NQO1, AMPK, histone H3, and GAPDH. The antigen-antibody complexes were detected by enhanced Super Signal West Pico Chemiluminescent Substrate (Thermo Scientific). Membranes were stripped with Restore TM PLUS stripping buffer (Thermo Scientific) and used for reprobing with other antibodies or loading controls.

2.5. Ablation of Nrf2 by siRNA. Thp1 cells cultured in RPMI 1640 medium containing 10% FBS were incubated with Nrf2-siRNA (120 nM) or siRNA negative control with HiPerFect Transfection Reagent as per the manufacturer's instructions (Qiagen, USA). The cells were incubated in a humidified CO_2 incubator for 48 h at 37°C. Silencing of Nrf2 was determined by Western blotting.

2.6. Quantitative RT-PCR Analysis of HO1 mRNA. Total RNA was isolated from the treated cells using TRIzol reagent and was quantified by using a nanodrop spectrophotometer (NanoDrop Technologies). TaqMan reverse transcription reagents kit was used for the synthesis of cDNA from total RNA (Life Technologies). Q-PCR amplifications (performed in triplicate) were performed by using 1 μl of cDNA using the iTaq Universal SYBR Green Supermix (Bio-Rad). Housekeeping gene *GAPDH* was used as a normalizer. ABI Prism 7500 Sequence detection system using forward: 5$'$-C GGGCCAGCAACAAAGTG-3$'$, and reverse: 5$'$-CCAGAA AGCTGAGTGTAAGGACC-3$'$ was used for qPCR analysis of *HO1* gene.

2.7. Determination of HO1 and Nrf2 in STZ-Induced Diabetic Mice. Seven-week-old C57BL/6 male mice were purchased from Envigo. Diabetes was induced in mice by injecting a single dose of streptozotocin (STZ; 165 mg/kg, i.p.) and blood glucose levels were measured by a glucometer (True Metrix). The mice with blood glucose levels >400 mg/dl were selected and randomly divided into diabetic and diabetic + fidarestat groups. Fidarestat (10 mg/kg/day, i.p.) was administered to diabetic mice, and the animals were euthanized on day 3.

2.8. Statistical Analysis. Data are presented as mean ± SD. The p values were determined using the unpaired Student's t-test (GraphPad Prism software) and a p value of <0.05 considered as statistically significant.

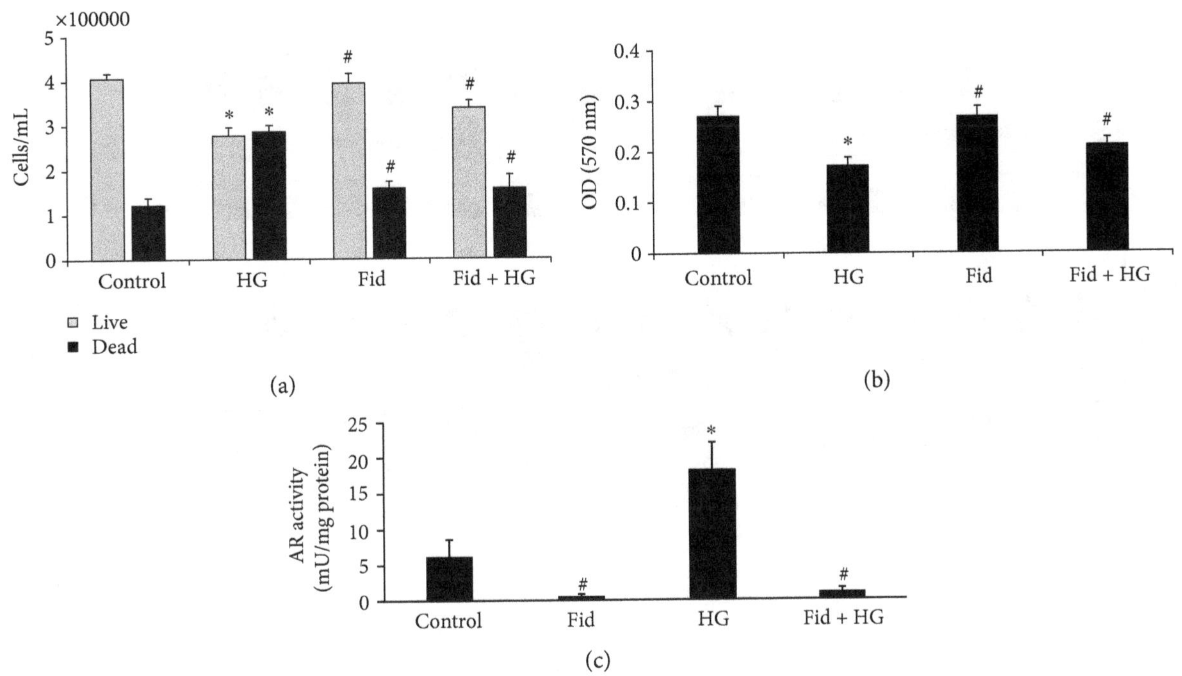

FIGURE 1: AR inhibition prevents HG-induced Thp1 cell viability. Thp1 cells (3000 cells/well) were pretreated with fidarestat for overnight followed by incubation with HG (25 mM) for another 48 h. (a) Cell viability was determined by MTT assay. (b) Live and dead cell counts were determined by staining with trypan blue using a hemocytometer. (c) AR activity was determined spectrophotometrically using glyceraldehyde as a substrate. Data represent mean ± SD ($n = 5$). $^*p < 0.01$ when compared with control, and $\#p < 0.05$ when compared with the HG-treated group.

3. Results

3.1. AR Inhibition Prevents HG-Induced Thp1 Cells Viability. The effect of AR inhibition on HG-induced Thp1 cells viability was examined by measuring the live and dead cell counts as well as MTT absorbance. The data shown in the Figure 1(a) indicates that HG treatment of Thp1 cells decreased the number of live cells and increased the number of dead cells indicating that HG decreases Thp1 cell viability. However, pretreatment of Thp1 cells with AR inhibitor prevented the HG-induced decrease in the Thp1 cell viability. Similar results were observed when we measured the cell viability by MTT assay (Figure 1(b)). The data shown in Figure 1(c) also indicates that AR activity was significantly increased in the HG-treated Thp1 cells and fidarestat prevented it. These results thus suggest that AR inhibition prevents HG-induced decrease in the cell viability of Thp1 cells.

3.2. AR Inhibitor Increases the Expression of Nrf2. To examine how pretreatment of cells with AR inhibitor prevents HG-induced decrease in Thp1 cell viability, we examined the effect of AR inhibitor on the expression of Nrf2. Pretreatment of Thp1 cells with fidarestat alone or HG alone induced Nrf2 expression in a time-dependent manner. Further, preincubation of cells with fidarestat followed by incubation with HG significantly augmented the HG-induced increase in the expression of Nrf2 (Figure 2(a)). Similarly, treatment of Thp1 cells with HG decreased the expression of Keap1, a negative regulator of Nrf2 and preincubation with fidarestat, followed by HG decreased the expression of the Keap1 protein (Figure 2(a)). We next examined the effect of AR inhibitor on Nrf2 DNA binding activity in Thp1 cells. Nrf2 transcriptional activity increased in the fidarestat-treated Thp1 cells in a time-dependent manner as compared to that in control cells (Figure 2(b)). Further, fidarestat augmented the HG-induced Nrf2 transcriptional activity in Thp1 cells. These results thus suggest that preincubation of cells with AR inhibitor prepares the cells against oxidative insult by inducing the expression of Nrf2.

3.3. AR Inhibition Increases the Antioxidative Protein Expressions in Thp1 Cells. We next examined the effect of AR inhibitor on the expression of various Nrf2-dependent antioxidative proteins. Results shown in Figure 3(a) indicate that fidarestat alone or HG alone increased the levels of antioxidant proteins such as HO1 and NQO1 in Thp1 cells. Further, pretreatment with fidarestat followed by HG synergistically increased the HO1 and NQO1 protein expressions in Thp1 cells (Figure 3(a)). Similarly, AR inhibitor also increased the levels of HO1 in Thp1 cell lysates (Figure 3(b)). Furthermore, mRNA expression of *HO1* increased significantly in cells treated with HG in the presence of fidarestat as compared to HG- or fidarestat-treated cells (Figure 3(c)). Furthermore, AR inhibitor also significantly increased the HG-induced SOD as well as catalase activities in Thp1 cells (Figures 3(d) and 3(e)). Thus, our results indicate that pretreatment of Thp1 cells with fidarestat enhances the antioxidant status of the cells as a defense against hyperglycemic stress.

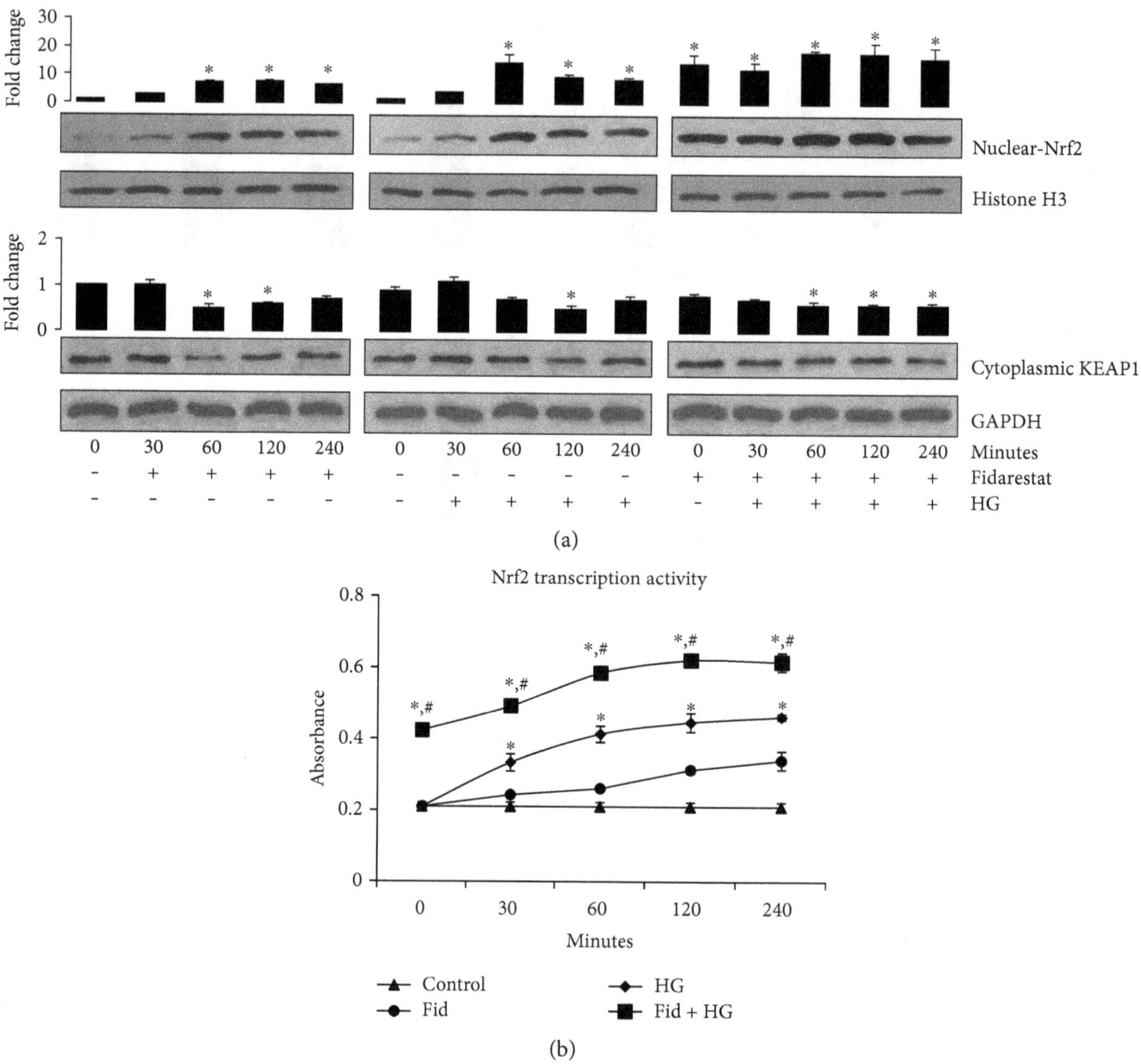

FIGURE 2: AR inhibition augments HG- induced Nrf2 activation in Thp1 cells. Thp1 cells were treated with fidarestat (10 μM) for indicated times. Subsequently, the cells were also pretreated with fidarestat for overnight followed by incubation with HG for 30, 60, 120, and 240 minutes. Equal amounts of nuclear and cytosolic proteins were subjected to Western blot analysis for the expression of Nrf2 and Keap1, respectively. Histone H3 and GAPDH served as loading controls for nuclear and cytosolic protein extract, respectively. A representative blot from three independent analyses is shown (a). Nrf2 transcription factor assay using the nuclear protein of treated Thp1 cells was carried out using an ELISA kit (b). Data represent mean ± SD ($n = 5$). $^*p < 0.05$ when compared with control, and $\#p < 0.05$ when compared with the HG-treated group.

3.4. Effect of AR Inhibitor on HG-Induced Cell Viability in Nrf-2-Knockdown Thp1 Cells. To examine the effect of Nrf2 on AR-regulated cell growth, we determined the Thp1 cell viability in the Nrf2-siRNA knockdown cells in the absence and presence of fidarestat. Incubation of Nrf2 knockdown cells with HG (25 mM) significantly increased cell death of Thp1 cells when compared to that of control cells (Figure 4). Further, fidarestat prevented the HG-induced Thp1 cell death in control siRNA-transfected cells but not in the Nrf2-siRNA-transfected cells, suggesting that fidarestat prevents Thp1 cell viability by increasing the Nrf2 expression.

3.5. AR Inhibitor Increases the Expression of Nrf2 and HO1 in Mouse Diabetic Heart and Kidney Tissues. We next examined the effect of fidarestat on the expression of antioxidant proteins, HO1, and Nrf2 in STZ-induced diabetic mouse heart and kidney tissues. Similar to data shown in the Thp1 cells, AR-inhibitor (fidarestat) also augmented the STZ-induced increase in the expression of Nrf2, HO1, and NQO1 in the heart and kidney homogenates of mice (Figure 5).

3.6. AR Inhibitor Regulates HG-Induced Phosphorylation of AMPK-α1 in Thp1 Cells. Since AMPK-α1 activation has been shown to activate Nrf2 signals, we next investigated the effect of fidarestat on HG-induced AMPK-α1 activation in Thp1 cells. Our results shown in Figure 6(a) indicate that fidarestat increased the HG-induced phosphorylation of AMPK-α1 in Thp1 cells. Further, to investigate the effect of Nrf2

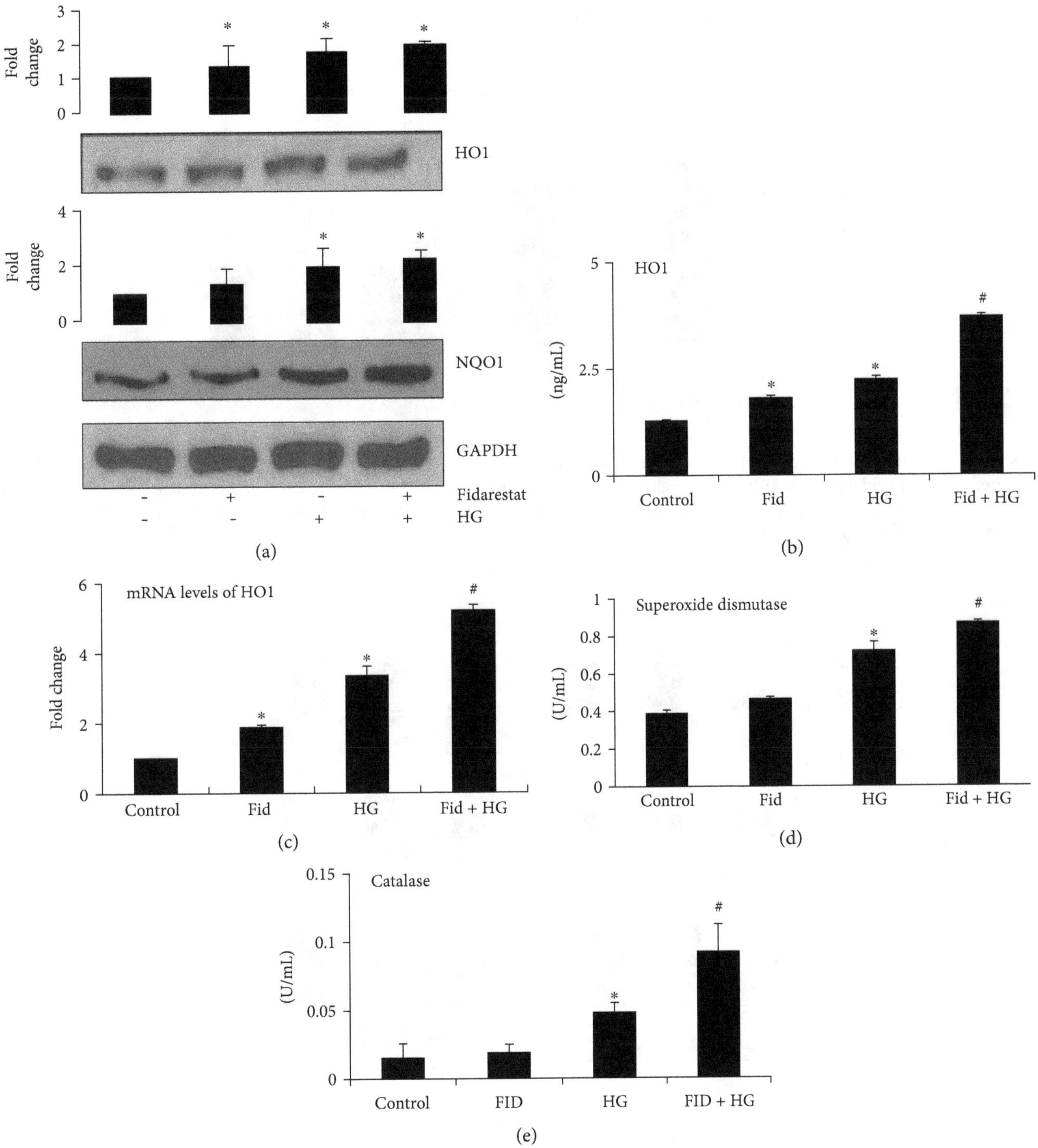

FIGURE 3: AR inhibitor induces the expression of Nrf2-dependent antioxidant enzymes in HG-treated Thp1 cells. Thp1 cells were pretreated with fidarestat for 14 h followed by incubation with HG (25 mM) for another 24 h. Equal amounts of proteins were subjected to Western blot analysis for the expression of HO1 and NQO1. Fold changes were determined after normalizing with loading control GAPDH. A representative blot from three independent analyses is shown (a). The HO1 levels in the cell lysates were determined by ELISA (b). The mRNA levels of the *HO1* gene in Thp1 cells were determined by RT-PCR as described in Section 2 (c). SOD and catalase activities were analyzed in Thp1 cell lysates by using specific kits as per the manufacturer's instructions (d and e). Data represent mean ± SD ($n = 5$). $^*p < 0.01$ versus control; $\#p < 0.05$ when compared with the HG-treated group or the Fidarestat alone-treated group.

on AMPK-α1 activation, Nrf2-siRNA-transfected Thp1 cells were stimulated with HG ± fidarestat and examined AMPK-α1 activation. The results shown in Figure 6 indicate that HG-induced increase in the phosphorylation of Nrf2 in the absence of fidarestat. However, pretreatment of fidarestat to the Nrf2 knockdown cells did not show any

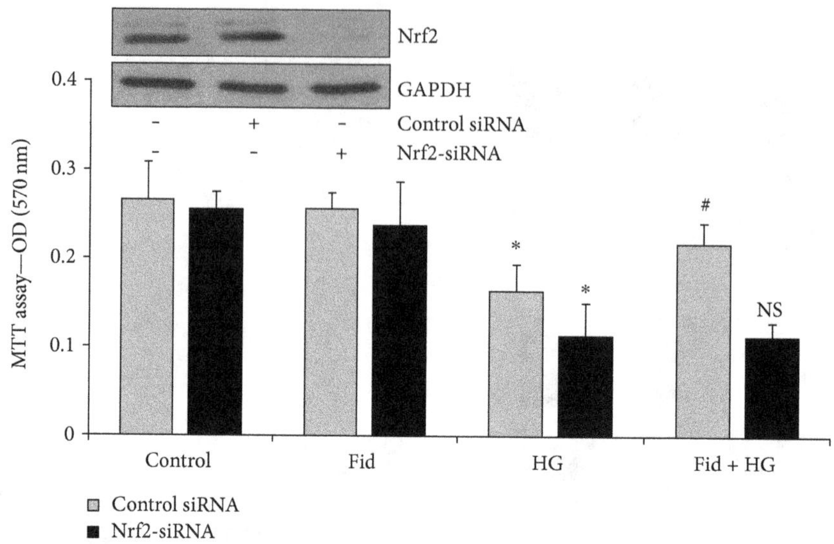

FIGURE 4: AR-inhibition regulates cell viability of Thp1 cells via Nrf2 activation. The control-siRNA and Nrf2-siRNA-transfected Thp1 cells were treated with HG ± fidarestat for 48 h, and the cell viability was determined by MTT assay. Data represent in mean ± SD ($n = 6$). $^*p < 0.01$ versus control; $\#p < 0.01$ versus HG; NS = nonsignificant versus HG-treated cells. The inset shows Western blots for Nrf2 in control and siRNA-transfected cells. GAPDH = loading control.

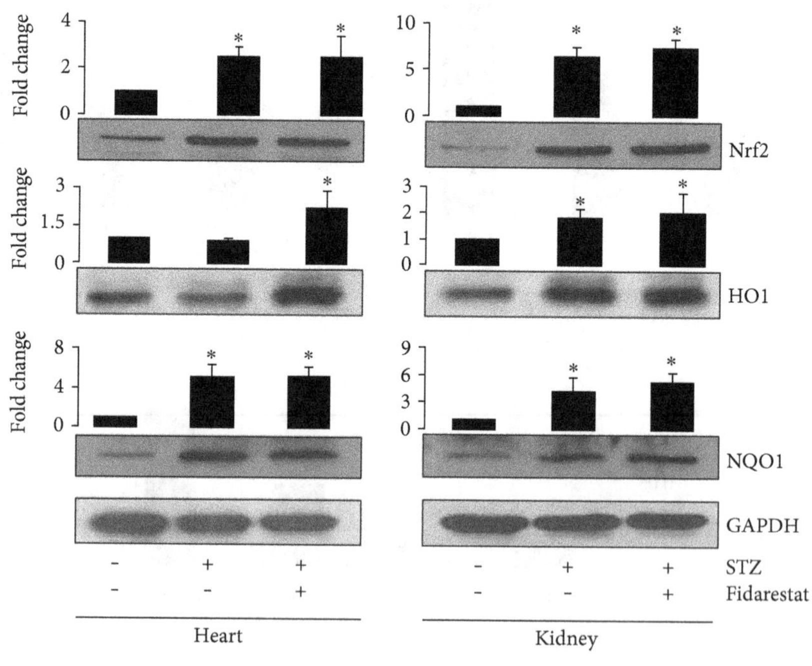

FIGURE 5: AR inhibitor induces the expression of Nrf2 and its dependent antioxidant enzymes in STZ-induced diabetic mice tissues. STZ-induced diabetic mice were treated without or with fidarestat as described in Section 2. An equal amount of proteins from the heart and kidney homogenates were subjected to Western blot analysis using specific antibodies against Nrf2, HO1, and NQO1. Fold changes were determined after normalizing with loading control, GAPDH. A representative blot from three independent analyses is shown. $^*p < 0.05$ when compared with control, and $\#p < 0.05$ when compared with the HG-treated group.

significant differences in the phosphorylation of AMPK-α1. These results suggest that by regulating the Nrf2-mediated AMPK-α1, AR inhibitor could modulate hyperglycemic stress in Thp1 cells.

4. Discussion

We have shown previously that pretreatment with AR inhibitors prevents cytokine-, chemokine-, HG-, and LPS-induced

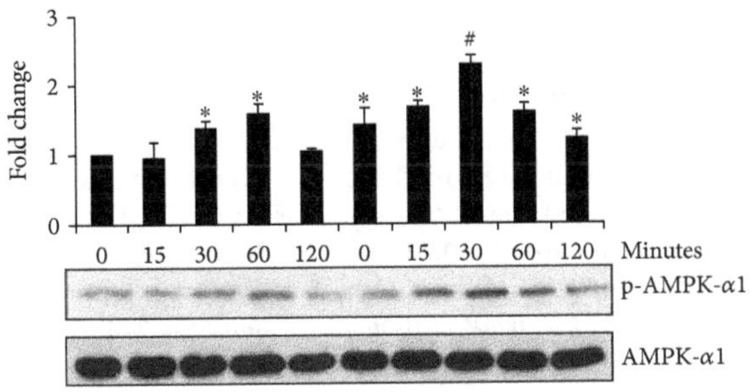

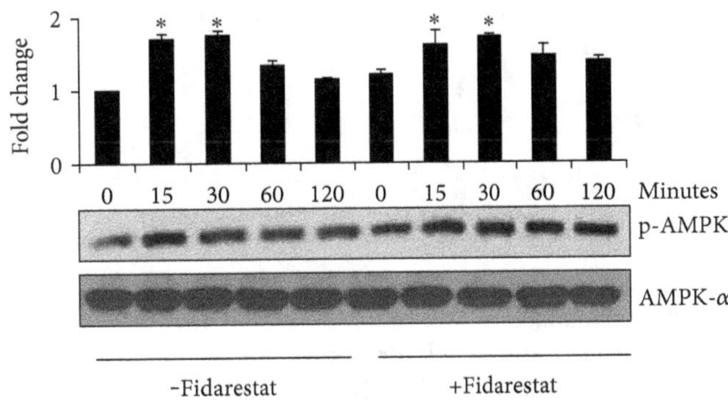

FIGURE 6: AR inhibition increases HG-induced phosphorylation of AMPK-α1 in Thp1 cells. (a) The Thp1 cells and (b) control and Nrf2-SiRNA-transfected cells were pretreated with fidarestat for overnight followed by incubation with HG for 15, 30, 60, and 120 min. Equal amounts of cytosolic proteins were subjected to Western blot analysis using antibodies against total and phospho-AMPK-α1. Fold changes were determined after normalizing with total AMPK-α1. A representative blot from three independent analyses is shown. $^*p < 0.05$ when compared with control, and $\#p < 0.05$ when compared with the HG-treated group.

inflammatory response mediated by NF-κB in various cellular studies [12–15]. Further, AR inhibitors prevent NF-κB-mediated proinflammatory pathways in vitro and in vivo models of hyperglycemia [12, 16]. However, it is not clear how pretreatment with AR inhibitors prepares cells against oxidative stress and activates Nrf2-mediated anti-inflammatory pathways. In this study, we have demonstrated that fidarestat induces Nrf2-mediated antioxidative and anti-inflammatory pathways in Thp1 monocytic cells. Further, fidarestat also augmented the HG-induced expression of Nrf2 and its downstream targets. These results suggest that preincubation with AR inhibitors prepares the cells to defend against pathological effects of hyperglycemia.

Nrf2 transcription factor regulates the expression of a number of cytoprotective antioxidative genes including *SOD*, catalase, *GSTs*, *AR*, *HO1*, *NQO1*, and so forth [9, 10]. Several studies indicate that antioxidants overexpress the Nrf2 pathway as a defense mechanism against various oxidative insults including hyperglycemia [17, 18]. Further, antioxidants such as flavonoids, triterpenoids, quinols, and tBHQ increase the activation of Nrf2 and protect against diabetes-induced nephropathy [19–23]. In addition, Nrf2 null mice are susceptible to the STZ-induced kidney injury [24]. Another study indicates that sulforaphane prevents metabolic dysfunction in hyperglycemia by increasing the expression of the Nrf2 pathway in human endothelial cells [25, 26]. Similarly, curcumin has been shown to decrease insulin resistance, improve pancreatic cell function, and reduce hyperglycemia-induced inflammatory response and complications by activating the Nrf2 pathway [27–29]. These studies suggest the significance of Nrf2 activation in diabetes complications. Consistent with these studies, our current data also suggest that treatment of Thp1 cells with fidarestat augmented the HG-induced Nrf2 activity indicating that fidarestat increases antioxidative balance in the cells and thereby regulates HG-induced cell viability. Furthermore, we have evaluated the effect of fidarestat on HG-induced Thp1 cell viability in Nrf2-ablated cells. Our results demonstrate that AR inhibitor prevented the HG-induced cell death in control cells but not in Nrf2-ablated cells suggesting that Nrf2-mediated antioxidative pathways are required for the actions of AR inhibitor.

Increased expression of Nrf2 leads to increased expression of enzymes linked to antioxidative (NQO1, GSTs, catalase, SOD) and anti-inflammatory (HO1, AR) functions that counteract against oxidative insults [10, 30]. HO1 is an anti-inflammatory protein, and its overexpression has been shown to prevent various inflammatory complications including diabetes [31]. Specifically, HO1 has been shown to protect against HG-induced retinal endothelial cells damage and also prevent vascular inflammatory response in hyperglycemia [32–34]. In this study, our results indicate that fidarestat increases the expression of HO1 and augments HG-induced HO1 in Thp1 cells as well as kidney and heart tissues of STZ-induced diabetic mice suggesting that anti-inflammatory activities of AR inhibition may be through activation of HO1. In addition, our studies also suggest that AR inhibitor increases the expression of SOD and catalase in Thp1 cells and HO1 and NQO1 proteins in STZ-induced diabetic mice heart and kidney tissues, indicating that AR inhibition prevents hyperglycemia-induced oxidative stress by overexpressing various antioxidative enzymes. Since activation of AMPK has been shown to be involved in the regulation of Nrf2 pathway [35], we have also examined the effect of AR inhibitor fidarestat on HG-induced changes in the phosphorylation of AMPK-α1 in Thp1 cells. Our results suggest that pretreatment with fidarestat stimulates phosphorylation of AMPK-α1 in HG-induced Thp1 cells. However, fidarestat pretreatment has no effect on the AMPK-α1 activation in Nrf2-ablated cells.

In conclusion, we have shown that AR inhibitor fidarestat prevents HG-induced Thp1 cell death by induction of Nrf2 expression; DNA binding activity; and expression of HO1, NQO1, SOD, and catalase via activation of AMPK-α1. This suggests that AR inhibition prevents hyperglycemia-induced complications by upregulating anti-inflammatory

Nrf2 pathway in addition to downregulating the proinflammatory NF-κB pathway.

Abbreviations

AR: Aldose reductase
FBS: Fetal bovine serum
Fid: Fidarestat
HG: High glucose
HO1: Hemeoxygenase 1
NQO1: NAD(P)H-quinone dehydrogenase 1
Nrf2: Nuclear factor erythroid 2- (NF-E2-) related factor 2
MTT: 3-(4,5-Dimethylthiazol-2-Yl)-2,5-diphenyltetrazolium bromide
SOD: Superoxide dismutase
STZ: Streptozotocin.

Conflicts of Interest

Authors declare no conflict of interest.

Acknowledgments

This study was supported by the funding from NIH/NIDDK, grant DK104786.

References

[1] P. Geraldes, J. Hiraoka-Yamamoto, M. Matsumoto et al., "Activation of PKC-δ and SHP-1 by hyperglycemia causes vascular cell apoptosis and diabetic retinopathy," *Nature Medicine*, vol. 15, no. 11, pp. 1298–1306, 2009.

[2] V. Busik, S. Mohr, and M. B. Grant, "Hyperglycemia-induced reactive oxygen species toxicity to endothelial cells is dependent on paracrine mediators," *Diabetes*, vol. 57, no. 7, pp. 1952–1965, 2008.

[3] S. K. Srivastava, K. V. Ramana, and A. Bhatnagar, "Role of aldose reductase and oxidative damage in diabetes and the consequent potential for therapeutic options," *Endocrine Reviews*, vol. 26, no. 3, pp. 380–392, 2005.

[4] K. V. Ramana, "Aldose reductase: new insights for an old enzyme," *Biomolecular Concepts*, vol. 2, no. 1-2, 2011.

[5] K. V. Ramana and S. K. Srivastava, "Aldose reductase: a novel therapeutic target for inflammatory pathologies," *The International Journal of Biochemistry & Cell Biology*, vol. 42, no. 1, pp. 17–20, 2010.

[6] K. V. Ramana, "Aldose reductase mediates mitogenic signaling in vascular smooth muscle cells," *Journal of Biological Chemistry*, vol. 277, no. 35, pp. 32063–32070, 2002.

[7] K. V. Ramana, B. Friedrich, S. Srivastava, A. Bhatnagar, and S. K. Srivastava, "Activation of nulcear factor-B by hyperglycemia in vascular smooth muscle cells is regulated by aldose reductase," *Diabetes*, vol. 53, no. 11, pp. 2910–2920, 2004.

[8] S. Srivastava, K. V. Ramana, R. Tammali, S. K. Srivastava, and A. Bhatnagar, "Contribution of aldose reductase to diabetic hyperproliferation of vascular smooth muscle cells," *Diabetes*, vol. 55, no. 4, pp. 901–910, 2006.

[9] T. Nguyen, P. Nioi, and C. B. Pickett, "The Nrf2-antioxidant response element signaling pathway and its activation by oxidative stress," *Journal of Biological Chemistry*, vol. 284, no. 20, pp. 13291–13295, 2009.

[10] Q. Ma, "Role of Nrf2 in oxidative stress and toxicity," *Annual Review of Pharmacology and Toxicology*, vol. 53, no. 1, pp. 401–426, 2013.

[11] R. Tammali, A. Saxena, S. K. Srivastava, and K. V. Ramana, "Aldose reductase inhibition prevents hypoxia-induced increase in hypoxia-inducible factor-1α (HIF-1α) and vascular endothelial growth factor (VEGF) by regulating 26 S proteasome-mediated protein degradation in human colon cancer cells," *Journal of Biological Chemistry*, vol. 286, no. 27, pp. 24089–24100, 2011.

[12] K. V. Ramana, B. Friedrich, R. Tammali, M. B. West, A. Bhatnagar, and S. K. Srivastava, "Requirement of aldose reductase for the hyperglycemic activation of protein kinase C and formation of diacylglycerol in vascular smooth muscle cells," *Diabetes*, vol. 54, no. 3, pp. 818–829, 2005.

[13] M. Shoeb, U. C. S. Yadav, S. K. Srivastava, and K. V. Ramana, "Inhibition of aldose reductase prevents endotoxin-induced inflammation by regulating the arachidonic acid pathway in murine macrophages," *Free Radical Biology and Medicine*, vol. 51, no. 9, pp. 1686–1696, 2011.

[14] S. K. Srivastava, U. C. S. Yadav, A. B. M. Reddy et al., "Aldose reductase inhibition suppresses oxidative stress-induced inflammatory disorders," *Chemico-Biological Interactions*, vol. 191, no. 1–3, pp. 330–338, 2011.

[15] S. Pandey, S. K. Srivastava, and K. V. Ramana, "A potential therapeutic role for aldose reductase inhibitors in the treatment of endotoxin-related inflammatory diseases," *Expert Opinion on Investigational Drugs*, vol. 21, no. 3, pp. 329–339, 2012.

[16] W. H. Tang, K. A. Martin, and J. Hwa, "Aldose reductase, oxidative stress, and diabetic mellitus," *Frontiers in Pharmacology*, vol. 3, 2012.

[17] J. B. de Haan, "Nrf2 activators as attractive therapeutics for diabetic nephropathy," *Diabetes*, vol. 60, no. 11, pp. 2683-2684, 2011.

[18] B. Li, S. Liu, L. Miao, and L. Cai, "Prevention of diabetic complications by activation of Nrf2: diabetic cardiomyopathy and nephropathy," *Experimental Diabetes Research*, vol. 2012, pp. 1–7, 2012.

[19] K. Liby, "The synthetic triterpenoids, CDDO and CDDO-Imidazolide, are potent inducers of Heme oxygenase-1 and Nrf2/ARE signaling," *Cancer Research*, vol. 65, no. 11, pp. 4789–4798, 2005.

[20] R. K. Thimmulappa, R. J. Fuchs, D. Malhotra et al., "Preclinical evaluation of targeting the Nrf2 pathway by triterpenoids (CDDO-Im and CDDO-me) for protection from LPS-induced inflammatory response and reactive oxygen species in human peripheral blood mononuclear cells and neutrophils," *Antioxidants & Redox Signaling*, vol. 9, no. 11, pp. 1963–1970, 2007.

[21] D. P. W. Wong, G. Wells, and T. Hagen, "Heteroaromatic 4-arylquinols are novel inducers of nuclear factor-erythroid 2-related factor 2 (Nrf2)," *European Journal of Pharmacology*, vol. 643, no. 2-3, pp. 188–194, 2010.

[22] H. Li, L. Zhang, F. Wang et al., "Attenuation of glomerular injury in diabetic mice with tert-butylhydroquinone through nuclear factor erythroid 2-related factor 2-dependent antioxidant gene activation," *American Journal of Nephrology*, vol. 33, no. 4, pp. 289–297, 2011.

[23] Y. Yang, G. Chen, X. Cheng et al., "Therapeutic potential of digitoflavone on diabetic nephropathy: nuclear factor erythroid

2-related factor 2-dependent anti-oxidant and anti-inflammatory effect," *Scientific Reports*, vol. 5, no. 1, 2015.

[24] T. Jiang, Z. Huang, Y. Lin, Z. Zhang, D. Fang, and D. D. Zhang, "The protective role of Nrf2 in streptozotocin-induced diabetic nephropathy," *Diabetes*, vol. 59, no. 4, pp. 850–860, 2010.

[25] M. Xue, Q. Qian, A. Adaikalakoteswari, N. Rabbani, R. Babaei-Jadidi, and P. J. Thornalley, "Activation of NF-E2-related factor-2 reverses biochemical dysfunction of endothelial cells induced by hyperglycemia linked to vascular disease," *Diabetes*, vol. 57, no. 10, pp. 2809–2817, 2008.

[26] Y. Bai, X. Wang, S. Zhao, C. Ma, J. Cui, and Y. Zheng, "Sulforaphane protects against cardiovascular disease via Nrf2 activation," *Oxidative Medicine and Cellular Longevity*, vol. 2015, pp. 1–13, 2015.

[27] Z. GHorbani, A. Hekmatdoost, and P. Mirmiran, "Anti-hyperglycemic and insulin sensitizer effects of turmeric and its principle constituent curcumin," *International Journal of Endocrinology and Metabolism*, vol. 12, no. 4, 2014.

[28] Y. Masuda, N. D. Vaziri, S. Li et al., "The effect of Nrf2 pathway activation on human pancreatic islet cells," *PLoS One*, vol. 10, no. 6, p. e0131012, 2015.

[29] D. Zhang, M. Fu, S. H. Gao, and J. L. Liu, "Curcumin and diabetes: a systematic review," *Evidence-Based Complementary and Alternative Medicine*, vol. 2013, pp. 1–16, 2013.

[30] E. Kang, G. Kim, H. Kim et al., "Nrf2 regulates curcumin-induced aldose reductase expression indirectly via nuclear factor-κB," *Pharmacological Research*, vol. 58, no. 1, pp. 15–21, 2008.

[31] G. Negi, V. Nakkina, P. Kamble, and S. S. Sharma, "Heme oxygenase-1, a novel target for the treatment of diabetic complications: focus on diabetic peripheral neuropathy," *Pharmacological Research*, vol. 102, pp. 158–167, 2015.

[32] Á. F. Castilho, C. A. Aveleira, E. C. Leal et al., "Heme oxygenase-1 protects retinal endothelial cells against high glucose- and oxidative/nitrosative stress-induced toxicity," *PLoS One*, vol. 7, no. 8, p. e42428, 2012.

[33] M. Li, D. H. Kim, P. L. Tsenovoy et al., "Treatment of obese diabetic mice with a heme oxygenase inducer reduces visceral and subcutaneous adiposity, increases adiponectin levels, and improves insulin sensitivity and glucose tolerance," *Diabetes*, vol. 57, no. 6, pp. 1526–1535, 2008.

[34] A. Saad, H. Ibrahim, W. Nazmy, and A. Hussein, "Induction of heme oxygenase-1 improves glucose tolerance and enhances insulin sensitivity in obese diabetic rats," *Journal of Advances in Medical and Pharmaceutical Sciences*, vol. 10, no. 3, pp. 1–11, 2016.

[35] M. S. Joo, W. D. Kim, K. Y. Lee, J. H. Kim, J. H. Koo, and S. G. Kim, "AMPK facilitates nuclear accumulation of Nrf2 by phosphorylating at serine 550," *Molecular and Cellular Biology*, vol. 36, no. 14, pp. 1931–1942, 2016.

2

Acute Elevated Glucose Promotes Abnormal Action Potential-Induced Ca^{2+} Transients in Cultured Skeletal Muscle Fibers

Erick O. Hernández-Ochoa, Quinton Banks, and Martin F. Schneider

Department of Biochemistry and Molecular Biology, University of Maryland School of Medicine, Baltimore, MD 21201, USA

Correspondence should be addressed to Erick O. Hernández-Ochoa; ehernandez-ochoa@som.umaryland.edu

Academic Editor: Mark A. Yorek

A common comorbidity of diabetes is skeletal muscle dysfunction, which leads to compromised physical function. Previous studies of diabetes in skeletal muscle have shown alterations in excitation-contraction coupling (ECC)—the sequential link between action potentials (AP), intracellular Ca^{2+} release, and the contractile machinery. Yet, little is known about the impact of acute elevated glucose on the temporal properties of AP-induced Ca^{2+} transients and ionic underlying mechanisms that lead to muscle dysfunction. Here, we used high-speed confocal Ca^{2+} imaging to investigate the temporal properties of AP-induced Ca^{2+} transients, an intermediate step of ECC, using an acute in cellulo model of uncontrolled hyperglycemia (25 mM, 48 h.). Control and elevated glucose-exposed muscle fibers cultured for five days displayed four distinct patterns of AP-induced Ca^{2+} transients (phasic, biphasic, phasic-delayed, and phasic-slow decay); most control muscle fibers show phasic AP-induced Ca^{2+} transients, while most fibers exposed to elevated D-glucose displayed biphasic Ca^{2+} transients upon single field stimulation. We hypothesize that these changes in the temporal profile of the AP-induced Ca^{2+} transients are due to changes in the intrinsic excitable properties of the muscle fibers. We propose that these changes accompany early stages of diabetic myopathy.

1. Introduction

Diabetes mellitus (DM), a complex metabolic syndrome, is due to the inability of the pancreas to produce and/or secrete insulin, referred as insulin deficiency or improper insulin signal transduction by tissues like hepatic, fat, and skeletal muscle, known as insulin resistance. In either insulin deficiency or resistance, the cells are unable to adequately metabolize the glucose, leading to hyperglycemia, the hallmark of the disease. Late complications of diabetes affect both the quality and quantity of life, resulting in major health costs [1]. The disease progression of both type 1 (T1D) and type 2 (T2D) diabetes are different, yet the clinical manifestations and complications are often similar [1]. During episodes of hyperglycemia, glucose levels reach abnormal elevated values ranging from 120 to 1200 mg/dL [2–4]. In addition to the change in glucose concentration, hyperglycemia is accompanied by significant changes in plasma osmolarity [2, 4, 5]. Individuals affected by long-term T2D repeatedly present modest but significant changes in glucose concentration and osmolarity, while patients with acute uncontrolled hyperglycemia (i.e., T1D) can exhibit even larger changes in osmolarity [2–5]. Consequently, it is anticipated that harmful effects of hyperglycemia and/or hyperglycemic-induced osmotic stress contributes to the progression of diabetic complications and comorbidities.

A common comorbidity of both T1D and T2D is sarcopenia and dynapenia—the loss of muscle mass and strength, respectively, and is termed diabetic myopathy [6, 7]. The adequate function of skeletal muscle is fundamental for body movement and glucose metabolism [8–10], and the development of diabetic myopathy, an understudied and commonly overlooked condition, is believed to worsen the metabolic status of the individual already affected with concurrent diabetic complications. Comprehensive studies involving large numbers of patients with chronic T2D have shown increased sarcopenia and dynapenia when contrasted to healthy individuals [11, 12]. Fatigue and weakness are also common findings in patients with acute episodes of hyperglycemia, particularly in patients with T2D [13]. There are numerous studies related to fatigue, sarcopenia, and dynapenia [14–18]; nevertheless, the precise cellular events linked with these muscular conditions in individuals afflicted by diabetes remain unidentified.

While previous studies have investigated the link between changes in skeletal muscle function and muscle mass [1, 7, 10–12, 14, 17–23], Ca^{2+} homeostasis and signaling in different models of long-term diabetes mellitus [24–27], few have examined the impact of relatively acute elevated glucose on action potential- (AP-) induced Ca^{2+} transients. Direct acute effects of hyperglycemia could have implications for the skeletal muscle myopathy seen in diabetes, especially in patients with poor glycemic control. In particular, studies of experimental diabetes in skeletal muscle have shown alterations in the excitation-contraction coupling (ECC)—a coordinated chain of cellular events that link membrane AP, intracellular Ca^{2+} release, and contractile machinery [28, 29]. We previously reported that muscle fibers exposed to elevated glucose display increased AP-evoked Ca^{2+} signals produced by single brief electric stimulation [25]. Yet, little is known about the consequences of acute elevated glucose on the temporal properties of AP-induced Ca^{2+} transients and the underlying ionic mechanisms that lead to muscle dysfunction. Here, we used ultra-high-speed confocal Ca^{2+} imaging to investigate the temporal properties of AP-induced Ca^{2+} transients, an intermediate step of ECC, using a cellular model of acute hyperglycemia. Our results reveal that elevated glucose-exposed fibers predominantly display abnormal AP-induced Ca^{2+} transients.

2. Methods

2.1. FDB Skeletal Muscle Fibers Culture. Studies were performed on skeletal muscle fibers enzymatically isolated from the *flexor digitorum brevis* (FDB) muscles of 4- to 5-week-old C57BL/6J mice as previously described [30–33]. Mice were euthanized by CO_2 exposure followed by cervical dislocation using protocols approved by the University of Maryland Institutional Animal Care and Use Committee. FDB skeletal muscle fibers were isolated, dissociated, and cultured in a humidified incubator at 37°C (5% CO_2) as previously described [30–33]. FDB muscles were dissected and maintained in minimum essential medium (MEM, Life Technologies, Carlsbad, CA, catalog number 11095080) and 2 mg/mL collagenase type I (Sigma-Aldrich, St. Louis, MO, catalog number C-0130) for 3 h. at 37 °C. Muscle fibers were plated on glass-bottomed culture dishes (Matek Inc., Ashland, MA, catalog number P35G-1.0-14-C) coated with laminin (Life Technologies, Carlsbad, CA, catalog number 23017015). After plating, cultures were incubated in MEM, containing 5.56 mM D-glucose, supplemented with 10% fetal bovine serum (FBS, Life Technologies, Carlsbad, CA, catalog number 10100139) and 50 $\mu g \cdot ml^{-1}$ gentamicin (Life Technologies, Carlsbad, CA, catalog number 15710064). This medium was used as a control isotonic condition (288 mOsm/kg). Two hours after plating, cultures were treated with cytosine β-D-arabinofuranoside (ara-C; Sigma-Aldrich, St. Louis, MO, catalog number C-1768; 10 μM for 24 h.) to reduce proliferating cells and to minimize fiber dedifferentiation [30, 33]. For fibers challenged with elevated extracellular glucose media, either D- or L-glucose (25 mM; 48 h.) was added to the control isotonic medium. Over an isotonic reference of 288 mOsm/kg, the addition of 25 mM D-glucose increased the osmolality to 313 mOsm/kg. Osmolarity of the culture media was measured in a Vapro-5520 Osmometer (Wescor Inc., Logan, UT). Here, muscle fiber cultures were 5 days old when used for acute experiments.

2.2. Ca^{2+} Imaging. Fluo-4 measurements were carried out on a high-speed confocal system (LSM 5 Live, Carl Zeiss, Jena, DE) as previously described [34, 35]. Muscle fibers were loaded with 1 μM fluo-4 AM (Life Technologies, Carlsbad, CA, catalog number F14201) in L-15 medium (Life Technologies, Carlsbad, CA, catalog number 21083027). The ionic composition of L-15 in mM is 137 NaCl, 5.7 KCl, 1.26 CaCl2, and 1.8 MgCl2, pH 7.4) supplemented with 0.25% *w/v* bovine serum albumin (BSA; Sigma-Aldrich, St. Louis, MO, catalog number A-7906) for 1 h. at room temperature. The dishes were rinsed once with L-15 medium for 5 min to remove residual fluo-4 AM. Individual muscle fibers were imaged with a 60×/1.3 NA water-immersion objective lens. Excitation for fluo-4 was provided by the 488 nm line of a 100 mW diode laser, and emitted light was collected at >505 nm. Action potential- (AP-) induced Ca^{2+} transients were triggered using a brief electrical field stimulus. External field stimulation and inclusion and exclusion criteria of the characteristics of muscle fibers used in this study were performed as previously described [25, 36]. Supramaximal field stimulation (1 ms square pulse, 30 V/cm) was produced by a custom pulse generator and applied via two platinum wires positioned perpendicular to the bottom of the dish, ~5 mm apart, to elicit action potentials. Muscle fibers were centrally positioned relative to the electrodes and to the field of view, at less than about a ±45° angle relative to an imaginary line between the tips of the electrodes, and only fibers exhibiting all or no activation and reproducible responses to field stimulation of alternating polarity were used for the analysis. A variable range of the cultured muscle fibers (3–7%) from the control group or from other groups challenged with elevated glucose did not respond to electrical stimulation of both polarities and were excluded from the analysis. Electrical field stimulation was synchronized relative to the beginning of acquisition. The field stimulus was applied 100 ms after the beginning of the scan sequence, providing control images before stimulation. Confocal line scanning was performed at the ends of the fibers and perpendicular to the long axis of the fibers. These line-scan confocal images were used to calculate the resting steady-state fluorescence level (F_0). The average intensity of fluorescence within selected regions of interest (ROIs; dashed rectangles shown in line-scan images in Figures 1 and 2) within a myofiber was measured with Zeiss LSM Image Examiner (Carl Zeiss, Jena, Germany). The ROIs were located in areas spanning the edge and center

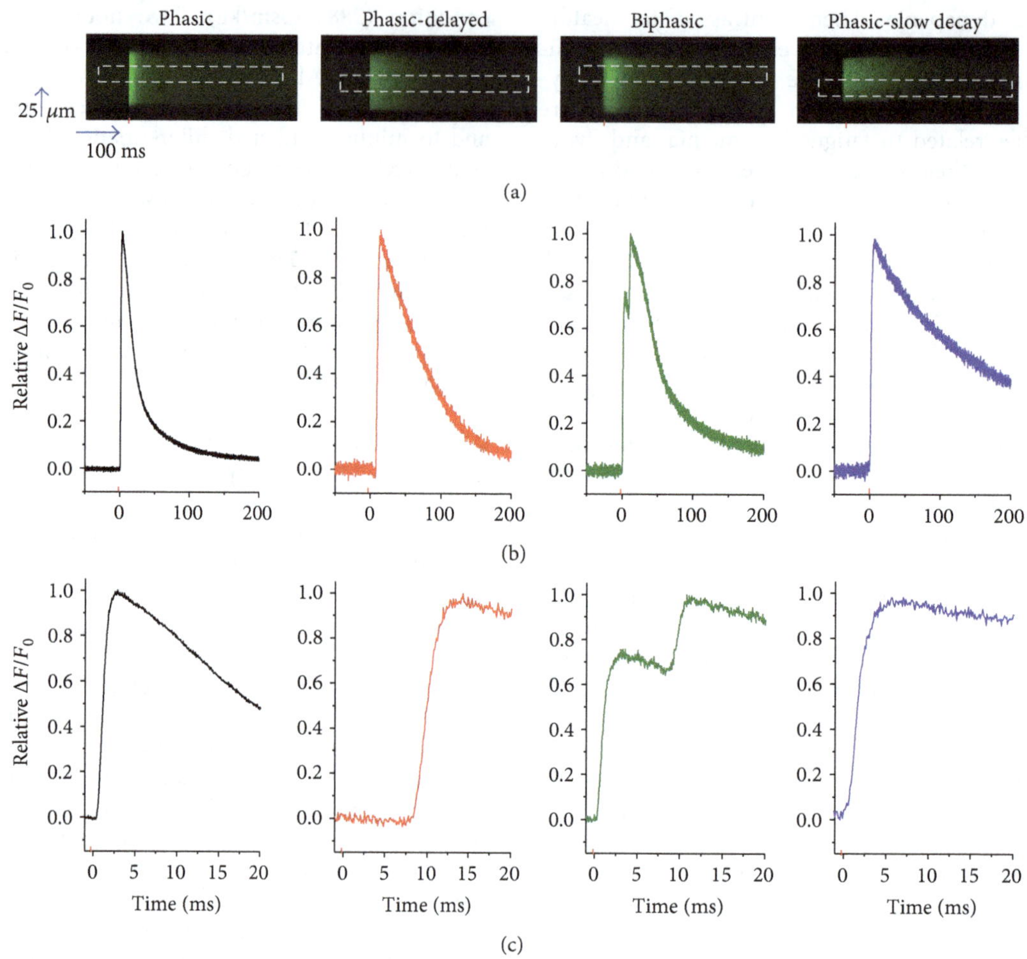

FIGURE 1: Muscle fibers cultured for 5 days exhibit multiple patterns of action potential (AP)-induced Ca^{2+} transients: control conditions. (a) Representative confocal line-scan images of AP-induced Ca^{2+} transients in 5-day-old cultured muscle fibers maintained in control medium. Note that four different patterns were identified: phasic, phasic-delayed, biphasic, and phasic-slow-decay. The red mark indicates the time when field electrical stimulus was applied, and the dashed rectangle illustrates the region of interest used to measure the time course of the Ca^{2+} transient. (b) Time course of the AP-induced Ca^{2+} transients shown in (a). (c) Zoomed-in versions of AP-induced Ca^{2+} transients shown in (b).

of the muscle fiber to monitor Ca^{2+} signals derived from subsarcolemmal and core regions of the fiber, or in regions covering the edges of the fiber to monitor the responses across the fiber width. Images in line-scan (x-t) mode (frame size: 512 × 10,000 pixels; scan speed: 100 μs/line for 1 s acquisition) were background corrected by subtracting an average value recorded outside the cell. The average F_0 value in each ROI before electrical stimulation was used to scale Ca^{2+} signals in the same ROI as $\Delta F/F_0$.

It is important to note that the temporal resolution of the Ca^{2+} transient is exclusively determined not only by the sampling rate but also by the kinetic properties of the dyes. Here, we used fluo-4, a high-affinity dye, instead of low-affinity dyes merely because in our imaging system this dye provides brighter responses than the low-affinity indicators. Based on our calibration data, fluo-4 was at most 40% saturated with Ca^{2+}. The length of the fibers used was 400–600 μm and the width was 25–80 μm. No attempts were made to distinguish muscle fiber types or to estimate the actual cytosolic Ca^{2+} concentration. Ca^{2+} imaging experiments were carried out at room temperature, 21–23°C.

2.3. Toxins and Channel Blockers. To assess the contribution of different ion channels to the development of the biphasic action potential Ca^{2+} transient, 5-day-old cultured fibers were exposed to either gadolinium (Axxora, San Diego, CA, catalog number 400-023-M500), apamin (Sigma-Aldrich, St. Louis, MO, catalog number A-1289), or Jingzhaotoxin-III (JZTX-III; Alomone Labs, Jerusalem, IL, catalog number STJ-200), blockers of mechanosensitivity, SK channels, and $Na_v1.5$ channels, respectively. Ion channel blockade treatment was carried out using semilocal perfusion. The working concentration of the blockers used here was based on maximal blocking effects described in previous reports [37–39]. Fibers with biphasic action potential-induced Ca^{2+} transient were first identified, then the time course of the Ca^{2+} profile was assessed before and 10 minutes after blocker application.

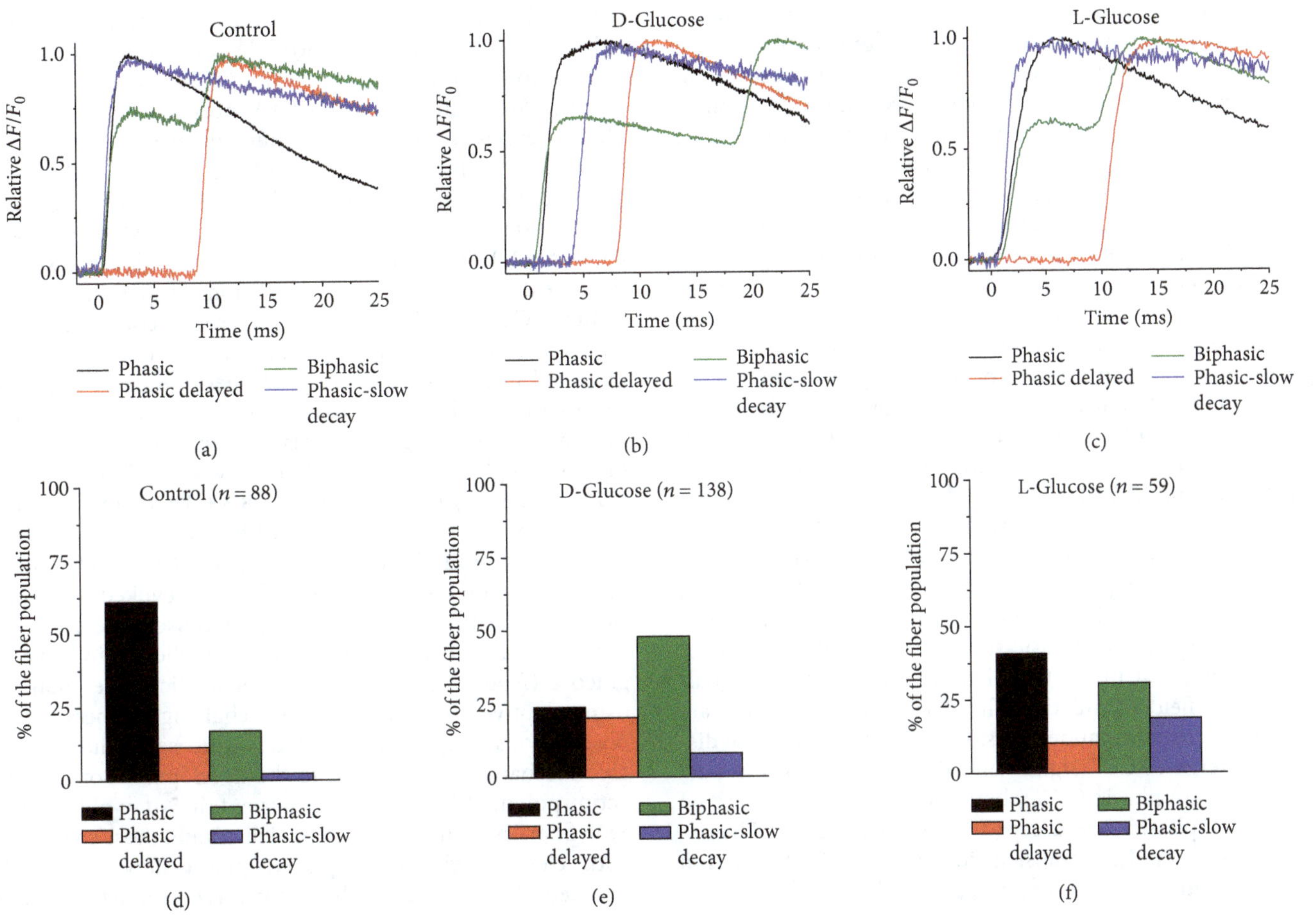

FIGURE 2: Sustained elevation of extracellular D-glucose modifies the distribution of AP-induced Ca^{2+} transients observed in 5-day-old cultured fibers. Zoomed-in and overlapped version of AP-induced Ca^{2+} transients for control (a), D-glucose (b), and L-glucose (c) challenged fibers. (d–f) Summary of distribution of AP-induced Ca^{2+} transients for fibers exposed to control isotonic medium (d), D-glucose (e), and L-glucose (f). Fibers exposed to D-glucose displayed a significantly larger proportion of biphasic action potential-induced Ca^{2+} transients when compared to control counterparts (X^2, $n = 286$, p value < 0.05).

2.4. Data Analysis. Images of arbitrarily selected muscle fibers were collected and evaluated blindly, using the same settings and enhancing parameters so that all images could be directly compared. Line-scan images were analyzed using LSM examiner (Carl Zeiss, Jena, DE). AP-induced Ca^{2+} signals and statistical analysis were conducted using Origin Pro 8 (OriginLab Corporation, Northampton, MA, USA) and SPSS for Windows ver. 24.0 (SPSS Inc., Chicago, IL, USA). Summary data were reported as mean ± SD. Normal distribution of data was assessed using the Kolmogorov-Smirnov test. Unpaired two-sample Student's *t*-test was used to test for differences between the means of the interspike interval of AP-induced Ca^{2+} transients from two different samples. For experiments that involved the measurements of AP-induced Ca^{2+} transients before or after the addition of ion channel blockers, the interspike interval was compared before and after the addition of blocker in the same muscle fiber. The statistical significance of interspike interval was analyzed using a paired Student's *t*-test on raw data. Cross-classifications and crosstabs were used to examine the relationship between two categorical variables. To test for significant differences, we compared the proportion in each variable, with condition (control and elevated glucose) as the independent variable and AP-induced Ca^{2+} transient pattern (phasic, biphasic, delayed, and slow decay) as the dependent variable, using Pearson chi-square (X^2). Differences were considered significant when p value < 0.05.

3. Results

3.1. Action Potential-Induced Ca^{2+} Transients in 5-Day-Old Cultured Control Fibers. Freshly dissociated or 1- to 3-day-old cultured FDB muscle fibers retain many properties of in situ fibers, including muscle contractions and Ca^{2+} transients that correlate with the number and frequency of field stimulation used. In response to a single 1 ms field stimulus, they respond with one single action potential, a single Ca^{2+} transient, and a single twitch) [30, 33], even when challenged with acute (1 h.) elevated glucose (see Supplementary Figure 1 available online at https://doi.org/10.1155/2017/1509048). In a previous study, we analyzed Ca^{2+} handling and action potential- (AP-) evoked Ca^{2+} transients in 5-day-old cultured control and high-glucose-exposed FDB fibers using a ratiometric Ca^{2+} dye and low temporal resolution [25]. To gain better time resolution of the Ca^{2+} transients, we next monitored fluo-4 transients during stimulation of FDB fibers using an ultra-high-speed (100 μs/line) confocal microscope in line-scan mode. Figure 1 illustrates representative *x-t* confocal line-scan images (Figure 1(a)) and corresponding fluo-4 Ca^{2+} transients (Figure 1(b)) of four different muscle fibers in control conditions and in response to a supramaximal single field stimulus. Confocal line scanning was performed at one end of the fiber and perpendicular to the long axis of the fiber. Successive vertical lines in each line-scan image reveal the time course of the fluorescence signal before and during repetitive stimulation at 100 μs resolution. At first glance, the line-scan images appear to display a single transient in the different fibers shown in Figure 1(a). However, fluo-4 Ca^{2+} profiles (Figure 1(b)) show the time course of the Ca^{2+} signals in more detail. In order to evaluate and compare the temporal profile of the Ca^{2+} signals elicited by action potentials, Ca^{2+} transients were normalized relative to peak maximum fluorescence. Using this approach, we identified four distinct and predominant AP-evoked Ca^{2+} transient profiles in 5-day-old cultured control fibers: phasic, phasic-delayed, biphasic, and phasic-slow decay. To further appreciate the temporal properties of these different Ca^{2+} signals elicited by field stimulation, the fluo-4 Ca^{2+} transients are shown in a time-expanded version in Figure 1(c). These distinct patterns of Ca^{2+} signals and their distributions in percentages were phasic (67%), biphasic (18%), phasic-delayed (12%), and phasic-slow decay (3%) (see Figure 2(d)). The rising phase of the Ca^{2+} transient following single stimulation occurred within ~1-2 ms of the applied field stimulus in muscle fibers with phasic responses (Figure 1). In contrast, muscle fibers with a rising phase starting >3 ms after the start of the stimulation were classified as delayed; the duration of this delay was variable (3–15 ms). Another group of fibers exhibited two summated Ca^{2+} transients in response to a single field stimulus, with the first response within 1-2 ms and the second response delayed as in the phasic-delayed fibers, and were classified as biphasic. Finally, another group of fibers exhibited a slow half-time of decay of >100 ms (not shown on the time scale of Figure 1), and were classified as phasic slow decay. These results indicate that 5-day-old cultured FDB fibers exhibit a heterogeneous fiber population that responds to single field stimulation different to freshly dissociated or 1-day-old cultured fibers [31, 35].

3.2. Action Potential-Induced Ca^{2+} Transients in 5-Day-Old Cultured Muscle Fibers Challenged with Elevated D-Glucose or L-Glucose. In another series of experiments, muscle fibers were challenged with elevated glucose (25 mM). We assessed the properties of AP-induced Ca^{2+} transients in fibers challenged with either D-glucose or L-glucose (Figure 2) using the same approach applied to 5-day-old cultured control fibers. Fibers exposed to elevated glucose displayed the same patterns of AP-induced Ca^{2+}observed in control fibers; however, the distribution of the patterns was different (Figure 2). In D-glucose exposed fibers (Figures 2(b) and 2(e)) the distribution was: biphasic (48%), phasic (24%), phasic-delayed (21%), and phasic-slow decay (7%). In L-glucose exposed fibers (Figures 2(c) and 2(f)) the distribution was: phasic (41%), biphasic (30%), phasic-slow decay (19%), and phasic-delayed (10%), whereas in control the distribution was phasic (67%), biphasic (18%), phasic-delayed (12%), and phasic-slow decay (3%) (Figures 2(a) and 2(d)). We tested whether elevated glucose-exposed fibers exhibit different distribution of patterns of AP-induced Ca^{2+} transients when compared to control counterparts. The two-sided asymptotic significance of the chi-square statistic was less than 0.05; X^2 (6, $n = 286$) 43.08 $p = 1.12E-7$, implying that elevated glucose-exposed fibers exhibit a different distribution of patterns of AP induced-Ca^{2+} transients when compared to control counterparts. Note that the biphasic pattern was more commonly observed in D-glucose challenged fibers, while in L-glucose exposed fibers the phasic pattern was predominant, as seen in control fibers (Figure 2). Also, the interspike interval in biphasic D-glucose challenged fibers was significantly longer (17.9 ± 4.2 ms in D-glucose versus 8.3 ± 3.4 ms in control or 9.1 ± 3.8 ms in L-glucose, in $n = 12$ fibers, 3 mice per group; $p = 0.09$, two-sample unpaired Student's *t*-test). The effects of D-glucose on the distribution of the AP-evoked Ca^{2+} transients were distinct to those observed in muscle fibers exposed with the same concentration of metabolically inactive L-glucose (Figure 2), suggesting a metabolic rather than an osmoadaptive effect in D-glucose challenged fibers. These observations suggest that elevated D-glucose facilitates excitable mechanism(s) that lead to the development of biphasic action potential-induced Ca^{2+} transients in 5-day-old cultured FDB fibers. Note that while control fibers and those challenged with elevated glucose displayed phasic-slow decay AP-induced Ca^{2+} transients, these fibers represented a variable but small fraction of the overall muscle fiber population and were not studied in detail in the present work.

3.3. Effect of Electrical Field Stimulation of Alternating Polarity in Fibers with Phasic or Delayed AP-Induced Ca^{2+} Transients. To examine the propagation time for AP-induced Ca^{2+} signals, fibers were subjected to suprathreshold field stimulation of alternate polarity. The Ca^{2+} transients in fibers with phasic responses occur with a similar short latency (<2 ms) in response to external stimulation of either polarity (Figure 3(a)), indicating AP-induced Ca^{2+} transients. The time course of the Ca^{2+} transients evaluated at two subsarcolemmal regions on opposite sides of the fiber (ROIs 1 and 2 in Figure 3(a)) reveals that suprathreshold pulses elicited synchronous AP-induced Ca^{2+} transients across the fiber width.

In fibers with phasic-delayed Ca^{2+} transients, the response can occur after a delay (3–15 ms) and could, in principle, result from alterations in AP propagation which translate into AP-induced Ca^{2+} propagation deficits (i.e., slow propagation). We wanted to evaluate whether the delay was caused by the absence of a direct response to stimulation at the site of imaging combined with a slow propagation of an AP from the fiber end away from the recording site and towards the recording site. If this were the case, then inverting the polarity of the stimulus applied to a phasic delayed fiber would trigger an AP-induced Ca^{2+} transient with a considerably shorter delay at the site of recording since propagation would no longer be required. Figure 3(b) shows AP-induced Ca^{2+} transients in a fiber with delayed responses

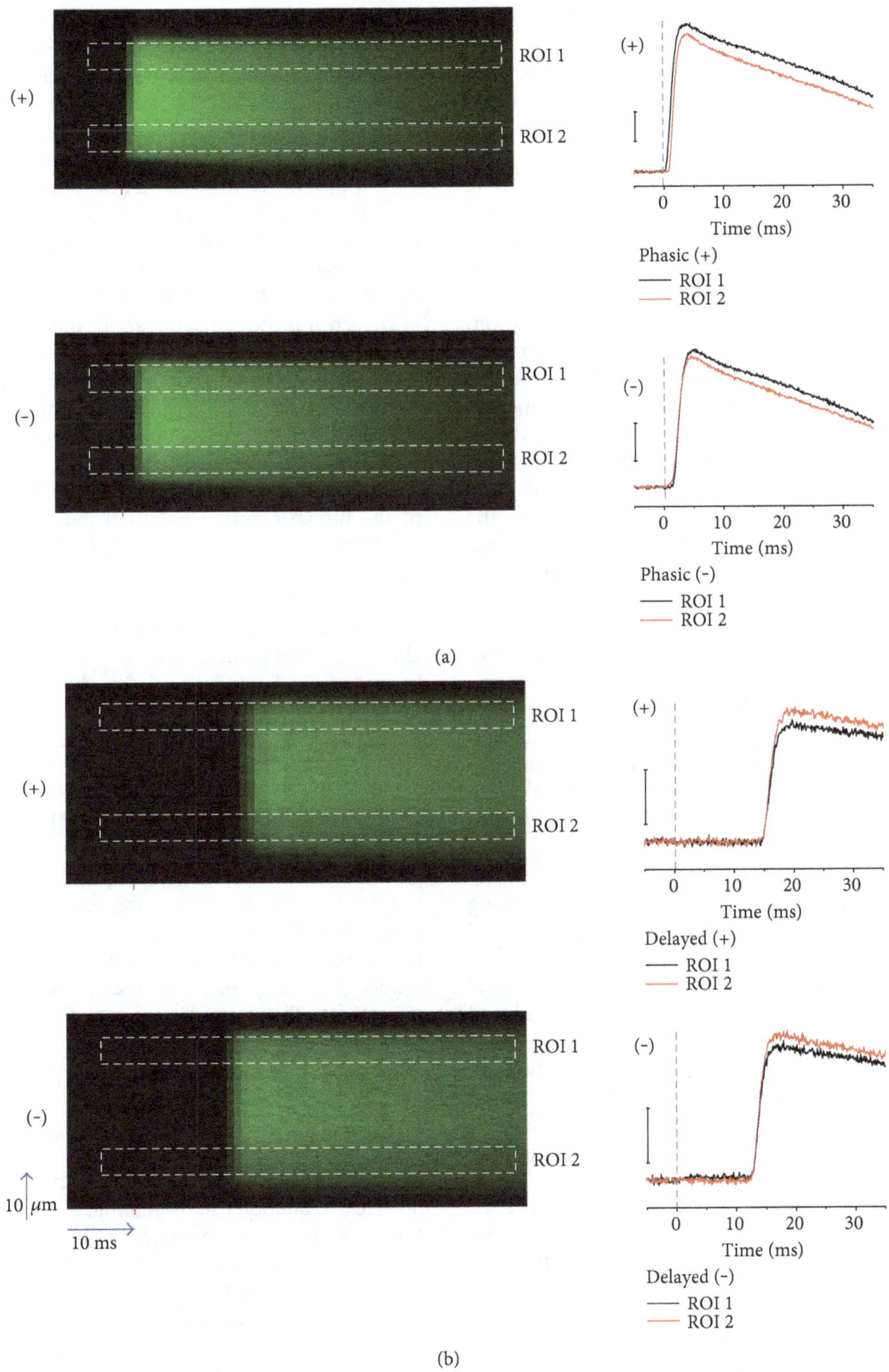

FIGURE 3: Effect of electrical field stimulation of alternating polarity in fibers with phasic and delayed AP-induced Ca^{2+} transients. (a) *Left*, line-scan images of *phasic* AP-induced Ca^{2+} transients elicited by field stimulation of alternate polarity and measured in two different regions of interest (ROIs); *right*, time course of the phasic AP-induced Ca^{2+} transients measured at two ROIs (ROI 1 and ROI 2) and elicited by the stimulus of positive (*upper traces*) or negative polarity (*lower traces*) at the fiber end where the recordings were made. (b) *Left*, line-scan images of *phasic-delayed* AP-induced Ca^{2+} transients elicited by field stimulation of alternate polarity and monitored in two ROIs; *right*, time course of the delayed AP-induced Ca^{2+} transients measured at two ROIs and elicited by the stimulus of positive (*upper traces*) or negative polarity (*lower traces*) at the fiber end where the recordings were made. The red mark in line-scan images indicates the time when the field stimulus was applied; the dashed rectangles illustrates the location of the ROIs.

using pulses of opposite polarity. As in the phasic fiber, suprathreshold pulses elicited synchronous AP-induced Ca^{2+} transients across the fiber width. The comparison of the time course of AP-induced Ca^{2+} transients measured at the same fiber end but with field stimuli of opposite polarity shows similar delayed time courses and only a modest shift (<3 ms) in their latency upon polarity change. This finding suggests that the Ca^{2+} transients are not delayed because of the time for propagation of the action potential or another signal from one end to the other end of the fiber. In that case, the signal recorded at the end of the fiber where the action potential is initiated would not exhibit the delay. However, this was *not* observed. Since the delay was similar for both polarities of stimulation (i.e., with the AP initiated either at the recording site or at the other end of the fiber), we conclude that the delay could be due to either a delay in the activation of the action potential (prior to its propagation along the fiber) or a delay in the activation of the Ca^{2+} transient after the action potential propagation along the fiber when the action potential is activated at the opposite end of the fiber where the recording is taking place. These possibilities are considered further in the discussion.

3.4. Blockers of Mechanosensitive Ion Channels, Ca^{2+}-Dependent K^+ Channels, and $Na_v1.5$ Channels Do Not Affect Biphasic Action Potential-Induced Ca^{2+} Transients Elicited by a Single Field Stimulus. Next, we investigated whether modifications of the excitable properties of the muscle fiber could account for the occurrence of the biphasic phenotype. We used blockers of ion channels known to modulate the membrane potential and AP properties of the skeletal muscle.

The mechanosensitive ion channels (MsC) in the skeletal muscle are activated by membrane stretch and strong membrane depolarization and are permeable to Na^+ and divalent cations [40]. Increased activity of MsC could cause elevated resting Ca^{2+} levels and/or membrane depolarization [37]. We hypothesized that MsC-induced depolarization would eventually trigger an ectopic AP-induced Ca^{2+} transient. To test whether the occurrence of the biphasic action potential-induced Ca^{2+} transient depended on MsC, the time course of fluo-4 Ca^{2+} elicited by field stimulation and a priori identified as a biphasic signal was measured in control external solution, followed by the addition of gadolinium (Gd^{3+}, 100 μM; Figure 4). Ten minutes after the application of Gd^{3+}, the Ca^{2+} signal was reassessed. The addition of Gd^{3+} did not affect the time course of the biphasic response. Gd^{3+} did not alter the interspike interval significantly ($n = 8$ fibers; $p > 0.05$, two-sample paired Student's t-test); although the amplitude of the Ca^{2+} signal was reduced after the Gd^{3+} addition, this effect was not further evaluated. After washout of Gd^{3+}, the amplitude of the Ca^{2+} transient remained reduced (data not shown). The above results suggest that MsC do not contribute to the occurrence of the biphasic action potential-induced Ca^{2+} transients in 5-day-old cultured muscle fibers.

The calcium-sensitive potassium channel with small potassium conductance, $K_{Ca}2.3$, is normally expressed at low level; however, its expression is markedly increased in denervated and myotonic dystrophy muscle [41]. $K_{Ca}2.3$ channel activity in the T-tubules of denervated skeletal muscle causes a local increase in potassium ion concentration that leads to hyperexcitability [38]. Because of their involvement in hyperexcitability, we next considered the possibility that $K_{Ca}2.3$ could be involved in the development of the biphasic action potential-induced Ca^{2+} transient. To test whether the occurrence of the biphasic Ca^{2+} transient involved $K_{Ca}2.3$ channels, the time course of fluo-4 Ca^{2+} elicited by field stimulation was measured in a control external solution, followed by the addition of apamin (1 μM) (Figure 4). $K_{Ca}2.3$ channels can be blocked by apamin [42]. Ten minutes after the application of apamin, the Ca^{2+} signal was measured again. As in the case of MsC, the addition of apamin did not alter the interspike interval significantly ($n = 8$ fibers; $p > 0.05$, two-sample paired Student's t-test), although a reduction in the amplitude of the Ca^{2+} signal was also observed (Figure 4). These results suggest that $K_{Ca}2.3$ channels do not contribute to the occurrence of the biphasic action potential-induced Ca^{2+} transients.

The expression of $Na_v1.5$ channels is low in 1- to 2-day-old cultured muscle fibers. However, $Na_v1.5$ expression increases in fibers cultured for over 3 days [43–45]. This $Na_v1.5$ increased expression could explain the occurrence of abnormal excitability and Ca^{2+} signals. To test whether increased $Na_v1.5$ function is involved in the altered action potential-induced Ca^{2+} signals seen in 5-day-old cultured fibers, we exposed the fibers to JZTX-III, a $Na_v1.5$ channel blocker [39, 46]. The addition of JZTX-III (1 μM; 10 min) to the external solution did not affect the time course of the biphasic response (Figure 4). JZTX-III caused a nonsignificant reduction in the interspike interval (17.3 ± 3.8 ms in D-glucose versus 15.8 ± 3.3 ms in D-glucose treated with JZTX-III, $n = 6$ fibers, 2 mice per group; $p = 0.509$, two-sample paired Student's t-test). Contrary to Gd^{3+} or apamin, the addition of JZTX-III to the recording solution did not reduce the amplitude of the AP-induced Ca^{2+} signals (Figure 4). These results suggest that $Na_v1.5$ channels do not contribute to the occurrence of the biphasic action potential-induced Ca^{2+} transients.

4. Discussion

Numerous studies have investigated how changes in skeletal muscle excitability, Ca^{2+} signaling, and contractility occur in acute and long-term hyperglycemia [12, 13, 20, 21, 47, 48]; however, few studies have examined the impact of diabetes mellitus on the excitability [22], contractility [49], and Ca^{2+} signaling [24] of the skeletal muscle at the cellular level. In particular, little is known about the temporal properties of AP-evoked Ca^{2+} signals during acute hyperglycemia. Using an in cellulo model and high-speed confocal Ca^{2+} imaging, we assessed the impact of acute elevated extracellular glucose (48 h.) on the temporal properties of AP-evoked Ca^{2+} signals. The present study shows that muscle fibers cultured in control medium (5 mM D-glucose) for 5 days display 4 distinct temporal waveforms of AP-induced Ca^{2+} transients: phasic, biphasic, phasic delayed, and phasic-slow decay, in order of predominance. Our study also shows that fibers challenged with elevated extracellular D-glucose (25 mM for 48 h; a condition

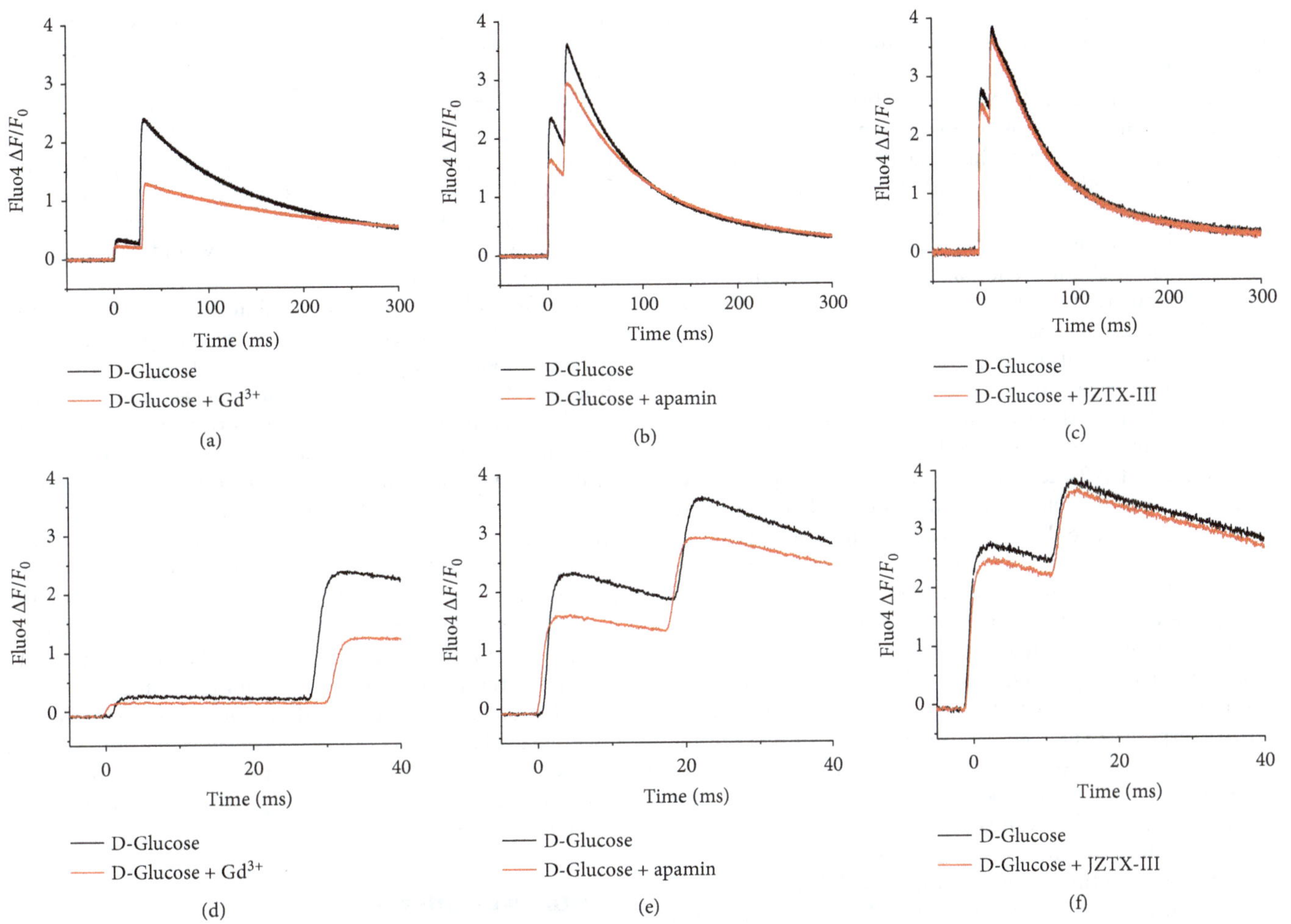

FIGURE 4: Inhibition of ion channels known to modulate the excitable properties of skeletal muscle: impact on biphasic AP-transients on 5-day old cultured fibers challenged with elevated glucose. Representative time course of a biphasic AP-induced Ca^{2+} transient (left panels) measured in fibers challenged with elevated D-glucose (25 mM; 48 h.) before (black traces) and 10 minutes after (red traces) the treatment with gadolinium (100 μM) (a), apamin (1 μM) (b), and JZTX-III (1 μM) (c). Panels (d–f) are zoomed-in versions of the records shown in (a–c) to better appreciate biphasic responses before and after channel blockers addition. No significant changes in time course of the Ca^{2+} transient (i.e., interspike interval) were found in fibers challenged with 25 mM D-glucose-exposed fibers and treated with gadolinium ($n = 8$ fibers; $p > 0.05$, two-sample paired Student's t-test), apamin ($n = 8$ fibers; $p > 0.05$, two-sample paired Student's t-test), or JZTX-III ($n = 6$ fibers; $p > 0.05$, two-sample paired Student's t-test), when compared to fibers challenged with D-glucose.

that could mimic severe uncontrolled hyperglycemia) also exhibit these 4 distinct patterns. However, under these conditions, the biphasic pattern is the predominant waveform, suggesting that elevated glucose promotes the biphasic responses. To our knowledge, this study is the first report of these abnormal AP-induced Ca^{2+} signals in relation to elevated glucose in fibers of normal morphology.

How was a short (1 ms) field stimulus capable of generating such delayed (>3 ms) or biphasic AP-induced Ca^{2+} transients? We have previously shown that the electrode array used in our study allows for the application of field pulses resulting in the depolarization of the end of the fiber close to the cathode, and hyperpolarization of the opposite end of the fiber (near the anode) [36]. In *phasic* fibers, pulses of alternating polarity elicited propagated AP-induced Ca^{2+} transients at the end of the fiber facing the cathode, near the recording site, and its longitudinal propagation along the fiber [36] (see Figure 3). The time to Ca^{2+} transient peak following single AP stimulation occurs in ~1-2 ms in phasic muscle fibers. The delayed responses (time to Ca^{2+} transient peak > 3 ms) and the second phase of biphasic responses were variable from fiber to fiber. We do not currently know the nature of this variation. We found that fibers with delayed AP-induced Ca^{2+} transient pulses of opposite polarity resulted in subtle latency changes of the Ca^{2+} transient (see Figure 3). This implies that the delay is *not* due to slow AP propagation through the T-tubule system [50, 51], which would cause a major delay for Ca^{2+} transients initiated at the opposite end from which the recordings are made, but not in responses initiated at the same end where recording occurs.

In the case of *phasic-delayed* fibers, we hypothesize that increased transient outward currents, like $K_v1.4$ and $K_v3.4$ type-A K^+ channels, channels expressed in skeletal muscle that oppose membrane depolarization [52, 53], will activate at the cathode near the recording site and will cause membrane potential to reach AP threshold with a delay longer than the stimulus. This delay in AP initiation will cause the observed delay of the AP-induced Ca^{2+} transients in the depolarized end of the fiber near the recording site. The fiber end undergoing hyperpolarization will only be depolarized after the delayed AP is initiated at the other end, followed by rapid propagation of the AP along the fiber. Thus, the (relatively long) delay will be similar at both ends of the fiber for a given polarity stimulation or at the same end of the fiber with alternating polarity stimulation (Figure 2(b)), as observed. Alternatively, AP initiation could have no delay at both ends of the fiber (and/or for both polarities of stimulation), but the Ca^{2+} release response could be delayed due to some as yet undetermined mechanism. In fibers with *biphasic* responses, the negative electrode induces an AP, which triggers the first AP-induced Ca^{2+} transient that propagates towards the positive electrode. The other end, subjected to hyperpolarization, could display voltage sags that counteract hyperpolarization and contribute to rebound membrane potential, triggering the second AP that will propagate toward the other end near to the recording site. Increased inward currents activated by hyperpolarization, such as Kir2.1 channels [54], could explain the membrane potential rebound. Thus, both fiber ends exhibit both a phasic and a delayed response. The Ca^{2+} transients seeing in *phasic-slow decay* fibers could arise from differences in Ca^{2+} binding and transport [55]. These possibilities, and others, require further experimental investigation.

Our results show that the inhibition of MsC with Gd^{3+} did not affect the time course of biphasic AP-induced Ca^{2+} transients during acute hyperglycemia. Note that Gd^{3+} is a nonspecific channel blocker; in addition to inhibiting MsC, it also blocks other ion channels such as voltage-gated K^+, Na^+, and L-type Ca^{2+} channels [56]. Fiber treatment with apamin, a K_{Ca} channel blocker [42], did not reverse the effects of elevated glucose on biphasic AP-induced Ca^{2+} transients. Similarly, JZTX-III, a $Na_v1.5$ channel blocker [39, 46], did not alter the occurrence of the biphasic responses in fibers challenged with elevated glucose. These findings suggest that neither MsCs, K_{Ca}, nor $Na_v1.5$ plays a role in the origin of the biphasic AP-induced Ca^{2+} transients. It is yet to be determined whether other ion channels play a role in the abnormal AP-induced Ca^{2+} transients in long-term cultures and/or exposure to elevated glucose.

Ca^{2+} signals are essential in numerous aspects of muscle function [57, 58]. A previous study reported the occurrence of local Ca^{2+} signals by acute (≤1 h.) hyperosmotic stress in the cell periphery of cultured muscle fibers [59]. Whether local Ca^{2+} signals are present in muscle fibers challenged with hyperosmotic stress induced by elevated glucose for more prolonged periods (>24 h.) remains to be determined.

Do these defects on AP-induced Ca^{2+} signals seen in long-term cultured fibers and experimental hyperglycemia occur in patients with diabetes? Most adults with diabetes have at least one coexisting condition, either acute or chronic [60]. Muscle weakness and fatigue are common complaints of diabetic patients during periods of acute [13] and long-term hyperglycemia [61] and are also common in muscle disuse atrophy [62, 63]. Because Ca^{2+} signals and excitable properties are critical for skeletal muscle function [52, 57], we hypothesize that if the changes in excitability and abnormal Ca^{2+} signals observed in five-day-old cultured fibers occur in vivo, these could contribute to the development of muscle weakness, fatigue, and diabetic myopathy. Further work exploring the underlying mechanisms and relationship between diabetes and skeletal muscle disuse (denervation/physical inactivity, etc.) would be of pathophysiological interest.

In this study, we used an in cellulo model of hyperglycemia using 25 mM glucose for 1-2 days. This paradigm is an extreme model of hyperglycemia, and it is restricted to a short spectrum of metabolic abnormalities and hormonal changes seen in diabetes (i.e., severe uncontrolled diabetes). The abnormalities in AP-induced Ca^{2+} signals that we observed may be influenced or caused by fiber disuse and/or denervation which may occur in long-term cultured muscle fibers [25, 64] and in some extent by in vitro dedifferentiation [33]. Both muscle disuse/denervation and dedifferentiation are characterized by abnormal excitability [33, 45]. Because ara-C treatments minimize the dedifferentiation process [25, 33] (see also Supplementary Figure 2), we believe that dedifferentiation could play a minor role in our observations. Nevertheless, the cultured muscle fibers used here represent a cellular model of muscle disuse/denervation [25, 65] and is a valuable alternative to animal studies to explore severe and acute effects of hyperglycemia on the function of skeletal muscle fibers.

Conflicts of Interest

The authors Erick O. Hernández-Ochoa, Quinton Banks, and Martin F. Schneider declare that they have no competing interests.

Authors' Contributions

Erick O. Hernández-Ochoa designed and performed the research and data analysis. Quinton Banks performed the research. Erick O. Hernández-Ochoa, Quinton Banks, and Martin F. Schneider edited and approved the manuscript. Erick O. Hernández-Ochoa wrote the paper.

Acknowledgments

This work was supported by NIH Grant R37-AR055099 to Martin F. Schneider from the National Institute of Arthritis and Musculoskeletal and Skin Diseases.

References

[1] J. M. Forbes and M. E. Cooper, "Mechanisms of diabetic complications," *Physiological Reviews*, vol. 93, no. 1, pp. 137–188, 2013.

[2] A. E. Kitabchi, G. E. Umpierrez, J. M. Miles, and J. N. Fisher, "Hyperglycemic crises in adult patients with diabetes," *Diabetes Care*, vol. 32, no. 7, pp. 1335–1343, 2009.

[3] A. L. Rosenbloom, "Hyperglycemic hyperosmolar state: an emerging pediatric problem," *The Journal of Pediatrics*, vol. 156, no. 2, pp. 180–184, 2010.

[4] A. Kratz, M. Ferraro, P. M. Sluss, and K. B. Lewandrowski, "Case records of the Massachusetts General Hospital. Weekly clinicopathological exercises. Laboratory reference values," *The New England Journal of Medicine*, vol. 351, no. 15, pp. 1548–1563, 2004.

[5] E. O. Hernandez-Ochoa and C. Vanegas, "Diabetic myopathy and mechanisms of disease," *Biochemistry Pharmacology Journals (Los Angel)*, vol. 4, no. 5, 2015.

[6] H. Andersen, P. C. Gadeberg, B. Brock, and J. Jakobsen, "Muscular atrophy in diabetic neuropathy: a stereological magnetic resonance imaging study," *Diabetologia*, vol. 40, no. 9, pp. 1062–1069, 1997.

[7] M. P. Krause, M. C. Riddell, C. S. Gordon, S. A. Imam, E. Cafarelli, and T. J. Hawke, "Diabetic myopathy differs between Ins2Akita+/– and streptozotocin-induced type 1 diabetic models," *Journal of Applied Physiology*, vol. 106, no. 5, pp. 1650–1659, 2009.

[8] E. Ferrannini, O. Bjorkman, G. A. Reichard Jr. et al., "The disposal of an oral glucose load in healthy subjects. A quantitative study," *Diabetes*, vol. 34, no. 6, pp. 580–588, 1985.

[9] E. Ferrannini, D. C. Simonson, L. D. Katz et al., "The disposal of an oral glucose load in patients with non-insulin-dependent diabetes," *Metabolism*, vol. 37, no. 1, pp. 79–85, 1988.

[10] B. B. Kahn, A. S. Rosen, J. F. Bak et al., "Expression of GLUT1 and GLUT4 glucose transporters in skeletal muscle of humans with insulin-dependent diabetes mellitus: regulatory effects of metabolic factors," *The Journal of Clinical Endocrinology Metabolism*, vol. 74, no. 5, pp. 1101–1109, 1992.

[11] S. W. Park, B. H. Goodpaster, J. S. Lee et al., "Excessive loss of skeletal muscle mass in older adults with type 2 diabetes," *Diabetes Care*, vol. 32, no. 11, pp. 1993–1997, 2009.

[12] S. W. Park, B. H. Goodpaster, E. S. Strotmeyer et al., "Decreased muscle strength and quality in older adults with type 2 diabetes: the health, aging, and body composition study," *Diabetes*, vol. 55, no. 6, pp. 1813–1818, 2006.

[13] H. Andersen, O. Schmitz, and S. Nielsen, "Decreased isometric muscle strength after acute hyperglycaemia in type 1 diabetic patients," *Diabetic Medicine*, vol. 22, no. 10, pp. 1401–1407, 2005.

[14] X. Wang, Z. Hu, J. Hu, J. Du, and W. E. Mitch, "Insulin resistance accelerates muscle protein degradation: activation of the ubiquitin-proteasome pathway by defects in muscle cell signaling," *Endocrinology*, vol. 147, no. 9, pp. 4160–4168, 2006.

[15] L. Larsson, B. Sjödin, and J. Karlsson, "Histochemical and biochemical changes in human skeletal muscle with age in sedentary males, age 22-65 years," *Acta Physiologica Scandinavica*, vol. 103, no. 1, pp. 31–39, 1978.

[16] B. E. Tomlinson, D. Irving, and J. J. Rebeiz, "Total numbers of limb motor neurones in the human lumbosacral cord and an analysis of the accuracy of various sampling procedures," *Journal of the Neurological Sciences*, vol. 20, no. 3, pp. 313–327, 1973.

[17] J. E. Morley, "Diabetes, sarcopenia, and frailty," *Clinics in Geriatric Medicine*, vol. 24, no. 3, pp. 455–469, 2008.

[18] K. F. Petersen, S. Dufour, D. Befroy, R. Garcia, and G. I. Shulman, "Impaired mitochondrial activity in the insulin-resistant offspring of patients with type 2 diabetes," *The New England Journal of Medicine*, vol. 350, no. 7, pp. 664–671, 2004.

[19] J. C. Anthony, A. K. Reiter, T. G. Anthony et al., "Orally administered leucine enhances protein synthesis in skeletal muscle of diabetic rats in the absence of increases in 4E-BP1 or S6K1 phosphorylation," *Diabetes*, vol. 51, no. 4, pp. 928–936, 2002.

[20] A. Chonkar, R. Hopkin, E. Adeghate, and J. Singh, "Contraction and cation contents of skeletal soleus and EDL muscles in age-matched control and diabetic rats," *Annals of the New York Academy of Sciences*, vol. 1084, pp. 442–451, 2006.

[21] M. McGuire and M. MacDermott, "The influence of streptozotocin diabetes and metformin on erythrocyte volume and on the membrane potential and the contractile characteristics of the extensor digitorum longus and soleus muscles in rats," *Experimental Physiology*, vol. 84, no. 6, pp. 1051–1058, 1999.

[22] E. van Lunteren and M. Moyer, "Altered diaphragm muscle action potentials in Zucker diabetic fatty (ZDF) rats," *Respiratory Physiology & Neurobiology*, vol. 153, no. 2, pp. 157–165, 2006.

[23] A. Verkhratsky and P. Fernyhough, "Mitochondrial malfunction and Ca2+ dyshomeostasis drive neuronal pathology in diabetes," *Cell Calcium*, vol. 44, no. 1, pp. 112–122, 2008.

[24] J. D. Bruton, A. Katz, J. Lännergren, F. Abbate, and H. Westerblad, "Regulation of myoplasmic Ca(2+) in genetically obese (ob/ob) mouse single skeletal muscle fibres," *Pflügers Archiv*, vol. 444, no. 6, pp. 692–699, 2002.

[25] E. O. Hernandez-Ochoa, P. Robison, M. Contreras, T. Shen, Z. Zhao, and M. F. Schneider, "Elevated extracellular glucose and uncontrolled type 1 diabetes enhance NFAT5 signaling and disrupt the transverse tubular network in mouse skeletal muscle," *Experimental Biology and Medicine (Maywood, New Jersey)*, vol. 237, no. 9, pp. 1068–1083, 2012.

[26] I. Kimura and M. Kimura, "Increase in electrically-stimulated Ca2+ release and suppression of caffeine response in diaphragm muscle of alloxan-diabetic mice compared with the denervation effect," *Diabetologia*, vol. 33, no. 2, pp. 72–76, 1990.

[27] G. Racz, A. Szabó, A. Vér, and E. Zádor, "The slow sarco/endoplasmic reticulum Ca2+ –ATPase declines independently of slow myosin in soleus muscle of diabetic rats," *Acta Biochimica Polonica*, vol. 56, no. 3, pp. 487–493, 2009.

[28] K. G. Beam, P. Horowicz, A. G. Engel, and C. Franzini-Armstrong, "Excitation-contraction coupling in skeletal muscle," vol. 1, McGraw-Hill, New York, 3rd Ed. Myology edition, 2004.

[29] M. F. Schneider and E. O. Hernandez-Ochoa, "Skeletal muscle excitation-contraction coupling in muscle: fundamental biology and mechanisms of disease," Academic Press, Elsevier, London UK, 2012.

[30] L. D. Brown, G. G. Rodney, E. Hernández-Ochoa, C. W. Ward, and M. F. Schneider, "Ca2+ sparks and T tubule reorganization in dedifferentiating adult mouse skeletal muscle fibers," *American Journal of Physiology - Cell Physiology*, vol. 292, no. 3, pp. C1156–C1166, 2007.

[31] Y. Liu, S. L. Carroll, M. G. Klein, and M. F. Schneider, "Calcium transients and calcium homeostasis in adult mouse fast-twitch skeletal muscle fibers in culture," *The American Journal of Physiology*, vol. 272, no. 6, Part 1, pp. C1919–C1927, 1997.

[32] Y. Liu, Z. Cseresnyés, W. R. Randall, and M. F. Schneider, "Activity-dependent nuclear translocation and intranuclear distribution of NFATc in adult skeletal muscle fibers," *The Journal of Cell Biology*, vol. 155, no. 1, pp. 27–39, 2001.

[33] L. D. Brown and M. F. Schneider, "Delayed dedifferentiation and retention of properties in dissociated adult skeletal muscle fibers in vitro," *In Vitro Cellular & Developmental Biology - Animal*, vol. 38, no. 7, pp. 411–422, 2002.

[34] B. L. Prosser, E. O. Hernández-Ochoa, R. M. Lovering et al., "S100A1 promotes action potential-initiated calcium release flux and force production in skeletal muscle," *American Journal of Physiology Cell Physiology*, vol. 299, no. 5, pp. C891–C902, 2010.

[35] B. L. Prosser, N. T. Wright, E. O. Hernãndez-Ochoa et al., "S100A1 binds to the calmodulin-binding site of ryanodine receptor and modulates skeletal muscle excitation-contraction coupling," *The Journal of Biological Chemistry*, vol. 283, no. 8, pp. 5046–5057, 2008.

[36] E. O. Hernandez-Ochoa, C. Vanegas, S. R. Iyer, R. M. Lovering, and M. F. Schneider, "Alternating bipolar field stimulation identifies muscle fibers with defective excitability but maintained local ca(2+) signals and contraction," *Skeletal Muscle*, vol. 6, no. 6, 2016.

[37] E. W. Yeung, S. I. Head, and D. G. Allen, "Gadolinium reduces short-term stretch-induced muscle damage in isolated mdx mouse muscle fibres," *The Journal of Physiology*, vol. 552, Part 2, pp. 449–458, 2003.

[38] T. R. Neelands, P. S. Herson, D. Jacobson, J. P. Adelman, and J. Maylie, "Small-conductance calcium-activated potassium currents in mouse hyperexcitable denervated skeletal muscle," *The Journal of Physiology*, vol. 536, Part 2, pp. 397–407, 2001.

[39] Y. Xiao, J. Tang, Y. Yang et al., "Jingzhaotoxin-III, a novel spider toxin inhibiting activation of voltage-gated sodium channel in rat cardiac myocytes," *The Journal of Biological Chemistry*, vol. 279, no. 25, pp. 26220–26226, 2004.

[40] A. Franco-Obregon Jr. and J. B. Lansman, "Mechanosensitive ion channels in skeletal muscle from normal and dystrophic mice," *The Journal of Physiology*, vol. 481, Part 2, pp. 299–309, 1994.

[41] J. F. Renaud, C. Desnuelle, H. Schmid-Antomarchi, M. Hugues, G. Serratrice, and M. Lazdunski, "Expression of apamin receptor in muscles of patients with myotonic muscular dystrophy," *Nature*, vol. 319, no. 6055, pp. 678–680, 1986.

[42] M. I. Behrens, P. Jalil, A. Serani, F. Vergara, and O. Alvarez, "Possible role of apamin-sensitive K+ channels in myotonic dystrophy," *Muscle & Nerve*, vol. 17, no. 11, pp. 1264–1270, 1994.

[43] Y. Fu, A. Struyk, V. Markin, and S. Cannon, "Gating behaviour of sodium currents in adult mouse muscle recorded with an improved two-electrode voltage clamp," *The Journal of Physiology*, vol. 589, Part 3, pp. 525–546, 2011.

[44] M. Midrio, "The denervated muscle: facts and hypotheses. A historical review," *European Journal of Applied Physiology*, vol. 98, no. 1, pp. 1–21, 2006.

[45] D. Purves and B. Sakmann, "Membrane properties underlying spontaneous activity of denervated muscle fibres," *The Journal of Physiology*, vol. 239, no. 1, pp. 125–153, 1974.

[46] Z. Liao, C. Yuan, K. Peng, Y. Xiao, and S. Liang, "Solution structure of Jingzhaotoxin-III, a peptide toxin inhibiting both Nav1.5 and Kv2.1 channels," *Toxicon*, vol. 50, no. 1, pp. 135–143, 2007.

[47] M. Cotter, N. E. Cameron, D. R. Lean, and S. Robertson, "Effects of long-term streptozotocin diabetes on the contractile and histochemical properties of rat muscles," *Quarterly Journal of Experimental Physiology*, vol. 74, no. 1, pp. 65–74, 1989.

[48] S. W. Park, B. H. Goodpaster, E. S. Strotmeyer et al., "Accelerated loss of skeletal muscle strength in older adults with type 2 diabetes: the health, aging, and body composition study," *Diabetes Care*, vol. 30, no. 6, pp. 1507–1512, 2007.

[49] G. M. Stephenson, A. O'Callaghan, and D. G. Stephenson, "Single-fiber study of contractile and biochemical properties of skeletal muscles in streptozotocin-induced diabetic rats," *Diabetes*, vol. 43, no. 5, pp. 622–628, 1994.

[50] J. N. Edwards, T. R. Cully, T. R. Shannon, D. G. Stephenson, and B. S. Launikonis, "Longitudinal and transversal propagation of excitation along the tubular system of rat fast-twitch muscle fibres studied by high speed confocal microscopy," *The Journal of Physiology*, vol. 590, no. 3, pp. 475–492, 2012.

[51] G. S. Posterino, G. D. Lamb, and D. G. Stephenson, "Twitch and tetanic force responses and longitudinal propagation of action potentials in skinned skeletal muscle fibres of the rat," *The Journal of Physiology*, vol. 527, Part 1, pp. 131–137, 2000.

[52] K. Jurkat-Rott, M. Fauler, and F. Lehmann-Horn, "Ion channels and ion transporters of the transverse tubular system of skeletal muscle," *Journal of Muscle Research and Cell Motility*, vol. 27, no. 5–7, pp. 275–290, 2006.

[53] C. C. Shieh, M. Coghlan, J. P. Sullivan, and M. Gopalakrishnan, "Potassium channels: molecular defects, diseases, and therapeutic opportunities," *Pharmacological Reviews*, vol. 52, no. 4, pp. 557–594, 2000.

[54] C. A. Leech and P. R. Stanfield, "Inward rectification in frog skeletal muscle fibres and its dependence on membrane potential and external potassium," *The Journal of Physiology*, vol. 319, pp. 295–309, 1981.

[55] S. L. Carroll, M. G. Klein, and M. F. Schneider, "Decay of calcium transients after electrical stimulation in rat fast- and slow-twitch skeletal muscle fibres," *The Journal of Physiology*, vol. 501, Part 3, pp. 573–588, 1997.

[56] O. P. Hamill and D. W. McBride Jr., "The pharmacology of mechanogated membrane ion channels," *Pharmacological Reviews*, vol. 48, no. 2, pp. 231–252, 1996.

[57] M. W. Berchtold, H. Brinkmeier, and M. Muntener, "Calcium ion in skeletal muscle: its crucial role for muscle function, plasticity, and disease," *Physiological Reviews*, vol. 80, no. 3, pp. 1215–1265, 2000.

[58] S. Schiaffino, M. Sandri, and M. Murgia, "Activity-dependent signaling pathways controlling muscle diversity and plasticity," *Physiology (Bethesda)*, vol. 22, pp. 269–278, 2007.

[59] S. Apostol, D. Ursu, F. Lehmann-Horn, and W. Melzer, "Local calcium signals induced by hyper-osmotic stress in mammalian skeletal muscle cells," *Journal of Muscle Research and Cell Motility*, vol. 30, no. 3-4, pp. 97–109, 2009.

[60] J. N. Struijs, C. A. Baan, F. G. Schellevis, G. P. Westert, and G. A. van den Bos, "Comorbidity in patients with diabetes mellitus: impact on medical health care utilization," *BMC Health Services Research*, vol. 6, no. 84, 2006.

[61] L. Bianchi and S. Volpato, "Muscle dysfunction in type 2 diabetes: a major threat to patient's mobility and independence," *Acta Diabetologica*, vol. 53, no. 6, pp. 879–889, 2016.

[62] S. Cohen, J. A. Nathan, and A. L. Goldberg, "Muscle wasting in disease: molecular mechanisms and promising therapies," *Nature Reviews Drug Discovery*, vol. 14, no. 1, pp. 58–74, 2015.

[63] S. S. Rudrappa, D. J. Wilkinson, P. L. Greenhaff, K. Smith, I. Idris, and P. J. Atherton, "Human skeletal muscle disuse atrophy: effects on muscle protein synthesis, breakdown, and insulin resistance-a qualitative review," *Frontiers in Physiology*, vol. 7, no. 361, 2016.

[64] A. Bekoff and W. Betz, "Properties of isolated adult rat muscle fibres maintained in tissue culture," *The Journal of Physiology*, vol. 271, no. 2, pp. 537–564, 1977.

[65] W. J. Duddy, T. Cohen, S. Duguez, and T. A. Partridge, "The isolated muscle fibre as a model of disuse atrophy: characterization using PhAct, a method to quantify f-actin," *Experimental Cell Research*, vol. 317, no. 14, pp. 1979–1993, 2011.

3

Renoprotective Effects of the Dipeptidyl Peptidase-4 Inhibitor Sitagliptin: A Review in Type 2 Diabetes

Cristina Mega,[1,2,3] **Edite Teixeira-de-Lemos,**[1,2] **Rosa Fernandes,**[3,4] **and Flávio Reis**[3,4]

[1]*Agrarian School of Viseu (ESAV), Polytechnic Institute of Viseu (IPV), 3500-606 Viseu, Portugal*
[2]*Centre for the Study of Education, Technologies and Health (CI&DETS), Polytechnic Institute of Viseu (IPV), 3500-606 Viseu, Portugal*
[3]*Institute of Pharmacology and Experimental Therapeutics and Institute for Biomedical Imaging and Life Sciences (IBILI), Faculty of Medicine, University of Coimbra, 3000-548 Coimbra, Portugal*
[4]*CNC.IBILI Research Consortium, University of Coimbra, 3004-504 Coimbra, Portugal*

Correspondence should be addressed to Rosa Fernandes; rcfernandes@fmed.uc.pt and Flávio Reis; freis@fmed.uc.pt

Academic Editor: Kim Connelly

Diabetic nephropathy (DN) is now the single commonest cause of end-stage renal disease (ESRD) worldwide and one of the main causes of death in diabetic patients. It is also acknowledged as an independent risk factor for cardiovascular disease (CVD). Since sitagliptin was approved, many studies have been carried out revealing its ability to not only improve metabolic control but also ameliorate dysfunction in various diabetes-targeted organs, especially the kidney, due to putative underlying cytoprotective properties, namely, its antiapoptotic, antioxidant, anti-inflammatory, and antifibrotic properties. Despite overall recommendations, many patients spend a long time well outside the recommended glycaemic range and, therefore, have an increased risk for developing micro- and macrovascular complications. Currently, it is becoming clearer that type 2 diabetes mellitus (T2DM) management must envision not only the improvement in glycaemic control but also, and particularly, the prevention of pancreatic deterioration and the evolution of complications, such as DN. This review aims to provide an overview of the current knowledge in the field of renoprotective actions of sitagliptin, namely, improvement in diabetic dysmetabolism, hemodynamic factors, renal function, diabetic kidney lesions, and cytoprotective properties.

1. Introduction

Type 2 diabetes mellitus (T2DM) is recognized as being a group of chronic diseases characterized by hyperglycaemia where the importance of protecting the body from excessive glucose circulation cannot be overstated. The central key features of T2DM are a defect in insulin resistance and/or insulin secretion, which lead to hyperglycaemia and disrupt the normal relationship between insulin sensitivity and pancreatic β-cell function [1]. Degeneration of Langerhans islets with β-cell loss is secondary to insulin resistance and is regarded as the most important lesion for disease progression [2–5]. Currently, eight central players are considered to be involved in T2DM pathophysiology—the ominous octet—composed by muscle/liver insulin resistance, β-cell failure, enhanced lipolysis, hyperglucagonaemia, dysregulation of hepatic glucose production, brain insulin resistance, increased renal glucose reabsorption, and incretin hormone [glucagon-like peptide 1 (GLP-1) and glucose-dependent insulinotropic polypeptide (GIP)] deficiency, all contributing to a persistent state of hyperglycaemia [6]. GLP-1 and GIP are peptide hormones that are involved in the physiologic regulation of glucose homeostasis. These hormones are secreted from the gastrointestinal tract after a meal and stimulate insulin secretion in a glucose-dependent manner [7]. In T2DM, there is an "incretin defect," manifested through the reduction in incretin bioavailability, which in part is due to their rapid inactivation by dipeptidyl peptidase-4 (DPP-4) [8]. It is now also acknowledged that biochemical pathways, such as apoptosis, low-grade inflammation, and oxidative stress, which are mainly fuelled by hyperglycaemia and hyperlipidaemia, are key mediators of insulin resistance and β-cell dysfunction and are involved in the overall aggravation of the diabetic state [3, 9–15]. The persistent dysfunction of these metabolic pathways in the "ominous octet" organs, through the direct and indirect effects of hyperglycaemia, seems to have an important role in the development of T2DM's major long-term complications [16, 17].

Generally, diabetic complications are divided into macrovascular (coronary artery disease, peripheral arterial disease, and stroke) and microvascular complications (nephropathy, retinopathy, and neuropathy). T2DM-induced micro- and macrovascular complications and their pathologies are major contributors to disease morbidity and mortality, respectively [18, 19]. It is now known that inflammation promotes development and progression of diabetic microangiopathy, which trigger extracellular matrix protein synthesis and capillary basement membrane thickening; these conditions contribute to the development of severe diabetic complications, such as nephropathy, retinopathy, and neuropathy [20–22].

Diabetic nephropathy (DN) originates insidious chronic kidney disease (CKD) and is recognized as the single most common cause of end-stage renal disease (ESRD) and one of the main causes of death in diabetic patients worldwide, being also acknowledged as an independent risk factor for cardiovascular disease (CVD) [23–25].

T2DM can generally be prevented with interventions such as change in dietary habits and physical activity. However, individuals with established diabetes should be treated with antidiabetic drugs [26, 27]. T2DM therapy has vastly improved in the last 10 years with the availability of new drugs and drug classes. These pharmacological agents improve glycaemic control by increasing insulin secretion, ameliorating insulin action, decreasing hepatic gluconeogenesis, and delaying the absorption of carbohydrates [28, 29]. Currently, T2DM can be managed with biguanides, sulfonylureas, meglitinide derivatives, alpha-glucosidase inhibitors, thiazolidinediones, selective sodium-glucose transporter-2 (SGLT2) inhibitors, insulins, amylinomimetics, bile acid sequestrants, dopamine agonists, and incretin-based therapies, which include glucagon-like peptide1 (GLP-1) agonists and DPP-4 inhibitors, of which sitagliptin was the first to be discovered and marketed [29, 30]. Moreover, these drugs may be used in various therapeutic combinations as an add-on therapy for improved management of hyperglycaemia [29].

Treatment regimens of T2DM that reduce the levels of HbA1c to near or below 7% are able to significantly reduce the risk of microvascular complications and diabetes-related death [31–36]. Current recommendations by the consensus of the American Diabetes Association (ADA) and European Association for the Study of Diabetes (EASD) justify the selection of appropriate treatment based on its capability to achieve and maintain desired glycaemic goals [36–38]. Despite all recomendations, many patients spend a long time well outside the target glycaemic range and, therefore, have an increased risk for developing micro- and macrovascular complications [6, 39]. Currently, it is becoming clearer that T2DM management must envision not only glycaemic control but also and particularly, the mechanisms behind progression of pancreatic deterioration and evolution of diabetic complications [40, 41].

The ground-breaking incretin-based therapies that encompass GLP-1 agonists and DPP-4 inhibitors seem to address a previously unmet need in diabetes by modulating glucose supply [42, 43]. In fact, DPP-4 inhibitors, and especially sitagliptin, have progressively increased their therapeutic prominence in the management of T2DM by their capability to potentiate incretin activity. Various studies have described many pleiotropic effects of sitagliptin on various organs and tissues. The knowledge that DPP-4 has the highest expression levels in the kidneys of mammals, which is additionally upregulated in DN [44], indicates that DPP-4 inhibition by sitagliptin is a plausible therapeutic target for management of diabetic nephropathy.

This review outlines the evidence found in previous studies regarding the renoprotective action of sitagliptin in DN, focusing on renal function and lesions, as well as kidney tissue cytoprotective properties, particularly its antiapoptotic, antifibrotic, anti-inflammatory, and antioxidant properties.

2. The Incretin System in Diabetic Nephropathy

2.1. Overview of DN Pathophysiology. The kidney, besides contributing to the aggravation of hyperglycaemia in T2DM through gluconeogenesis [45] and glucose reabsorption, does not remain unscathed through diabetic evolution, developing progressive lesions and functional impairments that lead to DN [46]. Dysmetabolism, with a central role for chronic hyperglycaemia, and hemodynamic factors, namely, overactivity of the renin-angiotensin-aldosterone system (RAAS) and vascular endothelial growth factor (VEGF) deficiency, have key roles in the pathophysiology of DN. Chronic hyperglycaemia and dyslipidaemia induce mitochondrial deregulation and oxidative stress in kidney cells, which activate several metabolic pathways, including protein kinase C [47], nonenzymatic glycation [48], oxidative stress [49–54], and inflammation [55, 59].

Inflammatory response is mediated by diverse types of inflammatory cells (including macrophages, monocytes, and leukocytes) and molecules (such as adhesion molecules, chemokines, and cytokines, namely, TNF-α and IL-1β) [55, 60]. Besides altering glomerular hemodynamics and promoting increased vascular permeability, TNF-α activates several signalling pathways leading to apoptosis and necrosis. IL-1β also modifies vascular permeability and increases the expression of chemokines that induce proliferation and synthesis of extracellular matrix in the mesangium [57]. As inflammation persists, renal tissues are damaged, occurring endothelial dysfunction, mesangial nodule formation (Kimmelstiel-Wilson bodies), renal fibrosis, and apoptosis [55, 60].

Hemodynamic factors [61, 62] predominantly mediated by angiotensin II play a role via overactivity of the RAAS and promotion of VEGF deficiency. Interaction of metabolic factors, such as obesity and chronic hyperglycaemia, alters vasoactive regulating mechanisms of afferent and efferent arteriolar tonus, leading to increased glomerular capillary hydrostatic pressure, hyperperfusion, hyperfiltration, and microalbuminuria. These early renal hemodynamic changes, combined with systemic hypertension, are important in the development and progression of renal disease in T2DM [63].

Albuminuria is mostly glomerular in origin, as albumin must cross the glomerular filtration assembly, which is composed of three main cellular barriers that are of utmost importance for the ultrafiltration process, the fenestrated glomerular endothelial cells, glomerular basement membrane (GBM), and glomerular epithelial cells or podocytes. Alterations in this three-layered structure, like increased intraglomerular pressure, loss of negatively charged glycosaminoglycans in the basement membrane, and further in disease evolution, and increase in basement membrane pore size, contribute to albuminuria [64]. An increasing number of proteins have been identified to be present in foot projections of podocytes. Nephrin is a zipper-like protein that plays a functional role in the structure of the slit diaphragm. The spaces between the teeth of the zipper allow selective transport of small molecules (such as glucose and water) retaining, however, large proteins. Evidence suggests that nephrin could play a key role in glomerular filtration barrier and development of proteinuria as it is found to be downregulated in kidney failure and in diabetic rats [51]. In diabetes, early flattening and retraction of podocytes' foot processes are associated with thickening of the GBM. Thickening of GBM, as well as accumulation of mesangial matrix, and increased numbers of mesangial cells are considered as initial microscopic abnormalities. As the disease progresses, there is a close relationship between mesangial expansion and declining of glomerular filtration. Mesangial expansion also correlates inversely with capillary filtration surface area, which itself correlates to glomerular filtration rate [64]. Long-term persistence of the previous factors ultimately induces histological abnormalities in glomeruli, tubules, interstitium, and renal vascular tissues, affecting basement membranes, podocytes, endothelial, and mesangial cells, which eventually become irreversible [64–68].

The cumulative presence of cooperative risk factors, namely, obesity, hypertension, insulin resistance, hyperglycaemia, dyslipidaemia, and microalbuminuria, appears to support not only the aggravation of CKD but also the development of CVD called the cardiorenal metabolic syndrome [69]. However, the underlying mechanisms of micro- and macrovascular complications of diabetes are not yet completely clarified. It seems that diabetic microangiopathy in conjunction with the aforementioned diabetogenic factors, together with neovascularization of *vasa vasorum,* can lead to macrovascular complications. Consequently, alterations in small arteries and capillaries may be responsible not only for the enduring microvascular complications but also for CVD in diabetes and, thus, may constitute one more link between DN and CVD [18].

2.2. The Role of the Incretin System in the Pathophysiology of DN. The presence of the incretin hormone GLP-1 and of its receptor (GLP-1R) in the kidneys suggests that the incretin system can play a role in the modulation of kidney function [70, 71]. Incretin dynamics, which are significantly altered in T2DM, seem also to be implicated in alteration of vascular tonus, natriuretic, and diuretic properties in the kidney [72]. The localization of GLP-1R in endothelial cells and in the proximal renal tubules plays a role in regulating the composition of urine. Stimulation of the GLP-1R in blood vessels results in relaxation of smooth muscle and increased renal blood flow [73].

In the normal kidney, stimulation of GLP-1R by GLP-1 results in inactivation of the Na^+/H^+ exchanger isoform 3 (NHE3) transporter, blocking Na^+ and other electrolytes retrieval from tubular fluid, thus resulting in natriuresis and water loss, and possibly, lowered blood pressure [74]. However, DPP-4 has its highest cellular expression in the kidneys of mammals, being found in the brush border of the proximal tubules, endothelium of the glomerular capillaries, and epithelium of Bowman's capsule [8, 44, 75]. In T2DM, DPP-4 is additionally upregulated in glomeruli of patients with DN, being implicated in the reduction of the half-life of GLP-1 in the kidney [44, 76] and altering its natriuretic and diuretic properties [76].

Other pathophysiological interventions by DPP-4 seem to involve its interaction with extracellular matrix proteins in the kidney during the development and evolution of DN, but there is still insufficient data demonstrating that selective DPP-4 inhibition is able to affect these independent interactions [75]. The association between DPP-4 and integrin $\beta1$ appears to promote endothelial-to-mesenchymal transition (EndMT) by negatively regulating endothelial viability signalling via suppression of the VEGF-receptor 2 and induction of VEGF-receptor 1 in endothelial cells. It seems that DPP-4 inhibition is capable of inhibiting EndMT and transforming growth factor-$\beta2$- (TGF-$\beta2$-) induced Smad3 phosphorylation, and thus, the progression to renal sclerosis. EndMT is a known contributor to the accumulation of activated fibroblasts and myofibroblasts in kidney fibrosis [77].

Furthermore, DPP-4 might be implicated in the inactivation of stromal-derived factor-1 alpha (SDF-1α), a chemokine linked to the migration of hematopoietic and endothelial progenitor cells (EPCs) to sites of ischemic injury, involved in tissue repair and in the response to tissue hypoxia [44]. It has been reported that DPP-4 inhibition is able to recruit EPCs to sites of [78].

Direct effects of DPP-4 on immune cells and indirect effects through GLP-1-dependent and GLP-1-independent pathways suggest that enzyme inhibition may have beneficial effects beyond glycaemic control, which may contribute to CKD and CVD outcomes [71].

3. Sitagliptin

3.1. Pharmacokinetic and Pharmacodynamic Properties of Sitagliptin. Sitagliptin is an oral antidiabetic drug with a recommended dose of 100 mg once a day. Oral absorption is not affected by food. Sitagliptin displays 87% of bioavailability and a reversible fraction bound to plasma proteins of 38% [79]; its half-life is around 12.4 hours; hepatic metabolism of sitagliptin is minimal, mainly by cytochrome P450 3A4, while excretion occurs mainly (70–80%) by the kidney in its unchanged form, with a renal clearance of approximately 350 ml/min [80]. In general, the pharmacokinetic profile of sitagliptin is similar in both healthy volunteers and T2DM patients. The pharmacokinetic properties of the drug have also been evaluated in special patient populations with varying grades of hepatic and renal dysfunction. As a result of its metabolism and elimination route, dose adjustment is only required in patients with severe renal insufficiency, being effective and safe in patients with mild/moderate renal or hepatic impairment [81–85]. No dosage adjustment is necessary related to age, gender and race, or body mass index. Sitagliptin also has a low propensity for pharmacokinetic drug interactions [7].

Sitagliptin is a potent and highly selective DPP-4 competitive inhibitor that does not affect the closely related enzymes DPP-8 or DPP-9 at therapeutic concentrations [75–86]. Sitagliptin acts by inhibiting over 80% of the activity of DPP-4 enzyme (at 12 h postdose for 50 mg/day and at 24 h postdose for ≥100 mg/day), which is responsible for degrading GLP-1, preventing therefore its inactivation. This increases and prolongs plasma concentrations of the active form of GLP-1, allowing the consequent stimulation of insulin synthesis and secretion from pancreatic β-cells in a glucose-dependent manner [87–90].

As T2DM patients exhibit relative resistance to the actions of GIP [91], the main goals of DPP-4 inhibitors are to prolong the beneficial effects of endogenous GLP-1 [92] in order to maintain its insulinotropic activity [93]. Glycaemic levels are then further regulated by the resulting higher insulin levels and glucagon suppression from the direct action of GLP-1 on pancreatic α-cells [94]. Sitagliptin reduces blood glucose levels, in either the postprandial or the fasting state. It works differently from the previous drugs available for diabetes treatment and is orally active [95, 96].

Clinical trials have demonstrated the efficacy of sitagliptin in terms of improving glycaemic control in T2DM patients, used as either monotherapy, initial combination therapy (usually with a fixed dose combination of sitagliptin/metformin) or add-on therapy to metformin or to other antihyperglycaemic drugs, with or without metformin. Sitagliptin showed efficacy in decreasing HbA1c, fasting plasma glucose (FPG), and postprandial plasma glucose (PPG) levels and also increasing the proportion of patients achieving target HbA1c levels (<7.0%), as shown in several clinical studies [79, 97–100].

3.2. Sitagliptin Affords Protection in Organs Targeted by Diabetes. Experimental studies performed in animal models of T2DM that were treated with sitagliptin showed remarkable beneficial effects on glucose and HbA1c levels, an improvement of insulin resistance, together with promotion of weight loss and amelioration of lipid profile [101–110]. Moreover, sitagliptin was able to consistently alleviate oxidative stress and inflammation, which are key players in diabetes pathophysiology and in the development of DN [51, 57, 103, 111].

Sitagliptin promotes a conjoined improvement in dyslipidaemia and hypertension, which are interactive factors for CKD and CVD [104, 107–111]. Sitagliptin attenuates the progress of atherosclerosis in apolipoprotein-E-knockout mice via AMPK- and MAPK-dependent mechanisms [110]. Several reports have corroborated the cardiovascular protective aspects and have also identified cytoprotective properties, such as a decrease in heart oxidative stress, inflammation, and apoptosis [19, 78, 103, 112–118]. Concerning the impact of sitagliptin on lipid profiles in T2DM patients, the majority of studies reported a beneficial effect on triglycerides (TGs), high-density lipoprotein cholesterol (HDL-c), and low-density lipoprotein cholesterol (LDL-c) [119, 120]. DPP-4 inhibition also appears to improve endothelial function in diabetic patients, in both a GLP-1-dependent and GLP-1-independent manner [121, 122]. Furthermore, sitagliptin was able to increase EPC levels in diabetic patients [78].

Our research group has extensively studied the protective effects of sitagliptin on various organs targeted by diabetes, namely, the pancreas, retina, and kidney, in an animal model of T2DM. Sitagliptin was able to prevent the aggravation of both endocrine and exocrine pancreatic histopathological lesions and presented antiapoptotic and anti-inflammatory properties, as well as decreased insulin resistance and pro-proliferative and angiogenic actions [103, 123]. In the retina, sitagliptin treatment prevented changes in the endothelial subcellular distribution of tight junction proteins and improved nitrosative stress and inflammatory and apoptotic states [124]. Later studies in type 1 diabetic rats revealed that sitagliptin could prevent the increase in blood-retinal barrier permeability and decrease the retinal inflammation state and neuronal apoptosis [125]. Our studies in the kidney also revealed protective properties [8, 126]. Other authors have also found diabetic lesion improvement in the pancreas associated to antiapoptotic, pro-proliferative [111, 127–131], and anti-inflammatory properties [132–134].

Besides decreasing insulin resistance [5, 135, 136] and improving hepatic insulin sensitivity, sitagliptin seems also to prevent steatosis [137] through GLP-1R signalling in the liver and reduction of endoplasmic reticulum stress [138]. GLP-1R has been found to be expressed in human hepatocytes [138]. However, other authors failed to detect GLP-1R mRNA transcripts in human, rat, or mouse liver [139]. Antiapoptotic effects on human hepatoma cells by DPP-4 inhibition have also been identified [140].

Treatment of nonobese diabetic mice with sitagliptin not only prevented linoleic acid-induced adipose tissue hypertrophy but also protected against adipose tissue inflammation [131, 137].

In T2DM rats with uncontrolled neuropathy, sitagliptin as add-on to insulin therapy produced neuroprotective effects and ameliorated hyperalgesia, oxidative stress, and inflammation, more than either drug alone [141].

4. Sitagliptin Affords Renoprotection in Diabetic Nephropathy

4.1. Effects of Sitagliptin on Renal Function. The effects of sitagliptin on DN, using the ZDF rat, noticeably reduced renal dysfunction and injury in this model. In fact, sitagliptin treatment was able to decrease blood urea nitrogen (BUN) levels to values identical to those observed in lean control rats, suggesting an amelioration of renal function [126]. Nevertheless, serum creatinine levels were unchanged between study groups, which are in accordance with others using the ZDF rat as an animal model [106, 142].

Direct vasodilator effects have also been described for DPP-4 inhibitors [143]. In this regard, interactions of angiotensin II and DPP-4/GLP-1 signalling have been proposed as one of the mechanisms for the blood pressure- (BP-) lowering effect of DPP-4 inhibition [144]. Sitagliptin seems to be able to lower BP in a GLP-1-dependent manner through GLP-1R localized in renal endothelial cells and in the proximal renal tubules, which play a role in regulating the composition of urine. DPP-4 inhibition by sitagliptin administration increases GLP-1 availability which stimulates GLP-1R in blood vessels, through the sequential activation of the PKA/LKB1/AMPKα/eNOS axis, thus inducing relaxation of smooth muscle and improvement of renal blood flow [143, 145].

There are solid evidences that the proximal tubules play a major role in microalbuminuria in DN, namely, in early stages of the disease [146, 147]. In addition, stimulation of GLP-1R in the proximal tubules results in increased loss of salt, water, and electrolytes in urine. The latter occurs as the GLP-1Rs situated in proximal convoluted tubules of the kidneys are functionally linked to NHE3 transporters. NHE3 promotes recovery of Na^+ and other electrolytes from the tubular fluid (and thus from urine), thereby returning them into the circulation. Activation of the GLP-1R by GLP-1 results in inactivation of NHE3, which leads to increased Na^+ loss in urine, consequentially, through osmotic effects, to increased fluid loss, and possibly, to lowered BP [74]. An association of NHE3 with DPP-4 was found in the proximal tubule, which might affect NHE3 surface expression and/or activity [148]. Furthermore, DPP-4 inhibition, in experimental models of obesity and heart failure, was able to upregulate megalin, a receptor that mediates endocytosis of proteins in the proximal tubule [149, 150]. DPP-4 inhibition improved kidney injury and proteinuria in obese rodent models [126, 150–152]. Consistently, Aroor et al. have demonstrated that increased DPP-4 activity, evoked by angiotensin II, suppresses megalin expression in mice, an effect that was partially abolished by using a DPP4 inhibitor [153].

Effects of GLP-1 on lowering BP have been reported in both animal and human studies [154, 155]. The natriuretic and diuretic properties of GLP-1 were proved in infusion studies in a rat model of salt sensitivity by chronic intravenous infusion of GLP-1 [72]. Although glycaemic levels affect renal pathophysiology, the previously mentioned effects of incretin protection appear to be independent of these levels, although the underlying mechanisms still remain to be clarified [156, 157]. Diuretic and natriuretic actions of DPP-4 inhibitors seem to offer renoprotection in the setting of hypertension and other disorders of sodium retention. However, in the case of sitagliptin, available data is not yet sufficient to confirm this protective effect [74, 76].

4.2. Effects of Sitagliptin on Renal Lesions. Although DN has been traditionally considered primarily a glomerular disease, it is now widely accepted that the rate of function deterioration correlates best with the degree of renal tubulointerstitial fibrosis. This suggests that although the primary event is a condition marked by glomerular changes resulting in proteinuria, the long-term outcome is determined by events in the renal interstitium [158, 159].

In preclinical studies, initial histopathological observations of DN focused mainly on glomerular lesions, alluding, only briefly, to tubulointerstitial lesions and considering their presence as a secondary lesion of DN [160, 161]. The description of vascular lesions in the kidney was absent in animal model studies and could be scarcely found in a few human DN reports. Thus envisioning evaluation conformity and better correlation between human nephropathy and renal lesions observed in animal models, the international histopathological classification, currently approved for human DN, should be adopted in these studies. This histological classification was established in 2010 and evaluates glomerular, tubulointerstitial, and vascular lesions in a semi-quantitative manner, according to their severity and tissue distribution [162].

In experimental animal models, diabetic glomerular lesions initially display thickening of the GBM and mesangial expansion, which are followed by the appearance of nodular sclerosis and vascular pole hyalinization, accompanied by glomerular hypertrophy. With disease aggravation, glomerulosclerosis and glomerular atrophy become evident (Figure 1(a)), confirming the link between diabetes (hyperglycaemia and hyperlipidaemia) and progressive renal injury [8, 126].

In the tubulointerstitium (Figure 1(a)), tubular hypertrophy and associated basement membrane alterations (thickening and irregularity) precede interstitial fibrosis, tubular atrophy (IFTA), and formation of hyaline cylinders, which accompany progressive renal dysfunction (Figure 1(a)). There seems to be a correlation between aggravation of tubulointerstitial and glomerular lesions, which is suggested by the aggravation of both glomeruli and interstitium [126]. Interstitial enlargement also correlates with glomerular filtration, albuminuria, and mesangial expansion. It has been suggested that the accumulation of protein in the cytoplasm of proximal tubular cells causes an inflammatory reaction which leads to tubulointerstitial lesions [64, 163].

Arteriolar hyalinosis and arteriosclerosis are the main vascular lesions found in human DN and also in some experimental animal models of diabetes (Figure 2(a)), and similarly, also aggravate with disease progression [126, 162]. Various studies have shown that DPP-4 inhibition is able to improve renal lesions in experimental animal models. In fact, in the obese diabetic ZDF rat, sitagliptin treatment ameliorated glomerular, tubulointerstitial (Figure 1(b)), and vascular lesions (Figure 2(b)) [126]. Other studies have also reported that suppression of DPP-4 activity and/or protein expression resulted in an amelioration of kidney fibrosis, which was correlated with inhibition of EndMT and reduction of inflammatory and fibrotic markers [164–166]. Similar histopathological improvements with incretin therapies have been disclosed by other studies [166–168].

4.3. Renal Cytoprotective Effects of Sitagliptin. Several authors have been postulating that gliptins could theoretically avoid or delay diabetic complications [40, 169–170], namely,

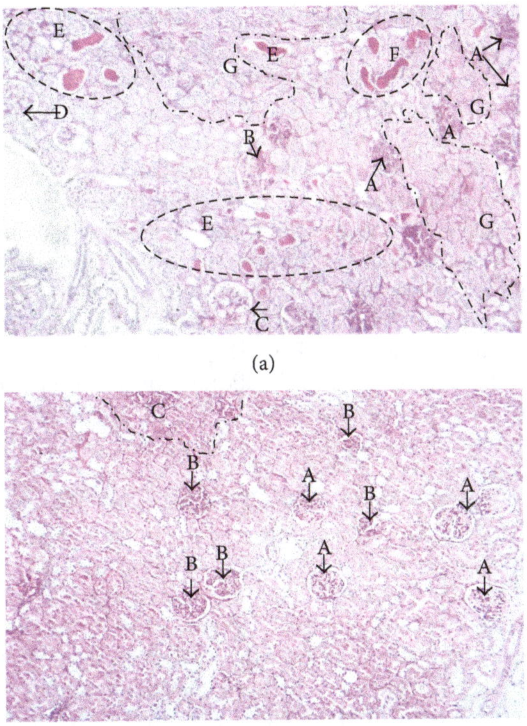

(a)

(b)

Figure 1: Effects of sitagliptin treatment on diabetic nephropathy lesions in an experimental model of type 2 diabetes. (a) Histopathological lesions in untreated diabetic nephropathy. *Glomerular lesions:* (A) glomerulosclerosis, (B) nodular sclerosis, (C) thickened capsule of Bowman, and (D) normal glomerulus. All other glomeruli on the image display various degrees of mesangial expansion. *Tubulointerstitial lesions:* (E) hyaline cylinders, (F) irregular shape of hyaline cylinders that indicates irregular tubular membranes, (G) various degrees of thickened and irregular tubular basement membranes a characteristic of interstitial fibrosis and tubular atrophy (IFTA). PAS staining of a kidney section from an obese diabetic untreated ZDF rat (original magnification ×100). (b) Improvement of histopathological lesions in sitagliptin-treated diabetic nephropathy. *Glomerular lesions:* Reduction of lesion severity, with global rise in (A) normal glomeruli and (B) the remainder showing various degrees of mesangial expansion, an early lesion of disease. *Tubulointerstitial lesions:* Most of the interstitium has normal appearance, showing only a focal patch of moderate interstitial fibrosis and tubular atrophy (IFTA); PAS staining of a kidney section from an obese diabetic sitagliptin-treated ZDF rat (original magnification ×100).

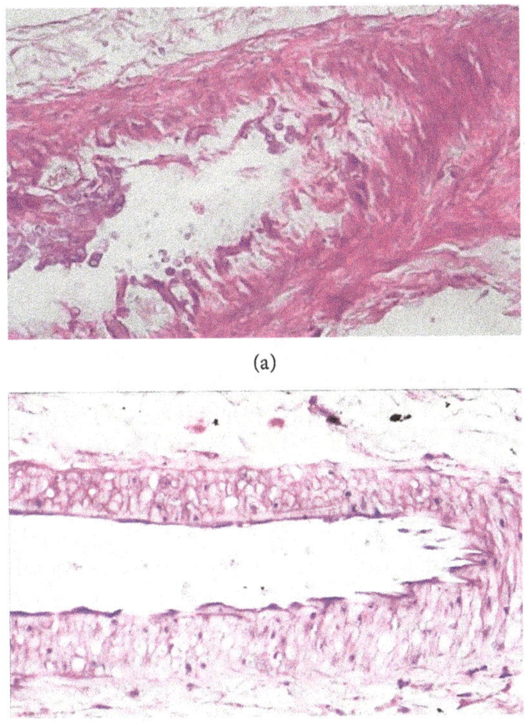

(a)

(b)

Figure 2: Effects of sitagliptin treatment on diabetic nephropathy vascular lesions in an experimental model of type 2 diabetes. (a) Histopathological lesions in untreated diabetic nephropathy: Renal arteries exhibiting marked hyperplastic arteriosclerosis and thickening and detachment of the intimal layer. Endothelial cells can no longer be identified; PAS staining of a kidney section from an obese diabetic untreated ZDF rat (original magnification ×400). (b) Improvement of histopathological vascular lesions in sitagliptin-treated diabetic nephropathy: A marked reduction in total wall and intimal layer thickening, showing normal endothelial cells; PAS staining of a kidney section from an obese diabetic sitagliptin-treated ZDF rat (original magnification ×400).

due to reduction of oxidative stress and inflammation, as well as by antiapoptotic and pro-proliferative properties on various organs and tissues, including the kidney [101–103, 138, 171, 172].

Considering that sitagliptin is not able to completely normalize hyperglycaemia in studies using low doses [8, 103, 126], an alternative mechanism for the beneficial effect on kidney function/lesions can occur by a direct tissue DPP-4 inhibition, via GLP-1-dependent and/or GLP-1-independent pathways. The GLP-1-dependent activity is reinforced by the expression of GLP-1R in the kidney. In fact, there are several mechanisms by which direct renoprotection could occur. GLP-1 has been associated with the protection of mesangial cells, as well as with the reestablishment of Na^+, acid-base and fluid homeostasis, which contributes to BP lowering and, collectively, to renoprotection [173–175]. The GLP-1-independent effects have been associated with other known substrates of DPP-4, such as high mobility group box 1 protein (HMGB1), meprin β, neuropeptide Y (NPY), and peptide YY (PYY) [76, 164].

It is known that DPP-4 exhibits its enzymatic activity in both membrane-anchored cell-surface peptidase and as a smaller soluble form in blood plasma [77, 131, 176]. In fact, there are some studies suggesting that microvascular endothelial cells are the main sources of endogenous DPP-4 [177, 178]. In addition, in vitro studies showed that both DPP-4 mRNA expression and enzyme activity were enhanced by exposure of human glomerular endothelial cells to high glucose concentrations [179–181]. In agreement, our research group has recently demonstrated that diabetic rats present an increased protein expression of DPP-4 in the kidney, when compared to nondiabetic animals [8].

Experimental studies in ZDF rats showed that chronic hyperglycaemia is associated with increased proinflammatory cytokines, namely, IL-1β and TNF-α in the kidney [8]. These outcomes are corroborated by other authors that described an increased expression of those proinflammatory cytokines in the diabetic kidney [58, 77, 182], leading to enhanced vascular permeability, oxidative stress, renal hypertrophy, and tubulointerstitial lesions. DPP-4 inhibition by low-dose sitagliptin has prevented the inflammatory profile and the proapoptotic state observed in the diabetic rat kidney, which might justify the improvement in renal function and tissular lesions (glomerular, tubulointerstitial, and vascular lesions). In fact, sitagliptin was able to prevent the increase in both mRNA and protein levels of the proinflammatory cytokines IL-1β and TNF-α in the diabetic kidneys of ZDF rats [8].

In Wistar rats treated with low- or high-dose sitagliptin during 16 weeks, urinary albumin excretion rate (UAER), serum creatinine, and kidney hypertrophy were significantly decreased. However, creatinine clearance rate and active GLP-1 levels were increased, with more pronounced changes in the high-dose sitagliptin-treated animals. Glomerular lesions were also improved following sitagliptin treatment. Protein and mRNA expression levels of podocalyxin and GLP-1R were significantly increased in both groups, while expression of signal-regulated kinases 1/2 (ERK1/2) and transforming growth factor-β1 (TGF-β1) was decreased [183]. Podocalyxin is a negatively charged transmembrane glycosaminoglycan that covers the secondary foot processes of the podocytes, which by electrical repellence keeps adjacent foot processes separated, maintaining the urinary filtration barrier open. Podocalyxin depletion is inversely correlated to albuminuria [64, 184]. These overall results also confirm a delay in DN progression promoted by sitagliptin, possibly via the inhibition of ERK1/2 signalling which seems to be activated by AGEs and is implicated in epithelial-myofibroblast transition [185]; by decreased TGF-β1 expression, a cytokine associated with inflammatory responses in T2DM, which has been recognized to be involved in the development of glomerulosclerosis and interstitial fibrosis; and by increasing the interaction between GLP-1 and the GLP-1R [186].

Recently, in a study involving 164 DN patients treated with metformin, sitagliptin (100 mg, once a day) was able to decrease UAER, which presented a close correlation with markers of renal fibrosis: TGF-β1 and platelet-derived growth factor-BB (PDGF-BB) [187]. Furthermore, PDGF-BB mRNA has been found to be overexpressed in diabetic patients and is considered a factor for mesangial cell proliferation and induction of TGF-β1, which shows a profibrotic action, being involved in the development of renal hypertrophy and accumulation of extracellular matrix in DN [188]. In addition, DPP-4 inhibition is known to downregulate TGF-β1 expression in mesangial cells [189]. Li et al. [190] suggest that the renoprotective mechanism of sitagliptin may be due to a reduction in protein kinase B (PKB)/Akt levels, which are involved in apoptosis pathways and restoration of adenosine monophosphate-activated protein kinase (AMPK) activity in diverse physiological processes, including ion transport, podocyte function and cell growth and cellular energy homeostasis, inhibition of TGF-β1, fibronectin, and p38/ERK MAPK signalling pathways involved in the regulation of ECM expression.

The activation of signalling pathways linked to cell death resulting from chronic hyperglycaemia and to a state of low-grade chronic inflammation contributes to an increase in apoptosis. A proapoptotic state seems to be favoured in the kidney of diabetic ZDF rats, which appears to be mediated by Bax and Bid. Sitagliptin prevented the Bax to Bcl-2 (mRNA and protein) ratio increase and reversed the increase in Bid and TUNEL-positive cells induced by chronic hyperglycaemia in the kidneys of this animal model [8]. In addition, sitagliptin was able to ameliorate serum TG content, thus reducing lipotoxicity-evoked apoptosis in the kidney [8, 190–193].

Additionally, it has been demonstrated that glucose-induced ROS production initiates podocyte apoptosis and its depletion in *vitro* and *in vivo*, leading to DN [49, 56, 194]. Therefore, the reduction of oxidative stress afforded by sitagliptin could eventually reduce ROS production and the consequent risk of cell death. A study on renal ischemia reperfusion damage in diabetic rats found sitagliptin to significantly decrease lipid peroxidation, xanthine oxidase activity, myeloperoxidase activity, and nitric oxide levels in renal tissue in comparison to those in untreated rats. Antioxidant enzymes like glutathione, glutathione peroxidase, superoxide dismutase, and catalase were significantly increased in sitagliptin-treated diabetic rats compared to those in the non-treated ones [195]. Other studies have demonstrated that GLP-1 receptor activation has also attenuated diabetic renal injury by reduction of kidney oxidative stress, inflammation, and apoptosis [196–199].

5. Concluding Remarks

The innovative class of DPP-4 inhibitors, such as sitagliptin, seem to address previously unmet needs in diabetes. In fact, DPP-4 has the highest expression levels in the kidneys of mammals, which is additionally upregulated in diabetic-induced CKD, indicating that DPP-4 inhibition by sitagliptin is a plausible therapeutic target for management of DN. In fact, several studies have been describing putative pleiotropic effects of sitagliptin on various organs and tissues. Sitagliptin showed not only the capacity to ameliorate diabetic dysmetabolism but also the potential to avert the decline of insulin secretion ability in pancreatic beta-cells through cytoprotective properties; these effects suggest a role in prevention of T2DM evolution and its complications. In the kidney, sitagliptin seems to provide renoprotection by restoring GLP-1 diuretic and natriuretic actions and by other mechanisms, including antiapoptotic, antifibrotic, anti-inflammatory, and antioxidant effects. However, additional studies are needed to clarify whether sitagliptin acts through indirect action via insulin secretion increment or through direct tissular DPP-4 inhibition. In addition, further research should also elucidate the contribution of GLP-1-dependent (which is sustained by expression of DPP-4 and GLP-1R in renal tissues) and/or GLP-1-independent pathways (reinforced by the existence of multiple DPP-4 substrates).

Due to its unique mechanism of action and pharmacological properties, DPP-4 inhibitors (including sitagliptin) have conquered their place in T2DM management. In addition, the low potential for interactions with other antidiabetic drugs allows its use in different combinations, with a low risk of hypoglycaemiac episodes. A fixed-dose combination with sodium/glucose cotransporter 2 (SLGT2) inhibitor ertugliflozin has been recently accepted and seems to contain the potential to exert further beneficial effects on the kidney, as both classes have been reported to lower UAER. Additional positive effects could be expected from the complementary mechanism of action of these drugs, with impact on both renal and cardiovascular systems. Disclosure of its protective actions on the diabetic kidney could open up the possibility of using sitagliptin therapy as a renoprotective strategy against the development and/or delay of DN.

Conflicts of Interest

The authors declare no conflicts of interest.

Authors' Contributions

Cristina Mega prepared the manuscript. Edite Teixeira-Lemos, Rosa Fernandes, and Flávio Reis equally contributed to the work and are colast authors and coresponsible for the manuscript. All authors read and approved the final manuscript.

Acknowledgments

The authors gratefully acknowledge the Portuguese Foundation for Science and Technology (FCT) through the projects PEst-C/SAU/UI3282/2013, CNC.IBILI Strategic Project (2015-UID/NEU/04539/2013), and the Operational Programme Competitiveness Factors (COMPETE-FEDER): FCOMP-01-0124-FEDER-028417 and POCI-01-0145-FEDER-007440, as well as Centro 2020 Regional Operational Programmes (CENTRO-01-0145-FEDER-000012: HealthyAging2020 and CENTRO-01-0145-FEDER-000008: BrainHealth 2020). Cristina Mega also thanks PROTEC grant by the Polytechnic Institute of Viseu (IPV) (PROTEC-SFRH/BD/50139/2009).

References

[1] M. Virally, J. F. Blicklé, J. Girard, S. Halimi, D. Simon, and P. J. Guillausseau, "Type 2 diabetes mellitus: epidemiology, pathophysiology, unmet needs and therapeutical perspectives," *Diabetic Medicine*, vol. 33, pp. 231–244, 2007.

[2] S. E. Kahn, "The importance of the β-cell in the pathogenesis of type 2 diabetes mellitus," *American Journal of Medicine*, vol. 108, pp. 2S–8S, 2000.

[3] P. Marchetti, R. Lupi, S. D. Guerra, M. Bugliani, L. Marselli, and U. Boggi, "The β-cell in human type 2 diabetes," *Advances in Experimental Medicine and Biology*, vol. 654, pp. 501–514, 2010.

[4] M. E. Cerf, "Beta cell dysfunction and insulin resistance," *Frontiers in Endocrinology*, vol. 4, p. 37, 2013.

[5] S. Yagihashi, W. Inaba, and H. Mizukami, "Dynamic pathology of islet endocrine cells in type 2 diabetes: b-cell growth, death, regeneration and their clinical implications," *Journal of Diabetes Investigation*, vol. 7, pp. 155–165, 2016.

[6] R. A. D. Fronzo, "From the triumvirate to the ominous octet: a new paradigm for the treatment of type 2 diabetes mellitus (banting lecture)," *Diabetes*, vol. 58, pp. 773–795, 2009.

[7] D. J. Drucker, "The biology of incretin hormones," *Cell Metabolism*, vol. 3, no. 3, pp. 153–165, 2006.

[8] C. Marques, C. Mega, A. Gonçalves et al., "Sitagliptin prevents inflammation and apoptotic cell death in the kidney of type 2 diabetic animals," *Mediators of Inflammation*, vol. 2014, Article ID 538737, 15 pages, 2014.

[9] M. K. Piya, P. G. McTernan, and S. Kumar, "Adipokine inflammation and insulin resistance: the role of glucose, lipids and endotoxin," *Journal of Endocrinology*, vol. 216, pp. T1–T15, 2013.

[10] S. Guo, "Insulin signaling, resistance, and metabolic syndrome: insights from mouse models into disease mechanisms," *Journal of Endocrinology*, vol. 220, pp. T1–T23, 2014.

[11] U. J. Jung and M.-S. Choi, "Obesity and its metabolic complications: the role of adipokines and the relationship between obesity, inflammation, insulin resistance, dyslipidemia and nonalcoholic fatty liver disease," *International Journal of Molecular Sciences*, vol. 15, no. 4, pp. 6184–6223, 2014.

[12] S. L. Lay, G. Simard, M. C. Martinez, and R. Andriantsitohaina, "Oxidative stress and metabolic pathologies: from an adipocentric point of view," *Oxidative Medicine and Cellular Longevity*, vol. 2014, Article ID 908539, 18 pages, 2014.

[13] L. Chen, R. Chen, H. Wang, and F. Liang, "Mechanisms linking inflammation to insulin resistance," *International Journal of Endocrinology*, vol. 2015, Article ID 508409, 9 pages, 2015.

[14] S. Tangvarasittichai, "Oxidative stress, insulin resistance, dyslipidemia and type 2 diabetes mellitus," *World Journal of Diabetes*, vol. 6, no. 3, pp. 456–480, 2015.

[15] K. N. Keane, V. F. Cruzat, R. Carlessi, P. I. H. de Bittencourt, and P. Newsholme, "Molecular events linking oxidative stress and inflammation to insulin resistance and β-cell dysfunction," *Oxidative Medicine and Cellular Longevity*, vol. 2015, Article ID 181643, 15 pages, 2015.

[16] E. J. Bae, "DPP-4 inhibitors in diabetic complications: role of DPP-4 beyond glucose control," *Archives of Pharmacal Research*, vol. 39, no. 8, pp. 1114–1128, 2016.

[17] L. A. Filla and J. L. Edwards, "Metabolomics in diabetic complications," *Molecular BioSystems*, vol. 12, pp. 1090–1105, 2016.

[18] A. Chawla, R. Chawla, and S. Jaggi, "Microvasular and macrovascular complications in diabetes mellitus: distinct or continuum?," *Indian Journal of Endocrinology and Metabolism*, vol. 20, no. 4, pp. 546–551, 2016.

[19] A. Mima, "Incretin-based therapy for prevention of diabetic vascular complications," *Journal of Diabetes Research*, vol. 2016, Article ID 1379274, 12 pages, 2016.

[20] T. S. Kern, "Contributions of inflammatory processes to the development of the early stages of diabetic retinopathy," *Journal of Diabetes Research*, vol. 2007, Article ID 95103, 14 pages, 2007.

[21] J. F. Navarro-González and C. Mora-Fernández, "The role of inflammatory cytokines in diabetic nephropathy," *Journal of the American Society of Nephrology*, vol. 19, pp. 433–442, 2008.

[22] A. M. Vincent, B. C. Callaghan, A. L. Smith, and E. L. Feldman, "Diabetic neuropathy: cellular mechanisms as therapeutic targets," *Nature Reviews Neurology*, vol. 7, pp. 573–583, 2011.

[23] M. Narres, H. Claessen, S. Droste et al., "The incidence of end-stage renal disease in the diabetic (compared to the non-diabetic) population: a systematic review," *PLoS One*, vol. 11, no. 1, article e0147329, 2016.

[24] J. A. J. G. Van den Brand, "Diabetes mellitus as a cause of end-stage renal disease in Europe: signs of improvement," *Clinical Kidney Journal*, vol. 9, no. 3, pp. 454–456, 2016.

[25] American Diabetes Association, "Standards of medical care in diabetes—2017," *Diabetes Care*, vol. 40, Supplement 1, 2017.

[26] M. Y. Donath, D. M. Schumann, M. Faulenbach, H. Ellingsgaard, A. Perren, and J. A. Ehses, "Islet inflammation in type 2 diabetes: from metabolic stress to therapy," *Diabetes Care*, vol. 31, no. 2, pp. S161–S164, 2008.

[27] W. J. Rejeski, E. H. Ip, A. G. Bertoni et al., "Lifestyle change and mobility in obese adults with type 2 diabetes," *New England Journal of Medicine*, vol. 366, no. 13, pp. 1209–1217, 2012.

[28] J. J. Marín-Peñalver, I. Martín-Timón, C. Sevillano-Collantes, and F. J. del Cañizo-Gómez, "Update on the treatment of type 2 diabetes mellitus," *World Journal of Diabetes*, vol. 7, no. 17, pp. 354–395, 2016.

[29] R. Khardori, "Type 2 diabetes mellitus medication," Medscape, May 2017, http://emedicine.medscape.com/article/117853-overview.

[30] R. Godinho, C. Mega, E. Teixeira-de-Lemos et al., "The place of dipeptidyl peptidase-4 inhibitors in type 2 diabetes therapeutics: a "me too" or "the special one" antidiabetic class?," *Journal of Diabetes Research*, vol. 2015, Article ID 806979, 28 pages, 2015.

[31] "International Diabetes Federation (IDF) 2014," https://www.idf.org/about-diabetes/what-is-diabetes.

[32] D. M. Nathan, P. McGee, M. W. Steffes, J. M. Lachin, and DCCT/EDIC Research Group, "Relationship of glycated albumin to blood glucose and HbA1c values and to retinopathy, nephropathy, and cardiovascular outcomes in the DCCT/EDIC study," *Diabetes*, vol. 63, pp. 282–290, 2014.

[33] National Institute for Health and Care Excellence (NICE), "Type 2 diabetes in adults: management. NICE guidelines [NG28] 2015," April 2017, https://www.nice.org.uk/guidance/ng28/chapter/1-recommendations.

[34] American Diabetes Association (ADA), "Strategies for Improving Care," *Diabetes Care*, vol. 39, Supplement 1, pp. S6–S12, 2016.

[35] S. Ayadurai, H. L. Hattingh, L. B. G. Tee, and S. N. Md Said, "A narrative review of diabetes intervention studies to explore diabetes care opportunities for pharmacists," *Journal of Diabetes Research*, vol. 2016, Article ID 5897452, 11 pages, 2016.

[36] G. Rayman, "Glycaemic control, glucose variability and the triangle of diabetes care," *British Journal of Diabetes*, vol. 16, Supplement 1, pp. S3–S6, 2016.

[37] S. E. Kahn, M. E. Cooper, and S. D. Prato, "Pathophysiology and treatment of type 2 diabetes: perspectives on the past, present, and future," *The Lancet*, vol. 383, pp. 1068–1083, 2014.

[38] S. E. Inzucchi, R. M. Bergenstal, J. B. Buse et al., "Management of hyperglycemia in type 2 diabetes: a patient-centered approach: position statement of the American Diabetes Association (ADA) and the European Association for the Study of Diabetes (EASD)," *Diabetes Care*, vol. 35, no. 6, pp. 1364–1379, 2012.

[39] M. Mata-Cases, D. Mauricio, and J. Franch-Nadal, "Clinical characteristics of type 2 diabetic patients on basal insulin therapy with adequate fasting glucose control who do not achieve HbA1c targets," *Journal of Diabetes*, vol. 9, no. 1, pp. 34–44, 2017.

[40] D. Russell-Jones and S. Gough, "Recent advances in incretin-based therapies," *Clinical Endocrinology*, vol. 77, no. 4, pp. 489–499, 2012.

[41] B. L. Wajchenberg, "β-cell failure in diabetes and preservation by clinical treatment," *Endocrine Reviews*, vol. 28, no. 2, pp. 187–218, 2017.

[42] W. T. Cefalu, "The physiologic role of incretin hormones: clinical applications," *Journal of the American Osteopathic Association*, vol. 110, no. 3, Supplement 2, pp. S8–S14, 2010.

[43] M. C. Riddle, "Glycemic management of type 2 diabetes: an emerging strategy with oral agents, insulins, and combinations," *Endocrinology and Metabolism Clinics of North America*, vol. 34, pp. 77–98, 2005.

[44] A. A. Hasan and B. Hocher, "Role of soluble and membrane-bound dipeptidylpeptidase-4 in diabetic nephropathy," *Journal of Molecular Endocrinology*, vol. 59, no. 1, pp. R1–R10, 2017.

[45] J. E. Gerich, "Role of the kidney in normal glucose homeostasis and in the hyperglycaemia of diabetes mellitus: therapeutic implications," *Diabetic Medicine*, vol. 27, no. 2, pp. 136–142, 2010.

[46] M. A. Nauck, "Update on developments with SGLT2 inhibitors in the management of type 2 diabetes," *Drug Design Development and Therapy*, vol. 8, pp. 1335–1380, 2014.

[47] H. Noh and G. L. King, "The role of protein kinase C activation in diabetic nephropathy," *Kidney International*, vol. 106, pp. S49–S53, 2007.

[48] N. Tanji, G. S. Markowitz, C. Fu et al., "Expression of advanced glycation end products and their cellular receptor RAGE in diabetic nephropathy and nondiabetic renal disease," *Journal of the American Society of Nephrology*, vol. 11, no. 9, pp. 1656–1666, 2000.

[49] K. Susztak, A. C. Raff, M. Schiffer, and E. P. Böttinger, "Glucose-induced reactive oxygen species cause apoptosis of podocytes and podocyte depletion at the onset of diabetic nephropathy," *Diabetes*, vol. 55, no. 1, pp. 225–233, 2006.

[50] J. M. Forbes, M. T. Coughlan, and M. E. Cooper, "Oxidative stress as a major culprit in kidney disease in diabetes," *Diabetes*, vol. 57, no. 6, pp. 1446–1454, 2008.

[51] Z. Cao and M. E. Cooper, "Pathogenesis of diabetic nephropathy," *Journal of Diabetes Investigation*, vol. 2, no. 4, pp. 243–247, 2011.

[52] D. K. Singh, P. Winocour, and K. Farrington, "Oxidative stress in early diabetic nephropathy: fueling the fire," *Nature Reviews Endocrinology*, vol. 7, no. 3, pp. 176–184, 2011.

[53] X. Chen, Z. Ren, W. Liang et al., "c-Abl mediates angiotensin II-induced apoptosis in podocytes," *Journal of Molecular Histology*, vol. 44, no. 5, pp. 597–608, 2013.

[54] V. P. Singh, A. Bali, N. Singh, and A. S. Jaggi, "Advanced glycation end products and diabetic complications," *The Korean Journal of Physiology & Pharmacology*, vol. 18, no. 1, pp. 1–14, 2014.

[55] A. Rivero, C. Mora, M. Muros, J. García, H. Herrera, and J. F. Navarro-González, "Pathogenic perspectives for the role of inflammation in diabetic nephropathy," *Clinical Science*, vol. 116, no. 6, pp. 479–492, 2009.

[56] P. Gao, F.-F. He, H. Tang et al., "NADPH oxidase-induced NALP3 inflammasome activation is driven by thioredoxin-interacting protein which contributes to podocyte injury in hyperglycemia," *Journal of Diabetes Research*, vol. 2015, Article ID 504761, 12 pages, 2015.

[57] K. Kanasaki, G. Taduri, and D. Koya, "Diabetic nephropathy: the role of inflammation in fibroblast activation and kidney fibrosis," *Frontiers in Endocrinology*, vol. 4, p. 7, 2013.

[58] M. B. Duran-Salgado and A. F. Rubio-Guerra, "Diabetic nephropathy and inflammation," *World Journal of Diabetes*, vol. 5, no. 3, pp. 393–398, 2014.

[59] S. Morano, R. Cipriani, C. Santangelo et al., "Angiotensin blockade and matrix synthesis by glomerular epithelial cells in high glucose: a further experimental insight into the pathophysiology of diabetic nephropathy," *Clinical Therapeutics*, vol. 159, no. 3, pp. 151–154, 2008.

[60] T. Chawla, D. Sharma, and A. Singh, "Role of the renin angiotensin system in diabetic nephropathy," *World Journal of Diabetes*, vol. 1, no. 5, pp. 141–145, 2010.

[61] M. H. A. Muskiet, M. M. Smits, L. M. Morsink, and M. Diamant, "The gut–renal axis: do incretin-based agents confer renoprotection in diabetes?," *Nature Reviews Nephrology*, vol. 10, pp. 88–103, 2014.

[62] S. M. Marshall, "Recent advances in diabetic nephropathy," *Postgraduate Medical Journal*, vol. 80, pp. 624–633, 2004.

[63] E. Bortoloso, D. D. Prete, M. Dalla Vestra et al., "Quantitative and qualitative changes in vascular endothelial growth factor gene expression in glomeruli of patients with type 2 diabetes," *European Journal of Endocrinology*, vol. 150, pp. 799–807, 2004.

[64] H. J. Baelde, M. Eikmans, D. W. Lappin et al., "Reduction of VEGF-A and CTGF expression in diabetic nephropathy is associated with podocyte loss," *Kidney International*, vol. 71, pp. 637–645, 2007.

[65] J. J. Li, S. J. Kwak, D. S. Jung et al., "Podocyte biology in diabetic nephropathy," *Kidney International*, vol. 106, pp. S36–S42, 2007.

[66] J. S. Lin and K. Susztak, "Podocytes: the weakest link in diabetic kidney disease?," *Current Diabetes Reports*, vol. 16, no. 5, p. 45, 2016.

[67] J. R. Sowers, A. Whaley-Connell, and M. R. Hayden, "The role of overweight and obesity in the cardiorenal syndrome," *Cardiorenal Medicine*, vol. 1, pp. 5–12, 2011.

[68] P. Schlatter, C. Beglinger, J. Drewe, and H. Gutmann, "Glucagon-like peptide 1 receptor expression in primary porcine proximal tubular cells," *Regulatory Peptides*, vol. 141, pp. 120–128, 2007.

[69] A. Aroor, S. McKarns, R. Nistala et al., "DPP-4 inhibitors as therapeutic modulators of immune cell function and associated cardiovascular and renal insulin resistance in obesity and diabetes," *Cardiorenal Medicine*, vol. 3, no. 1, pp. 48–56, 2013.

[70] M. Yu, C. Moreno, K. M. Hoagland et al., "Antihypertensive effect of glucagonlike peptide 1 in Dahl salt-sensitive rats," *Journal of Hypertension*, vol. 21, pp. 1125–1135, 2003.

[71] E. P. Jensen, S. S. Poulsen, H. Kissow et al., "Activation of GLP-1 receptors on vascular smooth muscle cells reduces the autoregulatory response in afferent arterioles and increases renal blood flow," *American Journal of Physiology - Renal Physiology*, vol. 308, no. 8, pp. F867–F877, 2015.

[72] T. A. Salles, L. dos Santos, V. G. Barauna, and A. C. C. Girardi, "Potential role of dipeptidyl peptidase IV in the pathophysiology of heart failure," *International Journal of Molecular Sciences*, vol. 16, no. 2, pp. 4226–4249, 2015.

[73] E. E. Mulvihill and D. J. Drucker, "Metabolic implications of DPP-4 inhibition," *Endocrine Reviews*, vol. 35, no. 6, pp. 992–1019, 2014.

[74] K. V. Websky, C. Reichetzedera, and B. Hochera, "Physiology and pathophysiology of incretins in the kidney," *Current Opinion in Nephrology and Hypertension*, vol. 23, no. 1, pp. 54–60, 2014.

[75] S. Shi, D. Koya, and K. Kanasaki, "Dipeptidyl peptidase-4 and kidney fibrosis in diabetes," *Fibrogenesis & Tissue Repair*, vol. 9, p. 1, 2016.

[76] G. P. Fadini, E. Boscaro, M. Albiero et al., "The oral dipeptidyl peptidase-4 inhibitor sitagliptin increases circulating endothelial progenitor cells in patients with type 2 diabetes mellitus. Possible role of stromal derived factor-1α," *Diabetes Care*, vol. 33, pp. 1607–1609, 2010.

[77] G. L. Plosker, "Sitagliptin: a review of its use in patients with type 2 diabetes mellitus," *Drugs*, vol. 74, pp. 223–242, 2014.

[78] G. A. Herman, C. Stevens, K. Van Dyck et al., "Pharmacokinetics and pharmacodynamics of sitagliptin, an inhibitor of dipeptidyl peptidase IV, in healthy subjects: results from two randomized, double-blind, placebo-controlled studies with single oral doses," *Journal of Clinical Pharmacology and Therapeutics*, vol. 78, no. 6, pp. 675–688, 2005.

[79] A. J. Bergman, J. Cote, B. Yi et al., "Effect of renal insufficiency on the pharmacokinetics of sitagliptin, a dipeptidyl peptidase-4 inhibitor," *Diabetes Care*, vol. 30, no. 7, pp. 1862–1864, 2007.

[80] E. M. Migoya, C. H. Stevens, A. J. Bergman et al., "Effect of moderate hepatic insufficiency on the pharmacokinetics of sitagliptin," *Canadian Journal of Clinical Pharmacology*, vol. 16, no. 1, pp. 165–170, 2009.

[81] J. C. Arjona Ferreira, M. Marre, N. Barzilai et al., "Efficacy and safety of sitagliptin versus glipizide in patients with type 2 diabetes and moderate-to-severe chronic renal insufficiency," *Diabetes Care*, vol. 36, no. 5, pp. 1067–1073, 2013.

[82] J. J. Neumiller and I. B. Hirsch, "Management of hyperglycemia in diabetic kidney disease," *Diabetes Spectrum*, vol. 28, no. 3, pp. 214–219, 2015.

[83] C. C. R. Betônico, S. M. O. Titan, M. L. C. Correa-Giannella, M. Nery, and M. Queiroz, "Management of diabetes mellitus in individuals with chronic kidney disease: therapeutic perspectives and glycemic control," *Clinics*, vol. 71, no. 1, pp. 47–53, 2016.

[84] D. Kim, L. Wang, M. Beconi et al., "2(2R)-4-oxo-4-[3-(trifluoromethyl)-5,6-dihydro[1, 2, 4]triazolo[4,3-a]pyrazin-7(8H)- yl]-1-(2,4,5-trifluorophenyl)butan-2-amine: a potent, orally active dipeptidyl peptidase IV inhibitor for the treatment of type 2 diabetes," *Journal of Medicinal Chemistry*, vol. 48, no. 1, pp. 141–151, 2005.

[85] S. E. Inzucchi and D. K. McGuire, "New drugs for the treatment of diabetes: part II. Incretin-based therapy and beyond," *Circulation*, vol. 117, no. 4, pp. 574–584, 2008.

[86] B. Ahrén, "Dipeptidyl peptidase-4 inhibitors: clinical data and clinical implications," *Diabetes Care*, vol. 30, no. 6, pp. 1344–1350, 2007.

[87] R. K. Campbell, "Rationale for dipeptidyl peptidase 4 inhibitors: a new class of oral agents for the treatment of type 2 diabetes mellitus," *Annals of Pharmacotherapy*, vol. 41, no. 1, pp. 51–60, 2007.

[88] J. Rosenstock and B. Zinman, "Dipeptidyl peptidase-4 inhibitors and the management of type 2 diabetes mellitus," *Current Opinion in Endocrinology, Diabetes, and Obesity*, vol. 14, no. 2, pp. 98–107, 2007.

[89] L. L. Baggio and D. J. Drucker, "Biology of incretins: GLP-1 and GIP," *Gastroenterology*, vol. 132, no. 6, pp. 2131–2157, 2007.

[90] J. F. Gautier, S. P. Choukem, and J. Girard, "Physiology of incretins (GIP and GLP-1) and abnormalities in type 2 diabetes," *Diabetes & Metabolism*, vol. 34, Supplement 2, pp. S65–S72, 2008.

[91] C. F. Deacon, P. Danielsen, L. Klarskov, M. Olesen, and J. J. Holst, "Dipeptidyl peptidase IV inhibition reduces the degradation and clearance of GIP and potentiates its insulinotropic and antihyperglycemic effects in anesthetized pigs," *Diabetes*, vol. 50, no. 7, pp. 1588–1597, 2001.

[92] G. A. Herman, A. Bergman, F. Liu et al., "Pharmacokinetics and pharmacodynamic effects of the oral DPP-4 inhibitor sitagliptin in middle-aged obese subjects," *Journal of Clinical Pharmacology*, vol. 46, no. 8, pp. 876–886, 2006.

[93] B. Ahrén, E. Simonsson, H. Larsson et al., "Inhibition of dipeptidyl peptidase IV improves metabolic control over a 4-week study period in type 2 diabetes," *Diabetes Care*, vol. 25, no. 5, pp. 869–875, 2002.

[94] B. Ahrén, "Insulin plus incretin: a glucose-lowering strategy for type 2-diabetes," *World Journal of Diabetes*, vol. 5, no. 1, pp. 40–51, 2014.

[95] A. J. Scheen, "Pharmacokinetics of dipeptidylpeptidase-4 inhibitors," *Diabetes Obesity and Metabolism*, vol. 12, no. 8, pp. 648–658, 2010.

[96] S. S. Engel, E. Round, G. T. Golm, K. D. Kaufman, and B. J. Goldstein, "Safety and tolerability of sitagliptin in type 2 diabetes: pooled analysis of 25 clinical studies," *Diabetes Therapy*, vol. 4, no. 1, pp. 119–145, 2013.

[97] K. Garg, C. D. Tripathi, and S. Kumar, "Clinical review of sitagliptin: a DPP-4 inhibitor," *Journal of the Association of Physicians of India*, vol. 61, pp. 57–61, 2013.

[98] K. Esposito, P. Chiodini, M. I. Maiorino, G. Bellastella, A. Capuano, and D. Giugliano, "Glycaemic durability with dipeptidyl peptidase-4 inhibitors in type 2 diabetes: a systematic review and meta-analysis of long-term randomised controlled trials," *BMJ Open*, vol. 4, article e005442, 2014.

[99] J. Mu, J. Woods, and Y. P. Zhou, "Chronic inhibition of dipeptidyl peptidase-4 with a sitagliptin analog preserves pancreatic β-cell mass and function in a rodent model of type 2 diabetes," *Diabetes*, vol. 55, no. 6, pp. 1695–1704, 2006.

[100] J. Mu, A. Petrov, G. J. Eiermann et al., "Inhibition of DPP-4 with sitagliptin improves glycemic control and restores islet cell mass and function in a rodent model of type 2 diabetes," *European Journal of Pharmacology*, vol. 623, pp. 148–154, 2009.

[101] L. Ferreira, E. Teixeira-de-Lemos, F. Pinto et al., "Effects of sitagliptin treatment on dysmetabolism, inflammation, and oxidative stress in an animal model of type 2 diabetes (ZDF rat)," *Mediators of Inflammation*, vol. 2010, Article ID 592760, 11 pages, 2010.

[102] M. Ji, L. Xia, J. Cao, and D. Zou, "Sitagliptin/metformin versus insulin glargine combined with metformin in obese subjects with newly diagnosed type 2 diabetes," *Medicine*, vol. 95, no. 11, article e2961, 2016.

[103] Y. Kondo, N. Harada, A. Hamasaki et al., "Sitagliptin monotherapy has better effect on insulinogenic index than glimepiride monotherapy in Japanese patients with type 2 diabetes mellitus: a 52-week, multicenter, parallel-group randomized controlled trial," *Diabetology & Metabolic Syndrome*, vol. 8, no. 15, 2016.

[104] X. Ren, G. Liu, Y. Wang et al., "Influence of dipeptidyl peptidase-IV inhibitor sitagliptin on extracellular signal-regulated kinases 1/2 signaling in rats with diabetic nephropathy," *Pharmacology*, vol. 100, pp. 1–13, 2017.

[105] B. Gallwitz, "Extra-pancreatic effects of incretin-based therapies," *Endocrine*, vol. 47, no. 2, pp. 360–371, 2014.

[106] E. J. Verspohl, "Novel therapeutics for type 2 diabetes: incretin hormone mimetics (glucagon-like-peptide-1 receptor agonists) and dipeptidyl peptidase-4 inhibitors," *Pharmacology & Therapeutics*, vol. 124, pp. 113–138, 2009.

[107] R. E. Van Genugten, D. H. van Raalte, and M. Diamant, "Dipeptidyl peptidase-4 inhibitors and preservation of pancreatic islet-cell function: a critical appraisal of the evidence," *Diabetes Obesity and Metabolism*, vol. 14, pp. 101–111, 2012.

[108] Y. Zeng, C. Li, M. Guan et al., "The DPP-4 inhibitor sitagliptin attenuates the progress of atherosclerosis in apolipoprotein-E-knockout mice via AMPK- and MAPK-dependent mechanisms," *Cardiovascular Diabetology*, vol. 13, no. 32, 2014.

[109] A. V. Matveyenko, S. Dry, H. I. Cox et al., "Beneficial endocrine but adverse exocrine effects of sitagliptin in the human islet amyloid polypeptide transgenic rat model of type 2 diabetes: interactions with metformin," *Diabetes*, vol. 58, no. 7, pp. 1604–1615, 2009.

[110] Y. S. Liu, Z. W. Huang, L. Wang et al., "Sitagliptin alleviated myocardial remodeling of the left ventricle and improved cardiac diastolic dysfunction in diabetic rats," *Journal of Pharmacological Sciences*, vol. 127, no. 3, pp. 260–274, 2015.

[111] L. M. McCormick, A. C. Kydd, P. A. Read et al., "Chronic dipeptidyl peptidase-4 inhibition with sitagliptin is associated with sustained protection against ischemic left ventricular dysfunction in a pilot study of patients with type 2 diabetes mellitus and coronary artery disease," *Circulation: Cardiovascular Imaging*, vol. 7, no. 2, pp. 274–281, 2014.

[112] N. Apaijai, H. Pintana, S. C. Chattipakorn, and N. Chattipakorn, "Effects of vildagliptin versus sitagliptin, on cardiac function, heart rate variability and mitochondrial function in obese insulin resistant rats," *British Journal of Pharmacology*, vol. 169, no. 5, pp. 1048–1057, 2013.

[113] B. Picatoste, E. Ramírez, A. Caro-Vadillo et al., "Sitagliptin reduces cardiac apoptosis, hypertrophy and fibrosis primarily by insulin-dependent mechanisms in experimental type-II diabetes. Potential roles of GLP-1 isoforms," *PLoS One*, vol. 8, no. 10, article e78330, 2013.

[114] P. A. Read, F. Z. Khan, P. M. Heck, S. P. Hoole, and D. P. Dutka, "DPP-4 inhibition by sitagliptin improves the myocardial response to dobutamine stress and mitigates

stunning in a pilot study of patients with coronary artery disease," *Circulation. Cardiovascular Imaging*, vol. 3, no. 2, pp. 195–201, 2010.

[115] M. T. Kelleni, E. F. Amin, and A. M. Abdelrahman, "Effect of metformin and sitagliptin on doxorubicin-induced cardiotoxicity in rats: impact of oxidative stress, inflammation, and apoptosis," *Journal of Toxicology*, vol. 2015, Article ID 424813, 8 pages, 2015.

[116] T. Mita, N. Katakami, T. Shiraiwa et al., "Sitagliptin attenuates the progression of carotid intima-media thickening in insulin-treated patients with type 2 diabetes: the sitagliptin preventive study of intima-media thickness evaluation (spike): a randomized controlled trial," *Diabetes Care*, vol. 39, no. 3, pp. 455–464, 2016.

[117] R. E. Amori, J. Lau, and A. G. Pittas, "Efficacy and safety of incretin therapy in type 2 diabetes: systematic review and meta-analysis," *Journal of the American Medical Association*, vol. 298, no. 2, pp. 194–206, 2007.

[118] M. Fan, Y. Li, and S. Zhang, "Effects of sitagliptin on lipid profiles in patients with type 2 diabetes mellitus: a meta-analysis of randomized clinical trials," *Medicine*, vol. 95, no. 2, pp. 1–9, 2016.

[119] P. C. M. Van Poppel, M. G. Netea, P. Smits, and C. Tack, "Vildagliptin improves endothelium-dependent vasodilatation in type 2 diabetes," *Diabetes Care*, vol. 34, no. 9, pp. 2072–2077, 2011.

[120] J. S. Yoon and H. W. Lee, "Understanding the cardiovascular effects of incretin," *Diabetes & Metabolism Journal*, vol. 35, no. 5, pp. 437–443, 2011.

[121] C. Mega, H. Vala, P. Rodrigues-Santos et al., "Sitagliptin prevents aggravation of endocrine and exocrine pancreatic damage in the Zucker diabetic fatty rat - focus on amelioration of metabolic profile and tissue cytoprotective properties," *Diabetology & Metabolic Syndrome*, vol. 6, no. 1, p. 42, 2014.

[122] A. Gonçalves, E. Leal, A. Paiva et al., "Protective effects of the dipeptidyl peptidase IV inhibitor sitagliptin in the blood-retinal barrier in a type 2 diabetes animal model," *Diabetes, Obesity and Metabolism*, vol. 14, no. 5, pp. 454–463, 2012.

[123] A. Gonçalves, C. Marques, E. Leal et al., "Dipeptidyl peptidase-IV inhibition prevents blood-retinal barrier breakdown, inflammation and neuronal cell death in the retina of type 1 diabetic rats," *Biochimica et Biophysica Acta (BBA) - Molecular Basis of Disease*, vol. 1842, no. 9, pp. 1454–1463, 2014.

[124] C. Mega, E. T. de Lemos, H. Vala et al., "Diabetic nephropathy amelioration by a low dose sitagliptin in an animal model of type 2 diabetes (Zucker diabetic fatty rat)," *Experimental Diabetes Research*, vol. 2011, Article ID 162092, 12 pages, 2011.

[125] A. Maida, T. Hansotia, C. Longuet, T. Seino, and D. J. Drucker, "Differential importance of glucose-dependent insulinotropic polypeptide vs glucagon-like peptide 1 receptor signaling for β cell survival in mice," *Gastroenterology*, vol. 137, pp. 2146–2157, 2009.

[126] J. A. Yeom, E. S. Kim, H. S. Park et al., "Both sitagliptin analogue & pioglitazone preserve the β-cell proportion in the islets with different mechanism in non-obese and obese diabetic mice," *BMB Reports*, vol. 44, no. 11, pp. 713–718, 2011.

[127] Y. Takeda, Y. Fujita, and J. Honjo, "Reduction of both beta cell death and alpha cell proliferation by dipeptidyl peptidase-4 inhibition in a streptozotocin-induced model of diabetes in mice," *Diabetologia*, vol. 55, no. 2, pp. 404–412, 2012.

[128] S. Karabulut, Z. M. Coskunb, and S. Bolkent, "Immunohistochemical, apoptotic and biochemical changes by dipeptidyl peptidase-4 inhibitor-sitagliptin in type-2 diabetic rats," *Pharmacological Reports*, vol. 67, no. 5, pp. 846–853, 2015.

[129] J. Shirakawa, T. Okuyama, M. Kyohara et al., "DPP-4 inhibition improves early mortality, β cell function, and adipose tissue inflammation in db/db mice fed a diet containing sucrose and linoleic acid," *Diabetology & Metabolic Syndrome*, vol. 8, no. 16, 2016.

[130] A. D. Dobrian, Q. Ma, J. W. Lindsay et al., "Dipeptidyl peptidase IV inhibitor sitagliptin reduces local inflammation in adipose tissue and in pancreatic islets of obese mice," *American Journal of Physiology: Endocrinology and Metabolism*, vol. 300, no. 2, pp. E410–E421, 2011.

[131] N. Satoh-Asahara, Y. Sasaki, H. Wada et al., "A dipeptidyl peptidase-4 inhibitor, sitagliptin, exerts anti-inflammatory effects in type 2 diabetic patients," *Metabolism*, vol. 62, no. 3, pp. 347–351, 2013.

[132] G. Derosa, A. Carbone, A. D'Angelo et al., "Variations in inflammatory biomarkers following the addition of sitagliptin in patients with type 2 diabetes not controlled with metformin," *Internal Medicine*, vol. 52, no. 19, pp. 2179–2187, 2013.

[133] F. Beguinot, "Tribbles homologue 3 (TRIB3) and the insulin-resistance genes in type 2 diabetes," *Diabetologia*, vol. 53, pp. 1831–1834, 2010.

[134] S. Prudente, D. Scarpelli, M. Chandalia et al., "The trib3 Q84R polymorphism and risk of early-onset type 2 diabetes," *Journal of Clinical Endocrinology & Metabolism*, vol. 94, no. 1, pp. 190–196, 2009.

[135] J. Shirakawa, H. Fujii, K. Ohnuma et al., "Diet-induced adipose tissue inflammation and liver steatosis are prevented by DPP-4 inhibition in diabetic mice," *Diabetes*, vol. 60, pp. 1246–1257, 2011.

[136] S. Oyadomari, H. P. Harding, Y. Zhang, M. Oyadomari, and D. Ron, "Dephosphorylation of translation initiation factor 2α enhances glucose tolerance and attenuates hepatosteatosis in mice," *Cell Metabolism*, vol. 7, pp. 520–532, 2008.

[137] V. Aviv, I. Meivar-Levy, I. H. Rachmut, T. Rubinek, E. Mor, and S. Ferber, "Exendin-4 promotes liver cell proliferation and enhances PDX-1-induced liver to pancreas transdifferentiation," *The Journal of Biological Chemistry*, vol. 284, no. 48, pp. 33509–33520, 2009.

[138] L. Gaetaniello, M. Fiore, S. de Filippo, N. Pozzi, S. Tamasi, and C. Pignata, "Occupancy of dipeptidyl peptidase IV activates an associated tyrosine kinase and triggers an apoptotic signal in human hepatocarcinoma cells," *Hepatology*, vol. 27, pp. 934–942, 1998.

[139] M. E. Kelany, T. M. Hakami, A. H. Omar, and M. A. Abdallah, "Combination of sitagliptin and insulin against type 2 diabetes mellitus with neuropathy in rats: neuroprotection and role of oxidative and inflammation stress," *Pharmacology*, vol. 98, pp. 242–250, 2016.

[140] B. F. Schrijvers, A. Flyvbjerg, R. G. Tilton, N. H. Lameire, and A. S. D. Vriese, "A neutralizing VEGF antibody prevents glomerular hypertrophy in a model of obese type 2 diabetes, the Zucker diabetic fatty rat," *Nephrology Dialysis Transplantation*, vol. 21, no. 2, pp. 324–329, 2006.

[141] L. Liu, J. Liu, W. T. Wong et al., "Dipeptidyl peptidase 4 inhibitor sitagliptin protects endothelial function in hypertension through a glucagon-like peptide 1-dependent mechanism," *Hypertension*, vol. 60, pp. 833–841, 2012.

[142] S. Kröller-Schön, M. Knorr, M. Hausding et al., "Glucose-independent improvement of vascular dysfunction in experimental sepsis by dipeptidyl-peptidase 4 inhibition," *Cardiovascular Research*, vol. 96, pp. 140–149, 2012.

[143] I. Kawasaki, Y. Hiura, A. Tamai et al., "Sitagliptin reduces the urine albumin-to-creatinine ratio in type 2 diabetes through decreasing both blood pressure and estimated glomerular filtration rate," *Journal of Diabetes*, vol. 7, no. 1, pp. 41–46, 2015.

[144] L. M. Russo, R. M. Sandoval, S. B. Campos, B. A. Molitoris, W. D. Comper, and D. Brown, "Impaired tubular uptake explains albuminuria in early diabetic nephropathy," *Journal of the American Society of Nephrology*, vol. 20, no. 3, pp. 489–494, 2009.

[145] G. B. Peres and Y. M. Michelacci, "The role of proximal tubular cells in the early stages of diabetic nephropathy," *Journal of Diabetes & Metabolism*, vol. 6, p. 551, 2015.

[146] A. C. Girardi, B. C. Degray, T. Nagy, D. Biemesderfer, and P. S. Aronson, "Association of Na^+-H^+ exchanger isoform NHE3 and dipeptidyl peptidase IV in the renal proximal tubule," *The Journal of Biological Chemistry*, vol. 276, no. 49, pp. 46671–46677, 2001.

[147] D. F. Arruda-Junior, F. L. Martins, R. Dariolli et al., "Dipeptidyl peptidase IV inhibition exerts renoprotective effects in rats with established heart failure," *Frontiers in Physiology*, vol. 7, p. 293, 2016.

[148] R. Nistala, J. Habibi, G. Lastra et al., "Prevention of obesity-induced renal injury in male mice by DPP4 inhibition," *Endocrinology*, vol. 155, no. 6, pp. 2266–2276, 2014.

[149] R. Nistala, J. Habibi, A. Aroor et al., "DPP4 inhibition attenuates filtration barrier injury and oxidant stress in the zucker obese rat," *Obesity*, vol. 22, no. 10, pp. 2172–2179, 2014.

[150] W. J. Liu, S. H. Xie, Y. N. Liu et al., "Dipeptidyl peptidase IV inhibitor attenuates kidney injury in streptozotocin-induced diabetic rats," *Journal of Pharmacology and Experimental Therapeutics*, vol. 340, pp. 248–255, 2012.

[151] A. Aroor, M. Zuberek, C. Duta et al., "Angiotensin II stimulation of DPP4 activity regulates megalin in the proximal tubules," *International Journal of Molecular Sciences*, vol. 17, no. 5, 2016.

[152] B. Hocher, C. Reichetzeder, and M. L. Alter, "Renal and cardiac effects of DPP-4 inhibitors – from preclinical development to clinical research," *Kidney and Blood Pressure Research*, vol. 36, pp. 65–84, 2012.

[153] B. P. Pacheco, R. O. Crajoinas, G. K. Couto et al., "Dipeptidyl peptidase IV inhibition attenuates blood pressure rising in young spontaneously hypertensive rats," *Journal of Hypertension*, vol. 29, pp. 520–528, 2011.

[154] S. Saha, Y. Li, and M. B. Anand-Srivastava, "Reduced levels of cyclic AMP contribute to the enhanced oxidative stress in vascular smooth muscle cells from spontaneously hypertensive rats," *Canadian Journal of Physiology and Pharmacology*, vol. 86, pp. 190–198, 2008.

[155] A. Avogaro and G. P. Fadini, "The effects of dipeptidyl peptidase-4 inhibition on microvascular diabetes complications," *Diabetes Care*, vol. 37, no. 10, pp. 2884–2894, 2014.

[156] A. A. Eddy, "Serine proteases, inhibitors and receptors in renal fibrosis," *Thrombosis and Haemostasis*, vol. 101, no. 4, pp. 656–664, 2009.

[157] G. Tramonti and Y. S. Kanwar, "Tubular biomarkers to assess progression of diabetic nephropathy," *Kidney International*, vol. 79, no. 10, pp. 1042–1044, 2011.

[158] S. Hoshi, Y. Shu, F. Yoshida et al., "Podocyte injury promotes progressive nephropathy in zucker diabetic fatty rats," *Laboratory Investigation*, vol. 82, no. 1, pp. 25–35, 2002.

[159] N. Gassler, M. Elger, B. Kränzlin et al., "Podocyte injury underlies the progression of focal segmental glomerulosclerosis in the fa/fa Zucker rat," *Kidney International*, vol. 60, no. 1, pp. 106–116, 2001.

[160] T. W. Tervaert, A. L. Mooyaart, K. Amann et al., "Pathologic classification of diabetic nephropathy," *Journal of the American Society of Nephrology*, vol. 21, no. 4, pp. 556–563, 2010.

[161] K. White, "Histological appearance of diabetic nephropathy," *Diapedia 7105002828 rev.*, no. 5, 2014.

[162] U. Panchapakesan and C. Pollock, "The role of dipeptidyl peptidase – 4 inhibitors in diabetic kidney disease," *Frontiers in Immunology*, vol. 6, p. 443, 2015.

[163] H. S. Min, J. E. Kim, M. H. Lee et al., "Dipeptidyl peptidase IV inhibitor protects against renal interstitial fibrosis in a mouse model of ureteral obstruction," *Laboratory Investigation*, vol. 94, no. 6, pp. 598–607, 2014.

[164] S. Shi, S. P. Srivastava, M. Kanasaki et al., "Interactions of DPP-4 and integrin $\beta 1$ influences endothelial-to-mesenchymal transition," *Kidney International*, vol. 88, no. 3, pp. 479–489, 2015.

[165] G. Tonolo and S. Cherchi, "Tubulointerstitial disease in diabetic nephropathy," *International Journal of Nephrology and Renovascular Disease*, vol. 7, pp. 107–115, 2014.

[166] P. Vavrinec, R. H. Henning, S. W. Landheer et al., "Vildagliptin restores renal myogenic function and attenuates renal sclerosis independently of effects on blood glucose or proteinuria in Zucker diabetic fatty rat," *Current Vascular Pharmacology*, vol. 12, pp. 836–844, 2014.

[167] I. Raz, M. Hanefeld, L. Xu et al., "Efficacy and safety of the dipeptidyl peptidase-4 inhibitor sitagliptin as monotherapy in patients with type 2 diabetes mellitus," *Diabetologia*, vol. 49, no. 11, pp. 2564–2571, 2006.

[168] V. Gupta and S. Kalra, "Choosing a gliptin," *Indian Journal of Endocrinology and Metabolism*, vol. 15, no. 4, pp. 298–308, 2011.

[169] Y. Wang, S. Landheer, W. H. van Gilst et al., "Attenuation of renovascular damage in Zucker diabetic fatty rat by NWT-03, an egg protein hydrolysate with ACE- and DPP-4-inhibitory activity," *PLoS One*, vol. 7, no. 10, article e46781, 2012.

[170] H. Y. Jin, W. J. Liu, J. H. Park, H. S. Baek, and T. S. Park, "Effect of dipeptidyl peptidase-IV (DPP-IV) inhibitor (vildagliptin) on peripheral nerves in streptozotocin-induced diabetic rats," *Archives of Medical Research*, vol. 40, pp. 536–544, 2009.

[171] Y. Ishibashi, S. Yamagishi, T. Matsui et al., "Pravastatin inhibits advanced glycation end products (AGEs)-induced proximal tubular cell apoptosis and injury by reducing receptor for AGEs (RAGE) level," *Metabolism*, vol. 61, pp. 1067–1072, 2012.

[172] T. Tanaka, Y. Higashijima, T. Wada, and M. Nangaku, "The potential for renoprotection with incretin-based drugs," *Kidney International*, vol. 86, pp. 701–711, 2014.

[173] J. L. Górriz, J. Nieto, J. F. Navarro-González, P. Molina, A. Martínez-Castelao, and L. M. Pallardó, "Nephroprotection by hypoglycemic agents: do we have supporting data?," *Journal of Clinical Medicine*, vol. 4, no. 10, pp. 1866–1889, 2015.

[174] W. S. Silva Júnior, A. F. Godoy-Matos, and L. G. Kraemer-Aguiar, "Dipeptidyl peptidase 4: a new link between diabetes mellitus and atherosclerosis?," *Biomedical Research International*, vol. 2015, Article ID 816164, 10 pages, 2015.

[175] V. Matheeussen, L. Baerts, G. De Meyer et al., "Expression and spatial heterogeneity of dipeptidyl peptidases in endothelial cells of conduct vessels and capillaries," *Biological Chemistry*, vol. 392, no. 3, pp. 189–198, 2011.

[176] T. Romacho, S. Vallejo, L. A. Villalobos et al., "Soluble dipeptidyl peptidase-4 induces microvascular endothelial dysfunction through proteinase-activated receptor-2 and thromboxane A2 release," *Journal of Hypertension*, vol. 34, no. 5, pp. 869–876, 2016.

[177] C. G. Yu, N. Zhang, S. S. Yuan et al., "Endothelial progenitor cells in diabetic microvascular complications: friends or foes?," *Stem Cells International*, vol. 2016, Article ID 1803989, 10 pages, 2016.

[178] R. H. Ahmed, H. Z. Huri, Z. Al-Hamodi, S. D. Salem, and S. Muniandy, "Serum levels of soluble CD26/dipeptidyl peptidase-IV in type 2 diabetes mellitus and its association with metabolic syndrome and therapy with antidiabetic agents in Malaysian subjects," *PLoS One*, vol. 10, no. 10, article e0140618, 2015.

[179] D. Röhrborn, N. Wronkowitz, and J. Eckel, "DPP-4 in diabetes," *Frontiers in Immunology*, vol. 6, p. 386, 2015.

[180] J. Donate-Correa, E. Martín-Núñez, M. Muros-de-Fuentes, C. Mora-Fernández, and J. F. Navarro-González, "Inflammatory cytokines in diabetic nephropathy," *Journal of Diabetes Research*, vol. 2015, Article ID 948417, 9 pages, 2015.

[181] J. F. Navarro and C. Mora, "Diabetes, inflammation, proinflammatory cytokines, and diabetic nephropathy," *The Scientific World Journal*, vol. 6, pp. 908–917, 2006.

[182] X. Ren, G. Liu, Y. Wang et al., "Influence of dipeptidyl peptidase-iv inhibitor sitagliptin on extracellular signal-regulated kinases 1/2 signaling in rats with diabetic nephropathy," *Pharmacology*, vol. 100, no. 1-2, pp. 1–13, 2017.

[183] J. S. Nielsen and K. M. McNagny, "Novel functions of the CD34 family," *Journal of Cell Science*, vol. 121, Part 22, pp. 3682–3692, 2008.

[184] J. H. Li, W. Wang, X. R. Huang et al., "Advanced glycation end products induce tubular epithelial-myofibroblast transition through the RAGE-ERK1/2 MAP kinase signaling pathway," *The American Journal of Pathology*, vol. 164, no. 4, pp. 1389–1397, 2004.

[185] K. B. Gomes, K. F. Rodrigues, and A. P. Fernandes, "The role of transforming growth factor-beta in diabetic nephropathy," *International Journal of Medical Genetics*, vol. 2014, Article ID 180270, 6 pages, 2014.

[186] F. Yang, T. Yu, K. Li, X. Jiang, J. Li, and J. Wang, "Sitagliptin reduces transforming growth factor-β1 and platelet derived growth factor-BB in regulation of UAER in type 2 diabetic nephropathy stage III patients," *Biomedical Research*, vol. 28, no. 6, pp. 2571–2577, 2017.

[187] S. S. Bessa, T. A. Hussein, M. A. Morad, and A. M. Amer, "Urinary platelet-derived growth factor-BB as an early marker of nephropathy in patients with type 2 diabetes: an Egyptian study," *Renal Failure*, vol. 34, no. 6, pp. 670–675, 2012.

[188] Y. Ishibashi, Y. Nishino, T. Matsui, M. Takeuchi, and S. I. Yamagishi, "Glucagon-like peptide-1 suppresses advanced glycation end product-induced monocyte chemoattractant protein-1 expression in mesangial cells by reducing advanced glycation end product receptor level," *Metabolism*, vol. 60, no. 9, pp. 1271–1277, 2011.

[189] J. Li, M. Guan, C. Li et al., "The dipeptidyl peptidase-4 inhibitor sitagliptin protects against dyslipidemia-related kidney injury in apolipoprotein E knockout mice," *International Journal of Molecular Sciences*, vol. 15, pp. 11416–11434, 2014.

[190] H. S. Lee, "Mechanisms and consequences of hypertriglyceridemia and cellular lipid accumulation in chronic kidney disease and metabolic syndrome," *Histology and Histopathology*, vol. 26, no. 12, pp. 1599–1610, 2011.

[191] A. R. Martins and S. Mas, "Lipotoxicity and kidney," *Portuguese Journal of Nephrology & Hypertension*, vol. 29, no. 4, pp. 306–315, 2015.

[192] S. J. Glastras, H. Chen, R. T. McGrath et al., "Effect of GLP-1 receptor activation on offspring kidney health in a rat model of maternal obesity," *Scientific Reports*, vol. 6, article 23525, 2016.

[193] F. A. Wagener, D. Dekker, J. H. Berden, A. Scharstuhl, and J. van der Vlag, "The role of reactive oxygen species in apoptosis of the diabetic kidney," *Apoptosis*, vol. 14, no. 12, pp. 1451–1458, 2009.

[194] M. D. Sanchez-Niño, A. Benito-Martin, and A. Ortiz, "New paradigms in cell death in human diabetic nephropathy," *Kidney International*, vol. 78, no. 8, pp. 737–744, 2010.

[195] J. Vaghasiya, N. Sheth, Y. Bhalodia, and R. Manek, "Sitagliptin protects renal ischemia reperfusion induced renal damage in diabetes," *Regulatory Peptides*, vol. 166, no. 1–3, pp. 48–54, 2011.

[196] H. Hendarto, T. Inoguchi, Y. Maeda et al., "GLP-1 analog liraglutide protects against oxidative stress and albuminuria in streptozotocin-induced diabetic rats via protein kinase A mediated inhibition of renal NAD(P)H oxidases," *Metabolism*, vol. 61, no. 10, pp. 1422–1434, 2012.

[197] R. Kodera, K. Shikata, T. Takasuta et al., "Dipeptidyl peptidase-4 inhibitor ameliorates early renal injury through its antiinflammatory action in a rat model of type 1 diabetes," *Biochemical and Biophysical Research Communications*, vol. 443, no. 3, pp. 828–833, 2014.

[198] S. Nakashima, T. Matsui, M. Takeuchi, and S. I. Yamagishi, "Linagliptin blocks renal damage in type 1 diabetic rats by suppressing advanced glycation end products-receptor axis," *Hormone and Metabolic Research*, vol. 46, pp. 717–721, 2014.

[199] T. Matsui, S. Nakashima, Y. Nishino et al., "Dipeptidyl peptidase-4 deficiency protects against experimental diabetic nephropathy partly by blocking the advanced glycation end products-receptor axis," *Laboratory Investigation*, vol. 95, no. 5, pp. 525–533, 2015.

4

Four Plasma Glucose and Insulin Responses to a 75g OGTT in Healthy Young Japanese Women

Kei Takahashi[1], **Hidetaka Nakamura**[1], **Hiroshi Sato**[1], **Hideto Matsuda**[2], **Kazuo Takada**[1] and **Tomiko Tsuji**[1]

[1]*Department of Health and Nutrition, Faculty of Health and Human Life, Nagoya Bunri University, 365, Maeda, Inazawa-Cho, Inazawa City, Aichi, Japan*
[2]*Department of Food and Nutrition, College of Nagoya Bunri University, 2-1, Sasazuka-Cho, Nishi-Ku, Nagoya, Aichi, Japan*

Correspondence should be addressed to Kei Takahashi; takahashi.kei@nagoya-bunri.ac.jp

Academic Editor: Ed Randell

The incidence of diabetes has been gradually increasing, not only in middle-aged individuals but also in young individuals. However, insulin and glucose patterns have not been investigated in apparently healthy young individuals, as they are typically grouped as controls. In this study, we investigated and classified glucose and insulin patterns in healthy young women. Sixty-two nonobese women without metabolic disease were recruited. The subjects underwent a 75 g oral glucose tolerance test (OGTT), physical measurements, and a biochemical examination. Two subjects displayed impaired glucose tolerance. The 62 subjects were categorized into four patterns by plasma glucose and insulin peak time during OGTT: normal type ($n = 39$), insulin-late type ($n = 11$), insulin- and glucose-late type ($n = 7$), and insulin-very late type ($n = 5$). OGTT glucose and insulin levels at all time points, insulinogenic index, HOMA-IR, and glucose area under the curve (AUC) significantly differed among the four groups. However, insulin AUC did not significantly differ. We did not detect significant differences in body condition or biochemical measurements. Our study demonstrated that some healthy young individuals might have delayed insulin secretion by OGTT. Early detection of altered glucose metabolism might be helpful to improve lifestyle choices and prevent progression to diabetes.

1. Introduction

Chronic diabetes mellitus is characterized by hyperglycemia, which promotes oxidative stress and leads to microangiopathy, such as retinopathy, nephropathy and neuropathy, and macroangiopathy, such as ischemic heart disease and cerebrovascular disease [1, 2]. Recently, it has been reported that not only fasting plasma glucose levels but also postchallenge glucose spikes are problematic in patients with diabetes [3, 4]. For example, cardiovascular disease risk in patients with hyperglycemia 120 min after a meal was higher than in patients with fasting hyperglycemia. Controlling postprandial hyperglycemia is beneficial for prevention and reduction of cardiovascular risks in patients with diabetes [5, 6]. Similarly, patients with type 2 diabetes display delayed early insulin secretion compared with that in healthy adults and are insulin resistant [7]. These reports indicate that postprandial plasma glucose and insulin curves are important.

The incidence of diabetes in younger individuals is gradually increasing [8]. However, there are few studies investigating healthy young subjects. In Japanese universities, most college students do not undergo medical examinations and are not aware of their carbohydrate metabolic conditions. In adults, fasting glucose levels are assessed during a medical examination, but fasting insulin secretion and postchallenge glucose levels are not. The Funagata Study [5], a large Japanese epidemiology study, investigated subjects over 40 years of age but did not include younger individuals. Furthermore, this study did not assess postchallenge insulin levels. Therefore, we believed that it was necessary to assess carbohydrate metabolism and prediabetes status in young healthy individuals.

Mitsui et al. [9] investigated the characteristics of diabetes with isolated fasting hyperglycemia (DM/IFH), with isolated postchallenge hyperglycemia (DM/IPH), and with both fasting and postchallenge hyperglycemia (DM/FPH) in Japanese men. Furthermore, in this study, the DM/IFH and DM/IPH groups were subdivided into two groups and compared. In contrast, young healthy individuals were used as a control group and were not divided into subgroups or analyzed in detail. In several studies investigating diabetes using 75 g oral glucose tolerance tests (OGTTs) [7, 10, 11], healthy individuals were the standard control group with which individuals with diabetes and prediabetes were compared. However, type 2 diabetes in Asia is an increasing epidemic, particularly in individuals at a relatively young age and with a low BMI [8, 12]. Furthermore, Fukushima et al. [13] reported that impaired early-phase insulin secretion played a very important role in the deterioration from normal glucose tolerance to impaired glucose tolerance (IGT) in Japanese middle-aged individuals. Therefore, we thought it necessary to show detailed insulin and glucose patterns in healthy young women during a 75 g OGTT.

In this study, we assessed prediabetes and diabetes by 75 g OGTTs in healthy undergraduates in Japan and investigated varying insulin and plasma glucose responses. In addition, we compared physical and biochemical parameters in the different insulin and glucose response groups.

2. Materials and Methods

Ethical approval was obtained from the Research Ethics Committee of the Nagoya Bunri University, and the study was conducted according to the principles expressed in the Declaration of Helsinki. Subjects were informed about the experimental procedures and purpose of the study prior to giving written consent.

Sixty-two female college students were recruited for this study from Nagoya Bunri University in Japan after receiving an explanation of the study. Inclusion criteria for the study were apparently healthy young adults between 19 and 23 years of age with no history of lifestyle-related disease (e.g., diabetes, hypertension, or lipid abnormalities).

The subjects received both physical and blood examinations. Body weight, bone mass, lean body mass, and percent body fat were measured by body composition analyzer InBody 720 (InBody Japan Inc., Tokyo), and body mass index (BMI) was calculated. Subjects underwent a 75 g OGTT according to the recommendations of the World Health Organization [14]. Venous blood samples were obtained directly before (0 min) and during the OGTT (30, 60, and 120 min) for determination of plasma glucose and insulin concentrations. Blood parameters were measured by FALCO Biosystems Ltd. (Kyoto, Japan). Plasma glucose and insulin concentrations were measured by the hexokinase glucose-6-phosphate dehydrogenase method and radioimmunoassay, respectively [15, 16]. Parameters related to protein and lipid metabolism, liver and kidney function, and blood characteristics were measured in blood collected following an overnight fast to confirm the absence of disease. Furthermore, to evaluate carbohydrate metabolism, we calculated homeostasis model assessment-insulin resistance (HOMA-IR), homeostasis model assessment for β-cell function (HOMA-β) [17], insulinogenic index (II) [18], quantitative insulin sensitivity check index (QUICKI) [19], and area under the curve of glucose (AUC-G) and insulin (AUC-I). HOMA-IR, HOMA-β, II, and QUICKI were calculated using the following formulas: $\text{insulin}_0 \times \text{glucose}_0/405$, $\text{insulin}_0 \times 360/(\text{glucose}_0 - 63)$, $\Delta\text{insulin}_{30}/\Delta\text{glucose}_{30}$, and $1/[\log(\text{insulin}_0) + \log(\text{glucose}_0)]$, respectively, with insulin expressed in μU/mL and glucose in mg/dL. The diagnostic criteria for diabetes from the Japanese Diabetes Society [20] and the World Health Organization [14] were used. The normal type in criteria for diabetes was evaluated at less than 110 mg/dL of fasting plasma glucose levels and 140 mg/dL of 120 min glucose levels. IGT was evaluated at less than 110 mg/dL of fasting plasma glucose levels and from 140 mg/dL to 199 mg/dL of 120 min glucose levels. The diabetes was evaluated with fasting glucose of 126 mg/dL and over or 120 min glucose of 200 mg/dL and over.

Glucose and insulin response types were determined based on the time of peak insulin and plasma glucose concentrations during a 75 g OGTT [21–24], and each parameter was compared. Values are expressed as means ± SD. All data analyses were conducted using Prism (version 5.01; obtained from GraphPad Software, San Diego, CA, USA), and p values < 0.05 were considered statistically significant. For the statistical evaluation, the significance of the differences in mean values between the four types were tested by one-way ANOVA followed by Dunn's multiple comparison tests.

3. Results

Two of 62 subjects (3.2%) displayed elevated 120 min plasma glucose levels (160 and 187 mg/dL) following oral glucose administration, despite fasting glucose levels below 110 mg/dL, and were, therefore, diagnosed with IGT. This 62 nondiabetic subjects were categorized into four groups based on plasma insulin and glucose peak times, which were the times with the highest insulin and glucose concentrations, respectively, during an OGTT (Figure 1). The four groups were as follows: the peak insulin and glucose times both occurred at 30 min (normal type; $n = 39$ (62.9%), Figure 1(a)); insulin and glucose peak times were 60 min and 30 min, respectively (insulin- (I-) late type; $n =$ 11 (17.7%), Figure 1(b)); both peak times occurred at 60 min (insulin- and glucose- (I&G-) late type; $n = 7$ (11.3%), Figure 1(c)); and insulin and glucose peak times were 120 min and 30 min, respectively (I-very late type; $n =$ 5 (8.1%), Figure 1(d)). In each group, insulin and plasma glucose concentrations at the peak time were higher than those at baseline (0 min).

Table 1 displays the ages and body conditions based on each OGTT response type. There were no significant between-type differences.

The comparisons of indexes of glucose metabolism in each group are summarized in Table 2. There were no significant differences in plasma glucose levels at 0 min among the

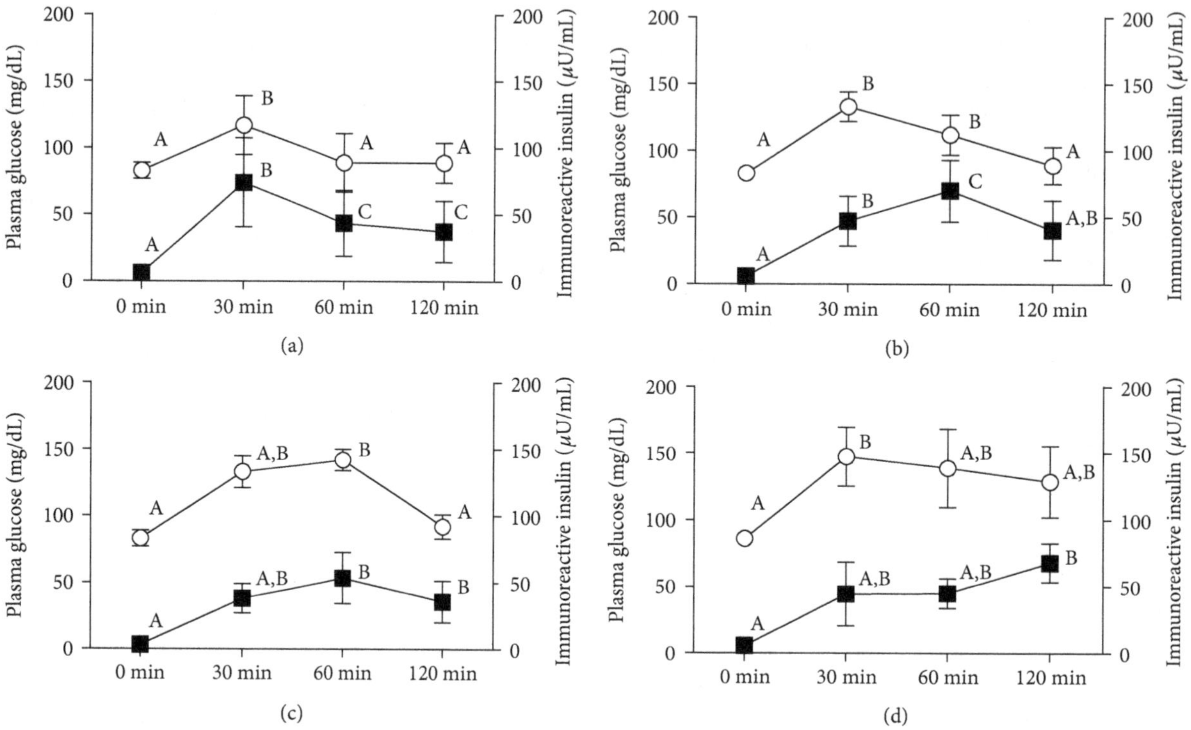

Figure 1: Relationship between plasma glucose levels and insulin reactivity during a 75 g oral glucose tolerance test. Squares: insulin levels. Open circles: plasma glucose levels. (a) Normal type ($n = 39$). (b) Insulin-late type ($n = 11$). (c) Insulin- and glucose-late type ($n = 7$). (d) Insulin-very late type ($n = 5$). Values are means ± SD. Values for each index with different superscript letters are statistically different at $p < 0.05$ by comparing different time points of each patterns, as determined by Dunn's multiple comparison test.

Table 1: Body condition of healthy women by insulin and glucose response type.

Type	Normal	Insulin-late	Insulin- & glucose-late	Insulin-very late
Number	39 (62.9%)	11 (17.7%)	7 (11.3%)	5 (8.1%)
Age (years)	20.6 ± 0.9	20.4 ± 1.0	19.9 ± 1.1	20.7 ± 0.5
Body weight (kg)	52.3 ± 6.9	53.1 ± 6.8	52.1 ± 6.2	53.3 ± 2.2
Height (cm)	158.0 ± 4.5	157.7 ± 5.1	160.9 ± 8.1	158.3 ± 1.7
Body mass index (kg/m^2)	20.9 ± 2.3	21.4 ± 1.0	20.1 ± 1.4	21.3 ± 1.0
Bone mass (kg)	2.23 ± 0.21	2.25 ± 0.11	2.18 ± 0.31	2.23 ± 0.11
Lean body mass (kg)	37.2 ± 3.3	37.8 ± 1.9	36.4 ± 5.6	38.2 ± 1.6
Percent body fat (%)	27.0 ± 4.8	27.5 ± 4.5	28.6 ± 4.7	29.6 ± 3.7

Values are means ± SD. There were no significant differences.

four groups. The 60 min plasma glucose concentrations in the I-late and I&G-late type groups were significantly higher than those in the normal type group, but there were no differences in 120 min glucose levels. In I-very late type group, the 30 min, 60 min, and 120 min glucose levels were significantly higher than those in normal type. In contrast, 0 min and 30 min immunoreactive insulin levels in the I&G-late type group were lower than those in the normal and I-late type groups. The 60 min insulin concentrations in the I-late type group were higher than those in the normal type group. And the 120 min insulin in I-very late group was higher than those in the normal. HOMA-IR and HOMA-β in the I&G-late type group was lower while QUICKI values were higher than those in the other groups. II values in the normal type group was higher than those in the other type groups. AUC-G in the I&G-late and I-very late type groups were higher than that in the normal type group, but there were no significant differences in AUC-I among the four groups.

Additional biochemical parameters are displayed in Table 3. There were no significant differences in any parameter among types.

4. Discussion

This study was performed in young healthy women without lifestyle-related diseases or other diseases. They underwent

Table 2: Glucose metabolism of women by insulin and glucose response type.

Type	Normal	Insulin-late	Insulin- & glucose-late	Insulin-very late
Number	39	11	7	5
Plasma glucose (mg/dL)				
0 min	83.4 ± 6.1	83.5 ± 4.5	83.0 ± 5.7	86.0 ± 3.0
30 min	117.0 ± 22.2^{a}	$133.2 \pm 10.9^{a,b}$	$133.1 \pm 12.0^{a,b}$	147.4 ± 22.1^{b}
60 min	89.2 ± 22.2^{a}	112.1 ± 14.5^{b}	142.0 ± 15.6^{b}	139.0 ± 29.4^{b}
120 min	89.3 ± 14.8^{a}	$88.8 \pm 13.5^{a,b}$	$92.0 \pm 9.4^{a,b}$	114.7 ± 24.8^{b}
Immunoreactive insulin (μU/mL)				
0 min	6.2 ± 2.7^{a}	5.7 ± 1.9^{a}	3.2 ± 0.8^{b}	$5.7 \pm 1.4^{a,b}$
30 min	74.1 ± 33.4^{a}	47.2 ± 18.6^{a}	38.1 ± 11.1^{b}	$44.5 \pm 24.0^{a,b}$
60 min	42.3 ± 23.7^{a}	65.9 ± 26.0^{b}	$53.5 \pm 19.2^{a,b}$	$45.0 \pm 12.9^{a,b}$
120 min	36.1 ± 21.5^{a}	$40.6 \pm 22.1^{a,b}$	$35.6 \pm 15.6^{a,b}$	68.0 ± 14.5^{b}
HbA1c (%)	5.18 ± 0.27	5.12 ± 0.22	5.05 ± 0.20	5.10 ± 0.17
HOMA-IR	1.32 ± 0.63^{a}	1.23 ± 0.43^{a}	0.66 ± 0.18^{b}	$1.20 \pm 0.26^{a,b}$
Insulinogenic index	2.50 ± 2.14^{a}	1.10 ± 0.94^{b}	0.76 ± 0.38^{b}	0.59 ± 0.25^{b}
HOMA-β	115 ± 47^{a}	$108 \pm 44^{a,b}$	65 ± 33^{b}	$92 \pm 35^{a,b}$
QUICKI	0.38 ± 0.03^{a}	0.38 ± 0.03^{a}	0.42 ± 0.02^{b}	$0.38 \pm 0.02^{a,b}$
AUC-glucose (hr·mg/dL)	191 ± 31^{a}	$216 \pm 21^{a,b}$	240 ± 11^{b}	253 ± 53^{b}
AUC-insulin (hr.μU/mL)	91.9 ± 44.8	94.7 ± 38.5	77.8 ± 27.3	88.0 ± 29.8

Values are means ± SD. HOMA-IR: homeostasis model assessment-insulin resistance; HOMA-β: homeostasis model assessment for β-cell function; QUICKI: quantitative insulin sensitivity check index; AUC: area under the curve. The values for each index with different superscript letters are statistically different at $p < 0.05$ by comparing different patterns of each time, as determined by Dunn's multiple comparison test.

Table 3: Biochemical status of woman by insulin and glucose response type.

Type	Normal	Insulin-late	Insulin- & glucose-late	Insulin-very late
Number	39	11	7	5
Total protein (g/dL)	7.67 ± 0.40	7.50 ± 0.45	7.28 ± 0.25	7.30 ± 0.43
Albumin (g/dL)	4.70 ± 0.25	4.79 ± 0.16	4.80 ± 0.22	4.63 ± 0.35
Albumin/globulin ratio	1.73 ± 0.25	1.84 ± 0.36	2.00 ± 0.32	1.75 ± 0.21
AST (U/L)	17.3 ± 3.2	17.6 ± 3.7	20.2 ± 6.1	15.5 ± 2.4
ALT (U/L)	13.3 ± 4.9	12.6 ± 5.8	14.8 ± 8.1	14.0 ± 6.8
γ-GTP (U/L)	17.7 ± 8.8	16.1 ± 4.9	16.2 ± 4.4	20.0 ± 8.4
LDL-C (mg/dL)	91.7 ± 21.3	90.0 ± 19.8	86.7 ± 13.8	105.3 ± 19.4
Triglyceride (mg/dL)	57.8 ± 22.7	43.0 ± 9.8	48.2 ± 16.1	68.5 ± 48.8
HDL-C (mg/dL)	68.9 ± 14.9	76.2 ± 7.8	73.3 ± 14.9	66.8 ± 13.7
Blood uric nitrogen (mg/dL)	11.7 ± 2.5	12.3 ± 4.5	10.3 ± 2.1	16.0 ± 6.7
Serum creatinine (mg/dL)	0.57 ± 0.08	0.58 ± 0.05	0.59 ± 0.08	0.55 ± 0.08
Serum uric acid (mg/dL)	4.18 ± 0.76	4.17 ± 0.74	4.18 ± 1.05	4.98 ± 0.87
White blood cell count ($\times 10^2/\mu$L)	60.7 ± 15.5	57.5 ± 11.7	55.1 ± 11.6	60.0 ± 14.3
Red blood cell count ($\times 10^4/\mu$L)	446 ± 28	451 ± 36	459 ± 27	444 ± 19
Hemoglobin (g/dL)	13.3 ± 0.9	13.3 ± 1.3	12.6 ± 2.7	13.3 ± 0.9
Hematocrit (%)	40.9 ± 2.2	40.1 ± 3.7	40.3 ± 6.5	40.6 ± 2.3
MCV (fL)	91.9 ± 3.5	90.6 ± 4.0	87.4 ± 11.4	91.4 ± 3.4
MCH (pg)	29.8 ± 1.8	29.4 ± 1.7	27.3 ± 5.3	30.0 ± 1.4
MCHC (%)	32.4 ± 1.2	32.5 ± 0.9	30.9 ± 2.7	32.8 ± 1.1
Platelet count ($\times 10^4/\mu$L)	26.6 ± 5.1	26.7 ± 6.0	24.7 ± 8.0	26.4 ± 4.2

Values are means ± SD. There were no significant differences.

a 75 g OGTT and were categorized in four groups based on peak times of plasma insulin and glucose. There were several studies categorized with insulin secretion time. Hayakawa [21] and Kai et al. [22] divided the two insulin types into type with peak time from 30 min to 60 min (normal) and those with peaks at 120 min. Sasaki et al. [23] and Tanabe et al. [24] divided the three insulin types into type with peak time at 30 min, 60 min, and 120 min, and we used this classification in this study. However, they divided the types without considering the peak time of plasma glucose levels. In this study, we divided the types considering not only insulin peak time but also plasma glucose peak, and as a result we could divide them into four types. There were no subjects with fever or menstruation on the day of the experiment. Even if there is a missing declaration, insulin secretion is more susceptible to pregnancy and aging than menstruation [25], so we think that it does not have a significant influence on grouping of subjects.

In this study, we were unable to investigate physical activity or food requirements. However, our subjects were studying nutritional science to become dietitians and might, therefore, have better exercise and dietary habits than general college students. The number of subjects in each group were not equal, and the statistical difference might be hard to confirm, especially for the I-very late type group. However, it was important to reveal patterns prior to the appearance of a carbohydrate metabolic disorder in young healthy women, because it might facilitate diabetes prevention.

We did not identify subjects with abnormal fasting plasma glucose levels or other blood characteristics but did identify two subjects with IGT and four distinct carbohydrate patterns in healthy subjects by OGTT. In the two subjects with IGT, BMIs were below 25 kg/m^2 and the insulin peak time was 120 min after glucose administration. The other biochemical parameters were normal, and they did not have a family medical history of diabetes in a relative within the second degree of relationship.

Relative to the normal group, insulin secretion was delayed in the I-late and I&G-late groups and even further delayed in the I-very late group. And the number of subjects with normal response patterns was greater while that with abnormal patterns was smaller. However, this might be because this study was conducted only with young healthy women. If we did it with a larger number of subjects including men middle aged and older, this ratio might have changed. In the normal type group (Figure 1(a)), insulin secretion increased until 30 min after glucose administration, at which time, plasma glucose and insulin levels gradually decreased. Therefore, only glucose values at 30 min, which also corresponded to the insulin peak time, were significantly higher than 0 min glucose values. Glucose levels at 60 and 120 min declined, returning to concentrations comparable to those at baseline. Compared with that of the normal group, the I-late and I&G-late type groups displayed intermediate impairment of carbohydrate metabolism. The subjects in these groups displayed delayed insulin secretion following glucose administration. In the I-late type group (Figure 1(b)), in which the peak time for insulin was 60 min and glucose was 30 min, insulin sensitivity might be normal, because the increase in insulin secretion from 30 to 60 min resulted in a decrease in glucose levels. In addition, insulin secretory capacity was normal, because HOMA-IR, HOMA-β, AUC-G, and AUC-I, which are indices of carbohydrate metabolism, were not significantly different from the normal type group (Table 2). The third group was the I&G-late type group (Figure 1(c)), characterized by peak insulin and glucose times at 60 min. This group displayed not only an insulin secretory delay but also a secretion shortage during fasting and the early stages of the OGTT. For example, immunoreactive insulin levels and HOMA-IR values, which were calculated using fasting glucose and insulin levels, were significantly lower than those in the control and I-late type groups (Table 2). II values, which were calculated using glucose and insulin levels at fasting and 30 min after glucose administration, were lower than those in the normal groups, because early insulin secretion after glucose administration was the lowest. However, although the 60 min insulin level was the peak value in the I&G-late group, it did not differ significantly from that in the normal type group. AUC-I values in the I&G-late type group did not differ from the other groups. These results suggest that fasting and early insulin secretion were lower than those in the normal group, but total secretion was comparable. The final group was the I-very late type group, characterized by a peak insulin time at 120 min and peak glucose time at 30 min. This insulin and glucose pattern was similar to subjects with IGT. Insulin secretion during the early stage was low, and glucose levels remained elevated above 110 mg/dL at 120 min post-glucose administration, despite maintained insulin secretion between 30 and 120 min (Table 2 and Figure 1(d)). This phenomenon was caused by a secretion delay and not insulin resistance, because HOMA-IR was not abnormal and AUC-I values did not significantly differ from those in the normal type group. Tanabe et al.'s study [24] in healthy people averaging 60 years old showed that the insulin peak at 120 min was 25 out of 680 (3.7%). Though we had 3 people (5.0%) in our I-very late type group without IGT subjects, it was more than that proportion. This phenomenon might be consistent with the gradually increasing number of young individuals with diabetes [8].

In this study, we did not detect differences in AUC-I levels between the four groups but did find differences in AUC-G levels and peak times. This result suggests that differences in carbohydrate metabolism in healthy young women were caused by different insulin secretion times and not secretory capacity or insulin resistance. However, the mechanisms underlying differences in secretion times remain unclear. For example, these differences might be caused by genetic background, obesity, exercise habits, skipping breakfast, having a midnight meal, and speed eating [12, 26–29]. However, in this study, there were subjects with BMIs above 25 kg/m^2 in the normal and I-late type groups but not in the I&G-late and I-very late type groups. In each group, there were subjects with a family medical history of diabetes in a relative within the second degree of relationship, and this did not differ between groups (data not shown). Biochemical parameters, including HOMA-IR and II, were normal. We did not investigate the other factors in this study. Kikuoka et al. demonstrated that 13.1% of subjects with impaired fasting glucose progressed to type 2 diabetes within 5 years [30]. Future studies will investigate lifestyle habits and conduct a follow-up survey of the four insulin and plasma glucose response groups.

Normal indices of carbohydrate metabolism (e.g., fasting plasma glucose, HOMA-IR, and II) did not allow us to classify the subjects into four groups. For example, if we classified only with peak insulin times, we might not have noticed the significant differences in HOMA-IR, QUICKI, and immunoreactive insulin levels between the I-late type and I&G-late type groups. If we classified subjects only according to peak glucose times, we might not have noticed the maintenance of hyperglycemia between 30 and 120 min in the I-very late type group. We revealed these differences by using both peak glucose and insulin times. In our study, about 37% of subjects had delayed insulin secretion. In a typical study, these individuals might be categorized into the control group. In our 60 subjects, excluding two IGT subjects, the average plasma glucose levels were 83.6 ± 5.6, 123.3 ± 21.3, 100.8 ± 27.0, and 90.8 ± 15.2 mg/dL at 0, 30, 60, and 120 min post-glucose administration, respectively. The average insulin levels were 5.8 ± 2.5, 68.1 ± 42.4, 52.4 ± 37.5, and 41.6 ± 30.8 μU/mL, respectively. These values were similar to normal type values in this study, and thus, individuals with delayed insulin secretion, who might be at risk for diabetes, would have been overlooked in the healthy control group. We believe that an understanding of one's own carbohydrate metabolism is important for type 2 diabetes prevention. OGTTs may allow us to assess glucose and insulin response types.

5. Conclusions

We revealed that insulin secretion and plasma glucose patterns could be categorized into four groups, despite all subjects being healthy young women, because postchallenge and fasting insulin secretion varied among individuals. The first group was the normal type group, in which insulin and glucose levels 30 min after glucose administration during an OGTT were highest and then gradually decreased. The second type displayed delayed postchallenge insulin secretion. However, other indices of carbohydrate metabolism (e.g., HOMA-IR, HOMA-β, AUC-I, and AUC-G) were not significantly different. The third group displayed delayed and reduced insulin secretion. In this group, fasting insulin levels were low, and the lack of additional insulin secretion caused a delay in peak plasma glucose levels. The fourth group displayed very late postchallenge insulin secretion, and this group contained IGT subjects. The delayed secretion caused persistent postprandial hyperglycemia until 120 min after glucose administration. Even in some healthy young women, insulin secretion was delayed after oral glucose administration, and they might, therefore, need improvements in their lifestyle habits. Confirmation of insulin secretion and plasma glucose patterns in young healthy individuals might be helpful for early type 2 diabetes prevention. Future studies should compare lifestyle habits among the groups and conduct a follow-up survey to identify subjects that develop IGT.

Conflicts of Interest

The authors have no conflicts of interest directly relevant to the content of this article.

Acknowledgments

The funding of this investigation was provided in part by Nagoya Bunri University.

References

[1] J. E. Gerich, "Clinical significance, pathogenesis, and management of postprandial hyperglycemia," *Archives of Internal Medicine*, vol. 163, no. 11, pp. 1306–1316, 2003.

[2] M. Brownlee, "The pathobiology of diabetic complications: a unifying mechanism," *Diabetes*, vol. 54, no. 6, pp. 1615–1625, 2005.

[3] T. S. Temelkova-Kurktschiev, C. Koehler, E. Henkel, W. Leonhardt, K. Fuecker, and M. Hanefeld, "Postchallenge plasma glucose and glycemic spikes are more strongly associated with atherosclerosis than fasting glucose or HbA1c level," *Diabetes Care*, vol. 23, no. 12, pp. 1830–1834, 2000.

[4] F. Anan, T. Masaki, T. Eto et al., "Postchallenge plasma glucose and glycemic spikes are associated with pulse pressure in patients with impaired glucose tolerance and essential hypertension," *Hypertension Research*, vol. 31, no. 8, pp. 1565–1571, 2008.

[5] M. Tominga, H. Eguchi, H. Manaka, K. Igarashi, T. Kato, and A. Sekikawa, "Impaired glucose tolerance is a risk factor for cardiovascular disease, but not impaired fasting glucose. The Funagata Diabetes Study," *Diabetes Care*, vol. 22, no. 6, pp. 920–924, 1999.

[6] DECODE Study Group and On behalf of the European Diabetes Epidemiology Group, "Glucose tolerance and cardiovascular mortality: comparison of fasting and 2-hour diagnostic criteria," *Archives of Internal Medicine*, vol. 161, pp. 397–405, 2001.

[7] C. Weyer, C. Bogardus, D. M. Mott, and R. E. Pratly, "The natural history of insulin secretory dysfunction and insulin resistance in the pathogenesis of type 2 diabetes mellitus," *The Journal of Clinical Investigation*, vol. 104, no. 6, pp. 787–794, 1999.

[8] J. C. N. Chan, V. Malik, W. Jia et al., "Diabetes in Asia: epidemiology, risk factors, and pathophysiology," *JAMA*, vol. 301, no. 20, pp. 2129–2140, 2009.

[9] R. Mitsui, M. Fukushima, Y. Nishi et al., "Factors responsible for deteriorating glucose tolerance in newly diagnosed type 2 diabetes in Japanese men," *Metabolism*, vol. 55, no. 1, pp. 53–58, 2006.

[10] C. Moris, C. O'Grada, M. Ryan et al., "Identification of differential responses to an oral glucose tolerance test in healthy adults," *PLoS ONE*, vol. 8, no. 8, article e72890, 2013.

[11] H. K. Yang, J. H. Lee, I. Y. Choi et al., "The insulin resistance but not the insulin secretion parameters have changed in the Korean population during the last decade," *Diabetes & Metabolism Journal*, vol. 39, no. 2, pp. 117–125, 2015.

[12] M. Fujii, H. Ohnishi, S. Saitho, M. Mori, and K. Shimamoto, "Comparison of the effect of abdominal obesity on new onset of type 2 diabetes in a general Japanese. Elderly population with that in a non-elderly population-the Tanno and Sobetsu Study (in Japanese)," *Nippon Ronen Igakkai Zasshi Japanese Journal of Geriatrics*, vol. 48, pp. 71–77, 2011.

[13] M. Fukushima, H. Suzuki, and Y. Seino, "Insulin secretion capacity in the development from normal glucose tolerance to type 2 diabetes," *Diabetes Research and Clinical Practice*, vol. 66, Supplement, pp. S37–S43, 2004.

[14] World Health Organization and Department of Noncommunicable Disease Surveillance, *Definition, Diagnosis and Classification of Diabetes Mellitus and its Complications: Report of a WHO Consultation. Part 1: Diagnosis and Classification of Diabetes Mellitus*, p. 59, World Health Organization, Geneva, 1999, WHO/NCD/NCS/99.2.

[15] J. L. B. Richard and C. M. Donna, "Evaluation of glucose 6 phosphate dehydrogenase from *Leuconostoc mesentroides* in the hexokinase method for determining glucose in serum," *Clinical Chemistry*, vol. 20, no. 5, pp. 586–590, 1974.

[16] J. D. M. Albano, R. P. Ekins, G. Maritz, and R. C. Tuner, "A sensitive, precise radioimmunoassay of serum insulin relying on charcoal separation of bound and free hormone moieties," *European Journal of Endocrinology*, vol. 70, pp. 487–509, 1972.

[17] D. R. Matthews, J. P. Hosker, A. S. Rudenski, B. A. Naylor, D. F. Treacher, and R. C. Turner, "Homeostasis model assessment: insulin resistance and β-cell function from fasting plasma glucose and insulin concentrations in man," *Diabetologia*, vol. 28, no. 7, pp. 412–419, 1985.

[18] Y. Seino, M. Ikeda, M. Yawata, and H. Imura, "The insulinogenic index in secondary diabetes," *Hormone and Metabolic Research*, vol. 7, no. 2, pp. 107–115, 1975.

[19] A. Katz, S. S. Nambi, K. Mather et al., "Quantitative insulin sensitivity check index: a simple, accurate method for assessing insulin sensitivity in humans," *The Journal of Clinical Endocrinology & Metabolism*, vol. 85, no. 7, pp. 2402–2410, 2000.

[20] Y. Seino, K. Nanjo, N. Tajima et al., "Report of the committee on the classification and diagnostic criteria of diabetes mellitus (revision for international harmonization of HbA1c in Japan) (in Japanese)," *Journal of the Japan Diabetes Society*, vol. 55, pp. 485–504, 2012.

[21] H. Hayakawa, "Dynamics of insulin secretion in liver disease (in Japanese)," *Japanese Journal of Gastroenterology*, vol. 67, no. 6, pp. 457–468, 1970.

[22] Y. Kai, R. Abe, S. Katono et al., "Plasma insulin response in the cases with a borderline 50g oral glucose tolerance test (in Japanese)," *Journal of the Japan Diabetes Society*, vol. 17, no. 1, pp. 16–22, 1974.

[23] A. Sasaki, K. Matsumiya, M. Arao, K. Hasegawa, and N. Horiuchi, "Evaluation of insulin response in subjects with normal and mildly impaired glucose tolerance (in Japanese)," *Journal of the Japan Diabes Society*, vol. 21, no. 11, pp. 983–992, 1978.

[24] M. Tanabe, Y. Arase, H. Tsuji et al., "Insulin secretory response to oral glucose in subjects with normal glucose intolerance (in Japanese)," *Ningen Dock*, vol. 26, no. 4, pp. 601–606, 2011.

[25] T. Okuyama and Y. Terauchi, "Blood glucose: gender-specific medicine in diabetes mellitus (in Japanese)," *Journal of the Japan Diabetes Society*, vol. 56, no. 8, pp. 522–524, 2013.

[26] Y. Azami, A. Ikota, K. Ito et al., "A multi-center study of young adults with type 2 diabetes mellitus: their clinical characteristics and the comparison of lifestyle and socioeconomic status with a nation-wide survey (in Japanese)," *Journal of the Japan Diabetes Society*, vol. 59, no. 2, pp. 95–104, 2016.

[27] T. Fukui, S. Yoshitaka, Y. Yamomoto, Y. Ayada, and T. Yasuda, "Dose lifestyle really affect insulin resistance? (in Japanese)," *Ningen Dock*, vol. 22, no. 1, pp. 51–58, 2007.

[28] Y. Soga, C. Shirai, and A. Ijichi, "Association between daily lifestyle and the risk of metabolic syndrome among young adults in Japan. An analysis of Kobe city young adult health examination data (in Japanese)," *Japanese Journal of Public Health*, vol. 60, no. 2, pp. 98–106, 2013.

[29] K. Funatsu, T. Yamashita, M. Honma et al., "Relationship between fatty liver and insulin resistance in non-obese and obese subjects (in Japanese)," *Ningen Dock*, vol. 26, no. 1, pp. 37–43, 2011.

[30] H. Kikuoka, H. Tatsuta, K. Yasuwaki et al., "Risk factors for progression from IFG to type 2 diabetes - follow-up at health examination (in Japanese)," *Journal of the Japan Diabetes Society*, vol. 47, no. 9, pp. 723–726, 2004.

5

Upregulations of Clcn3 and P-Gp Provoked by Lens Osmotic Expansion in Rat Galactosemic Cataract

Lixia Ji,[1] Lixia Cheng,[2] and Zhihong Yang[1]

[1]*Department of Pharmacology, School of Pharmacy, Qingdao University, Qingdao, China*
[2]*Department of Endocrinology, People's Hospital of Weifang, Weifang, China*

Correspondence should be addressed to Lixia Ji; lixiaji@163.com

Academic Editor: Hiroshi Okamoto

Objective. Lens osmotic expansion, provoked by overactivated aldose reductase (AR), is the most essential event of sugar cataract. Chloride channel 3 (Clcn3) is a volume-sensitive channel, mainly participating in the regulation of cell fundamental volume, and P-glycoprotein (P-gp) acts as its modulator. We aim to study whether P-gp and Clcn3 are involved in lens osmotic expansion of galactosemic cataract. *Methods and Results.* In vitro, lens epithelial cells (LECs) were primarily cultured in gradient galactose medium (10–60 mM), more and more vacuoles appeared in LEC cytoplasm, and mRNA and protein levels of AR, P-gp, and Clcn3 were synchronously upregulated along with the increase of galactose concentration. In vivo, we focused on the early stage of rat galactosemic cataract, amount of vacuoles arose from equatorial area and scattered to the whole anterior capsule of lenses from the 3rd day to the 9th day, and mRNA and protein levels of P-gp and Clcn3 reached the peak around the 9th or 12th day. *Conclusion.* Galactosemia caused the osmotic stress in lenses; it also markedly leads to the upregulations of AR, P-gp, and Clcn3 in LECs, together resulting in obvious osmotic expansion in vitro and in vivo.

1. Introduction

Sugar cataract is the major ocular complication of diabetes, which seriously impairs the ocular function of diabetic subjects [1]. Hyperglycemia is thought to be the underlying factor of diabetic cataractogenesis [2]. Lens osmotic expansion, a crucial and reversible process, greatly triggers the rapid onset and accelerates the maturation of true cataract [3]; thus, this is the critical stage for the prevention of diabetic cataract. Cell swelling is the main feature of lens osmotic expansion; several proteins such as AR, P-gp, and Clcn3 are proposed to participate in this pathological mechanism.

AR catalyzes the NADPH-dependent reductions of a broad variety of aldehydes or ketones to their corresponding alcohols [4–6]. AR is the rate-limiting enzyme of polyol pathway; its overactivation induced by hyperglycemia is the blasting fuse of diabetic cataract [6]. Both galactose and glucose belong to AR substrates, but AR has higher affinity to galactose than to glucose, and galactitol is even more difficult to be further metabolized than sorbitol, so galactosemic cataract formed more rapidly than diabetic cataract model [3, 7, 8]. Although galactosemic cataract and diabetic cataract are together called "sugar cataract" [7], most researchers prefer to use galactose-induced cataract model to study the pathological mechanism of lens osmotic expansion [1, 9–11].

In lenses, AR is primarily located in LECs, and its biologic activity in LECs is approximately 21-fold of that in cortical fibers [12]. In physiological conditions, almost no glucose enters polyol pathway; but it will be markedly activated by hyperglycemia and even more than 30% glucose enters polyol pathway when blood glucose level is over 11.1 mmol/l [4, 13]. Activated AR converts amount of glucose to sorbitol, and the later does not readily diffuse across cell membrane and is poorly further reduced by sorbitol dehydrogenase [4, 13]. Therefore, more and more hypertonic sorbitol accumulates in cytoplasm and absorbs water, leading to gradual swelling of lenticular cells [13]. In lenses, perhaps AR activation originally acts as homeostatic regulation against the high osmolality of extracellular glucose; nothing but the overactivation of AR causes the accumulation of a large majority of sorbitol accompanied by influx of much water, so LECs gradually swell and eventually cause cell rupture.

Modulation of cell volume is highly conservative in evolution to maintain constant cellular volume by regulating internal ingredients to cope with the changed osmolarity [14, 15]. Despite a matter of debate existed, most investigators thought that modulation of cell volume mainly depended on the coordination of P-gp and Clcn3 [15, 16].

P-gp, a highly conserved membrane protein, is a member of ATP-binding cassette (ABC) transporter protein super family [17–19]. In humans, P-gp is encoded by the multidrug resistance gene 1 (MDR 1); in rodents, mdr1a and mdr1b genes are homologous to human MDR1 [17–19]. P-gp has already been approved to have bimodal functions; it not only serves as the transmembrane transporter being responsible for the efflux of multidrugs in isotonic condition but also switches to a modulator of Clcn3 in hyperosmotic environment [20, 21]. Reversible phosphorylation is the possible mechanism for functional shuttle of P-gp [16]. Upregulation of P-gp is closely linked to overactivated Clcn3 [10, 16], which is a volume-regulated chloride channel. Clcn3 is highly associated with the regulation of fundamental volume in response to cell swelling or shrinking [15]. The opening of Clcn3 allows the efflux of diverse osmolytes such as several amino acids and polyols, leading to concomitant decrease of cell volume [16, 22]. Anti-P-gp monoclonal antibody could directly combine distinct epitopes of P-gp and obviously inhibited Cl^- conductance induced by cell swelling [23]. P-gp also expressed in lens [24] and was markedly upregulated in LEC layer isolated from 30% galactose-fed rats on the 4th and 7th days [10]. Besides, P-gp transgenic hamsters could develop cataracts resembling those in mice with congenital osmotic cataract [25]. P-gp should be considered as a modulator in lens osmotic expansion of sugar cataract [24]. However, administration of AR inhibitors to galactose-fed rats could reverse the upregulation of P-gp, indicating a potential pathophysiological linkage between the osmotic stress and P-gp stimulation [10].

On the basis of the previous theories and results, we hypothesize that lens osmotic expansion, imposed by AR overactivation, would stimulate Clcn3 and its modulator P-gp to delay the lenticular swelling.

2. Materials and Methods

2.1. Primary Culture of Beagle Dog LECs. The whole eyeballs were immediately enucleated from beagle dogs after being sacrificed; we soaked them into 75% ethanol for 10 minutes, carefully isolated the lens by posterior method, and cut the lens capsule into two parts at the equatorial zone. Due to the specific distribution of monolayer LECs below the anterior capsule of lens, all anterior capsules were collected, cut into tiny fractions, moved into a flask, and gently shook to spread evenly on the bottom. In order to increase the adherence, the flask was firstly cultivated in 100% bovine fetal serum (FBS; Gibco, Auckland, New Zealand) in an erect position for 4 hours, then followed by being positioned horizontally. 24 hours later, we added 5 ml Dulbecco's modified Eagle medium (DMEM; Hyclone, Beijing, China) supplemented with 15% FBS, 2 mM glutamine, 100 μg/ml streptomycin, and 100 U/ml penicillin. Another 24 hours later, we observed that many LECs were growing below or around the capsule tissue fractions, the 3rd to 8th passages of LECs were used in following studies.

2.2. Osmotic Expansion of LECs Induced by Gradient Galactose. The LECs were harvested and seeded on 6-well plates (20,000/well); 24 hrs later, galactose was added to final concentrations of 0, 10, 20, 30, 40, 50, and 60 mM. After 48-hour cultivation, we observed LECs' morphology under inverted microscope and harvested them. One part was used to extract total mRNA and detect mRNA expression by real-time RT-PCR; another part was used to extract total protein and measure targeted genes' protein level by Western blot. For the assessment of cell viability, LEC cultivation was carried out on 96-well plates, and cell viability was monitored by using CCK-8 reagent (Dojindo, Japan).

2.3. Induction of Rat Galactosemic Cataract and Assessment of Lens Opacification [26]. Male Sprague-Dawley rats (21 days old) with average body weight of 40 ± 4.07 g were purchased from the laboratory animal center at Qingdao Food and Drug Administration (SCXK-Lu-20140001; Qingdao, China). They were treated according to the ARVO statement for the Use of Animals in Ophthalmic and Vision Research. All the rats were randomized into two groups ($n = 24$), and they had free access to AIN-93 stock diet. While animals drank different water, rats in normal group drank pure water, but rats in control group drank 12.5% galactose solution in the first 7 days and 10% galactose solution from the 8th day to the end; the whole duration was 18 days. Every 3 days, lens opacification was evaluated (without anesthesia) by using a hand-held slit lamp (SL-15; Cowa, Japan) proceeded after full mydriasis with tropicamide hydrochloride. Cataract severity was scored by the same experienced observer who was blinded to the identity of each individual animal. Lens opacification was graded into five stages as follows [8, 26]: grade 0, clear normal lenses; grade 1, vacuoles, located in the cortex, cover less than one-third of the lens anterior segment, forming a subcapsular cataract; grade 2, vacuoles cover approximately two-thirds of the lens anterior segment; grade 3, diffuse opacity in cortex with/without some vacuoles; grade 4, diffuse opacity in cortex and moderate nuclear opacity; grade 5, mature milky cataract is observed as a dense opacity in both cortex and nucleus. After assessment of sugar cataract, four rats of each group were sacrificed with CO_2 on the day of 3, 6, 9, 12, 15, and 18, respectively. Each time, we promptly isolated the intact lenses by posterior approach, weighed them, and observed the lens shape and transparency in vitro. At last, all the lens samples were thrown into lipid nitrogen and stored at −80°C until further assay.

2.4. mRNA Expressions of AR, P-Gp, and Clcn3 in LECs and Lenses. Total RNA was extracted from LECs or lenses with TRIzol reagent (TaKaRa, Dalian, China) on the basis of manufacturer's protocol. To avoid amplification of genomic DNA sequences, all RNA samples were treated with DNase I and diluted to 100 ng/μl. 2.5 μg total RNA of each sample was reverse-transcribed into first strand cDNA with the iScript cDNA Synthesis Kit (Invitrogen, Waltham, MA, America) as described by the manufacturer. mRNA quantification was performed by using SYBR Green PCR Kit (TaKaRa, Dalian, China); all reactions were carried out in a single tube reaction setup on the ARI7000 real-time PCR system. The temperature profile was as follows: stage 1, 10 s at 95°C for denaturation of cDNA/RNA hybrid; stage 2, 40 cycles of 5 s at 95°C and 34 s at 61°C; and stage 3, 15 s at 95°C, 1 min at 60°C and 15 s at 95°C. β-Actin, a housekeeping gene, was chosen as an internal control to normalize the expressions of target genes. A control PCR reaction involving only Taq polymerase and the primer combination was used as a negative PCR control. Specific primers were designed based on published sequences (GenBank), β-actin sense, 5′-ACTCTTCCAGC CTTCCTTC-3′, and antisense, 5′ATCTCCTTCTGCATCC TGTC-3′; AR sense, 5′-GTG ACC GAG GCT GTG AA-3′, and antisense, 5′-AGA GGG TTG AAG TTG GAG A-3′; P-gp sense, 5′-GCC CAT CCT GTT TGA CTG-3′, and antisense, 5′-CGC TTC CTG GAC GAC CTT-3′; and Clcn3 sense, 5′-ACA CTG ACG GGA TTG G-3′, and antisense, 5′-AGG CAT ACG GAG CAA-3′. Results were expressed as fold change of target genes versus β-actin by ΔΔCt method.

2.5. Protein Detection of AR, P-Gp, and Clcn3 by Western Blot. LECs or lens capsules were homogenized in ice-cold lysate buffer containing 2 mM EDTA, 50 mM Tris-phosphate, 150 mM NaCl, 1% NP-40, 0.5% sodium deoxycholate, 0.1% SDS, 1 mM PMSF, and 1% protease inhibitor cocktail (Nakarai Tesque, Kyoto, Japan). Tissue samples were firstly subjected for sonication (40 W, 30 minutes) on ice and then subsequently harvested the supernatants after centrifugation at 20,000*g* for 40 minutes at 4°C. Protein level was determined by bicinchoninic acid (BCA) method. Proteins (100 mg per sample) were run on a 10% gradient sodium dodecylsulfate-polyacrylamide electrophoresis gel, then transferred on polyvinylidene difluoride (PVDF) membrane (Bio-Rad, Hercules, CA, America). After blocking by TBS-T (0.01 mol/l TBS with 0.1% Tween 20) containing 5% (*w*/*v*) nonfat milk, the blots were incubated with specific primary antibodies at 4°C, such as 12 hrs with anti-goat polyclonal AR antibody (sc17736, dilution 1 : 1000; Santa Cruz, CA, America), or 48 hrs with anti-mouse monoclonal P-gp antibody (sc59593, dilution 1 : 200; Santa Cruz), or 12 hrs with anti-mouse monoclonal Clcn3 antibody (sc390010, dilution 1 : 1000; Santa Cruz). After washing by TBS-T, the membranes were incubated with anti-goat/mouse/rabbit IgG-labeled with horseradish peroxidase (dilution 1 : 2000; Santa Cruz) for 60 min at room temperature. These membranes were washed again with TBS-T and visualized by the enhanced chemiluminescence method using LAS-3000 imaging system (Fuji Photo Film, Tokyo, Japan). Exposure times ranged from 20 to 120 sec based on different proteins.

2.6. Statistical Analysis. All the data were presented as mean ± standard deviation (SD); the grade of sugar cataract was analyzed by Mann–Whitney test, and other data were evaluated with one-way ANOVA (two-tailed test). p value less than 0.05 was considered to be statistically significant.

3. Results

3.1. Effects of Galactose on LECs' Morphology. In primary culture, fractions of lens anterior capsule were tightly attached to the flask bottom in 24 hours; some LECs were growing below or around lens capsule fractions after 48-hour cultivation (Figure 1(a)). Most oval LECs had typical epithelial-like structure with big nuclear and abundant cytoplasm. In the following passages, several LECs would switch to shuttle-like fiber cells, so we only used the 3rd to 8th passages of LECs in further studies. As to the osmotic expansion of LECs (Figure 1(c)), lots of tiny vacuoles appeared around the nucleus in the LEC cytoplasm under the coincubation with galactose in 48 hours. The higher the galactose concentration was the more the tiny vacuoles appeared. This phenomenon never appeared in normal LECs in 48-hour incubation. Our results were consistent with similar observations reported in dog LECs cultured in medium containing 3-fluoro-3-deoxy-galactoseactose [27]. As to cell viability (Figure 1(b)), only high-level galactose (>40 mM) could significantly inhibit the cell viability compared with the normal level.

3.2. mRNA Expressions and Protein Levels of AR, P-g, and Clcn3 in LECs Induced by Galactose. As shown in Figure 2(a), CT value of AR mRNA expression was about 18.5 in normal group cultivated in DMEM containing 1000 mg/l glucose, but the expressions of P-gp and Clcn3 mRNA were almost undetected. In comparison with the normal level, AR initially increased to 1.51-fold at 30 mM galactose ($p < 0.05$), then gradually increased to 2.24-fold at 50 mM ($p < 0.001$) and kept the peak at 60 mM. 30 mM galactose markedly increased the mRNA level of Clcn3 to 1.62-fold ($p < 0.05$) and it arrived at 4.15-fold peak at 60 mM ($p < 0.001$). As to P-gp, the modulator of Clcn3, its mRNA level obviously increased to 2.01-fold at 40 mM ($p < 0.05$) and reached the peak of 3.89-fold at 60 mM ($p < 0.001$). On cellular level, AR, P-gp, and Clcn3 could be activated by high level galactose and their responses to galactose were almost consistent.

Protein levels of AR, P-gp, and Clcn3 were summarized in Figure 2(b). Although LECs were incubated in gradient galactose levels, β-actin expressed very stably. Proteins of AR, P-gp, and Clcn3 expressed weakly in normal medium with glucose (1000 mg/l), but they were followed by consistent rises as the galactose concentration gradually increased from 0 to 60 mM. In normal group, protein levels of AR, P-gp, and Clcn3 were only 0.50-fold, 0.39-fold, and 0.43-fold of β-actin, respectively, and they gradually increased to 1.71-fold, 1.10-fold, and 1.64-fold of β-actin in 60 mM galactose incubation, respectively.

3.3. Onset and Formation of Galactosemic Cataract in Rats. As shown in Figures 3(a) and 3(b), normal lenses had always been at grade 0 and isolated lenses were transparent in the whole duration, but lens opacification of galactose group gradually increased by almost one grade every 3 days. In early six days, more and more tiny vacuoles continually appeared in the periphery of lens, subsequently extended to the whole

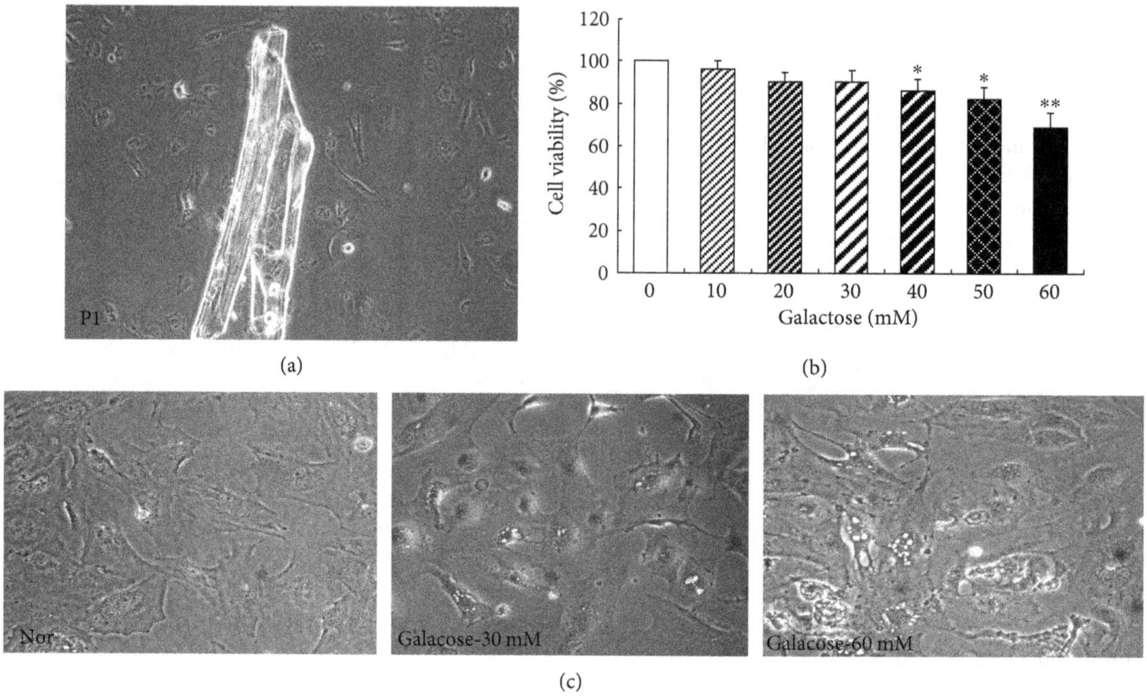

FIGURE 1: Primary culture of LECs and osmotic expression induced by gradient galactose. (a) Primary culture of beagle dog LECs (×100), P1 means the 1st passage of LECs; (b) effects of galactose on LEC viability, galactose concentration is 10, 20, 30, 40, 50, and 60 mM; (c) morphological characteristics of LECs induced by gradient galactose (×200). $^{*}p < 0.05$, $^{**}p < 0.01$ versus normal group.

anterior capsule with or without expanded "Y" in the central area. By the 6th day, tiny vacuoles occupied over two-thirds of the anterior capsule; the average cataract grade was 2.27, and we observed that isolated galactosemic lenses began to be blurry. Although we decreased galactose concentration from 12.5% to 10% from the 8th day, lens opacification was persistently aggravated in the following days. At the 9th day, slight nuclear opacification appeared in about 80% lenses of the control group. And at the end of the 18th day, more than 85% lenses of control group were milky both in the lens cortex and in the nuclear; most of galactosemic lenses were at stage 5.

As to the ratio of lens weight to body weight (Figure 3(c)), the ratio of normal 21-day SD rat was about 3.37×10^{-4}; it slowly decreased as normal rats grew up, but the ratio of cataractous rats obviously increased in the first 6 days and gradually decreased in the following 9 days. The maximal ratio of galactosemic rats was 5.51×10^{-4} on the 6th day, but the normal level was only 2.76×10^{-4}; the control ratio was still higher (2.76×10^{-4}) than the normal level (1.98×10^{-4}) at the end of day 18.

3.4. mRNA Expressions and Protein Levels of AR, P-Gp, and Clcn3 in Rat Lenses. mRNA expressions of AR, P-gp, and Clcn3 were summarized in Figure 4(a). AR, a key enzyme of polyol pathway, was gradually upregulated from the 3rd day (1.11-fold) to the peak (2.21-fold) at the 9th day, and then, it slowly reduced to 1.57-fold at the end of 18 days. These results almost coincided with our previous study [26]. The mRNA changes of P-gp and Clcn3 were similar, both P-gp and Clcn3 were gradually upregulated from the beginning to the highest level of 2.36-fold and 2.25-fold at the 12th day, respectively; then, they maintained their high levels to the end.

Since elevation of gene transcription was not always coincident with gene translation, we further examined the protein levels of target genes including AR, P-gp, and Clcn3 by Western blot (Figure 4(b)). Our analysis revealed that protein level of β-actin had been always on the similar level for the whole duration. On day 0, AR protein was about 0.66-fold of β-actin, but only faint protein expressions of P-gp and Clcn3 were detected in rat lenses; they were 0.20-fold and 0.34-fold of β-actin, respectively. P-gp and Clcn3 could be significantly upregulated along with the accumulation of galactitol. Protein level of AR obviously increased to 1.18-fold of β-actin by the 9th day, and it kept on rising to the peak of 1.26-fold of β-actin on the 12th day. Clcn3 and P-gp also continuously increased to the highest levels of 0.89-fold (day 12) and 0.73-fold (day 9), respectively. Based on the above results, the increased protein expressions of AR, P-gp, and Clcn3 were associated with their elevated mRNA levels.

4. Discussion

Diabetes is predicted to be about 552 million up to 2030 [28]; the majority of diabetic subjects are susceptible to develop sugar cataract over 10 years later. Differing from aging cataract, lens osmotic expansion occurring in early stage is the key pathological mechanism of diabetic cataract [2].

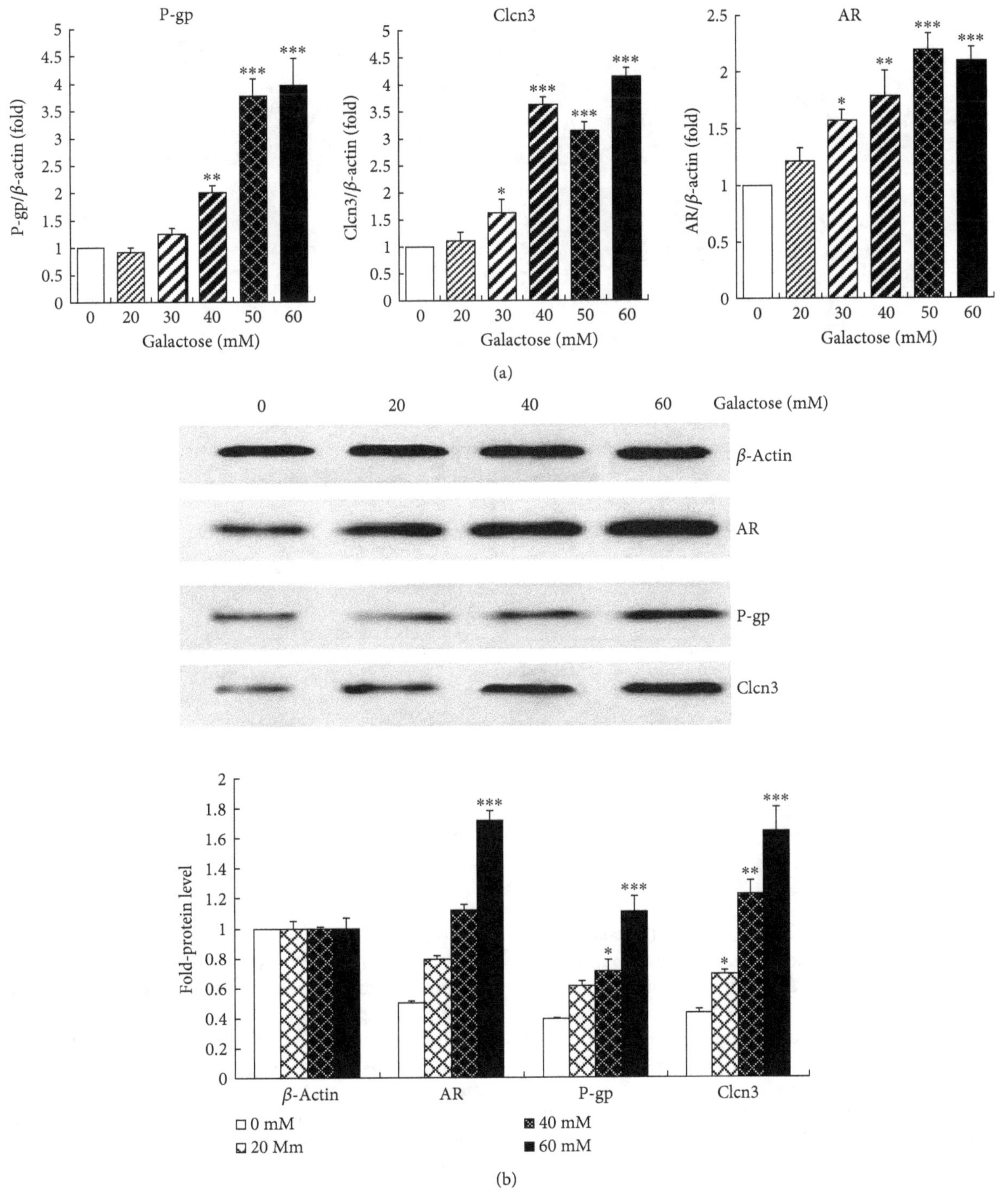

FIGURE 2: mRNA expressions and protein levels of AR, P-gp, and Clcn3 in LECs' osmotic expansion induced by gradient galactose. (a) mRNA expressions of target genes including AR, P-gp, and Clcn3; (b) Western blot and analysis of AR, P-gp, and Clcn3. $^{*}p < 0.05$, $^{**}p < 0.01$, and $^{***}p < 0.001$ versus the normal level of the same day.

Furthermore, lens osmotic expansion also induces serious oxidative stress, accelerating the maturation of sugar cataract. In fact, overactivation of AR in lenses resulted from hyperglycemia is the original cause, which leads to the accumulation of sorbitol and severe imbalances of electrolyte and water and further stimulates homeostasis system to reverse the swelling volume of lenticular cells. The related proteins involved in osmotic expansion are AR, Clcn3, and its modulator P-gp.

On cellular level, high level of galactose (≥40 mM) could induce more tiny vacuoles appearing in cytoplasm of LECs with decreased cell viability. The severity of vacuoles was tightly associated with galactose concentration. Similar phenomenon also existed in the lenses of rat galactosemic

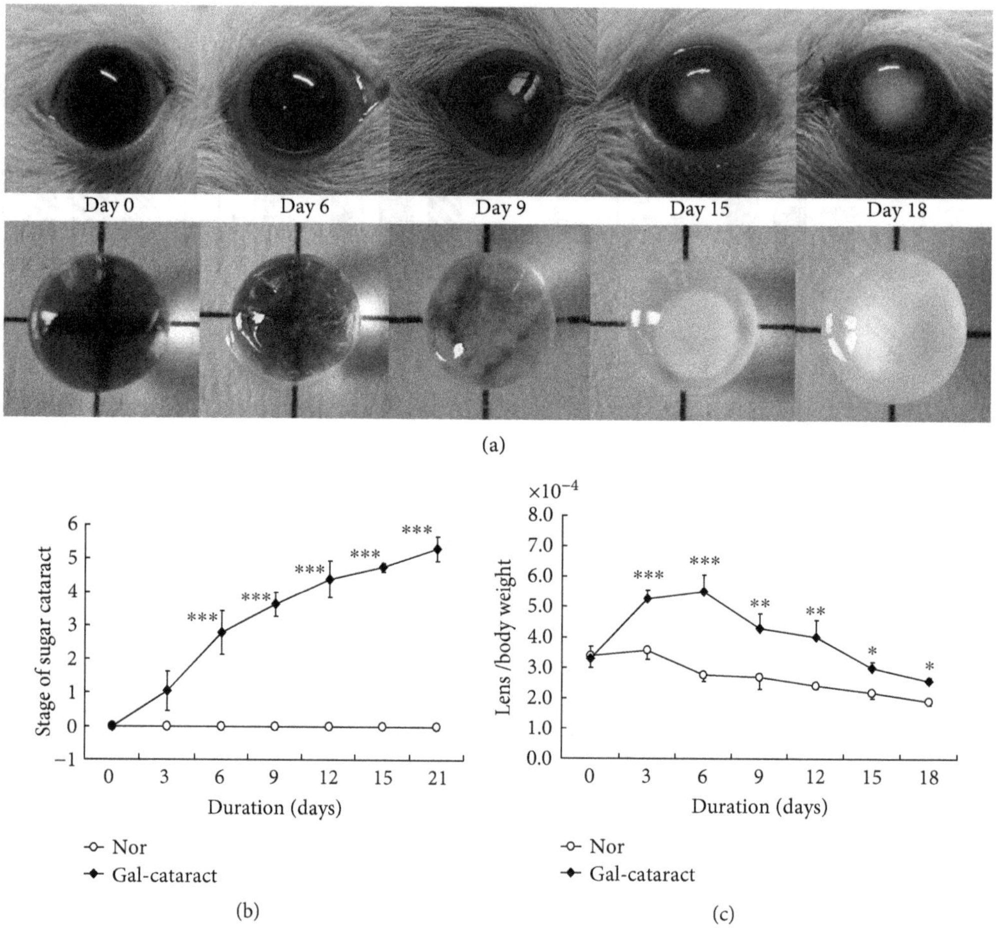

FIGURE 3: Onset and formation of rat sugar cataract induced by galactose. (a) Lens opacification of galactosemic cataract on the day of 0, 6, 9, 15, and 18; (b) grade of rat galactosemic cataract; and (c) the ratio of lens weight to body weight. $^{*}p < 0.05$, $^{**}p < 0.01$, and $^{***}p < 0.001$ versus normal level.

cataract model in vivo, and lots of vacuoles initially appeared around the lens equator and continuously expanded to anterior capsule during the early stage of sugar cataract. These were the factual manifests of lens osmotic expansion induced by galactose in vitro and in vivo; the following observations of mRNA and protein expressions demonstrated the potential mechanism.

But why did vacuoles firstly appear in LECs around the lens equator in rat galactose-induced cataract model? Perhaps it is related to the distribution of LECs. LECs are a monolayer of cubical epithelial cells located below the anterior capsule of the lens; they can consistently differentiate into fiber cells at the equatorial area. LECs in the equator are more active with stronger viability of proliferation and differentiation than other LECs. Therefore, they are more sensitive to hyperglycemia to form amount of dense vacuole clusters, initiating the development of sugar cataract. Above of them are just our speculation, the precise mechanism requires further investigations.

As to rat galactosemic cataract model, few tiny vacuoles arose around the equatorial area from the 3rd day; subsequently, dense clusters of vacuoles began to expand to the anterior capsule by day 6. Meanwhile, the ratio of lens weight to body weight increased dramatically to a crazy level, which indicated that an obvious osmotic expansion came into being in galactosemic lenses. RT-PCR results also presented the significant upregulations of AR, P-gp, and Clcn3 mRNA levels at the 6th day. Along with the ongoing of galactosemic cataract, most galactosemic rats began to enter the stage of nuclear opacification from the 12th day, so the early stage was the key period to investigate the dysregulations of AR, P-gp, and Clcn3 associated with lens osmotic expansion.

Maintenance of constant volume is the physiological function of Clcn3 in many types of mammalian cells [15, 16]. The followed cell swelling results from sorbitol accumulation in LECs; lenticular cells try to restore their original volume by activating chloride conductance [15]. P-gp, as the regulator of Clcn3, participates in the regulation of Clcn3 activity [16]. The present study showed that the dysregulations of Clcn3 and P-gp were almost synergetic in response to the lenticular swelling in LEC osmotic expansion and onset of rat galactosemic cataract. Although Clcn3 and P-gp expressed faintly in normal lens anterior capsules under physiological condition, both were predominantly upregulated in galactosemia, and the early stage was a key period of lens osmotic expansion.

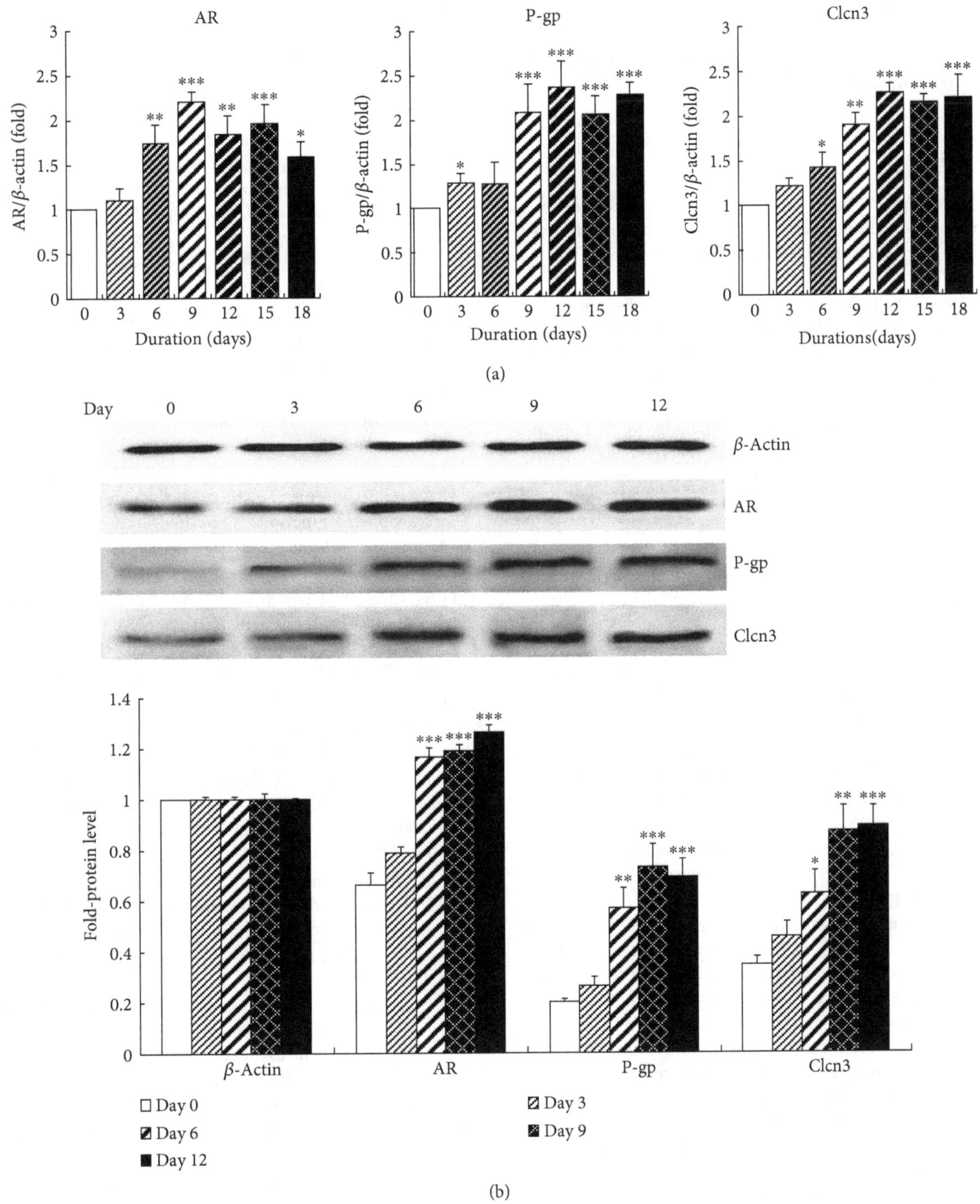

FIGURE 4: mRNA expressions and protein levels of AR, P-gp, and Clcn3 in lenses of galactosemic cataract rats. (a) mRNA expressions of target genes including AR, P-gp, and Clcn3 and (b) Western blot and analysis of AR, P-gp, and Clcn3. $^{*}p < 0.05$, $^{**}p < 0.01$, and $^{***}p < 0.001$ versus the normal level of same day.

In conclusion, AR was overactivated by galactosemia and led to severe osmotic expansion in lenticular cells; subsequently, P-gp and Clcn3 were both upregulated due to lenticular cell swelling and tried to maintain the osmotic balance within galactosemic lenses. AR, P-gp, and Clcn3 participated in the onset and formation of lens osmotic expansion in early stage of sugar cataract. We expect that dysregulations of the above genes can provide some information for rational development of drugs against galactosemic or diabetic cataract.

Conflicts of Interest

The authors declare that there is no conflict of interest regarding the publication of this article.

Acknowledgments

This study was supported by the Medical and Health Development Project of Shandong Province (2013WS2057).

References

[1] P. F. Kador, M. Wyman, and P. J. Oates, "Aldose reductase, ocular diabetic complications and the development of topical Kinostat®," *Progress in Retinal and Eye Research*, vol. 54, pp. 1–29, 2016.

[2] A. S. Grewal, S. Bhardwaj, D. Pandita, V. Lather, and B. S. Sekhon, "Updates on aldose reductase inhibitors for management of diabetic complications and non-diabetic diseases," *Mini Reviews in Medicinal Chemistry*, vol. 16, no. 2, pp. 120–162, 2016.

[3] P. Zhang, K. Xing, J. Randazzo, K. Blessing, M. F. Lou, and P. F. Kador, "Osmotic stress, not aldose reductase activity, directly induces growth factors and MAPK signaling changes during sugar cataract formation," *Experimental Eye Research*, vol. 101, pp. 36–43, 2012.

[4] P. Anil Kumar and G. Bhanuprakash Reddy, "Focus on molecules: aldose reductase," *Experimental Eye Research*, vol. 85, no. 6, pp. 739-740, 2007.

[5] N. Oishi, S. Morikubo, Y. Takamura et al., "Correlation between adult diabetic cataracts and red blood cell aldose reductase levels," *Investigative Ophthalmology & Visual Science*, vol. 47, no. 5, pp. 2061–2064, 2006.

[6] D. M. Kanchan, S. S. Kale, G. S. Somani, A. A. Kaikini, and S. Sathaye, "Thymol, a monoterpene, inhibits aldose reductase and high-glucose-induced cataract on isolated goat lens," *Journal of Pharmacy & Bioallied Sciences*, vol. 8, no. 4, pp. 277–283, 2016.

[7] J. H. Kinoshita, "Mechanisms initiating cataract formation. Proctor lecture," *Investigative Ophthalmology & Visual Science*, vol. 13, no. 10, pp. 713–724, 1974.

[8] P. Suryanarayana, M. Saraswat, T. Mrudula, T. P. Krishna, K. Krishnaswamy, and G. B. Reddy, "Curcumin and turmeric delay streptozotocin-induced diabetic cataract in rats," *Investigative Ophthalmology & Visual Science*, vol. 46, no. 6, pp. 2092–2099, 2005.

[9] C. S. Kim, J. Kim, Y. M. Lee, E. Sohn, and J. S. Kim, "Esculetin, a coumarin derivative, inhibits aldose reductase activity in vitro and cataractogenesis in galactose-fed rats," *Biomolecules & Therapeutics*, vol. 24, no. 2, pp. 178–183, 2016.

[10] T. Miyazawa, E. Kubo, Y. Takamura, and Y. Akagi, "Up-regulation of P-glycoprotein expression by osmotic stress in rat sugar cataract," *Experimental Eye Research*, vol. 84, no. 2, pp. 246–253, 2007.

[11] P. Suryanarayana, K. Krishnaswamy, and G. B. Reddy, "Effect of curcumin on galactose-induced cataractogenesis in rats," *Molecular Vision*, vol. 9, pp. 223–230, 2003.

[12] S. Hayman and J. H. Kinoshita, "Isolation and properties of lens aldose reductase," *The Journal of Biological Chemistry*, vol. 240, pp. 877–882, 1965.

[13] Z. Kyselova, M. Stefek, and V. Bauer, "Pharmacological prevention of diabetic cataract," *Journal of Diabetes and its Complications*, vol. 18, no. 2, pp. 129–140, 2004.

[14] M. E. Chamberlin and K. Strange, "Anisosmotic cell volume regulation: a comparative view," *American Journal of Physiology - Cell Physiology*, vol. 257, no. 2, pp. C159–C173, 1989.

[15] A. Sardini, J. S. Amey, K. H. Weylandt, M. Nobles, M. A. Valverde, and C. F. Higgins, "Cell volume regulation and swelling-activated chloride channels," *Biochimica et Biophysica Acta (BBA) - Biomembranes*, vol. 1618, no. 2, pp. 153–162, 2003.

[16] H. T. Idriss, Y. A. Hannun, E. Boulpaep, and S. Basavappa, "Regulation of volume-activated chloride channels by P-glycoprotein: phosphorylation has the final say!," *The Journal of Physiology*, vol. 524, no. 3, pp. 629–636, 2000.

[17] J. A. Endicott and V. Ling, "The biochemistry of P-glycoprotein-mediated multidrug resistance," *Annual Review of Biochemistry*, vol. 58, no. 1, pp. 137–171, 1989.

[18] M. M. Gottesman and I. Pastan, "Biochemistry of multidrug resistance mediated by the multidrug transporter," *Annual Review of Biochemistry*, vol. 62, no. 1, pp. 385–427, 1993.

[19] L. Saaby and B. Brodin, "A critical view on *in vitro* analysis of P-glycoprotein (P-gp) transport kinetics," *Journal of Pharmaceutical Sciences*, vol. 106, no. 9, pp. 2257–2264, 2017.

[20] G. M. Mintenig, M. A. Valverde, F. V. Sepulveda et al., "Specific inhibitors distinguish the chloride channel and drug transporter functions associated with the human multidrug resistance P-glycoprotein," *Receptors & Channels*, vol. 1, no. 4, pp. 305–313, 1993.

[21] H. Idriss, V. Urquidi, and S. Basavappa, "Selective modulation of P-glycoprotein's ATPase and anion efflux regulation activities with PKC α and PKC ε in Sf9 cells," *Cancer Chemotherapy and Pharmacology*, vol. 46, no. 4, pp. 287–292, 2000.

[22] S. Basavappa and J. C. Ellory, "The role of swelling-induced anion channels during neuronal volume regulation," *Molecular Neurobiology*, vol. 13, no. 2, pp. 137–153, 1996.

[23] C. G. Vanoye, G. A. Altenberg, and L. Reuss, "P-glycoprotein is not a swelling-activated Cl- channel; possible role as a Cl- channel regulator," *The Journal of Physiology*, vol. 502, no. 2, pp. 249–258, 1997.

[24] B. R. Merriman-Smith, M. A. Young, M. D. Jacobs, J. Kistler, and P. J. Donaldson, "Molecular identification of P-glycoprotein: a role in lens circulation?," *Investigative Ophthalmology & Visual Science*, vol. 43, no. 9, pp. 3008–3015, 2002.

[25] I. Dunia, J. J. Smit, M. A. van der Valk, H. Bloemendal, P. Borst, and E. L. Benedetti, "Human multidrug resistance 3-P-glycoprotein expression in transgenic mice induces lens membrane alterations leading to cataract," *The Journal of Cell Biology*, vol. 132, no. 4, pp. 701–716, 1996.

[26] L. Ji, C. Li, N. Shen et al., "A simple and stable galactosemic cataract model for rats," *International Journal of Clinical and Experimental Medicine*, vol. 8, no. 8, pp. 12874–12881, 2015.

[27] E. F. Secchi, M. J. Lizak, S. Sato, and P. F. Kador, "3-Fluoro-3-deoxy-D-galactose: a new probe for studies on sugar cataract," *Current Eye Research*, vol. 18, no. 4, pp. 277–282, 1999.

[28] D. R. Whiting, L. Guariguata, C. Weil, and J. Shaw, "IDF diabetes atlas: global estimates of the prevalence of diabetes for 2011 and 2030," *Diabetes Research and Clinical Practice*, vol. 94, no. 3, pp. 311–321, 2011.

6

Effects of High Glucose on the Expression of LAMA1 and Biological Behavior of Choroid Retinal Endothelial Cells

Guangwei Song,[1,2] Da Lin,[1,2] Licheng Bao,[1,2] Qi Jiang,[1,2] Yinan Zhang,[1,2] Haihua Zheng,[1,2] and Qianying Gao[1,2]

[1]*The Second Affiliated Hospital and Yuying Children's Hospital of Wenzhou Medical University, Wenzhou 325027, China*
[2]*The Second School of Medicine, Wenzhou Medical University, Wenzhou 325027, China*

Correspondence should be addressed to Haihua Zheng; eyezhh@126.com and Qianying Gao; gaoqy@mail.sysu.edu.cn

Academic Editor: Érika Bevilaqua Rangel

Hyperglycemia is one of the main causes of proliferative diabetic retinopathy (PDR) characterized by thickening of the vascular basement membrane. Laminin alpha 1 (LAMA1) is a primary component of laminin, a major protein constituent of the basement membrane. In this study, we investigated the role of LAMA1 in the development of PDR. Retinal choroidal vascular endothelial cells (RF/6A line) were exposed to glucose at different concentrations (5 mM, 15 mM, 25 mM, and 35 mM) and analyzed for cell growth, migration, proliferation, and adhesion. LAMA1 expression was examined 24 and 48 h following glucose treatment using Western blotting, RT-PCR, and immunofluorescence. The results showed that the proliferation, migration, and adhesion of RF/6A cells were increased by high glucose, whereas LAMA1 expression was slightly higher at 15 mM but decreased at 25 mM and 35 mM glucose compared to control. Thus, the changes in the biological behavior of high glucose-exposed retinal vascular endothelial cells correspond to variations in LAMA1 expression, indicating a possibility for LAMA1 involvement in PDR development. Our findings suggest that LAMA1 may play a role in PDR and, thus, may serve as a potential target for DR diagnosis and/or treatment.

1. Introduction

Diabetic retinopathy (DR) is one of the major microvascular complications caused by long-term hyperglycemia, and is also one of the most serious causes of blindness worldwide [1]. It is estimated that about one third of diabetic patients can develop DR [2] as a result of long-term accumulation of damaged small retinal vessels due to chronically poor blood glucose control [3]. Hyperglycemia is associated with the formation of advanced glycation end products, oxidative stress, inflammation, and neovascularization. These processes induce changes in the microvascular system, such as increased synthesis of extracellular matrix (ECM) proteins and thickening of the capillary basement membrane, which are the main pathological features of diabetic microangiopathy [4, 5].

DR is characterized by endothelial cell dysfunction, basement membrane thickening, increased fibrogenesis, and retinal detachment caused by fiber membrane retraction; in the advanced or proliferative (PDR) stage, blood vessels proliferate, resulting in neovascularization [6]. The thickened basement membrane is considered to be the consequence of upregulated expression of vascular basement membrane components such as type IV collagen, fibronectin, and laminin [5]. Oxidative damage is an important factor in endothelial cell dysfunction, and high glucose can cause excessive generation of reactive oxygen species (ROS) and activation of the protein kinase C (PKC)-beta pathway, leading to increased expression of ECM proteins and vascular endothelial growth factor (VEGF), and changes in endothelial cell permeability [7]. The ECM provides a scaffold required for vascular endothelial cells to form blood vessels, whereas adhesion to specific ECM components via integrins triggers intracellular signaling critically required for endothelial cell proliferation, migration, survival, and tube morphogenesis [8]. Thus, changes in the ECM are involved in endothelial dysfunction, basement membrane thickening, and neovascularization.

Laminin is one of the major ECM components participating in basement membrane formation. By binding to cell surface receptors, laminin induces different signal transduction pathways, which influence cell behavior such as adhesion, differentiation, migration, phenotype stability, and resistance to anoikis [9]. A previous study has shown that serum laminin can be used as a biomarker of DR associated with vascular endothelial dysfunction [10]. Laminin is a trimeric glycoprotein consisting of three chains, alpha, beta, and gamma and has been found in at least 16 different isoforms [11]. It was reported that the expression of laminin chains is regulated both spatially and temporally [12], suggesting that different laminin isoforms have distinct functional roles. A number of laminin isoforms are expressed in the basement membrane of retinal blood vessels and where they could influence vascular development [13].

Laminin α 1 (LAMA1), the most conserved subunit in all laminin isoforms, plays an essential role in embryonic development and promotes neurite outgrowth [14]. In mice, LAMA1 was shown to be expressed in the internal limiting membrane (ILM) between the retina and the vitreous body and in Bruch's membrane of the choroid, and it was reported that LAMA1 deficiency could cause abnormal cell adhesion and migration, leading to altered retinal angiogenesis, persistent vitreal fibroplasias, epiretinal membrane formation, and peripheral retinal degeneration [15, 16]. Epiretinal membranes were described in both of these mutants (LAMA1 knockout mice) which had characteristics similar to human persistent fetal vasculature (PFV) and proliferative vitreoretinopathy (PVR).

The aim of this study was to examine the role of LAMA1 in the development of PDR. As vascular endothelial cells play an important role in DR development [6], we used retinal choroidal vascular endothelial cells, which were exposed to different glucose concentrations and analyzed for cell behavior and LAMA1 expression.

2. Materials and Methods

2.1. Reagents and Antibodies. Rabbit anti-human LAMA1 antibody (sc-5582) was from Santa Cruz Biotechnology (Dallas, TX, USA). Mouse anti-human GAPDH antibody, goat anti-rabbit IgG H&L (ab150077), and goat anti-mouse IgG H&L were purchased from Abcam (Cambridge, MA, USA). TRIzol reagent and DAPI (4′,6-diamidino-2-phenylindole) were obtained from Invitrogen (Carlsbad, CA, USA). The PrimeScript RT reagent kit with gDNA Eraser and SYBR Premix Ex Taq™ II (Tli RNaseH Plus) kit were from Takara Clontech (Kyoto, Japan). Cell Counting Kit-8 (CCK-8) was from Dojindo (Kumamoto, Japan), and 4-well culture inserts were from Ibidi (cat. number 80469; Martinsried, Germany).

2.2. Cell Culture. Rhesus choroid retinal endothelial cells (RF/6A line; Chi Scientific, Jiangsu, China) were cultured in DMEM (Gibco, Life Technologies, NY, USA) supplemented with 10% fetal bovine serum (FBS; Gibco) and 1% penicillin/streptomycin (Gibco) at 37°C in a humidified incubator with 95% air-5% CO_2. Cells reaching at least 80% confluence were lifted by treatment with 0.25% trypsin/0.02% EDTA and passaged. To model hyperglycemic conditions, cells were grown in medium supplemented with 15 mmol/L, 25 mmol/L, and 35 mmol/L glucose for different times; control cells were grown at 5 mmol/L glucose.

2.3. Western Blotting. LAMA1 protein expression was assessed by Western blotting. RF/6A cells were washed twice with PBS and lysed with cold radioimmunoprecipitation assay (RIPA) buffer containing protease inhibitor phenylmethylsulfonyl fluoride (PMSF; Shanghai Beyotime Biotech Co., China). Lysed cells were collected using a cell scraper, transferred to Eppendorf tubes, and centrifuged for 30 min at 12,000 rpm (4°C) to obtain supernatants. A BCA protein assay kit (Shanghai Beyotime Biotech Co.) was used to determine protein concentrations. Protein samples (20 μg protein/well) were subjected to sodium dodecyl sulfate polyacrylamide gel electrophoresis (SDS-PAGE) and transferred to polyvinylidene difluoride (PVDF) membranes, which were blocked in 5% BSA for 2 h at room temperature. After that, the membranes were incubated with antibodies to LAMA1 (1:1000) overnight, washed three times with Tris-buffered saline containing 0.05% Tween 20 for 30 min each, and incubated with HRP-conjugated secondary antibodies for 2 h at room temperature. Specific bands were visualized using Immobilon Western Chemiluminescent HRP Substrate reagents (Millipore Corporation, MA, USA) in a transilluminator (ChemiDoc; Bio-Rad, Hercules, CA, USA). Band densities were quantified using the Image-Pro Plus software.

2.4. Real-Time PCR. LAMA1 mRNA expression in glucose-treated RF/6A cells was detected by real-time PCR. Total RNA was extracted using TRIzol according to the manufacturer's instructions, and its concentration was assessed by spectrophotometry; an $A_{260/280}$ ratio of 1.8–2.0 was considered acceptable. cDNA was synthesized using the PrimeScript RT reagent kit with gDNA Eraser according to the manufacturer's protocol and used as a template for PCR amplification. LAMA1 primers were synthesized by Sangon Corporation (Shanghai, China). Real-time PCR (SYBR Green) was performed according to the manufacturer's instructions in a LightCycler 480 system (Roche, Basel, Switzerland) in a volume of 20 μL containing SYBR Premix Ex Taq II (Takara RR820A), cDNA, and specific primers. Relative mRNA expression of LAMA1 was quantified by the comparative $2^{-\Delta\Delta ct}$ method after normalization to that of GAPDH. Primer sequences are shown in Table 1.

2.5. Immunofluorescence Staining. RF/6A cells were seeded onto glass coverslips, incubated at 37°C and 5% CO_2 until 80% confluence, fixed with 4% paraformaldehyde for 15 min at room temperature, washed three times with PBS, permeabilized with 0.1% Triton X-100 for 4 min, blocked in 3% BSA for 1 h, and incubated with anti-LAMA1 antibodies (1:50) overnight at 4°C. Cells were washed three times in PBS and incubated with goat anti-rabbit secondary antibodies for 1 h at 37°C followed by

TABLE 1: Primer sequences used for PCR.

Gene	Sequence	Length
LAMA1 (forward)	5′- GTT TCG AAC CTC CTC GCA GA-3′	88 bp
LAMA1 (reverse)	5′- CTT GCC GTC CAC AAG CTC TAG T-3′	
GAPDH (forward)	5′- GAT TCC ACC CAT GGC AAA TT-3′	103 bp
GAPDH (reverse)	5′- TCT CGC TCC TGG AAG ATG GT-3′	

DAPI staining for 10 min to visualize nuclei. Fluorescence images were obtained under a fluorescence microscope (model DM6000; Leica, Wetzlar, Germany).

2.6. Cell Growth Assay. RF/6A cells were cultured in normal glucose medium (5 mM) for 24 h to allow cell adherence; then, the medium was removed, and cell monolayers were washed once with PBS and incubated in medium supplemented with different concentrations of glucose. The bottom was marked to determine the position of observed cells; the growth of cells at the same position was observed at different time points (0, 1, 2, 3, and 4 days) under a microscope (Axio Observer A1; Carl Zeiss, Oberkochen, Germany).

2.7. Cell Proliferation Assay. Cell proliferation was measured using the CCK-8 method in accordance with the manufacturer's protocol. Briefly, RF/6A cells (7×10^3 cells/100 μL/well) were seeded into 96-well plates overnight and then cultured at different glucose concentrations for 96 h; normal glucose (5 mM) served as control. Cell proliferation was assessed every 24 h after addition of 10 μL of the CCK-8 solution for 90 min at 37°C and subsequent measuring of absorbance at 450 nm using a microplate reader (Synergy H1; BioTek, Winooski, VT, USA). The optical density reflected the proliferation of RF/6A cells. Each experiment was performed in five replicates, and detection was repeated three times per group to ensure accuracy of measurements. The experiment was repeated independently three times, and the mean values obtained in each experiment were used for statistical analysis.

2.8. Wound Healing Assay. Cell migration ability was assessed using wound healing assay by 4 Well Insert (Ibidi cat. number 80469). The Culture-Insert 4 Well consists of four wells, representing the four quarters of the round Culture-Insert. The wells are separated by a wall of 500 μm. When the wells are filled with adherent cells, a cell-free gap of approx. 500 μm is created between the adjacent wells after removing the Culture–Insert 4 Well. RF/6A cells (4×10^5 cells/mL) were plated into the four wells of a culture insert located at the center of a 35 mm culture dish. After 24 h, when the cells reached 90% confluence, the culture insert was removed to reveal the wound gap, and micrographs (baseline time 0) were taken at ×10 magnification using a digital camera attached to an inverted microscope (Axio Observer A1). Then, cells were washed with PBS to remove floating cells, fresh medium containing different glucose concentrations (5 mM, 15 mM, 25 mM, or 35 mM) was added, and cells were cultured for 72 h. Wound healing was monitored by taking micrographs at the same coordinates every 24 h. Quantitative analysis was performed by measuring the gap size of the wound using the Image-Pro Plus software and the results were presented as the percentage of the wound coverage; complete coverage was defined as 100%. Experiments were repeated three times.

2.9. Cell Adhesion Assay. Cell adhesion ability was measured using the modified CCK-8 method. Cell suspension (7×10^4 cells/mL) was prepared in medium containing different concentrations of glucose, and 100 μL of cell suspension was placed into each well of 96-well plates, which were then placed in 37°C incubator for 2, 4, 6, and 8 h. Then, cell monolayers were washed twice with PBS to remove unattached cells, and 100 μL of fresh culture medium containing 10 μL CCK-8 solution was added for 2 h. The assay was performed with five replicates. The absorbance was measured in a microplate reader; higher absorbance values reflected higher number of adhered cells.

2.10. Statistical Analysis. Each experiment was repeated at least three times and the data are presented as the mean ± standard deviation (SD). To assess the significance of differences between groups in multiple comparisons, one-way ANOVA was used; two-sided P values less than <0.05 indicated statistical significance. All statistical analyses were performed using the Prism 6.0 software (GraphPad Software, San Diego, CA, USA).

3. Results

3.1. Effects of High Glucose on the Growth of RF/6A Cells. RF/6A cells were cultured with different glucose concentrations and their growth was analyzed at 1, 2, 3, and 4 days after treatment. After 1 day of culture, no significant difference in cell growth was observed compared with control (normal glucose concentration, 5 mM); however, further culture in hyperglycemic conditions induced cell growth in a glucose concentration-dependent manner (Figure 1).

3.2. Effects of High Glucose on LAMA1 Expression in RF/6A Cells

3.2.1. Localization of LAMA1 Expression. Immunocytochemistry analysis indicated that LAMA1 was expressed mainly in the cytoplasm. LAMA1 expression was not affected by the treatment with 15 mM glucose for 24 h and 48 h, but was reduced by that with 25 mM and 35 mM glucose compared with control (5 mM) (Figure 2).

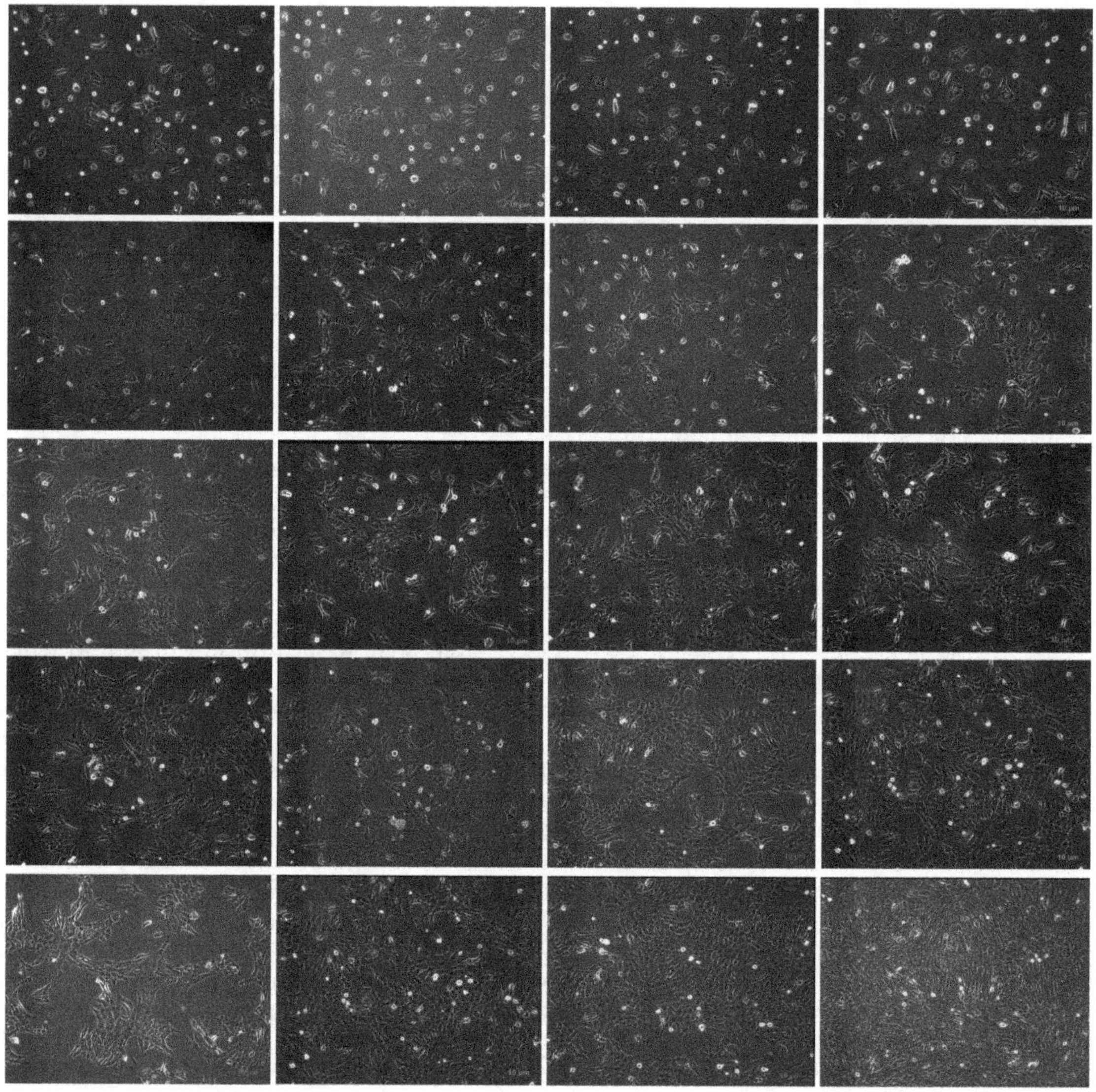

FIGURE 1: Effects of high glucose on the growth of RF/6A cells. RF/6A cells were grown in medium supplemented with different concentrations of glucose for the indicated times.

3.2.2. LAMA1 Protein Expression. The expression of LAMA1 protein was examined by Western blotting, which showed that 15 mM glucose slightly induced LAMA1 expression, but the difference with control (5 mM) was not statistically significant ($P > 0.05$). However, the increase in glucose concentration significantly downregulated LAMA1 protein expression, especially in the 35 mM group ($P < 0.05$), and the effect was more pronounced after 48 h exposure to high glucose (Figure 3).

3.2.3. LAMA1 mRNA Expression. Real-time PCR analysis of LAMA1 transcription in RF/6A cells showed that the exposure to 35 mM glucose significantly decreased LAMA1 mRNA levels compared to control (5 mM) ($P < 0.05$). There was also a slight decrease by 25 mM glucose, but the difference with control did not reach statistical significance ($P > 0.05$). These results are consistent with LAMA1 protein expression detected by Western blotting (Figure 4).

3.3. Effects of High Glucose on the Migration Ability of RF/6A Cells. The effect of high glucose concentration on retinal endothelial cell migration ability was analyzed by the wound healing assay. The results showed that wound healing was accelerated by high glucose in a concentration-dependent manner, indicating the induction of cell migration ability. At 24 h, the healed area was increased to $37.12 \pm 4.83\%$ (15 mM), $45.52 \pm 4.37\%$ (25 mM), and $49.77 \pm 2.35\%$ (35 mM) compared to $26.4 \pm 5.91\%$ in the control group (5 mM), and the difference was statistically significant ($P < 0.05$). At 48 h, the healed area was increased to $63.42 \pm 2.98\%$ (15 mM), $75.01 \pm 3.49\%$ (25 mM), and $80.79 \pm 5.53\%$ (35 mM) compared to $44.96 \pm 4.56\%$ in the control

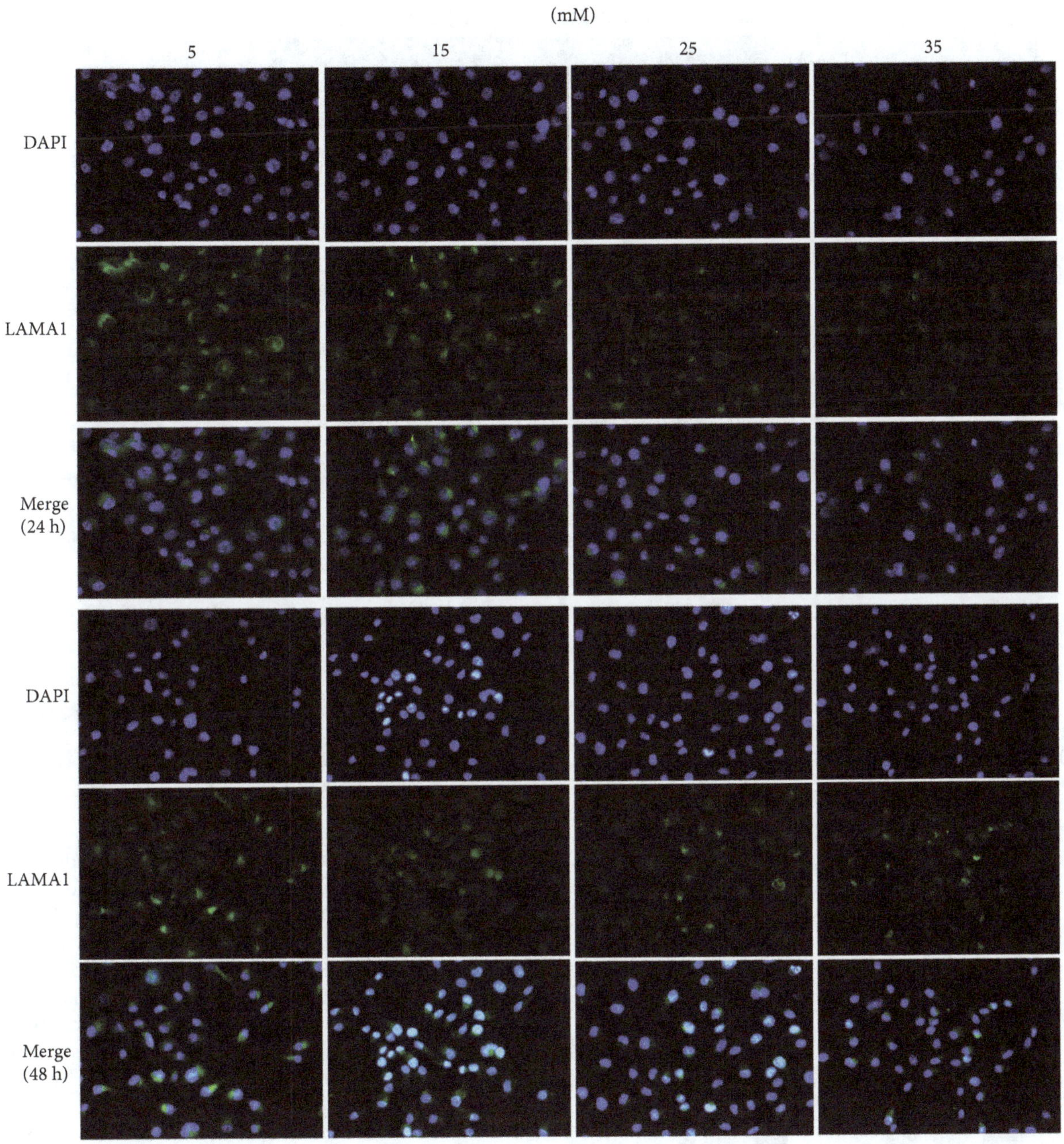

FIGURE 2: Immunocytochemistry analysis of LAMA1 expression in RF/6A cells treated with different concentrations of glucose for 24 and 48 h.

group (5 mM), and the difference was statistically significant ($P < 0.05$). After 72 h, the healed area in the control group was 71.44 ± 5.29, which was significantly lower ($P < 0.05$) than that in high glucose groups (100%) (Figure 5).

3.4. Effects of High Glucose on the Proliferation of RF/6A Cells. The CCK-8 assay showed that RF/6A cell proliferation in high glucose-supplemented medium was induced compared to control (5 mM), which was consistent with microscopic observations of cell growth. At 24 h, there was no statistically significant difference between the groups. However, at 48 h, an increase in cell proliferation compared to control was detected in the 25 mM group ($P < 0.05$), whereas at 72 h, it was revealed in the 25 mM and 35 mM groups ($P < 0.05$), and at 96 h, it was observed in all cells exposed to high glucose ($P < 0.05$) (Figure 6).

3.5. Effects of High Glucose on the Adhesion Ability of RF/6A Cells. The adhesion of cells cultured at the elevated glucose concentrations showed a trend for increase compared to control, and the difference between control and 25 mM and 35 mM glucose-treated cells was statistically significant at 6 and 8 h ($P < 0.05$; Figure 7).

4. Discussion

DR is one of the leading complications of diabetes worldwide and the primary cause of blindness in developed countries

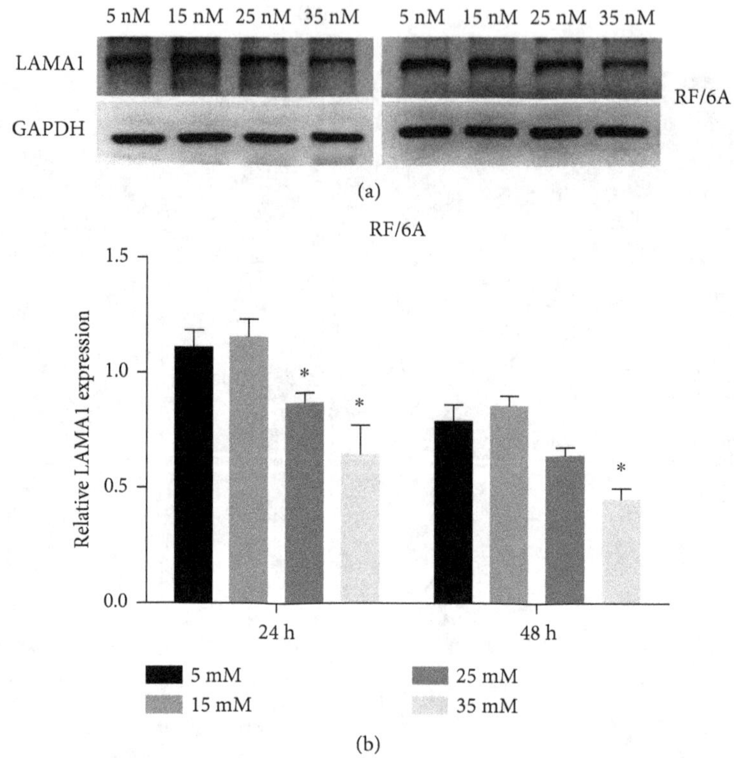

Figure 3: Expression of LAMA1 protein in RF/6A cells. RF/6A cells were treated with different concentrations of glucose for 24 and 48 h and LAMA1 expression was analyzed by Western blotting; GAPDH was used as loading control. (a) Representative gel images. Left, 24 h; right, 48 h. (b) Quantitative analysis of LAMA1 expression performed using the ImageJ software. The data are presented as the mean ± SD of three independent experiments; $^*P < 0.05$.

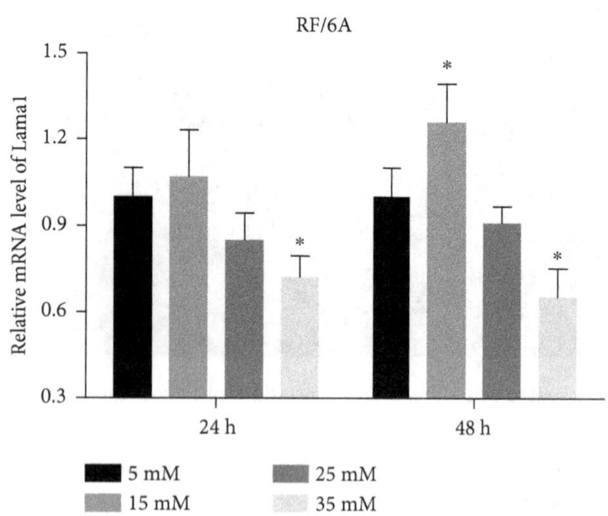

Figure 4: LAMA1 mRNA expression. RF/6A cells were treated with different concentrations of glucose for 24 and 48 h and analyzed for LAMA1 mRNA levels by real-time PCR. There was a significant decrease of LAMA1 mRNA expression in cells exposed to 35 mM glucose both at 24 and 48 h. The data are presented as the mean ± SD of three independent experiments; $^*P < 0.05$.

[17]. DR incidence is expected to grow in the next few years, and the disease is predicted to affect nearly 600 million people by the year 2035 [18]. However, the exact pathogenesis of DR is still unclear and is considered to be induced through several mechanisms: (1) polyol pathway, (2) advanced glycation end products, (3) PKC activation, (4) genetic factors, (5) inflammation, and (6) oxidative stress [6, 19]. Each mechanism can cause endothelial cell dysfunction, resulting in a series of physiological and biochemical abnormalities such as retinal ischemia, vascular permeability change, macular edema, VEGF upregulation, and neovascularization, which eventually lead to PDR [20]. Therefore, it is important to study the reaction of retinal endothelial cells to hyperglycemic condition characteristic for diabetes.

In recent years, research on PDR has been focused on the role of growth factors, especially VEGF-A, in ocular angiogenesis [21, 22], whereas less attention has been paid to the ECM, which is important for the development of retinal vessels and pathological neovascularization [8, 23]. Endothelial cells secrete proteases that degrade the original vascular basement membrane and cause its components to diffuse from the blood vessels to the surrounding ECM [24]. Laminin is one of the important ECM components that, together with collagen, form the basement membrane. In 1992, Ingber et al. [25] found that interactions between endothelial cells through basement membrane components play a critical role in angiogenesis. Among ECM proteins, LAMA1 is highly expressed in the eye structures, especially in retinal vessels and the lens [26]. Interestingly, several studies indicate that high glucose can induce the secretion of ECM proteins (collagen IV, fibronectin, and laminin) through signaling pathways such as TGF-β/Smad and PI3K/AKT [27–29];

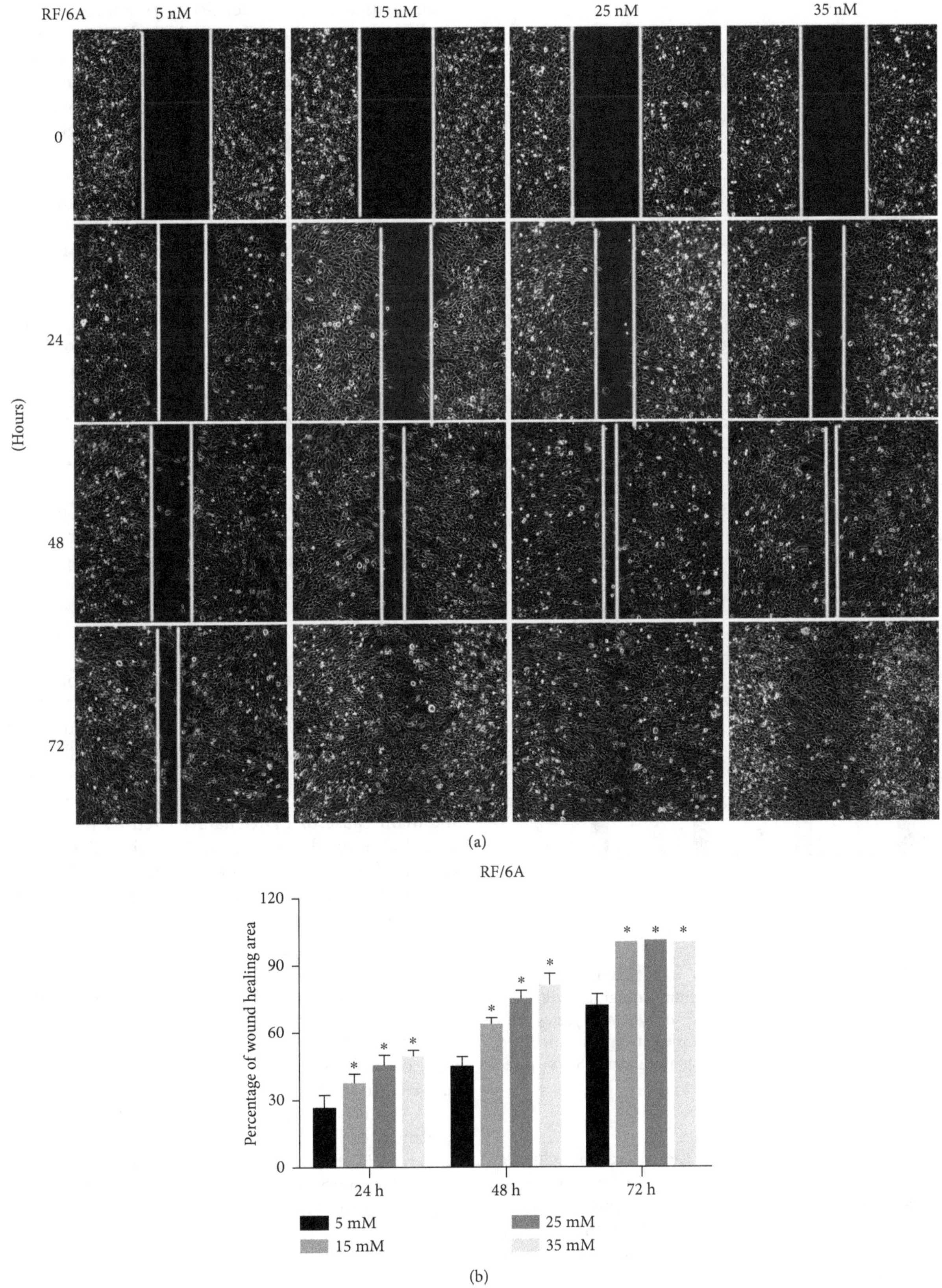

Figure 5: Cell migration ability. RF/6A cells grown at different concentrations of glucose for 24, 48, and 72 h were analyzed by the wound healing assay. (a) Representative microscopic images of wound healing. (b) Quantitative analysis of the gap size measured using the Image-Pro Plus software; $^*P < 0.05$.

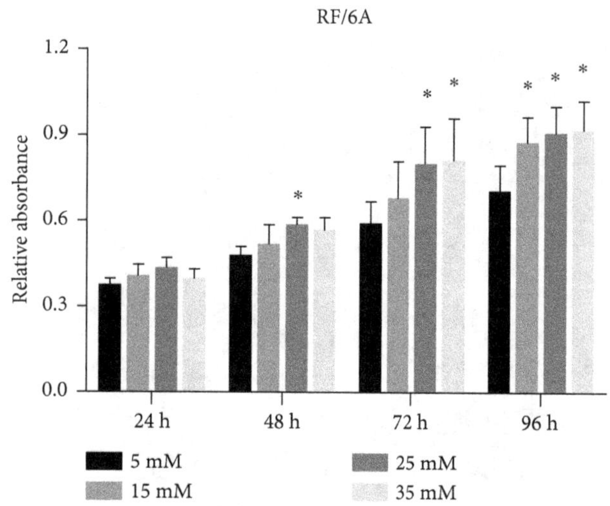

FIGURE 6: Proliferation of RF/6A cells exposed to high glucose concentrations. RF/6A cells grown at different concentrations of glucose for 96 h were analyzed for cell proliferation every 24 h using the CCK-8 assay. The data are presented as the mean ± SD of three independent experiments; $^*P < 0.05$.

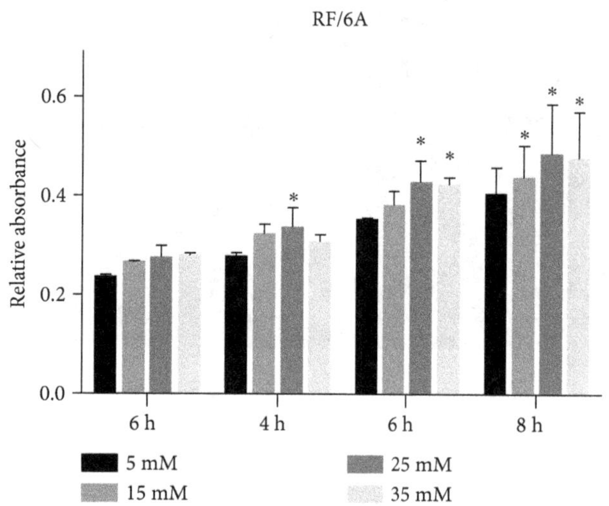

FIGURE 7: Adhesion ability of RF/6A cells exposed to high glucose. RF/6A cells suspended in medium containing different concentrations of glucose were seeded in 96-well plates and analyzed for adhesion after indicated times using the modified CCK-8 method. The data are presented as the mean ± SD of three independent experiments; $^*P < 0.05$.

however, our results showed that at the increase of glucose concentration, LAMA1 expression was only slightly upregulated and then showed a marked downward trend. Ning et al. [30] found that LAMA1 plays a critical role in the function and aging of the kidneys by regulating the mesangial cell population and mesangial matrix deposition through TGF-β/Smad signaling. TGF-β is a secreted signaling molecule with a fibrogenic effect that regulates diverse cellular processes, including proliferation, differentiation, migration, and apoptosis, and is being recognized as an important contributor to DR pathogenesis [31]. As in vitro and in vivo studies indicate that LAMA1 deficiency promotes mesangial cell proliferation and that this pathological change is very similar to diabetic nephropathy [30], we hypothesize that hyperglycemia can influence the proliferation of retinal endothelial cells through the LAMA1-TGF-β axis. LAMA1 expression could be first increased by high glucose through a compensatory mechanism and then start to decline, which would negatively regulate TGF-β signaling, inducing cell proliferation and migration. However, our present findings cannot confirm this hypothesis, which should be tested in further studies. The decrease of LAMA1 expression in RF/6A cells under high glucose conditions suggests that LAMA1 may serve as a protective factor in DR. Studies in mice indicate that mütations in the Lama1 gene promoted the formation of vitreoretinal blood vessels and the epiretinal membrane, supported persistence of fetal vasculature, and could cause vitreal fibroplasia and abnormal vascular development [15, 32]. Taken together, these and our data indicate that LAMA1 deficiency plays a role in DR pathogenesis.

Our study shows that high glucose promotes the growth and proliferation of endothelial cells and accelerates their migration, providing a material basis for angiogenesis and fiber proliferation. These results are consistent with a report by Beltramo et al. [33] that in the early stages of DR, hyperglycemia can cause a loss of pericytes, reducing their association with endothelial cells and increasing vascular permeability and endothelial cell proliferation, which ultimately leads to neovascularization. In contrast, other studies showed that high glucose inhibited endothelial cell proliferation and promoted apoptosis, causing endothelial damage, which results in diabetes-related vascular complications [34, 35]. However, it is well known that hyperglycemia is the main cause of PDR characterized by pathological neovascularization due to cell proliferation. Therefore, diverse effects of high glucose on endothelial cells suggest the existence of multiple molecular mechanisms underlying the development of PDR.

In summary, our study indicates that glucose at high concentration downregulates the expression of LAMA1, which corresponds to increased adhesion, proliferation, and migration of choroid retinal endothelial cells, suggesting that LAMA1 may exert a protective effect against DR. Thus, LAMA1 may be used as a new target for diagnosis and/or treatment of DR, providing a new direction for DR clinical research. Further studies are required to address specific molecular mechanisms and signaling pathways underlying LAMA1 role in DR development.

Conflicts of Interest

The authors declare that there is no conflict of interests regarding the publication of this paper.

Authors' Contributions

Guangwei Song and Da Lin contributed equally to this work.

Acknowledgments

This study was supported by all the members of the ophthalmology department of the Second Affiliated Hospital of Wenzhou Medical University and by the Zhejiang Natural Science Foundation (LY18H120009). The authors also thank Professor Qianying Gao from the State Key Laboratory of Sun Yat-sen University.

References

[1] R. A. Gangwani, J. X. Lian, S. McGhee, D. Wong, and K. K. Li, "Diabetic retinopathy screening: global and local perspective," *Hong Kong Medical Journal*, vol. 22, no. 5, pp. 486–495, 2016.

[2] C. Hernández, A. Simó-Servat, P. Bogdanov, and R. Simó, "Diabetic retinopathy: new therapeutic perspectives based on pathogenic mechanisms," *Journal of Endocrinological Investigation*, vol. 40, no. 9, pp. 925–935, 2017.

[3] H. Khalil, "Diabetes microvascular complications-a clinical update," *Diabetes & Metabolic Syndrome: Clinical Research & Reviews*, vol. 11, Supplement 1, pp. S133–S139, 2017.

[4] A. Chawla, R. Chawla, and S. Jaggi, "Microvasular and macrovascular complications in diabetes mellitus: distinct or continuum?," *Indian Journal of Endocrinology and Metabolism*, vol. 20, no. 4, pp. 546–551, 2016.

[5] S. Cherian, S. Roy, A. Pinheiro, and S. Roy, "Tight glycemic control regulates fibronectin expression and basement membrane thickening in retinal and glomerular capillaries of diabetic rats," *Investigative Ophthalmology & Visual Science*, vol. 50, no. 2, pp. 943–949, 2009.

[6] N. Cheung, P. Mitchell, and T. Y. Wong, "Diabetic retinopathy," *The Lancet*, vol. 376, no. 9735, pp. 124–136, 2010.

[7] S. V. Gogula, Department of IT, GITAM University, Patancheru Mandal, Medak Dist-502329, C. Divakar, C. Satyanarayana, Y. P. Kumar, and V. S. Lavanaya, "Computational investigation of pkcβ inhibitors for the treatment of diabetic retinopathy," *Bioinformation*, vol. 9, no. 20, pp. 1040–1043, 2013.

[8] P. N. Bishop, "The role of extracellular matrix in retinal vascular development and preretinal neovascularization," *Experimental Eye Research*, vol. 133, pp. 30–36, 2015.

[9] A. Domogatskaya, S. Rodin, and K. Tryggvason, "Functional diversity of laminins," *Annual Review of Cell and Developmental Biology*, vol. 28, no. 1, pp. 523–553, 2012.

[10] D. S. W. Ting, K.-A. Tan, V. Phua, G. S. W. Tan, C. W. Wong, and T. Y. Wong, "Biomarkers of diabetic retinopathy," *Current Diabetes Reports*, vol. 16, no. 12, p. 125, 2016.

[11] M. Durbeej, "Laminins," *Cell and Tissue Research*, vol. 339, no. 1, pp. 259–268, 2010.

[12] B. Byström, I. Virtanen, P. Rousselle, D. Gullberg, and F. Pedrosa-Domellöf, "Distribution of laminins in the developing human eye," *Investigative Ophthalmology & Visual Science*, vol. 47, no. 3, pp. 777–785, 2006.

[13] M. M. Edwards and O. Lefebvre, "Laminins and retinal vascular development," *Cell Adhesion & Migration*, vol. 7, no. 1, pp. 82–89, 2013.

[14] N. Ichikawa-Tomikawa, J. Ogawa, V. Douet et al., "Laminin $\alpha 1$ is essential for mouse cerebellar development," *Matrix Biology*, vol. 31, no. 1, pp. 17–28, 2012.

[15] M. M. Edwards, E. Mammadova-Bach, F. Alpy et al., "Mutations in *Lama1* disrupt retinal vascular development and inner limiting membrane formation," *Journal of Biological Chemistry*, vol. 285, no. 10, pp. 7697–7711, 2010.

[16] T. Vilboux, M. C. V. Malicdan, Y. M. Chang et al., "Cystic cerebellar dysplasia and biallelic *LAMA1* mutations: a laminopathy associated with tics, obsessive compulsive traits and myopia due to cell adhesion and migration defects," *Journal of Medical Genetics*, vol. 53, no. 5, pp. 318–329, 2016.

[17] R. S. Eshaq, A. M. Z. Aldalati, J. S. Alexander, and N. R. Harris, "Diabetic retinopathy: breaking the barrier," *Pathophysiology*, vol. 24, no. 4, pp. 229–241, 2017.

[18] A. Nanditha, R. C. W. Ma, A. Ramachandran et al., "Diabetes in Asia and the Pacific: implications for the global epidemic," *Diabetes Care*, vol. 39, no. 3, pp. 472–485, 2016.

[19] E. J. Duh, J. K. Sun, and A. W. Stitt, "Diabetic retinopathy: current understanding, mechanisms, and treatment strategies," *JCI Insight*, vol. 2, no. 14, article e93751, 2017.

[20] T. Y. Wong, C. M. G. Cheung, M. Larsen, S. Sharma, and R. Simó, "Diabetic retinopathy," *Nature Reviews Disease Primers*, vol. 2, article 16012, 2016.

[21] M. W. Stewart, "Treatment of diabetic retinopathy: recent advances and unresolved challenges," *World Journal of Diabetes*, vol. 7, no. 16, pp. 333–341, 2016.

[22] N. Ved, R. P. Hulse, S. M. Bestall, L. F. Donaldson, J. W. Bainbridge, and D. O. Bates, "Vascular endothelial growth factor-A_{165}b ameliorates outer-retinal barrier and vascular dysfunction in the diabetic retina," *Clinical Science*, vol. 131, no. 12, pp. 1225–1243, 2017.

[23] T. Nakama, S. Yoshida, K. Ishikawa et al., "Different roles played by periostin splice variants in retinal neovascularization," *Experimental Eye Research*, vol. 153, pp. 133–140, 2016.

[24] T. P. Lozito, J. M. Taboas, C. K. Kuo, and R. S. Tuan, "Mesenchymal stem cell modification of endothelial matrix regulates their vascular differentiation," *Journal of Cellular Biochemistry*, vol. 107, no. 4, pp. 706–713, 2009.

[25] D. E. Ingber, "Extracellular matrix as a solid-state regulator in angiogenesis: identification of new targets for anti-cancer therapy," *Seminars in Cancer Biology*, vol. 3, no. 2, pp. 57–63, 1992.

[26] N. S. Zinkevich, D. V. Bosenko, B. A. Link, and E. V. Semina, "*laminin alpha 1*gene is essential for normal lens development in zebrafish," *BMC Developmental Biology*, vol. 6, no. 1, p. 13, 2006.

[27] D. Qin, G. M. Zhang, X. Xu, and L. Y. Wang, "The PI3K/Akt signaling pathway mediates the high glucose-induced expression of extracellular matrix molecules in human retinal pigment epithelial cells," *Journal of Diabetes Research*, vol. 2015, Article ID 920280, 11 pages, 2015.

[28] S. H. Ko, O. K. Hong, J. W. Kim et al., "High glucose increases extracellular matrix production in pancreatic stellate cells by activating the renin–angiotensin system," *Journal of Cellular Biochemistry*, vol. 98, no. 2, pp. 343–355, 2006.

[29] J. H. Li, X. R. Huang, H. J. Zhu, R. Johnson, and H. Y. Lan, "Role of TGF-β signaling in extracellular matrix production under high glucose conditions," *Kidney International*, vol. 63, no. 6, pp. 2010–2019, 2003.

[30] L. Ning, H. Kurihara, S. de Vega et al., "Laminin α1 regulates age-related mesangial cell proliferation and mesangial matrix accumulation through the TGF-β pathway," *The American Journal of Pathology*, vol. 184, no. 6, pp. 1683–1694, 2014.

[31] S. E. Wheeler and N. Y. Lee, "Emerging roles of transforming growth factor β signaling in diabetic retinopathy," *Journal of Cellular Physiology*, vol. 232, no. 3, pp. 486–489, 2016.

[32] M. M. Edwards, D. S. McLeod, R. Grebe, C. Heng, O. Lefebvre, and G. A. Lutty, "*Lama1* mutations lead to vitreoretinal blood vessel formation, persistence of fetal vasculature, and epiretinal membrane formation in mice," *BMC Developmental Biology*, vol. 11, no. 1, p. 60, 2011.

[33] E. Beltramo, T. Lopatina, E. Berrone et al., "Extracellular vesicles derived from mesenchymal stem cells induce features of diabetic retinopathy in vitro," *Acta Diabetologica*, vol. 51, no. 6, pp. 1055–1064, 2014.

[34] H. Kang, X. Ma, J. Liu, Y. Fan, and X. Deng, "High glucose-induced endothelial progenitor cell dysfunction," *Diabetes and Vascular Disease Research*, vol. 14, no. 5, pp. 381–394, 2017.

[35] A. W. Stitt, T. M. Curtis, M. Chen et al., "The progress in understanding and treatment of diabetic retinopathy," *Progress in Retinal and Eye Research*, vol. 51, pp. 156–186, 2016.

7

Trajectories of Postload Plasma Glucose in the Development of Type 2 Diabetes in Japanese Adults

Rie Oka,[1,2] Kyoko Shibata,[3] Masaru Sakurai,[4] Mitsuhiro Kometani,[2] Masakazu Yamagishi,[2] Kenichi Yoshimura,[3] and Takashi Yoneda[2]

[1]*Department of Internal Medicine, Hokuriku Central Hospital, Kanazawa University Hospital, Kanazawa, Japan*
[2]*Department of Cardiovascular and Internal Medicine, Kanazawa University Graduate School of Medicine, Kanazawa, Japan*
[3]*Department of Biostatistics, Innovative Clinical Research Center (iCREK), Kanazawa University Hospital, Kanazawa, Japan*
[4]*Department of Social and Environmental Medicine, Kanazawa Medical University, Kanazawa, Japan*

Correspondence should be addressed to Rie Oka; ririoka@goo.jp

Academic Editor: Ed Randell

We aimed to clarify how the trajectories of 1-hour postload plasma glucose (PG) and 2-hour PG were different in the development of type 2 diabetes. Using data of repeated health checkups in Japanese workers from April 2006 to March 2016, longitudinal changes of fasting, 1-hour, and 2-hour PG on the oral glucose tolerance test were analyzed with a linear mixed effects model. Of the 1464 nondiabetic subjects at baseline, 112 subjects progressed to type 2 diabetes during the observation period (progressors). In progressors, 1-hour PG and 2-hour PG showed gradual increases with slopes of 1.33 ± 0.2 and 0.58 ± 0.2 mg/dL/year, respectively, followed by a steep increase by which they attained diabetes. Until immediately before the diabetes transition, age- and sex-adjusted mean level of 2-hour PG was 149 ± 2.7 mg/dL, 34 ± 2.7 (30%) higher compared to nonprogressors, while that of 1-hour PG was 206 ± 4.1 mg/dL, 60 ± 4.3 mg/dL (41%) higher compared to nonprogressors. In conclusion, diabetes transition was preceded by a mild elevation of 2-hour PG for several years or more. The elevation in 1-hour PG was larger than that of 2-hour PG until immediately before the transition to diabetes.

1. Introduction

Postload hyperglycemia is one of the early manifestations of impaired glucose metabolism. Conventionally, investigators defined postload hyperglycemia by 2-hour plasma glucose (PG) on the oral glucose tolerance test (OGTT) and demonstrated that the intervention at the stage of impaired glucose tolerance (IGT) was effective to prevent or delay the incidence of type 2 diabetes [1–3]. However, it has been recently reported that 1-hour PG has a superior predictive ability to 2-hour PG in three Western cohort studies [4–6] and in two Asian cohort studies [7, 8]. Cross-sectional investigations have also revealed that elevated 1-hour PG rather than 2-hour PG showed a stronger correlation with decreased insulin secretion assessed by insulinogenic index [4, 5, 7] or acute insulin response on the intravenous glucose tolerance test (IVGTT) [9]. The measurement of 1-hour PG cannot be ignored to detect the individuals with impairment of postload glucose metabolism.

In a few studies on trajectories of postload PG in the development of type 2 diabetes, 2-hour PG showed a gradual linear increase for more than 10 years, followed by a rapid deterioration before the diagnosis [10–12]. They reported that 2-hour PG on average was regulated within the normal range (<140 mg/dL) until 2 years before the onset of diabetes [10, 12]. They and any other investigators have not reported the trajectory of 1-hour PG. We hypothesized that 1-hour PG might increase earlier than 2-hour PG in those who later developed diabetes, which made its predictive ability better.

The aim of this study, therefore, was to depict trajectories of postload PG levels during the development of type 2 diabetes, with an interest in the difference of 1-hour PG from 2-hour PG. The optimal cutoff point of 1-hour PG in this population was also estimated.

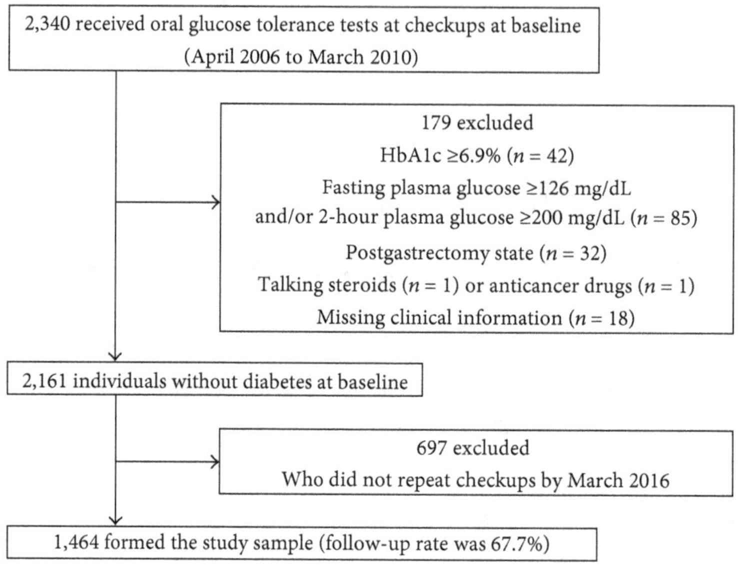

FIGURE 1: Study sample.

2. Methods

2.1. Study Subjects. A historical cohort study was conducted using data from the medical checkups of public school employees collected in the Hokuriku Central Hospital [7]. During April 2006 and March 2010 (baseline period), 2340 employees underwent an OGTT at a checkup [13]. If employees received more than one checkup during the baseline period, the initial checkup data were used. After those who had fasting PG ≥ 126 mg/dL and/or 2-hour PG ≥ 200 mg/dL ($n = 85$), who had HbA1c values ≥6.9% (52 mmol/mol) ($n = 42$), who had undergone gastrectomy ($n = 32$), who were taking steroids ($n = 1$), who were taking anticancer drugs ($n = 1$), or who had any missing data ($n = 18$) were excluded, we selected 2161 nondiabetic individuals. Of the 2161 thus selected, 1464 individuals repeated checkups at least once by March 2016 and comprised our study sample (Figure 1). The subjects were followed until they developed diabetes; if they remained free of diabetes, follow-up ended at the time of the last checkup. The remaining 697 subjects did not repeat checkups, which meant a follow-up rate of 67.7%. An OGTT was performed at all checkups during the follow-up period; but in the last two years (from April 2014 to March 2016), an OGTT was performed on 1191 subjects and the measurement of fasting PG only was performed in the remaining 273 subjects due to the financial reason of the mutual aid association. Information on smoking and drinking habits and medical history was obtained through a questionnaire. Subjects were considered current smokers if they smoked at least one cigarette per day. Alcohol use was defined by the number of days per week for drinking regardless of the amount consumed. Signed informed consent was obtained from all subjects, and the hospital review board approved the study protocol. The study was registered on the University Hospital Medical Information Network Clinical Trials Registry (UMIN-CTR, UMIN ID: UMIN000017662).

2.2. Diagnosis of Diabetes and Blood Sampling. Diabetes was diagnosed if fasting PG ≥ 126 mg/dL, 2-hour PG ≥ 200 mg/dL, and/or receiving treatments for type 2 diabetes based on the World Health Organization criteria (WHO) [14]. All the evaluations were performed at the health check department of the Hokuriku Central Hospital. Subjects were asked to visit the hospital between 8:00 a.m. and 9:00 a.m. after an overnight fast. At the baseline visit, an OGTT (75 g dextrose monohydrate in 250 ml water) with 0, 30, 60, and 120 min sampling to determine PG and insulin levels was performed on all subjects [13]. HbA1c assay was conducted at the central clinical laboratory in our hospital by a high-performance liquid chromatography (HPLC) method using ADAMS HA-8170 (ARKRAY, Kyoto). The following indices of insulin secretion and insulin sensitivity were calculated in this study: insulinogenic index = $(Ins_{30} - Ins_0[mU/L])/(Gluc_{30} - Gluc_0[mg/dL])$, where Ins_y and Glu_y represent values at time y min during the OGTT [15] and homeostatic model assessment of insulin resistance (HOMA) = $Glu_0(mg/dL) \times Ins_0(mU/L)/405$ [16].

2.3. Statistical Analysis. Analyses were conducted using SPSS software version 17.0 for Windows (SPSS Inc. Chicago, USA). Data are presented as the mean ± SD or the median with the interquartile range for continuous variables or as a frequency for categorical variables. Subjects were divided into two groups, those who progressed to diabetes (progressors) and those who did not (nonprogressors). The differences in the baseline characteristics were tested using Student's t-test or Mann–Whitney U tests for continuous variables or χ^2 test for categorical values. The mixed effects model was used to estimate the trajectories of fasting PG, 1-hour PG, and 2-hour PG [17]; this technique takes into account within-subject correlations from repeated measurements with unequal numbers of observations per subjects and unequal intervals between measurements. As fixed effects, we entered time with sex and age as covariates into the model. We set a timeline with 0 year at the year of diagnosis for progressors or at the last checkup for nonprogressors, and time of prior measurements was coded backward, giving minus values. As a random effect, we included the participant's identification number. We used SPSS to calculate the annual estimated levels of PG and used *R* to fit the model explaining the PG trajectories. The difference of the slopes of increase by time between progressors and nonprogressors was examined by the interaction between a dummy variable for progression (0 = nonprogressors; 1 = progressors) and time in the model. Finally, to identify the optimal cutoff point for progression of type 2 diabetes, subjects were divided by their baseline data at 140 mg/dL of 2-hour PG based on the cutoff value for IGT [14], at 155 mg/dL of 1-hour PG based on the prior study by Abdul-Ghani et al. [18], and at 180 mg/dL of 1-hour PG based on the committee report of Japan Diabetes Society [19]. Then the hazard ratio (HR) of the development of diabetes of those over versus those below the cutoff point was calculated by Cox proportional hazard regression analysis. The HR was calculated using three models: Model 1, the multivariable-adjusted model, with covariates including age, sex, BMI, fasting PG, HbA1c, smoking status (three-level variable: current/former/never smoker), alcohol use (three-level variable: drinking everyday/drinking 1–6 days per week/drinking less than 1 day per week), taking antihypertensive drugs (yes or no), and taking lipid-lowering drugs (yes or no); Model 2, in which Model 1 was additionally adjusted for the other PG values (i.e., 2-hour PG value for the division by 1-hour PG and 1-hour PG value for the division by 2-hour PG); and Model 3, in which Model 2 was further adjusted for insulinogenic index and HOMA index. A p value <0.05 was considered statistically significant.

3. Results

3.1. Characteristics of Subjects. The study subjects were composed of 1464 subjects with a mean age of 52.0 ± 7.0 years and a mean BMI of 23.9 ± 3.2 kg/m^2 at baseline. Of these, 112 subjects developed type 2 diabetes during the observation, diagnosed by fasting PG ≥ 126 mg/dL ($n = 51$), 2-hour PG ≥ 200 mg/dL ($n = 72$), and/or receiving treatments for type 2 diabetes ($n = 2$). The remaining 1352 subjects stayed free of diabetes until follow-up. Table 1 presents the baseline characteristics of the two study groups: progressors and nonprogressors. Progressors included a higher proportion of men and had higher BMI, higher PG and insulin concentrations during OGTT, higher HbA1c, higher HOMA index, and lower insulinogenic index compared with nonprogressors ($p < 0.05$). Because 75 subjects had insulinogenic index values ≤0, the analysis including insulinogenic index was performed on 1389 subjects.

3.2. Mixed Effects Model Analysis. A mixed effects model was used as this enables effective use of repeated measurements even when numbers and intervals of observations were different per subjects. The number of observations in each year was shown at the bottom of Figure 2. Fasting PG in nonprogressors showed a slight increase from 95 ± 0.5 mg/dL to 98 ± 0.2 mg/dL during the 9 years of observation. In progressors, fasting PG showed a gradual increase until >1 year, followed by a steep increase immediately before the diagnosis (from 112 ± 2.6 to 124 ± 1.7 mg/dL) (Figure 2(a)). A steep increase immediately before the diagnosis in progressors was also observed for 1-hour PG (from 220 ± 5.4 to 249 ± 3.9 mg/dL) (Figure 2(b)) and for 2-hour PG (from 155 ± 5.4 to 221 ± 3.9 mg/dL) (Figure 2(c)). Compared to >9 years, the estimated level was not significantly different in any other year but 0 year for 1-hour PG ($p < 0.01$) and for 2-hour PG ($p < 0.001$). Age- and sex-adjusted mean level of 1-hour PG until >1 year was 206 ± 4.1 mg/dL, 60 ± 4.3 mg/dL (41%) higher compared to nonprogressors ($p < 0.001$), and that of 2-hour PG was 149 ± 2.7 mg/dL, 34 ± 2.7 mg/dL (30%) higher compared to nonprogressors ($p < 0.001$). In 112 progressors, between the final and prefinal measurements of glucose concentrations, 42 (38.5%) had a 1-year interval, 31 (28.4%) had a 2-year interval, and the remaining 39 (33.1%) had a 3 years or more interval, with a median value being 2 years in all progressors. When mixed effects model analysis was conducted in 28 progressors whose annual consecutive data were available until the diagnosis of diabetes, steep increases in 1-hour PG and 2-hour PG were also demonstrated (Supplementary Figure available online).

To test this statistically, we fit a model including time as a continuous variable plus a dummy variable for 0 year (1 = 0 year; 0 = from −9 to −1 year). The model including this dummy variable (piecewise model) fits better than the model with only continuous time variable (linear model) as assessed by Akaike information criterion (AIC). As shown in Table 2,

Table 1: Baseline characteristics of the subjects.

	Nonprogressors	Progressors
n	1352	112
Age (years)	52 ± 7	53 ± 7
Sex (% male)	69	79*
Body mass index (kg/m^2)	23.8 ± 3.1	25.2 ± 3.7*
Fasting plasma glucose (mg/dL)	95 ± 7	108 ± 9*
30 min plasma glucose (mg/dL)	149 ± 29	185 ± 29*
1-hour plasma glucose (mg/dL)	144 ± 41	209 ± 32*
2-hour plasma glucose (mg/dL)	113 ± 25	148 ± 31*
Fasting insulin (mU/L)	2.8/3.8/5.1	2.9/4.3/7.2*
30 min insulin (mU/L)	19.2/28.6/45.2	12.5/22.7/35.3*
HbA1c (%)	5.0/5.2/5.4	5.4/5.6/5.9*
Insulinogenic index ($n = 1389$)	0.30/0.50/0.88	0.14/0.24/0.43*
HOMA index	0.66/0.90/1.26	0.80/1.11/1.98*
Current smokers (%)	19.9	26.8*
Drinkers (%)	64.3	59.8
Antihypertensive medications (%)	13.2	19.6*
Lipid-lowering medications (%)	6.8	8.0

Data are expressed as mean ± SD, 25/50/75th percentile value, or number (%). *$p < 0.05$. HOMA: homeostasis model assessment of insulin resistance.

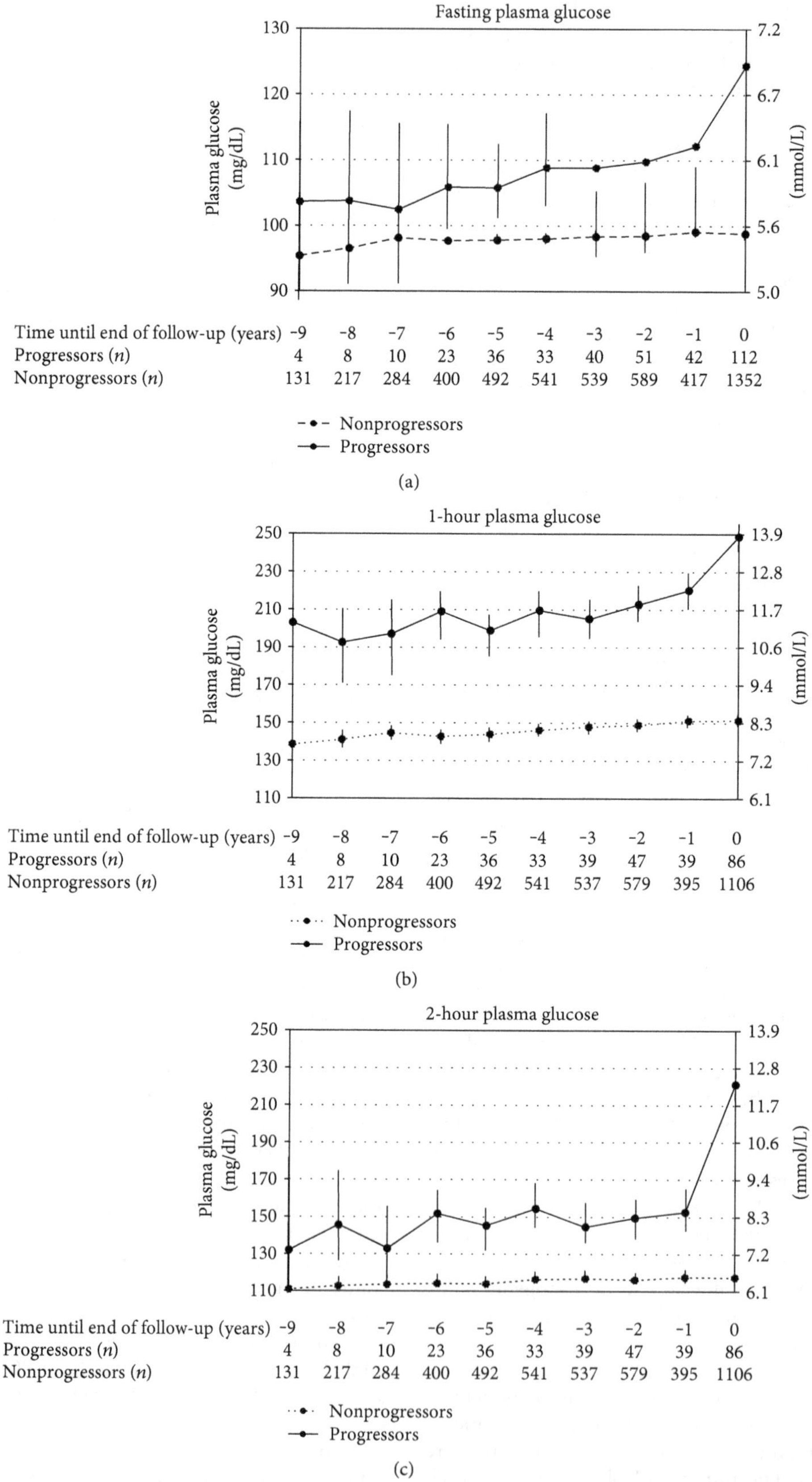

FIGURE 2: Trajectories of fasting (a), 1-hour (b), and 2-hour (c) plasma glucose until the incidence of type 2 diabetes in 112 progressors compared to 1352 nonprogressors. Analyses were adjusted for age and sex in mixed effects models. Error bars show 95% confidence intervals for the estimated levels.

Table 2: Fixed effects in the mixed effects models for changes of fasting, 1-hour, and 2-hour plasma glucose values in 112 progressors compared to 1352 nonprogressors.

	Fasting PG (mg/dL) Regression coefficient	SE	1-hour PG (mg/dL) Regression coefficient	SE	2-hour PG (mg/dL) Regression coefficient	SE
Intercept	89.9	0.9	105.2	4.2	101.6	2.7
Time (per year)	0.22	0.0	1.33	0.2	0.58	0.2
Progression	—	—	49.9	7.9	29.0	5.7
Progression × time	1.23	0.2	—	—	—	—
Progression × year 0	10.1	1.1	28.3	4.9	67.6	3.9

Piecewise mixed effects modeling adjusted for age and sex. Time = a continuous variable set at the year of diagnosis for progressors or at the last checkup for nonprogressors with 0; progression = a dummy variable, 1 for progressors and 0 for nonprogressors; all coefficients are significant, $p < 0.001$.

Table 3: Hazard ratios (HR) for the development of diabetes by different cutoff points of 1-hour PG and 2-hour PG.

Cutoff point	Sensitivity (%)	Specificity (%)	Crude HR (95% CI)	Adjusted HR (95% CI) Model 1	Model 2	Model 3
1-hour PG ≥155 mg/dL (8.6 mmol/L) (yes versus no)	92.9	60.3	18.2 (8.9–37.4)	7.7 (3.6–16.3)	5.9 (2.7–12.7)	5.1 (2.2–11.8)
1-hour PG ≥180 mg/dL (10.0 mmol/L) (yes versus no)	83.0	78.3	15.9 (9.7–26.0)	6.8 (3.9–11.9)	5.2 (2.9–9.4)	4.3 (2.3–8.1)
2-hour PG ≥140 mg/dL (7.8 mmol/L) (yes versus no)	60.7	83.4	7.3 (5.0–10.8)	3.1 (2.0–4.8)	1.6 (1.0–2.6)	1.6 (1.0–2.6)

Model 1: adjusted for age, sex, body mass index, fasting PG, HbA1c, smoking status, alcohol use, taking antihypertensive drugs, and taking lipid-lowering drugs. Model 2: adjusted for Model 1 variables plus the other PG (i.e., 2-hour PG for cutoff of 1-hour PG and 1-hour PG for cutoff of 2-hour PG). Model 3: adjusted for Model 2 variables plus insulinogenic index and HOMA index.

large regression coefficients for progression (49.9 for 1-hour PG and 29.0 for 2-hour PG) indicated the difference between progressors and nonprogressors throughout the observation. The interaction term progression × 0 year but not progression × time was significant both for 1-hour and 2-hour PG, indicating that the slope of increase was not significantly different between progressors and nonprogressors until >1 year. When diabetes was defined only by fasting PG ≥ 126 mg/dL and/or receiving treatments for type 2 diabetes; that is, individuals with isolated postload hyperglycemia were excluded from progressors, the results were similar (data not shown).

3.3. Predictive Abilities of Different Cutoff Points for 1-Hour PG and 2-Hour PG. Table 3 shows the HR for the development of diabetes of those over versus those below the three different cutoff points. The HR of those with 1-hour PG ≥ 155 mg/dL versus 1-hour PG< 155 mg/dL and the HR of those with 1-hour PG ≥ 180 mg/dL versus 1-hour PG< 180 mg/dL were significantly elevated even after adjusted for 2-hour PG, insulinogenic index, and HOMA index. The elevated HR of those with 2-hour PG ≥ 140 mg/dL versus 2-hour PG< 140 mg/dL was significant ($p < 0.05$) but was attenuated after further adjustments for 1-hour PG.

4. Discussion

In this study, we depicted trajectories of postload plasma glucoses during the development of type 2 diabetes in Japanese workers. In agreement with prior studies [10–12], diabetes transition was preceded by a mild elevation of 2-hour PG for many years where the slopes of increase were not significantly different between progressors and nonprogressors. The difference between progressors and nonprogressors was relatively large in 1-hour PG rather than 2-hour PG until immediately before the diagnosis. These trajectories help to understand why 1-hour PG better predicts the future development of type 2 diabetes than 2-hour PG.

A rapid glucose rise in 2-hour PG immediately before the onset of diabetes (from −1 to 0 year) confirmed in this study was consistent with several cohort studies [10–12, 20, 21]. In the Pima longitudinal study which comprised 20 years before the development of diabetes, an exponential increase in the 2-hour glucose levels occurred during the final 4 years preceding the onset [10]. Ferrannini et al. also reported that the natural history of diabetes was marked by a steep increase in 2-hour plasma glucose in 3 years or shorter time frame, in which they discussed instability paradigm, in individuals who are destined to become diabetic; insulin sensitivity and insulin secretion are more or less altered, generating a critical state of instability [11]. In such an unstable condition, a relatively small further change would result in a large, rapid rise in glucose concentrations. In the Whitehall II Study, the magnitude of this rapid increase in 2-hour PG was larger than 70 mg/dL from >2 to 0 year [12], which was comparable to ours (68 mg/dL from >1 to 0 year). As diabetes was attained by such a rapid rise in the short time frame, the difference of 2-hour PG between progressors and nonprogressors does not become large until just before the diagnosis.

Mild elevation in 2-hour PG levels continued for several years or more until just before the aforementioned rapid rise. During this period, the slope in 2-hour PG as well as 1-hour PG was not significantly different between progressors and nonprogressors, in agreement with the results from the Whitehall II Study [12]. Therefore, contrary to our hypothesis, 1-hour PG did not increase earlier or faster than 2-hour PG, but the difference between progressors and nonprogressors present at the commencement of the observation was maintained for many years. As the difference in 1-hour PG was relatively larger rather than 2-hour PG until immediately before the diagnosis, it would be natural that progressors and nonprogressors were better discriminated by 1-hour PG than 2-hour PG.

Higher 1-hour PG than 2-hour PG is common in nondiabetic people as demonstrated by the studies on the shape of glucose curve during the OGTT [22–24]; about half of the study subjects had monophasic glucose curves, with a peak during 30–90 min followed by a decrease during 90–120 min. The second popular type was biphasic, who had a nadir by 90 min and an increase again during 90–120 min. Compared to subjects with biphasic shape, monophasic subjects had a worse insulin sensitivity, lower insulin secretion, higher 1-hour PG [22–24], and higher risk for type 2 diabetes [25]. The elevation of 1-hour PG might reflect the characteristic of these monophasic type of subjects. Whether the elevation of 1-hour PG is acquired or inherent is not known, but elevated 1-hour PG is likely to be present in the very early years in the natural course of the development of type 2 diabetes.

The cutoff point of 155 mg/dL for 1-hour PG was first proposed by Abdul-Ghani et al. [18] and has been demonstrated to be useful to identify the individuals at higher risk for type 2 diabetes in other independent cohort studies from Finnish [5], Jewish [8], and Asian Indian populations [26]. Abdul-Ghani et al. set 155 mg/dL based on the result that the sum of sensitivity and specificity was maximal (0.75 and 0.79 for sensitivity and specificity, resp.), and they also reported that the optimal cutoff point for fasting PG was as low as 94 mg/dL applying the same method [18]. Indeed, the HR for future diabetes was significantly elevated both in NGT and IGT with 1-hour PG $155 \leq$ mg/dL in this study. However, 44% of our study subjects had 1-hour PG $155 \leq$ mg/dL at baseline. Such a lower cutoff point might bring problems with socioeconomic costs as the new definition of "prediabetes" did so [27, 28]. As Asians have greater glycaemic excursions after taking glucose than Europeans [29], the ethnicity may also be taken into account to set the optimal cutoff point for 1-hour PG.

The strength of our study is the longitudinal observation of postload plasma glucoses, which allow for the comparison between the trajectory of 1-hour and that of 2-hour PG. However, several limitations of this study should be considered. First, data on subjects who did not receive checkups during the follow-up period were not available. Subjects who missed checkups might be less conscious about their health, which biased the study subjects toward metabolically healthy people. However, baseline characteristics including BMI, glucose, and insulin concentrations between the subjects who were followed and those who were missed were not significantly different. Second, 60 out of 112 progressors were diagnosed as diabetes only by 2-hour PG $200 \leq$ mg/dL with normal fasting PG (<126 mg/dL), and the estimated value of fasting PG at the diagnosis (0 year) in progressors was relatively low compared to the prior studies. Our results may reflect more the character of isolated postload hyperglycemia rather than combined fasting and postload hyperglycemia. However, when diagnosis of diabetes was conducted only by fasting PG and/or receiving treatments, the results were similar. Third, the measurement of PG concentrations relied on a single OGTT, which is known to have within-subject variability [30].

In conclusion, longitudinally observed, diabetes transition was preceded by a mild elevation of 2-hour PG for many years. The difference in 1-hour PG between progressors and nonprogressors was relatively large until immediately before the diagnosis.

Conflicts of Interest

The authors declare that there are no conflicts of interest associated with this manuscript.

Acknowledgments

The authors thank the subjects and the staff at the Health Check Department of Hokuriku Central Hospital, Dr. Toru Aizawa at Aizawa Hospital for his thoughtful comments, and Dr. Kota Suzuki at Aichi Medical University for the advice on statistical analyses.

References

[1] W. C. Knowler, E. Barrett-Connor, S. E. Fowler et al., "Reduction in the incidence of type 2 diabetes with lifestyle intervention or metformin," *The New England Journal of Medicine*, vol. 346, pp. 393–403, 2002.

[2] J. Tuomilehto, J. Lindstrom, J. G. Eriksson et al., "Prevention of type 2 diabetes mellitus by changes in lifestyle among subjects with impaired glucose tolerance," *The New England Journal of Medicine*, vol. 344, pp. 1343–1350, 2001.

[3] E. M. Balk, A. Earley, G. Raman, E. A. Avendano, A. G. Pittas, and P. L. Remington, "Combined diet and physical activity promotion programs to prevent type 2 diabetes among persons at increased risk: a systematic review for the community preventive services task force," *Annals of Internal Medicine*, vol. 163, pp. 437–451, 2015.

[4] M. A. Abdul-Ghani, K. Williams, R. A. DeFronzo, and M. Stern, "What is the best predictor of future type 2 diabetes?," *Diabetes Care*, vol. 30, pp. 1544–1548, 2007.

[5] M. A. Abdul-Ghani, V. Lyssenko, T. Tuomi, R. A. DeFronzo, and L. Groop, "Fasting versus postload plasma glucose concentration and the risk for future type 2 diabetes: results from the Botnia Study," *Diabetes Care*, vol. 32, pp. 281–286, 2009.

[6] A. Alyass, P. Almgren, M. Akerlund et al., "Modelling of OGTT curve identifies 1 h plasma glucose level as a strong predictor of incident type 2 diabetes: results from two prospective cohorts," *Diabetologia*, vol. 58, pp. 87–97, 2015.

[7] R. Oka, T. Aizawa, S. Miyamoto, T. Yoneda, and M. Yamagishi, "One-hour plasma glucose as a predictor of the development of type 2 diabetes in Japanese adults," *Diabetic Medicine*, vol. 33, pp. 1399–1405, 2016.

[8] M. Bergman, A. Chetrit, J. Roth, R. Jagannathan, M. Sevick, and R. Dankner, "One-hour post-load plasma glucose level during the OGTT predicts dysglycemia: observations from the 24year follow-up of the Israel Study of glucose intolerance, obesity and hypertension," *Diabetes Research and Clinical Practice*, vol. 120, pp. 221–228, 2016.

[9] M. A. Marini, E. Succurro, S. Frontoni et al., "Insulin sensitivity, β-cell function, and incretin effect in individuals with elevated 1-hour postload plasma glucose levels," *Diabetes Care*, vol. 35, pp. 868–872, 2012.

[10] C. C. Mason, R. L. Hanson, and W. C. Knowler, "Progression to type 2 diabetes characterized by moderate then rapid glucose increases," *Diabetes*, vol. 56, pp. 2054–2061, 2007.

[11] E. Ferrannini, M. Nannipieri, K. Williams, C. Gonzales, S. M. Haffner, and M. P. Stern, "Mode of onset of type 2 diabetes from normal or impaired glucose tolerance," *Diabetes*, vol. 53, pp. 160–165, 2004.

[12] A. G. Tabak, M. Jokela, T. N. Akbaraly, E. J. Brunner, M. Kivimaki, and D. R. Witte, "Trajectories of glycaemia, insulin sensitivity, and insulin secretion before diagnosis of type 2 diabetes: an analysis from the Whitehall II study," *Lancet*, vol. 373, pp. 2215–2221, 2009.

[13] R. Oka, K. Yagi, M. Sakurai et al., "Insulin secretion and insulin sensitivity on the oral glucose tolerance test (OGTT) in middle-aged Japanese," *Endocrine Journal*, vol. 59, pp. 55–64, 2012.

[14] World Health Organization ID, *Definition and Diagnosis of Diabetes Mellitus and Intermediate Hyperglycaemia: Report of a WHO/IDF Consultation*, World Health Organization, Geneva, 2006.

[15] K. Kosaka, T. Kuzuya, R. Hagura, and H. Yoshinaga, "Insulin response to oral glucose load is consistently decreased in established non-insulin-dependent diabetes mellitus: the usefulness of decreased early insulin response as a predictor of non-insulin-dependent diabetes mellitus," *Diabetic Medicine*, vol. 13, no. 9, Supplement 6, pp. S109–S119, 1996.

[16] D. R. Matthews, J. P. Hosker, A. S. Rudenski, B. A. Naylor, D. F. Treacher, and R. C. Turner, "Homeostasis model assessment: insulin resistance and beta-cell function from fasting plasma glucose and insulin concentrations in man," *Diabetologia*, vol. 28, pp. 412–419, 1985.

[17] G. M. L. N. Fitzmaurice and J. H. Ware, *Applied Longitudinal Analysis*, John Wiley & Sons, New York, 2011.

[18] M. A. Abdul-Ghani, T. Abdul-Ghani, N. Ali, and R. A. DeFronzo, "One-hour plasma glucose concentration and the metabolic syndrome identify subjects at high risk for future type 2 diabetes," *Diabetes Care*, vol. 31, no. 8, pp. 1650–1655, 2008.

[19] Committee of the Japan Diabetes Society on the Diagnostic Criteria of Diabetes Mellitus, Y. Seino, K. Nanjo et al., "Report of the committee on the classification and diagnostic criteria of diabetes mellitus," *Journal of Diabetes Investigation*, vol. 1, no. 5, pp. 212–228, 2010.

[20] A. H. Xiang, C. Wang, R. K. Peters, E. Trigo, S. L. Kjos, and T. A. Buchanan, "Coordinate changes in plasma glucose and pancreatic beta-cell function in Latino women at high risk for type 2 diabetes," *Diabetes*, vol. 55, pp. 1074–1079, 2006.

[21] E. Laspa, A. Christen, Z. Efstathiadou, D. G. Johnston, and I. F. Godsland, "Long-term changes and variability in diabetes risk factors prior to the development of impaired glucose homeostasis," *Diabetic Medicine*, vol. 24, no. 11, pp. 1269–1278, 2007.

[22] M. Kanauchi, K. Kimura, K. Kanauchi, and Y. Saito, "Beta-cell function and insulin sensitivity contribute to the shape of plasma glucose curve during an oral glucose tolerance test in non-diabetic individuals," *International Journal of Clinical Practice*, vol. 59, pp. 427–432, 2005.

[23] O. Tschritter, A. Fritsche, F. Shirkavand, F. Machicao, H. Häring, and M. Stumvoll, "Assessing the shape of the glucose curve during an oral glucose tolerance test," *Diabetes Care*, vol. 26, no. 4, pp. 1026–1033, 2003.

[24] A. Tura, U. Morbiducci, S. Sbrignadello, Y. Winhofer, G. Pacini, and A. Kautzky-Willer, "Shape of glucose, insulin, C-peptide curves during a 3-h oral glucose tolerance test: any relationship with the degree of glucose tolerance?," *American Journal of Physiology. Regulatory, Integrative and Comparative Physiology*, vol. 300, pp. R941–R948, 2011.

[25] M. A. Abdul-Ghani, V. Lyssenko, T. Tuomi, R. A. Defronzo, and L. Groop, "The shape of plasma glucose concentration curve during OGTT predicts future risk of type 2 diabetes," *Diabetes/Metabolism Research and Reviews*, vol. 26, pp. 280–286, 2010.

[26] M. Priya, R. M. Anjana, F. S. Chiwanga, K. Gokulakrishnan, M. Deepa, and V. Mohan, "1-hour venous plasma glucose and incident prediabetes and diabetes in Asian Indians," *Diabetes Technology & Therapeutics*, vol. 15, pp. 497–502, 2013.

[27] T. M. Dall, W. Yang, P. Halder et al., "The economic burden of elevated blood glucose levels in 2012: diagnosed and undiagnosed diabetes, gestational diabetes mellitus, and prediabetes," *Diabetes Care*, vol. 37, pp. 3172–3179, 2014.

[28] J. S. Yudkin and V. M. Montori, "The epidemic of pre-diabetes: the medicine and the politics," *BMJ*, vol. 349, article g4485, 2014.

[29] M. Kataoka, B. J. Venn, S. M. Williams, L. A. Te Morenga, I. M. Heemels, and J. I. Mann, "Glycaemic responses to glucose and rice in people of Chinese and European ethnicity," *Diabetic Medicine*, vol. 30, pp. e101–e107, 2013.

[30] K. M. Utzschneider, R. L. Prigeon, J. Tong et al., "Within-subject variability of measures of beta cell function derived from a 2 h OGTT: implications for research studies," *Diabetologia*, vol. 50, no. 12, pp. 2516–2525, 2007.

8

High Intensity Aerobic Exercise Training Improves Deficits of Cardiovascular Autonomic Function in a Rat Model of Type 1 Diabetes Mellitus with Moderate Hyperglycemia

Kenneth N. Grisé,[1] T. Dylan Olver,[2] Matthew W. McDonald,[1] Adwitia Dey,[1] Mao Jiang,[1] James C. Lacefield,[3] J. Kevin Shoemaker,[2,4,5] Earl G. Noble,[1,5] and C. W. James Melling[1]

[1]*Exercise Biochemistry Laboratory, School of Kinesiology, Faculty of Health Sciences, Western University, London, ON, Canada N6A 3K7*

[2]*Neurovascular Research Laboratory, School of Kinesiology, Faculty of Health Sciences, Western University, London, ON, Canada N6A 3K7*

[3]*Department of Electrical and Computer Engineering, Department of Medical Biophysics and Robarts Research Institute, Western University, London, ON, Canada N6A 3K7*

[4]*Department of Physiology and Pharmacology, Western University, London, ON, Canada N6A 3K7*

[5]*Lawson Health Research Institute, London, ON, Canada N6C 2R5*

Correspondence should be addressed to C. W. James Melling; jmelling@uwo.ca

Academic Editor: Mark A. Yorek

Indices of cardiovascular autonomic neuropathy (CAN) in experimental models of Type 1 diabetes mellitus (T1DM) are often contrary to clinical data. Here, we investigated whether a relatable insulin-treated model of T1DM would induce deficits in cardiovascular (CV) autonomic function more reflective of clinical results and if exercise training could prevent those deficits. Sixty-four rats were divided into four groups: sedentary control (C), sedentary T1DM (D), control exercise (CX), or T1DM exercise (DX). Diabetes was induced via multiple low-dose injections of streptozotocin and blood glucose was maintained at moderate hyperglycemia (9–17 mM) through insulin supplementation. Exercise training consisted of daily treadmill running for 10 weeks. Compared to C, D had blunted baroreflex sensitivity, increased vascular sympathetic tone, increased serum neuropeptide Y (NPY), and decreased intrinsic heart rate. In contrast, DX differed from D in all measures of CAN (except NPY), including heart rate variability. These findings demonstrate that this T1DM model elicits deficits and exercise-mediated improvements to CV autonomic function which are reflective of clinical T1DM.

1. Introduction

A common and serious complication of Type 1 diabetes mellitus (T1DM) is diabetic autonomic neuropathy [1, 2]. Cardiovascular autonomic neuropathy (CAN) is a subset of diabetic autonomic neuropathy characterized by impaired autonomic control of the cardiovascular (CV) system [3]. CAN is also consistently associated with increased mortality. For instance, CAN has been reported to increase the mortality of diabetic patients by a factor of 3.45 [4]. Clinically, the most common methods for assessing CAN are heart rate variability (HRV) analysis and baroreflex sensitivity (BRS) [3, 5, 6]. In T1DM, aspects of the baroreflex arc can be impaired [7], such that both baroreceptor activity and excitability are blunted [8, 9] and the aortic depressor nerves undergo axonal atrophy [8]. As well, autonomic efferents, primarily of the parasympathetic nervous system (PSNS), have decreased activity, reduced responsiveness, and decreased neurochemical activity in the heart [10, 11]. Impairment of central nervous system regions has also been reported as the limiting factor of BRS [12, 13]. Reduced heart rate variability (HRV) is often the earliest symptom of CAN [14]. Whether measured by time domain analysis or by frequency domain analysis and whether in clinical or experimental T1DM, HRV is consistently reported to be reduced in T1DM [5, 14–17].

Exercise has been demonstrated to be an effective means of improving deficits in HRV and BRS in both clinical and experimental T1DM [18–21]. Such improvements have been attributed to improved insulin sensitivity, increased endogenous antioxidant and anti-inflammatory mediators, and improved autonomic control of the CV system [22–24]. Despite similar reductions in HRV and BRS, there are marked differences in early-stage changes to other CV parameters between clinical and experimental T1DM [25]. Specifically, in clinical T1DM, increases in heart rate (HR) and blood pressure (BP) are commonly reported in early autonomic neuropathy [1, 3, 14, 24, 26–28]. In contrast, experimental STZ-induced T1DM is regularly associated with decreased BP and HR, beginning shortly after diabetes induction [15, 16, 29–31]. Due to these opposing initial changes in BP and HR, exercise training is often observed to produce contrasting outcomes on CV parameters in experimental and clinical T1DM, namely, increased BP and HR in experimental T1DM and decreased BP and HR in clinical T1DM [19, 25, 32–34]. As a result, both the increase and decrease of these CV factors are concurrently cited as exercise-mediated improvements to CAN with little consideration of the fact that the changes are opposed between these two contexts of T1DM [25]. This is important because if animal models do not accurately reproduce T1DM pathology, then the outcomes of experimental studies may not translate to the treatment of human CAN, as the mechanisms underlying the pathology and exercise modifications may differ.

Another important difference between experimental and clinical T1DM is the common omission of insulin treatment in experimental diabetes leading to severe hyperglycemia ranging from roughly 17 to 25 mM blood glucose concentrations ([BG]) [15, 16, 29, 30]. As the severity and duration of hyperglycemia have been shown to influence the degree of diabetic neuropathy, acute and steep elevations of [BG] in STZ-induced T1DM may not only cause early onset neuropathy to the PSNS but also cause acute neuropathy of the sympathetic nervous system (SNS) and directly affect the sinoatrial (SA) node. These changes may mediate the observed reduction in BP and HR that arise acutely in experimental T1DM and in late-stage clinical T1DM [2, 35–38]. Indeed, intensive insulin therapy has been shown to restore BP and HR to non-T1DM levels in STZ-induced T1DM rats [25, 39].

Yet, despite the use of insulin therapy in clinical T1DM, it is often the case that chronic, moderate hyperglycemia is maintained as a result of difficulties in regulating [BG] in response to dynamic influences on glycemic control, such as food intake and exercise [40, 41]. This is often resultant of a tendency to err on the side of moderate hyperglycemia in order to circumvent the acute discomfort and danger associated with hypoglycemic episodes, which occur more frequently with diabetic neuropathy due to the impairment of the glucagon response [40, 42, 43]. To address this, our laboratory established a model of T1DM using a multiple low-dose STZ-treatment and insulin therapy to replicate the moderate hyperglycemia observed in clinical T1DM [44]. In our previous studies that employed this model, we observed impairments in glucose tolerance, vascular responsiveness, cardiac function, and bone health, which were improved with high intensity aerobic exercise training [44–47].

The purpose of the current study was to investigate whether our model of multiple low-dose STZ-induced T1DM with insulin therapy would induce deficits in cardiovascular autonomic function more representative of clinical T1DM, and if high intensity aerobic training could prevent those deficits. We hypothesised that (1) our model of STZ-induced T1DM would elicit indices of CAN, including a blunted BRS (bradycardia and tachycardia response), lowered HRV and intrinsic heart rate, increased vascular sympathetic tone, and increased mean arterial pressure, and (2) high intensity aerobic exercise training would prevent or ameliorate the indications of CAN.

2. Materials and Methods

2.1. Ethics Approval. The protocols used in this investigation were approved by the University of Western Ontario Council on Animal Care and conformed to the guidelines of the Canadian Council on Animal Care.

2.2. Animals. Eight-week-old male Sprague-Dawley rats were obtained from Charles River Laboratories Canada (Saint-Constant, Quebec). The rats were housed in pairs and maintained on a 12-hour dark/light cycle at a constant temperature (20±1°C) and relative humidity (50%). Rats were allowed access to standard rat chow and water *ad libitum*.

2.3. Experimental Groups. Sixty-four rats were randomly assigned to one of four groups as follows: (1) sedentary control (C, n = 16); (2) exercised control (CX, n = 16); (3) sedentary T1DM (D, n = 16); (4) exercised T1DM (DX, n = 16). All functional and blood endpoint measures were acquired 24 hours after the final exercise bout.

2.4. T1DM Induction and Insulin Dose. Upon arrival rats were acclimatized to the laboratory setting for five days. Subsequently, T1DM was induced over five consecutive days by multiple intraperitoneal (IP) injections of 20 mg/kg streptozotocin (STZ, Sigma-Aldrich) dissolved in a citrate buffer (0.1 M, pH 4.5). Diabetes was confirmed by blood glucose measurements greater than or equal to 18 mM on two consecutive days. If necessary, subsequent 20 mg/kg STZ injections were administered until diabetes was confirmed. Following the confirmation of diabetes, insulin pellets (1 pellet; 2 U insulin/day; Linplant, Linshin Canada, Inc., Toronto, Ontario, Canada) were implanted subcutaneously in the abdominal region. Insulin pellet doses were then monitored for 1 week and adjusted (±0.5 pellets) in order to obtain daily nonfasting blood glucose concentrations in the moderate hyperglycemic range of 9–17 mM. Insulin dose was determined by multiplying the total quantity of pellet implanted (0.5 pellet increments) by the amount of insulin released per pellet (2 units of insulin/day/pellet) divided by the body weight (Kg) of the rat.

2.5. Body Weight and Blood Glucose Concentration. Body weights and nonfasting blood glucose concentrations were obtained weekly. Blood was obtained from the saphenous vein by venous puncture with a 30-gauge needle and measured via Freestyle Lite Blood Glucose Monitoring System (Abbott Diabetes Care Inc., Mississauga, Ontario, Canada).

2.6. Intravenous Glucose Tolerance Test. Intravenous glucose tolerance tests (IVGTT) were performed on all animals prior to T1DM induction (pre-T1DM) and at the end of week 10 of the exercise training period. Rats were fasted for approximately 8 to 12 hours prior to the assay and did not perform exercise on the day of their IVGTT. A sterile-filtered dextrose solution (50% dextrose, 50% ddH_2O) was injected (1 g/kg) into the lateral tail vein of the conscious rat. Following dextrose infusion, blood glucose was measured at 5 minutes, at 10 minutes, and then at 10-minute intervals thereafter until blood glucose levels plateaued.

2.7. Exercise Protocol. Prior to the initiation of the exercise training program, rats were familiarized with the exercise equipment on two consecutive days. The familiarization consisted of two 15-minute sessions of running at progressive treadmill speeds up to 30 meters per minute (m/min). The treadmill was a custom-built apparatus fabricated by the physical plant at University of Western Ontario and has been used in many previous studies [44–47]. The exercise training program consisted of 1 hour of motor-driven treadmill running per day at 27 m/min with a 6-degree incline, 5 days per week, for 10 weeks. The exercise intensity was determined based on earlier research that investigated oxygen uptake in rats at various treadmill speeds. The chosen intensity was found to represent approximately 75–85% VO_{2max} [48, 49].

2.8. Preparative Surgery and Instrumentation. To achieve a surgical plane of anesthesia, rats were placed in an induction chamber circulating 4% isoflurane (96% O_2). Once motor reflexes were undetectable, rats were transferred to a nosecone delivering 3% isoflurane (97% O_2) and placed on a hot water pad (37°C). Rats were cannulated with saline-infused polyethylene (PE90) catheters in the right jugular vein and carotid artery and each catheter was attached to a three-way stopcock. The jugular vein catheter was used for drug infusions and the carotid artery catheter was connected in series with a pressure transducer (PX272, Edwards Life Sciences, Irvine, California, USA) for arterial blood pressure measurements.

At the end of the preparative surgery, rats were injected IP with a 25 mg/Kg "cocktail" of urethane (16 mg/mL) and α-chloralose (100 mg/mL), an anesthetic cocktail that has been shown to have the least inhibition of baseline CV control and autonomic function [50]. A total of 10 mL of urethane/α-chloralose was made, 5 mL of which was diluted to 50% with ddH_2O and was used as needed to maintain anesthesia throughout data collection. Isoflurane anesthesia was gradually removed, whereby urethane/α-chloralose was the primary anesthesia used during data collection.

2.9. Basal Heart Rate, Systolic Blood Pressure, and Mean Arterial Pressure. Heart rate (HR), systolic blood pressure (SBP), and mean arterial pressure (MAP) were determined from the blood pressure pulse waveform and were collected while the rats were under urethane/α-chloralose anesthesia in the supine position. The pressure transducer was calibrated using a standard analog manometer. Data were obtained using a PowerLab data acquisition system, digitized, and recorded at 1000 Hz using the bundled LabChart 7 Pro software (ADInstruments, Colorado Springs, CO, USA).

2.10. Heart Rate Variability. Prior to drug infusions, 5 minutes of spontaneous electrocardiogram data was sampled at 1000 Hz and analyzed with LabChart HRV analysis software (ADInstruments). Time domain analysis of the standard deviation between normal peak pulses of the pressure pulse waveform (SDNN) was quantified as a measure of the total variability of the HR. Frequency domain analysis of the high frequency (HF) band of the Fast Fourier Transform (FFT) of the data was assessed as an index of parasympathetically mediated HRV.

2.11. Baroreflex Sensitivity. Baroreflex sensitivity (BRS) was assessed using the modified Oxford technique [51, 52]. The BRS was quantified using the slope of the linear regression line representing the linear portion of the sigmoidal heart rate-systolic blood pressure relationship (ΔHR {BPM}/ ΔSBP $\{mmHg\}^{-1}$) after rapid bolus injections (~5 s) of phenylephrine (PE, 12 μg/Kg, 10 μg/mL) and sodium nitroprusside (SNP, 60 μg/Kg, 110 μg/mL) dissolved in ddH_2O. The rationale for this method is detailed by Studinger et al. (2007) [54]. For each drug, the catheter was first filled with a 0.2 mL volume to ensure accuracy of the drug dose. After a stable baseline was obtained, a bolus injection of SNP was rapidly infused and the reflex SNS mediated tachycardia response was measured. The analysis began at the onset of SBP decrease after SNP infusion and ended when SBP reached its nadir. This was followed by a saline flush to washout any remaining SNP in the catheter. After a stable baseline was reestablished, this same procedure was then followed using PE to measure PSNS mediated reflex bradycardia, except that analysis began at the onset of SBP increase and ended when SBP reached its zenith. Responses to PE and SNP were plotted separately and only regression lines (slopes) with correlation coefficients (r) $\geq$ 0.70 and $p < 0.05$ were accepted [53, 54].

2.12. Vascular Sympathetic Tone. To measure the sympathetic contribution to baseline vascular resistance, MAP was assessed before and after a bolus injection of the α-adrenergic receptor blocker, prazosin (85 μg/Kg, 500 μg/mL). Following this protocol, animals were euthanized via exsanguination while still under urethane/α-chloralose anesthesia.

2.13. Neuropeptide Y ELISA. To ensure physiological testing did not confound serum neuropeptide Y concentration

[NPY] measurement, a subset of animals from each group did not undergo surgery for heart rate variability, baroreflex sensitivity, mean arterial pressure, or vascular sympathetic tone measurements. Rather, at the end of the 10-week exercise training period these animals were anesthetized via intraperitoneal injection of sodium pentobarbital (65 mg/kg) and blood serum samples for [NPY] measurement were collected upon euthanasia. Serum [NPY] was measured using an NPY ELISA kit (USCN Life Sciences Inc.) according to the manufacturer's instructions.

2.14. Intrinsic Heart Rate. A Langendorff preparation was used to measure intrinsic heart rate. Following the euthanasia of animals for blood [NPY] measurement, hearts were extracted and immediately arrested by placing them in ice cold Krebs-Henseleit buffer (KHB). Hearts were cannulated for unpaced retrograde aortic constant flow perfusion (15 mL/min) of coronary arteries with KHB (containing 120 mM NaCl, 4.63 M KCl, 1.17 mM KH_2PO_4, 1.25 mM $CaCl_2$, 1.2 mM $MgCl_2$, 20 mM $NaHCO_3$, and 8 mM glucose gassed with 95% O_2 and 5% CO_2) that was maintained at 37°C [55]. Hearts were equilibrated for 30 min to determine baseline intrinsic heart rate.

2.15. Data Analysis and Statistics. Body weight and blood glucose concentrations were compared using a two-way repeated measures ANOVA, while endpoint measures were compared by two-way ANOVA, with the exception of endpoint insulin dose, which was compared using a one-tailed t-test. When significance was found, pairwise comparisons were made using the Fisher LSD post hoc test. Data are represented as mean ± standard error, with a significance level set at $p < 0.05$.

3. Results

3.1. Animal Characteristics. All groups increased in body weight over the course of the study ($p < 0.05$, Figure 1(a)). At the end of the study, the body weights of the T1DM groups (D and DX) were lower than non-T1DM groups (C and CX), and exercised groups (CX and DX) weighed less than their nonexercised counterparts (C and D; $p < 0.05$). Following the confirmation of diabetes, weekly [BG] was mostly maintained in the targeted range of 9–17 mM; however, the [BG] did move outside of this range periodically. The [BG] in the T1DM groups were elevated in comparison to the non-T1DM groups ($p < 0.05$; Figure 1(b)). Within the non-T1DM and T1DM groups, there was no difference in [BG] between nonexercised and exercised groups (C versus CX and D versus DX; $p > 0.05$).

3.2. Intravenous Glucose Tolerance Test and Insulin Dosages. The glucose clearance rate (K_G) of the diabetic groups (D and DX) decreased from pre-T1DM to week 10 of training ($p < 0.05$), whereas K_G of the CX group increased ($p < 0.05$; Figure 2(a)). Both diabetic groups had significantly lower K_G values than both the control groups (C and CX) at week 10 ($p < 0.05$; Figure 2(a)). However, there was not a significant interaction between diabetes and exercise on K_G. The amount of insulin supplementation that the DX group received was significantly less than the amount the D group received at week 10 ($p < 0.05$; Figure 2(b)).

3.3. Mean Arterial Pressure, Heart Rate, and Intrinsic Heart Rate. For resting HR and MAP, there was not a significant difference between groups at week 10 (Figures 3(a) and 3(b), resp.). However, for the intrinsic heart rate (IHR), there was main effect of both exercise and T1DM, where T1DM decreased the IHR, while exercise increased IHR ($p < 0.05$, Figure 3(c)). Further, within the T1DM groups (D and DX), exercise increased IHR, while within the nonexercised groups (C and D) T1DM decreased IHR ($p < 0.05$).

3.4. Heart Rate Variability. Total HRV at week 10, as measured by the standard deviation of the normal pulse wave peaks (SDNN), was not significantly different between groups (Figure 4(a)). However, there was a main effect of exercise on the HF contribution to HRV, where exercise increased HF HRV ($p < 0.05$, Figure 4(b)). Particularly, within the T1DM groups (D and DX), exercise increased HF HRV ($p < 0.05$).

3.5. Baroreflex Sensitivity. In response to SNP infusion, there was not a significant difference between groups in the tachycardia BRS response (Figure 5(a)). However, a significant interaction between T1DM and exercise was observed for BRS during the bradycardia response to phenylephrine ($p < 0.05$, Figure 5(b)). More specifically, within the T1DM groups (D and DX) exercise prevented the reduction in BRS that was observed in the D group ($p < 0.05$).

3.6. Vascular Sympathetic Tone and Serum NPY. An interaction between T1DM and exercise was observed for the prazosin-induced change in MAP ($p < 0.05$, Figure 6(a)). Within the nonexercised groups (C and D), T1DM resulted in an increased change in MAP ($p < 0.05$). Within the T1DM groups (D and DX) exercise prevented the increased change in MAP observed in the D group ($p < 0.05$). There was also a main effect of T1DM on [NPY] ($p < 0.05$, Figure 6(b)). Within the nonexercised groups (C and D) and exercised groups (CX and DX), serum [NPY] was increased by T1DM ($p < 0.05$).

4. Discussion

This study demonstrated that a multiple low-dose STZ model with moderate hyperglycemia, maintained using insulin therapy, produced deficits in cardiovascular autonomic function without inducing the resting bradycardia or hypotension typical of other STZ models. This study also showed that high intensity aerobic exercise training can prevent deficits of cardiovascular autonomic function caused by T1DM. Furthermore, because [BG] was held within a moderate hyperglycemic range, the observed exercise-mediated improvements to indications of CAN were independent of changes in [BG] and, instead, may primarily have been the result of

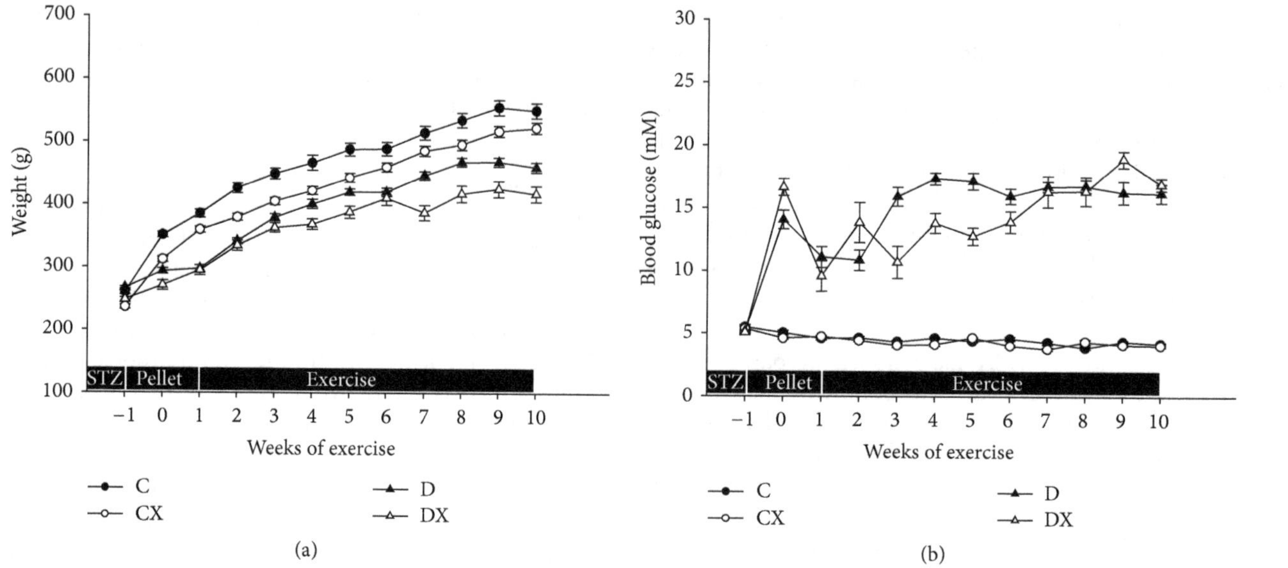

FIGURE 1: (a) Weekly body weights: C, sedentary control ($n = 16$); CX, control exercise ($n = 16$); D, sedentary T1DM ($n = 15$); DX, T1DM exercise ($n = 12$). (b) Weekly blood glucose concentrations: C ($n = 16$); CX ($n = 15$); D ($n = 15$); DX ($n = 13$). STZ, pellet, and exercise indicate the periods of STZ injection, insulin pellet implantation, and aerobic exercise, respectively. Significantly different groups ($p < 0.05$). Data are mean ± SE. There was significant difference in body weight between T1DM and non-T1DM groups, while a significant difference was evident between exercised and nonexercised groups. The blood glucose concentrations in the T1DM groups were significantly different than non-T1DM groups.

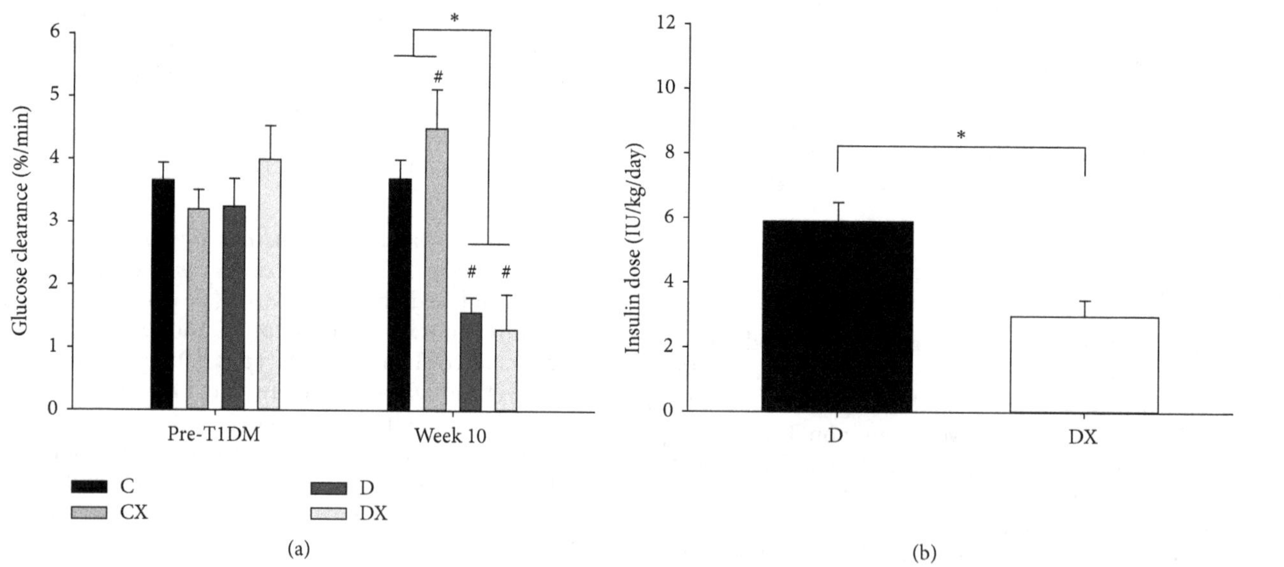

FIGURE 2: (a) IVGTT glucose clearance rate (K_G) values prior to T1DM induction (pre-T1DM) and week 10 of exercise training: C, sedentary control ($n = 16$); CX, control exercise ($n = 15$); D, sedentary T1DM ($n = 15$); DX, T1DM exercise ($n = 15$). (b) Insulin dosages at week 10: D ($n = 16$); DX ($n = 16$). *Significantly different groups ($p < 0.05$). #Significantly different from week 1. Data are mean ± SE.

improvements to other aspects of glucoregulation and/or the preservation of autonomic nervous system function.

Although we found time domain analysis of total HRV, as measured by the SDNN, did not demonstrate differences between groups, frequency domain analysis exposed a reduction in the HF power in the D group compared with the DX group. Since the HF power corresponds to the level of vagally mediated parasympathetic HRV, these results demonstrate not only the detrimental effects of T1DM on autonomic cardiac control but also the benefits of exercise training toward ameliorating those effects. These findings are similar to those of other experiments of both experimental [16, 21] and clinical diabetes [18, 56, 57]. For example, Mostarda et al. (2009) reported that STZ-induced T1DM reduced the HF component of HRV, which was improved by exercise [21]. Also, they found that the vagal tonus of the control exercised

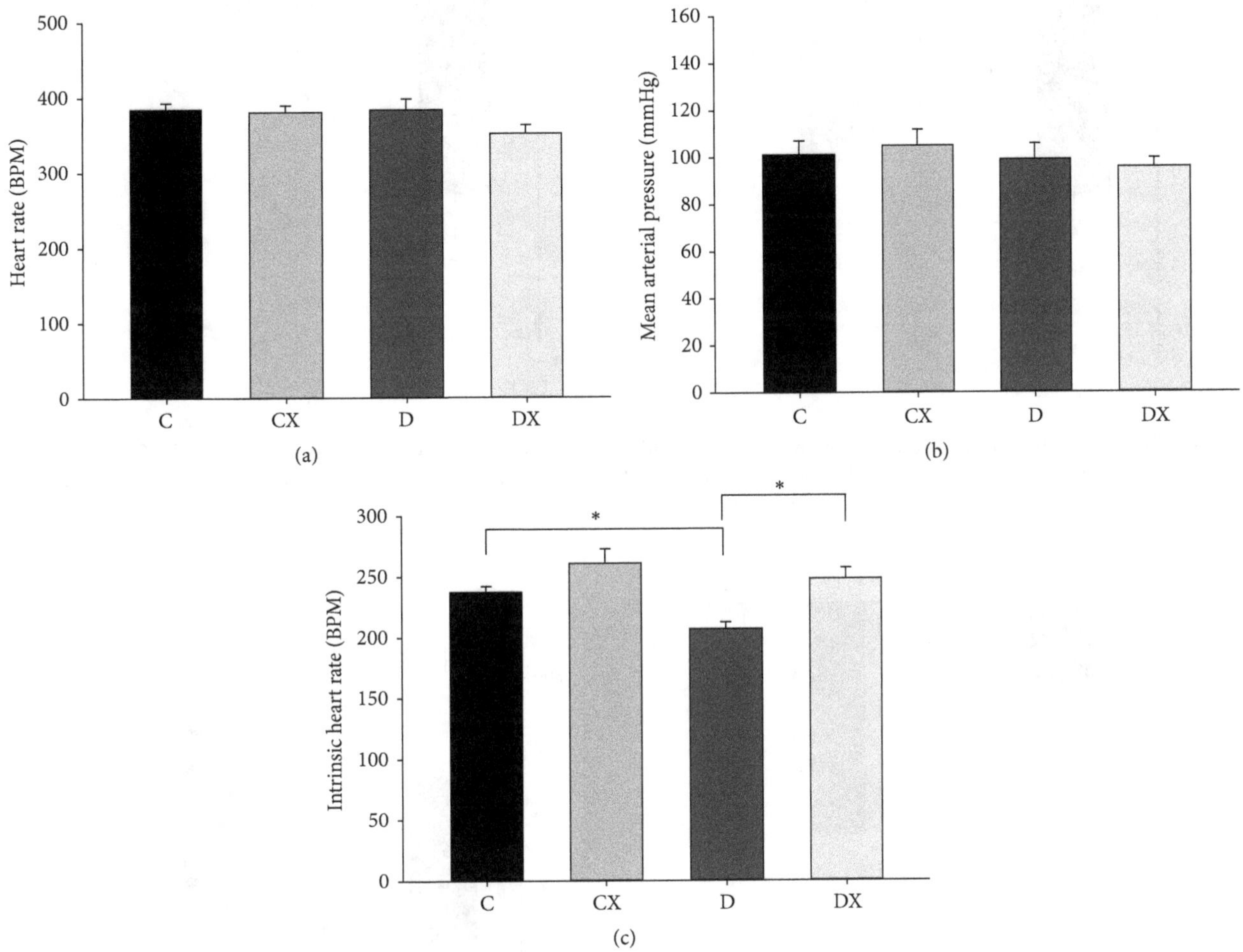

FIGURE 3: (a) Heart rate (beats per minute) and (b) mean arterial pressure at week 10. C, sedentary control (n = 7); CX, control exercise (n = 7); D, sedentary T1DM (n = 8); DX, T1DM exercise (n = 10). (c) Intrinsic heart rate (IHR) at week 10. C (n = 10); CX (n = 11); D (n = 12); DX (n = 9). *Significantly different groups ($p < 0.05$). Data are mean ± SE.

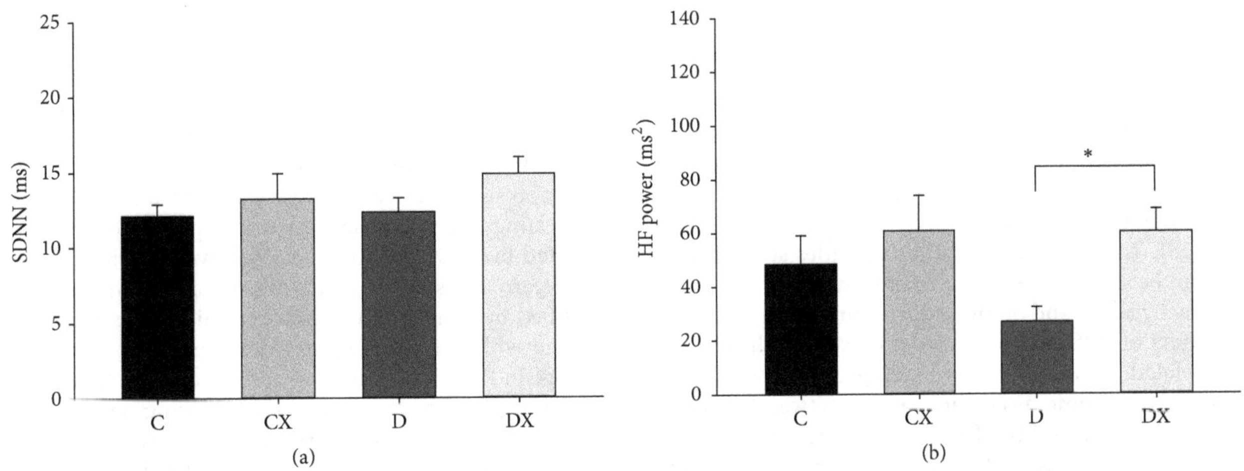

FIGURE 4: (a) Total HRV (SDNN) at week 10: C, sedentary control (n = 5); CX, control exercise (n = 7); D, sedentary T1DM (n = 8); DX, T1DM exercise (n = 8). (b) High Frequency (HF, parasympathetic) HRV component at week 10: C (n = 6); CX (n = 7); D (n = 8); DX (n = 8). *Significantly different groups ($p < 0.05$). Data are mean ± SE.

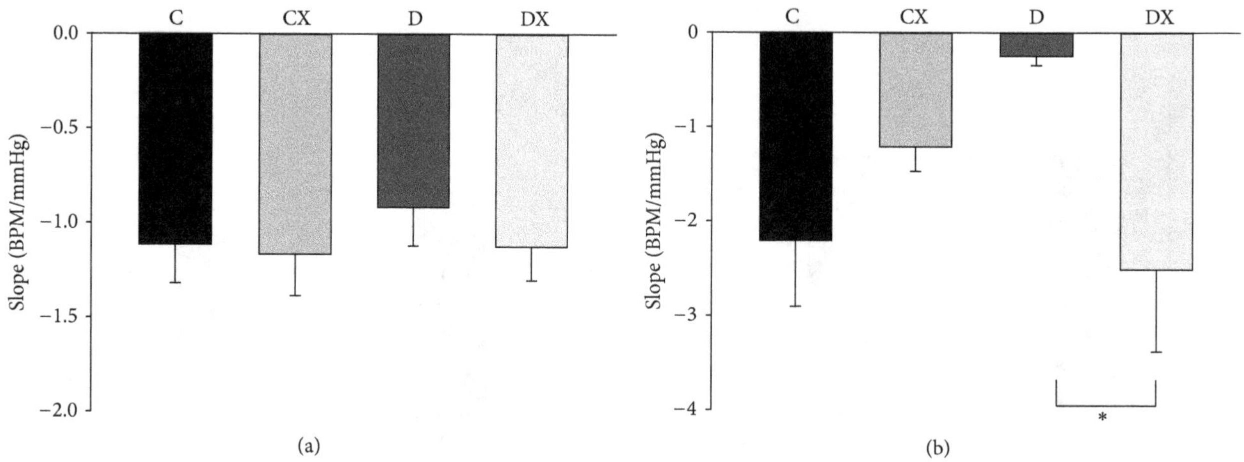

FIGURE 5: (a) Tachycardia baroreflex response sensitivity to sodium nitroprusside at week 10: C, sedentary control ($n = 7$); CX, control exercise ($n = 6$); D, sedentary T1DM ($n = 6$); DX, T1DM exercise ($n = 10$). (b) Bradycardia baroreflex response to phenylephrine at week 10: C ($n = 7$); CX ($n = 5$); D ($n = 7$); DX ($n = 10$). *Significantly different groups ($p < 0.05$). Data are mean ± SE.

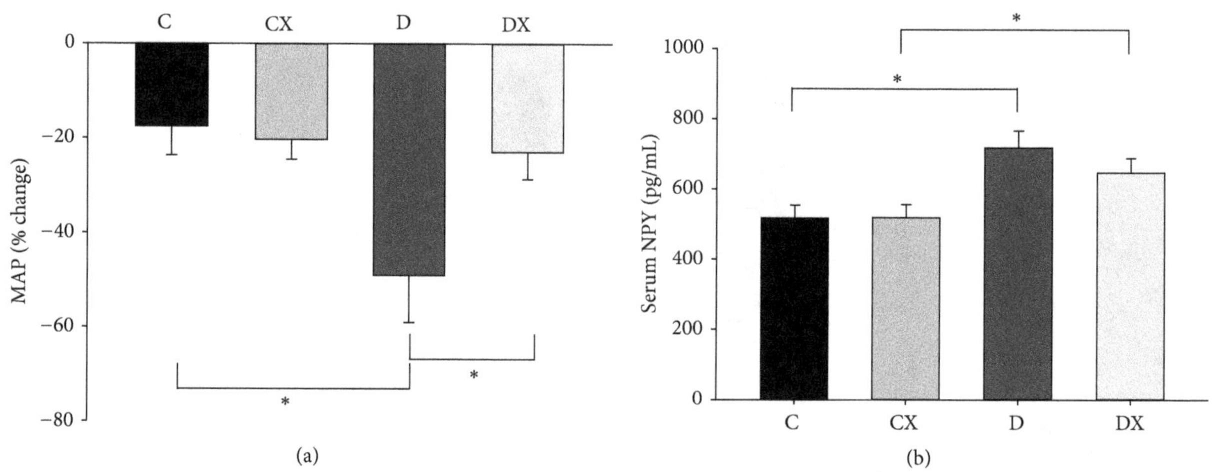

FIGURE 6: (a) Vascular sympathetic tone (VST) at week 10. This was determined by measuring the percent change in MAP after prazosin treatment at week 10: C, sedentary control ($n = 8$); CX, control exercise ($n = 7$); D, sedentary T1DM ($n = 5$); DX, T1DM exercise ($n = 7$). (b) Serum NPY at week 10: C ($n = 6$); CX ($n = 6$); D ($n = 6$); DX ($n = 6$). *Significantly different groups ($p < 0.05$). Data are mean ± SE.

rats did not differ from sedentary controls [21]. Likewise, Chen et al. (2008) reported that children with T1DM who performed a high level of physical activity did not differ from controls in HRV; however, children with T1DM who had low level of physical activity had significantly reduced HRV compared to both active children with T1DM and non-T1DM children [18]. Thus, the current study provides support that exercise can be an effective means to improve HRV in T1DM.

Both tachycardia and bradycardia responses were studied in the context of BRS analysis in order to explore the control features related to unloading or loading of the baroreceptors, respectively. Some discrepancy exists between different experimental models of T1DM and their impact on BRS measures. Investigations using the hyperglycemic Non-Obese Diabetic (NOD) T1DM mouse model have shown elevations in BRS measures rather than attenuated responses [58]. In contrast, tachycardic-SNP and bradycardic-PE responses have been shown to be lower in STZ-induced T1DM hyperglycemic rats in comparison to non-T1DM controls [21] but were improved with exercise training [59]. In the current study, the slope of the hypotensive tachycardia response was not significantly different between any of the groups suggesting that responses to baroreceptor unloading are not affected by T1DM or exercise. However, T1DM reduced the bradycardia response to baroreceptor loading, which was nullified by concurrent exercise training. These findings are in line with previous reports demonstrating a bradycardia change in PE-BRS without an accompanying change in SNP-BRS [60], which was improved following aerobic exercise [61]. Discrepancies in BRS responses in T1DM models seem to be closely associated with both the duration and the severity of diabetes. A recent study examining the time-course of BRS changes in response to STZ-induced hyperglycemia reported that alteration of the SNP-BRS was not evident until 12 weeks of diabetes, while a change in PE-BRS was evident as early as 4 weeks after induction [62]. Interestingly, the animals in the aforementioned study were moderately hyperglycemic (16–18 mM), suggesting that the severity of the hyperglycemia may play a role in the progression of this neuropathy. This relationship has also been demonstrated in humans. Vinik and Ziegler (2007) reported that poor glycemic control [63] and duration of diabetes [64] play a central role in progression of cardiovascular autonomic neuropathy. Yet, it is not clear what role insulin therapy may play in the neuropathy. Insulin supplementation to STZ-induced T1DM rats can modify the changes in BRS sensitivity evident at 48 weeks of T1DM [65]. Indeed, in clinical T1DM patients, intensive therapy is well documented to slow the progression and delay the appearance of abnormal autonomic function [66].

However, the current study provides evidence that the ability of exercise to ameliorate cardiovascular autonomic dysfunction may be independent of its ability to reduce [BG], which challenges the direct relationship between [BG] and CAN suggested by previous studies [67–69]. The IVGTT performed at the conclusion of the 10-week exercise period demonstrated an increased glucose clearance rate (K_G) and therefore glucose tolerance, in the CX group compared to the preexercise training period. However, in both the sedentary and exercise diabetic groups there was an equal decline in K_G to nearly the same rate. This decrease was significantly different from pre-T1DM values and the week 10 values of the C and CX groups. While this would normally indicate that both of the diabetic groups developed equally impaired glucose tolerance, it was also the case that the DX group required approximately half of the dosage of exogenous insulin compared to the D group to maintain their [BG] in the 9–17 mM range. With double the insulin dose, it is likely that the total serum insulin over a given time during IVGTT would have been greater in the D than DX group, and with their K_G being equal, that would indicate that there was a greater insulin sensitivity in the diabetic exercise group [70, 71]. Together, these IVGTT results demonstrate that exercise training improved glucose tolerance and insulin sensitivity [67]. Furthermore, since the [BG] of the diabetic groups in this study was held in a constant range, any abovementioned exercise-induced improvements to CV autonomic function would not have been mediated through a reduction in systemic [BG] but may have been the result of improvements in insulin sensitivity and glucose utilization [72, 73]. This should be borne in mind when considering the effects of diabetes and exercise on indices of CV autonomic function, such as HRV and BRS.

An alternative mechanism by which exercise can influence BRS was reported by Bernardi et al. (2011), who elucidated the importance of tissue oxygenation in T1DM [74]. They demonstrated that a reduced parasympathetic BRS in patients with T1DM was improved by both oxygen supplementation and deep breathing to the same degree, which indicated the increased respiration and oxygen delivery resultant of exercise could have been mediating increases in BRS. This led the authors to suggest that hypoxia in T1DM functionally restrains parasympathetic activity. However, reduced BRS could also be attributed to defects in the baroreceptors, baroreceptor afferent nerves, CNS structures, or efferent fibres of the baroreflex circuit [7, 8, 61]. In the present study, the finding that the tachycardia response of the baroreflex was unimpaired by T1DM, while the bradycardia response was, suggests that the afferent arm and central regulators of the baroreflex were not dysfunctional and that the observed decrement of baroreflex bradycardia may have been caused partly by alterations in efferent parasympathetic outflow [8, 29]. The smaller HF HRV in the D group is consistent with this interpretation.

Another interesting outcome of the current study was the alteration of sympathetic vasomotor control in the D group, which was also modified by concurrent exercise training. In this study, prazosin treatment resulted in a drop in MAP that was approximately twofold greater in the D group compared to the C and DX groups, which is indicative of a much greater sympathetic contribution to the maintenance of baseline vascular resistance [75, 76]. Similarly, Martinez-Nieves and Dunbar (1999) reported that male T1DM rats had a greater decrease in MAP after a bolus injection of prazosin compared to their control cohorts [77]. However, they postulated that an elevated prazosin response could be the result of increased α_1-adrenergic receptor sensitivity [77]. Yet, in this study, the finding that treatment with PE, an α_1-adrenergic receptor agonist, did not result in a greater peak SBP, nor a greater percent increase in SBP from baseline in the T1DM group (data not shown), argues against a receptor-based sensitivity mechanism and, rather, suggests that efferent sympathetic outflow may have been elevated in the D group. However, we cannot determine the mechanism that resulted in prazosin showing a preferential decrease in MAP in the D group versus DX or C based on the data in this study. Yet, in line with the current results, such elevations in resting sympathetic activity would make activation of the BRS response to SNP-induced hypotension more difficult.

The conclusion above regarding sympathetic hyperactivity in the D group is supported by measurements of neuropeptide Y [NPY] obtained in this study. [NPY] is coreleased with norepinephrine from perivascular and cardiac sympathetic nerve terminals during sympathetic activation [78, 79]. In clinical T1DM, a diabetes-related decrease in [NPY] is attributed to impaired sympathetic function, whereas increased [NPY] is attributed to sympathetic overactivity [79–81]. In the current study, serum [NPY] was greater in both of the T1DM groups in comparison to their control groups. This finding is consistent with elevated sympathetic outflow in clinical T1DM [81]. Interestingly, no major impact of exercise was observed on serum [NPY]. Thus, despite the ability of exercise to preserve reflex cardiac function in T1DM, hyperglycemia itself appears to have impacted basal vascular adrenergic activity in both T1DM groups. This observation is consistent with the sympathoexcitatory effect of hyperglycemia [82]. As both T1DM groups were maintained at equally elevated [BG], there may have been a correspondingly similar stimulation of peripheral sympathetic activation and NPY release [79, 82, 83].

Despite improvements by exercise training to deficits of cardiovascular autonomic function, no observable statistical differences in either MAP or HR were evident between any of the groups. Indeed, it has been shown that alterations in autonomic function occur before or without alterations in MAP and HR and are uncorrelated to changes in sympathetic tone [84]. The observed changes in basal sympathetic activity may assist in the maintenance of blood pressure, ventricular function, and cardiac output during the early stage of diabetes, which is supported by our findings that inhibition of sympathetic activity results in a greater decrease in MAP in diabetic rats than normal rats [85]. In that respect, we previously reported that although T1DM animals demonstrated significant alterations in myocardial dimensions and structure, measurements of cardiac performance (ejection fraction, fractional shortening, and cardiac output measurements) were unchanged [44].

To evaluate the heart rate of these animals without neural influence, we measured the beat rate of denervated hearts using the isolated Langendorff technique. We found that the IHR of the D group was lower than both C and DX groups, which would support the notion that decreased IHR masked the effects of sympathetic overactivity in the current study. Further, it supports evidence that STZ-induced diabetes may have a direct effect on heart rate by modifying the heart itself [86, 87]. Interestingly, in some studies, insulin therapy was only able to partially reverse bradycardia and it was shown that STZ-treatment itself could lengthen the action potential duration in the SA node, slowing the HR [88]. However, if hyperglycemia or STZ directly affected cardiac muscle or the SA node and caused a decreased IHR in the D group, it is also the case that exercise training rescued or prevented the deficit, as the IHR of the DX group was not different from the CX group. Thus, previous experimental T1DM studies that reported that STZ-induced bradycardia and hypotension were caused by CAN, and that exercise-induced normalization of HR and BP was evidence of improvements in autonomic function, may really have been observing changes in intrinsic cardiac function which were independent of autonomic control. Such changes could instead have been due to depressed sarcoplasmic reticulum function or impaired calcium handling [87, 89, 90]. Therefore, the direct effects of STZ on the heart and IHR require further examination and should be taken into consideration in future studies that investigate the autonomic regulation of CV function in STZ-induced T1DM models.

An important consideration regarding the design of the current study was the use of anesthetized rats. In order to accurately reflect cardiovascular parameters in such a state, we selected an anaesthetic regime that provides the lowest level of influence on baseline and reflexive CV control attainable in rodent models [50]. A light plane anesthesia 0.5–1.2 g/kg has been shown to maintain the integrity of the cardiovascular system, where higher doses of urethane (above 1.5 g/kg) can produce hypotension and bradycardia, as well as high rates of mortality [91, 92]. In the current study we used a minimal dose of 25 mg/kg, which was reported in previous studies by our laboratory to have little influence on neurovascular blood flow measures [93–95]. That being said, it cannot be determined to what extent, if at all, the autonomic nervous system was augmented by the urethane-chloralose treatment in comparison to conscious animals. Further work examining a comparison of our anesthesia regime with freely moving conscious animals (using telemetry devices) will better address this matter.

5. Conclusions

In this study, T1DM induced indications of parasympathetic withdrawal, sympathetic overactivity, and, despite a decreased IHR, no change in resting MAP or HR. However, concurrent exercise training with T1DM maintained the sensitivity of the parasympathetically mediated baroreflex bradycardia, prevented an increase in vascular sympathetic tone, maintained a higher bodyweight, and prevented a decrease in IHR. The ability of exercise training to preserve parasympathetic function in this model of T1DM indicates that the exercise-mediated improvements to parasympathetic function are independent of alterations in [BG]. However, the finding that [NPY] remained elevated suggests that hyperglycemia has a direct impact on adrenergic activity. Taken together, our T1DM model of progressive STZ induction and insulin treatment induced autonomic impairments similar to those observed in clinical T1DM and demonstrates the novelty of this model for investigating the effectiveness of high intensity aerobic exercise training as a means to prevent the progression of CAN in T1DM. Thus, although not examined in this study, the mechanisms that underlie the physiological changes caused by T1DM and exercise can be the focus of future investigations using this model.

Abbreviations

BG: Blood glucose
BP: Blood pressure
BRS: Baroreflex sensitivity
C: Sedentary control
CAN: Cardiovascular autonomic neuropathy
CX: Exercised control
CV: Cardiovascular
D: Sedentary T1DM
DX: Exercised T1DM
HF: High frequency
HR: Heart rate
HRV: Heart rate variability
IHR: Intrinsic heart rate
MAP: Mean arterial pressure
NPY: Neuropeptide Y
PE: Phenylephrine
SBP: Systolic blood pressure
SNP: Sodium nitroprusside
SNS: Sympathetic nervous system
STZ: Streptozotocin
T1DM: Type 1 diabetes mellitus.

Conflict of Interests

The authors declare that there is no conflict of interests regarding the publication of this paper.

Authors' Contribution

Kenneth N. Grisé contributed to the study design, data collection, data analysis, and writing. T. Dylan Olver, Matthew W. McDonald, Adwitia Dey, and Mao Jiang contributed to the study design and data collection. James C. Lacefield and Earl G. Noble facilitated the data collection. J. Kevin Shoemaker provided data analysis and writing. C. W. James Melling contributed to the study design, data analysis, and writing.

Acknowledgments

This study was supported by the Canadian Institute of Health Research Grant (nos. CCT-83029 and 217532) and the Natural Sciences and Engineering Council Discovery Grant (RGPGP-2015-00059).

References

[1] A. I. Vinik, R. E. Maser, B. D. Mitchell, and R. Freeman, "Diabetic autonomic neuropathy," *Diabetes Care*, vol. 26, no. 5, pp. 1553–1579, 2003.

[2] S. V. P. Fazan, C. C. A. De Vasconcelos, M. M. Valencia, R. Nessler, and K. C. Moore, "Diabetic peripheral neuropathies: a morphometric overview," *International Journal of Morphology*, vol. 28, no. 1, pp. 51–64, 2010.

[3] M. Kuehl and M. J. Stevens, "Cardiovascular autonomic neuropathies as complications of diabetes mellitus," *Nature Reviews Endocrinology*, vol. 8, no. 7, pp. 405–416, 2012.

[4] R. E. Maser, B. D. Mitchell, A. I. Vinik, and R. Freeman, "The association between cardiovascular autonomic neuropathy and mortality in individuals with diabetes," *Diabetes Care*, vol. 26, no. 6, pp. 1895–1901, 2003.

[5] M. Lishner, S. Akselrod, V. M. Avi, O. Oz, M. Divon, and M. Ravid, "Spectral analysis of heart rate fluctuations. A non-invasive, sensitive method for the early diagnosis of autonomic neuropathy in diabetes mellitus," *Journal of the Autonomic Nervous System*, vol. 19, no. 2, pp. 119–125, 1987.

[6] A. Boysen, M. A. G. Lewin, W. Hecker, H. E. Leichter, and F. Uhlemann, "Autonomic function testing in children and adolescents with diabetes mellitus," *Pediatric Diabetes*, vol. 8, no. 5, pp. 261–264, 2007.

[7] Y. Li, "Cardiovascular autonomic dysfunction in diabetes as a complication: cellular and molecular mechanisms," in *Type 1 Diabetes Complications*, D. Wagner, Ed., 2011.

[8] H. C. Salgado, R. Fazan Júnior, V. P. Fazan, V. J. Da Silva, and A. A. Barreira, "Arterial baroreceptors and experimental diabetes," *Annals of the New York Academy of Sciences*, vol. 940, no. 55, pp. 20–27, 2001.

[9] Y.-L. Li, T. P. Tran, R. Muelleman, and H. D. Schultz, "Blunted excitability of aortic baroreceptor neurons in diabetic rats: involvement of hyperpolarization-activated channel," *Cardiovascular Research*, vol. 79, no. 4, pp. 715–721, 2008.

[10] C. Y. Maeda, T. G. Fernandes, H. B. Timm, and M. C. Irigoyen, "Autonomic dysfunction in short-term experimental diabetes," *Hypertension*, vol. 26, no. 6, part 2, pp. 1100–1104, 1995.

[11] D. D. Lund, A. R. Subieta, B. J. Pardini, and K. S. K. Chang, "Alterations in cardiac parasympathetic indices in STZ-induced diabetic rats," *Diabetes*, vol. 41, no. 2, pp. 160–166, 1992.

[12] H. Gu, P. N. Epstein, L. Li, R. D. Wurster, and Z. J. Cheng, "Functional changes in baroreceptor afferent, central and efferent components of the baroreflex circuitry in type 1 diabetic mice (OVE26)," *Neuroscience*, vol. 152, no. 3, pp. 741–752, 2008.

[13] H.-Y. Chen, J.-S. Wu, J.-J. Chen, and J.-T. Cheng, "Impaired regulation function in cardiovascular neurons of nucleus tractus solitarii in streptozotocin-induced diabetic rats," *Neuroscience Letters*, vol. 431, no. 2, pp. 161–166, 2008.

[14] M. Schönauer, A. Thomas, S. Morbach, J. Niebauer, U. Schönauer, and H. Thiele, "Cardiac autonomic diabetic neuropathy," *Diabetes & Vascular Disease Research*, vol. 5, no. 4, pp. 336–344, 2008.

[15] F. C. Howarth, M. Jacobson, O. Naseer, and E. Adeghate, "Short-term effects of streptozotocin-induced diabetes on the electrocardiogram, physical activity and body temperature in rats," *Experimental Physiology*, vol. 90, no. 2, pp. 237–245, 2005.

[16] B. D. Schaan, P. Dall'Ago, C. Y. Maeda et al., "Relationship between cardiovascular dysfunction and hyperglycemia in streptozotocin-induced diabetes in rats," *Brazilian Journal of Medical and Biological Research*, vol. 37, no. 12, pp. 1895–1902, 2004.

[17] B. Yang and K. H. Chon, "Assessment of diabetic cardiac autonomic neuropathy in type I diabetic mice," in *Proceedings of the Annual International Conference of the IEEE Engineering in Medicine and Biology Society (EMBC '11)*, pp. 6560–6563, Boston, Mass, USA, August 2011.

[18] S.-R. Chen, Y.-J. Lee, H.-W. Chiu, and C. Jeng, "Impact of physical activity on heart rate variability in children with type 1 diabetes," *Child's Nervous System*, vol. 24, no. 6, pp. 741–747, 2008.

[19] B. K. Pedersen and B. Saltin, "Evidence for prescribing exercise as therapy in chronic disease," *Scandinavian Journal of Medicine and Science in Sports*, vol. 16, supplement 1, pp. 3–63, 2006.

[20] H. Komine, J. Sugawara, K. Hayashi, M. Yoshizawa, and T. Yokoi, "Regular endurance exercise in young men increases arterial baroreflex sensitivity through neural alteration of baroreflex arc," *Journal of Applied Physiology*, vol. 106, no. 5, pp. 1499–1505, 2009.

[21] C. Mostarda, A. Rogow, I. C. M. Silva et al., "Benefits of exercise training in diabetic rats persist after three weeks of detraining," *Autonomic Neuroscience: Basic and Clinical*, vol. 145, no. 1-2, pp. 11–16, 2009.

[22] S. Golbidi, M. Badran, and I. Laher, "Antioxidant and anti-inflammatory effects of exercise in diabetic patients," *Experimental Diabetes Research*, vol. 2012, Article ID 941868, 16 pages, 2012.

[23] E. J. Henriksen and V. Saengsirisuwan, "Exercise training and antioxidants: relief from oxidative stress and insulin resistance," *Exercise and Sport Sciences Reviews*, vol. 31, no. 2, pp. 79–84, 2003.

[24] A. I. Vinik, R. E. Maser, and D. Ziegler, "Autonomic imbalance: prophet of doom or scope for hope?" *Diabetic Medicine*, vol. 28, no. 6, pp. 643–651, 2011.

[25] K. K. Hicks, E. Seifen, J. R. Stimers, and R. H. Kennedy, "Effects of streptozotocin-induced diabetes on heart rate, blood pressure and cardiac autonomic nervous control," *Journal of the Autonomic Nervous System*, vol. 69, no. 1, pp. 21–30, 1998.

[26] A. R. Lafferty, G. A. Werther, and C. F. Clarke, "Ambulatory blood pressure, microalbuminuria, and autonomic neuropathy in adolescents with type 1 diabetes," *Diabetes Care*, vol. 23, no. 4, pp. 533–538, 2000.

[27] J. J. Chillarón, M. P. Sales, J. A. Flores-Le-Roux et al., "Insulin resistance and hypertension in patients with type 1 diabetes," *Journal of Diabetes and its Complications*, vol. 25, no. 4, pp. 232–236, 2011.

[28] F. Collado-Mesa, H. M. Colhoun, L. K. Stevens et al., "Prevalence and management of hypertension in type 1 diabetes mellitus in Europe: the EURODIAB IDDM complications study," *Diabetic Medicine*, vol. 16, no. 1, pp. 41–48, 1999.

[29] P. Dall'Ago, V. O. K. Silva, K. L. D. De Angelis, M. C. Irigoyen, R. Fazan Jr., and H. C. Salgado, "Reflex control of arterial pressure and heart rate in short-term streptozotocin diabetic rats," *Brazilian Journal of Medical and Biological Research*, vol. 35, no. 7, pp. 843–849, 2002.

[30] R. Fazan Jr., G. Ballejo, M. C. O. Salgado, M. F. D. Moraes, and H. C. Salgado, "Heart rate variability and baroreceptor function in chronic diabetic rats," *Hypertension*, vol. 30, no. 3, part 2, pp. 632–635, 1997.

[31] K. C. Tomlinson, S. M. Gardiner, R. A. Hebden, and T. Bennett, "Functional consequences of streptozotocin-induced diabetes mellitus, with particular reference to the cardiovascular system," *Pharmacological Reviews*, vol. 44, no. 1, pp. 103–150, 1992.

[32] D. Lucini and M. Pagani, "Exercise: should it matter to internal medicine?" *European Journal of Internal Medicine*, vol. 22, no. 4, pp. 363–370, 2011.

[33] A. D. Harthmann, K. De Angelis, L. P. Costa et al., "Exercise training improves arterial baro- and chemoreflex in control and diabetic rats," *Autonomic Neuroscience*, vol. 133, no. 2, pp. 115–120, 2007.

[34] K. L. D. De Angelis, A. R. Oliveira, P. Dall'Ago et al., "Effects of exercise training on autonomic and myocardial dysfunction in streptozotocin-diabetic rats," *Brazilian Journal of Medical and Biological Research*, vol. 33, no. 6, pp. 635–641, 2000.

[35] Y. Harati, "Diabetic neuropathies: unanswered questions," *Neurologic Clinics*, vol. 25, no. 1, pp. 303–317, 2007.

[36] T. J. Orchard, C. E. Lloyd, R. E. Maser, and L. H. Kuller, "Why does diabetic autonomic neuropathy predict IDDM mortality? An analysis from the Pittsburgh Epidemiology of Diabetes Complications study," *Diabetes Research and Clinical Practice*, vol. 34, supplement 1, pp. S165–S171, 1996.

[37] K. L. De Angelis, B. D. Schaan, C. Y. Maeda, P. Dall'Ago, R. B. Wichi, and M. C. Irigoyen, "Cardiovascular control in experimental diabetes," *Brazilian Journal of Medical and Biological Research*, vol. 35, no. 9, pp. 1091–1100, 2002.

[38] G. Monckton and E. Pehowich, "Autonomic neuropathy in the streptozotocin diabetic rat," *Canadian Journal of Neurological Sciences*, vol. 7, no. 2, pp. 135–142, 1980.

[39] F. C. Howarth, M. Jacobson, M. Shafiullah, and E. Adeghate, "Long-term effects of streptozotocin-induced diabetes on the electrocardiogram, physical activity and body temperature in rats," *Experimental Physiology*, vol. 90, no. 6, pp. 827–835, 2005.

[40] W. H. Polonsky, C. L. Davis, A. M. Jacobson, and B. J. Anderson, "Hyperglycaemia, hypoglycaemia, and blood glucose control in diabetes: symptom perceptions and treatment strategies," *Diabetic Medicine*, vol. 9, no. 2, pp. 120–125, 1992.

[41] J. J. Valletta, A. J. Chipperfield, G. F. Clough, and C. D. Byrne, "Metabolic regulation during constant moderate physical exertion in extreme conditions in type 1 diabetes," *Diabetic Medicine*, vol. 29, no. 6, pp. 822–826, 2012.

[42] G. J. Taborsky and T. O. Mundinger, "Minireview: the role of the autonomic nervous system in mediating the glucagon response to hypoglycemia," *Endocrinology*, vol. 153, no. 3, pp. 1055–1062, 2012.

[43] D. J. Cox, L. A. Gonder-Frederick, J. A. Shepard, L. K. Campbell, and K. A. Vajda, "Driving safety: concerns and experiences of parents of adolescent drivers with type 1 diabetes," *Pediatric Diabetes*, vol. 13, no. 6, pp. 506–509, 2012.

[44] C. W. J. Melling, K. N. Grisé, C. P. Hasilo et al., "A model of poorly controlled type 1 diabetes mellitus and its treatment with aerobic exercise training," *Diabetes & Metabolism*, vol. 39, no. 3, pp. 226–235, 2013.

[45] K. E. Hall, M. W. McDonald, K. N. Grisé, O. Campos, E. G. Noble, and C. W. J. Melling, "he role of resistance and aerobic exercise training on insulin sensitivity measures in STZ-induced Type 1 diabetic rodents," *Metabolism*, vol. 62, no. 10, pp. 1485–1494, 2013.

[46] J. M. Murias, K. N. Grise, M. Jiang, H. Kowalchuk, C. W. J. Melling, and E. G. Noble, "Acute endurance exercise induces changes in vasorelaxation responses that are vessel-specific," *The American Journal of Physiology: Regulatory, Integrative and Comparative Physiology*, vol. 304, no. 7, pp. R574–R580, 2013.

[47] J. M. Murias, A. Dey, O. A. Campos et al., "High-intensity endurance training results in faster vessel-specific rate of vasorelaxation in type 1 diabetic rats," *PLoS One*, vol. 8, no. 3, Article ID e59678, 2013.

[48] T. G. Bedford, C. M. Tipton, N. C. Wilson, R. A. Oppliger, and C. V. Gisolfi, "Maximum oxygen consumption of rats and its changes with various experimental procedures," *Journal of Applied Physiology*, vol. 47, no. 6, pp. 1278–1283, 1979.

[49] B. Rodrigues, D. M. Figueroa, C. T. Mostarda, M. V. Heeren, M.-C. Irigoyen, and K. De Angelis, "Maximal exercise test is a useful method for physical capacity and oxygen consumption determination in streptozotocin-diabetic rats," *Cardiovascular Diabetology*, vol. 6, article 38, 2007.

[50] C. W. Usselman, L. Mattar, J. Twynstra, I. Welch, and J. K. Shoemaker, "Rodent cardiovascular responses to baroreceptor unloading: effect of plane of anaesthesia," *Applied Physiology, Nutrition and Metabolism*, vol. 36, no. 3, pp. 376–381, 2011.

[51] B. Gribbin, T. G. Pickering, P. Sleight, and R. Peto, "Effect of age and high blood pressure on barorefiex sensitivity in man," *Circulation Research*, vol. 29, no. 4, pp. 424–431, 1971.

[52] B. E. Hunt, L. Fahy, W. B. Farquhar, and A. Taylor J, "Quantification of mechanical and neural components of vagal baroreflex in humans," *Hypertension*, vol. 37, no. 6, pp. 1362–1368, 2001.

[53] L. Rudas, A. A. Crossman, C. A. Morillo, J. R. Halliwill, U. O. Kari, and T. A. Kuusela, "Human sympathetic and vagal baroreflex responses to sequential nitroprusside and phenylephrine," *The American Journal of Physiology—Heart and Circulatory Physiology*, vol. 76, no. 5, part 2, pp. H1691–H1698, 1999.

[54] P. Studinger, R. Goldstein, and J. A. Taylor, "Mechanical and neural contributions to hysteresis in the cardiac vagal limb of the arterial baroreflex," *The Journal of Physiology*, vol. 583, part 3, pp. 1041–1048, 2007.

[55] Z. Paroo, J. V. Haist, M. Karmazyn, and E. G. Noble, "Exercise improves postischemic cardiac function in males but not females: consequences of a novel sex-specific heat shock protein 70 response," *Circulation Research*, vol. 90, no. 8, pp. 911–917, 2002.

[56] G. Zoppini, V. Cacciatori, M. L. Gemma et al., "Effect of moderate aerobic exercise on sympatho-vagal balance in Type 2 diabetic patients," *Diabetic Medicine*, vol. 24, no. 4, pp. 370–376, 2007.

[57] S.-R. Chen, Y.-J. Lee, H.-W. Chiu, and C. Jeng, "Impact of glycemic control, disease duration, and exercise on heart rate

variability in children with type 1 diabetes mellitus," *Journal of the Formosan Medical Association*, vol. 106, no. 11, pp. 935–942, 2007.

[58] V. Gross, J. Tank, H.-J. Partke et al., "Cardiovascular autonomic regulation in Non-Obese Diabetic (NOD) mice," *Autonomic Neuroscience: Basic and Clinical*, vol. 138, no. 1-2, pp. 108–113, 2008.

[59] K. A. D. S. Silva, R. D. S. Luiz, R. R. Rampaso et al., "Previous exercise training has a beneficial effect on renal and cardiovascular function in a model of diabetes," *PLoS ONE*, vol. 7, no. 11, Article ID e48826, pp. 1–10, 2012.

[60] T. M. Murça, T. C. S. Almeida, M. K. Raizada, and A. J. Ferreira, "Chronic activation of endogenous angiotensin-converting enzyme 2 protects diabetic rats from cardiovascular autonomic dysfunction," *Experimental Physiology*, vol. 97, no. 6, pp. 699–709, 2012.

[61] L. Jorge, D. Y. da Pureza, D. da Silva Dias, F. F. Conti, M.-C. Irigoyen, and K. De Angelis, "Dynamic aerobic exercise induces baroreflex improvement in diabetic rats," *Experimental Diabetes Research*, vol. 2012, Article ID 108680, 5 pages, 2012.

[62] L.-Z. Hong, Y.-C. Chan, M.-F. Wang et al., "Modulation of baroreflex function by rosiglitazone in prediabetic hyperglycemic rats," *Physiological Research*, vol. 61, no. 5, pp. 443–452, 2012.

[63] A. I. Vinik and D. Ziegler, "Diabetic cardiovascular autonomic neuropathy," *Circulation*, vol. 115, no. 3, pp. 387–397, 2007.

[64] D. Ziegler, "Diabetic cardiovascular autonomic neuropathy: prognosis, diagnosis and treatment," *Diabetes/Metabolism Reviews*, vol. 10, no. 4, pp. 339–383, 1994.

[65] K. S. Chang and D. D. Lund, "Alterations in the baroreceptor reflex control of heart rate in streptozotocin diabetic rats," *Journal of Molecular and Cellular Cardiology*, vol. 18, no. 6, pp. 617–624, 1986.

[66] R. Pop-Busui, P. A. Low, B. H. Waberski et al., "Effects of prior intensive insulin therapy on cardiac autonomic nervous system function in type 1 diabetes mellitus: the diabetes control and complications trial/epidemiology of diabetes interventions and complications study (DCCT/EDIC)," *Circulation*, vol. 119, no. 22, pp. 2886–2893, 2009.

[67] G. Tancrede, S. Rousseau-Migneron, and A. Nadeau, "Beneficial effects of physical training in rats with a mild streptozotocin-induced diabetes mellitus," *Diabetes*, vol. 31, no. 5, part 1, pp. 406–409, 1982.

[68] J. A. Wegner, D. D. Lund, J. M. Overton, J. G. Edwards, R. P. Oda, and C. M. Tipton, "Select cardiovascular and metabolic responses of diabetic rats to moderate exercise training.," *Medicine & Science in Sports & Exercise*, vol. 19, no. 5, pp. 497–503, 1987.

[69] S. Chipkinn, S. Klugh, and L. Chasan-Taber, "Exercise and diabetes," *Cardiology Clinics*, vol. 19, no. 3, pp. 489–505, 2001.

[70] A. Tura, S. Sbrignadello, E. Succurro, L. Groop, G. Sesti, and G. Pacini, "An empirical index of insulin sensitivity from short IVGTT: validation against the minimal model and glucose clamp indices in patients with different clinical characteristics," *Diabetologia*, vol. 53, no. 1, pp. 144–152, 2010.

[71] R. G. Hahn, S. Ljunggren, F. Larsen, and T. Nyström, "A simple intravenous glucose tolerance test for assessment of insulin sensitivity," *Theoretical Biology and Medical Modelling*, vol. 8, no. 1, article 12, 2011.

[72] J. Paulson, J. Dennis, R. Mathews, and J. Bow, "Metabolic effects of treadmill exercise training on the diabetic heart," *Journal of Applied Physiology*, vol. 73, no. 1, pp. 265–271, 1992.

[73] T. L. Broderick, P. Poirier, and M. Gillis, "Exercise training restores abnormal myocardial glucose utilization and cardiac function in diabetes," *Diabetes/Metabolism Research and Reviews*, vol. 21, no. 1, pp. 44–50, 2005.

[74] L. Bernardi, M. Rosengård-Bärlund, A. Sandelin, V. P. Mäkinen, C. Forsblom, and P.-H. Groop, "Short-term oxygen administration restores blunted baroreflex sensitivity in patients with type 1 diabetes," *Diabetologia*, vol. 54, no. 8, pp. 2164–2173, 2011.

[75] I. Rodríguez-Gómez, Y. Baca, J. M. Moreno et al., "Role of sympathetic tone in BSO-induced hypertension in mice," *American Journal of Hypertension*, vol. 23, no. 8, pp. 882–888, 2010.

[76] D. S. DeLorey, J. B. Buckwalter, S. W. Mittelstadt, M. M. Anton, H. A. Kluess, and P. S. Clifford, "Is tonic sympathetic vasoconstriction increased in the skeletal muscle vasculature of aged canines?" *The American Journal of Physiology—Regulatory Integrative and Comparative Physiology*, vol. 299, no. 5, pp. R1342–R1349, 2010.

[77] B. Martinez-Nieves and J. Dunbar, "Vascular dilatatory responses to sodium nitroprusside (SNP) and alpha-adrenergic antagonism in female and male normal and diabetic rats," *Proceedings of the Society for Experimental Biology and Medicine*, vol. 222, no. 2, Article ID 44433, pp. 90–98, 1999.

[78] J. M. Lundberg, A. Franco-Cereceda, J. S. Lacroix, and J. Pernow, "Neuropeptide Y and sympathetic neurotransmission," *Annals of the New York Academy of Sciences*, vol. 611, pp. 166–174, 1990.

[79] C. Wahlestedt, R. Hakanson, C. A. Vaz, and Z. Zukowska-Grojec, "Norepinephrine and neuropeptide Y: vasoconstrictor cooperation in vivo and in vitro," *The American Journal of Physiology—Regulatory Integrative and Comparative Physiology*, vol. 258, no. 3, pp. R736–R742, 1990.

[80] A. Ejaz, F. W. LoGerfo, and L. Pradhan, "Diabetic neuropathy and heart failure: role of neuropeptides," *Expert Reviews in Molecular Medicine*, vol. 13, article e26, 2011.

[81] P. C. Perin, S. Maule, and R. Quadri, "Sympathetic nervous system, diabetes, and hypertension," *Clinical and Experimental Hypertension*, vol. 23, no. 1-2, pp. 45–55, 2001.

[82] S. Villafaña, F. Huang, and E. Hong, "Role of the sympathetic and renin angiotensin systems in the glucose-induced increase of blood pressure in rats," *European Journal of Pharmacology*, vol. 506, no. 2, pp. 143–150, 2004.

[83] D. Giugliano, R. Marfella, L. Coppola et al., "Vascular effects of acute hyperglycemia in humans are reversed by L-arginine. Evidence for reduced availability of nitric oxide during hyperglycemia," *Circulation*, vol. 95, no. 7, pp. 1783–1790, 1997.

[84] M. Pagani, G. Malfatto, S. Pierini et al., "Spectral analysis of heart rate variability in the assessment of autonomic diabetic neuropathy," *Journal of the Autonomic Nervous System*, vol. 23, no. 2, pp. 143–153, 1988.

[85] L. Zhang, X.-Q. Xiong, Z.-D. Fan, X.-B. Gan, X.-Y. Gao, and G.-Q. Zhu, "Involvement of enhanced cardiac sympathetic afferent reflex in sympathetic activation in early stage of diabetes," *Journal of Applied Physiology*, vol. 113, no. 1, pp. 47–55, 2012.

[86] M. A. Malone, D. D. Schocken, S. K. Hanna, X. Liang, and J. I. Malone, "Diabetes-induced bradycardia is an intrinsic metabolic defect reversed by carnitine," *Metabolism*, vol. 56, no. 8, pp. 1118–1123, 2007.

[87] S. Penpargkul, F. Fein, E. Sonnenblick, and J. Scheur, "Sarcoplasmic from diabetic reticular rats function," *Journal of Molecular and Cellular Cardiology*, vol. 13, no. 3, pp. 303–309, 1981.

[88] F. C. Howarth, R. Al-Sharhan, A. Al-Hammadi, and M. A. Qureshi, "Effects of streptozotocin-induced diabetes on action

potentials in the sinoatrial node compared with other regions of the rat heart," *Molecular and Cellular Biochemistry*, vol. 300, no. 1-2, pp. 39–46, 2007.

[89] P. K. Ganguly, G. N. Pierce, K. S. Dhalla, and N. S. Dhalla, "Defective sarcoplasmic reticular calcium transport in diabetic cardiomyopathy," *The American Journal of Physiology*, vol. 244, no. 6, pp. E528–E535, 1983.

[90] L. Ligeti, O. Szenczi, C. M. Prestia et al., "Altered calcium handling is an early sign of streptozotocin-induced diabetic cardiomyopathy," *International Journal of Molecular Medicine*, vol. 17, no. 6, pp. 1035–1043, 2006.

[91] W. B. Severs, L. C. Keil, P. A. Klase, and K. C. Deen, "Urethane anesthesia in rats. Altered ability to regulate hydration," *Pharmacology*, vol. 22, no. 4, pp. 209–226, 1981.

[92] K. J. Field, W. J. White, and C. M. Lang, "Anaesthetic effects of chloral hydrate, pentobarbitone and urethane in adult male rats," *Laboratory Animals*, vol. 27, no. 3, pp. 258–269, 1993.

[93] T. D. Olver, M. W. McDonald, K. N. Grisé, A. Dey, M. D. Allen, P. J. Medeiros et al., "Exercise training enhances insulin-stimulated nerve arterial vasodilation in rats with insulin-treated experimental diabetes," *The American Journal of Physiology: Regulatory, Integrative and Comparative Physiology*, vol. 306, no. 12, pp. R941–R950, 2014.

[94] T. D. Olver, L. Mattar, K. N. Grise et al., "Glucose-stimulated insulin secretion causes an insulin-dependent nitric oxide-mediated vasodilation in the blood supply of the rat sciatic nerve," *The American Journal of Physiology: Regulatory, Integrative and Comparative Physiology*, vol. 305, no. 2, pp. R157–R163, 2013.

[95] T. D. Olver, K. N. Grisé, M. W. McDonald, A. Dey, M. D. Allen, C. L. Rice et al., "The relationship between blood pressure and sciatic nerve blood flow velocity in rats with insulin-treated experimental diabetes," *Diabetes and Vascular Disease Research*, vol. 11, no. 4, pp. 281–289, 2014.

9

The Nrf2/Keap1/ARE Pathway and Oxidative Stress as a Therapeutic Target in Type II Diabetes Mellitus

Joshua A. David, William J. Rifkin, Piul S. Rabbani, and Daniel J. Ceradini

Hansjörg Wyss Department of Plastic and Reconstructive Surgery, New York University School of Medicine, 430 East 29th Street, New York, NY 10016, USA

Correspondence should be addressed to Daniel J. Ceradini; daniel.ceradini@nyumc.org

Academic Editor: Joseph F. Ndisang

Despite improvements in awareness and treatment of type II diabetes mellitus (TIIDM), this disease remains a major source of morbidity and mortality worldwide, and prevalence continues to rise. Oxidative damage caused by free radicals has long been known to contribute to the pathogenesis and progression of TIIDM and its complications. Only recently, however, has the role of the Nrf2/Keap1/ARE master antioxidant pathway in diabetic dysfunction begun to be elucidated. There is accumulating evidence that this pathway is implicated in diabetic damage to the pancreas, heart, and skin, among other cell types and tissues. Animal studies and clinical trials have shown promising results suggesting that activation of this pathway can delay or reverse some of these impairments in TIIDM. In this review, we outline the role of oxidative damage and the Nrf2/Keap1/ARE pathway in TIIDM, focusing on current and future efforts to utilize this relationship as a therapeutic target for prevention, prognosis, and treatment of TIID.

1. Introduction

The worldwide prevalence of diabetes mellitus (DM) was estimated at 8.5% in 2014, and the morbidity resulting from the microvascular and macrovascular complications of this disease is enormous [1]. Costs attributable to DM in 2013 were $101.4 billion in the United States alone, making it the most expensive medical condition by a significant margin [2–4]. The chronic hyperglycemia and impairments in insulin secretion and action that characterize type II diabetes mellitus (TIIDM) are associated with long-term damage, dysfunction, and failure of many organs, including the eyes, kidneys, nerves, heart, and blood vessels [5]. Decades of scientific research, randomized human trials, and clinical experience have demonstrated that a combination of lifestyle modifications and pharmaceutical interventions has the capacity to prevent or delay the onset of TIIDM and many of its devastating complications [6]. Consequently, major therapeutic advances, coupled with increased diabetes awareness and the implementation of national programs and guidelines for diabetes prevention, have helped alleviate disease-related morbidity and mortality [7]. Despite these improvements, this disease continues to pose a tremendous burden in the US, and the prevalence, deaths, and costs attributable to TIIDM are expected to continue increasing drastically [8]. As we gain further insight into the molecular underpinnings of this disease and its destructive sequelae, we advance the opportunity to develop novel, targeted approaches for diabetes treatment, prognosis, and, ultimately, prevention. In recent years, the Nrf2/Keap1/ARE antioxidant pathway has emerged as one such promising avenue of research. In this review, we summarize the roles of oxidative stress and the Nrf2/Keap1/ARE pathway in TIIDM, as well as the current state of efforts aimed at exploiting this relationship in order to minimize the devastating impact of this disease across the globe.

2. Oxidative Stress and Diabetes Mellitus

Oxidative stress occurs when free radical production overwhelms the endogenous antioxidant ability to neutralize these highly reactive chemical compounds. The ensuing cellular damage, such as DNA cross-linking and apoptosis, is a hallmark of oxidative stress and is a fundamental pathological process in cancer, aging, and a variety of chronic diseases [9–12]. In TIIDM, dysfunctional redox homeostasis has long been known to play a role in the pathogenesis of the disease and its complications through a variety of mechanisms, and diabetic patients have been shown to possess increased cellular levels of reactive oxygen species (ROS) and ROS-induced DNA damage [13–15]. Landmark studies by Giacco and Brownlee showed that the increased glycemic load in diabetes overwhelms the Krebs cycle, resulting in the inhibition of election transfer within the mitochondrial membrane and the accumulation of free radicals [14]. In particular, these free radicals include the highly reactive superoxide and hydroxyl compounds [16]. As ROS production increases, upregulation of four biochemical pathways occurs: polyol flux, intracellular advanced glycosylation end product (AGE) formation, protein kinase C activation, and hexosamine pathway flux [14]. These perturbations result in a variety of downstream effects known to underlie the pathogenesis and progression of TIIDM, including the depletion of natural antioxidant molecules and damage to vascular cells, as well as alterations in gene and protein expression, blood flow, and endothelial cell permeability [13, 17, 18].

3. The Nrf2/Keap1/ARE Pathway

Knowledge of the relationship between oxidative stress and TIIDM has precipitated intense investigation into the failure of the diabetic system to appropriately respond to increased oxidative loads. Regulation of cellular redox homeostasis under both stressed and nonstressed conditions occurs primarily at the transcriptional level, and the Nrf2/Keap1/ARE pathway is the primary mediator of this response. This signaling pathway regulates the expression of over 100 genes and functions related to oxidative stress and cell survival, including direct antioxidant proteins, phase I and II electrophile detoxification enzymes, the transport of toxic solutes, free radical metabolism, inhibition of inflammation, glutathione homeostasis, proteasome function, and the recognition of DNA damage, as well as the expression of various related growth factors and transcription factors [19] (Figure 1).

The principal mediator of this response is nuclear factor E2-related factor 2 (Nrf2), a master transcription factor. Upon binding the upstream cis-regulatory antioxidant response element (ARE) sequence located in the promoter regions of cytoprotective genes, Nrf2 triggers the transcriptional induction of multiple detoxifying enzymes [20]. Under nonstressed conditions, Nrf2 activity is suppressed by its native repressor Kelch-like ECH-associated protein 1 (Keap1), through interactions with a hairpin motif in the C terminus of the Nrf2-ECH homologous domain (Neh2) phosphorylation site on Nrf2. Keap1 is a cytoplasmic, actin cytoskeleton-associated adapter protein of the Cullin3-(Cul3-) based E3-ligase complex, which tags Nrf2 for ubiquitination and subsequent proteosomal degradation within the cytoplasm [21]. This signaling pathway has been established as the major mechanism of cellular defense against oxidative stress both physiologically and in a wide array of disease models [19]. First isolated in cloning studies in 1994 [22], the critical role of Nrf2, a member of the cap'n'collar family of basic leucine zipper transcription factors, in both constitutive and inducible ARE gene expression was soon elucidated both *in vitro* [23] and *in vivo* [20, 21, 24]. The precise molecular mechanisms of Nrf2 and Keap1 interaction are a topic of debate, particularly given the distinct subcellular locations of these two molecules [25]. It is nonetheless understood that modification of cysteine residues in the primary structure of Keap1, which act as cellular sensors for inducers of environmental stress, by thiol-reactive chemical species during states of excess oxidative or electrophilic stress results in the disruption of the Nrf2-Keap1 dimer and stabilization of Nrf2 [26]. Nrf2, once stabilized, is no longer repressed by Keap1 and becomes free to heterodimerize with members of the Maf family of transcription factors. With the assistance of a nuclear localization sequence, the Nrf2 heterodimer can rapidly translocate into the nucleus and bind to the ARE, resulting in the recruitment of elements required for the transcriptional activation of a variety of genes such as glutathione S-transferase A2 (GSTA2), NADPH quinone oxidoreductase (NQO-1), superoxide dismutase (SOD1), and heme oxygenase-1 (Ho-1) [19, 20, 27]. These antioxidant enzymes function to transform free radicals into less toxic substances through four primary mechanisms: (1) oxidation and reduction reactions, in which functional groups on hydrophobic molecules are exposed, (2) nucleophilic trapping processes, (3) transporter efflux of toxic metabolites, and (4) maintenance of reduced conditions by thiol-containing molecules [19, 28]. This protective stress recognition mechanism by Keap1 dually ensures suppression of Nrf2 during nonstressed conditions and an appropriate antioxidant response during periods of excessive cellular stress.

Given the intimate relationship between TIIDM and oxidative damage, the involvement of the Nrf2/Keap1/ARE pathway in this unsolved clinical problem has become a topic of great interest. We now know that dysfunction of this master antioxidant pathway is associated with the pathophysiology of diabetes and a wide range of its complications, such as diabetic nephropathy and impaired cutaneous wound healing, in both animal and human models [29–31] (Figure 2).

While the mechanism or mechanisms of this dysfunction in diabetes have only begun to be elucidated, therapies targeting the Nrf2/Keap1/ARE pathway represent a promising avenue in current research. As a critical upstream mediator of not only the global antioxidant response but also of anti-inflammatory genes and transcription factors involved in mitochondrial function, the Nrf2/Keap1/ARE pathway represents an ideal target in treating the widespread oxidative damage implicated in pancreatic damage, insulin resistance and sensitivity, and the progression of a broad spectrum of diabetic complications. Additionally, the inducible nature of this signaling pathway allows Keap1 to uniquely both sense the cellular redox state and responsively modify the degree of Nrf2 degradation via ubiquitination in response to this oxidative stress. This allows for modulation of cellular redox homeostasis via highly specific transcriptional activation of only those genes containing an ARE in the promoter region [32]. Furthermore, the Nrf2-mediated oxidative response may also possess aspects that are specific to diabetes. The activation of the aforementioned pathways underlying the

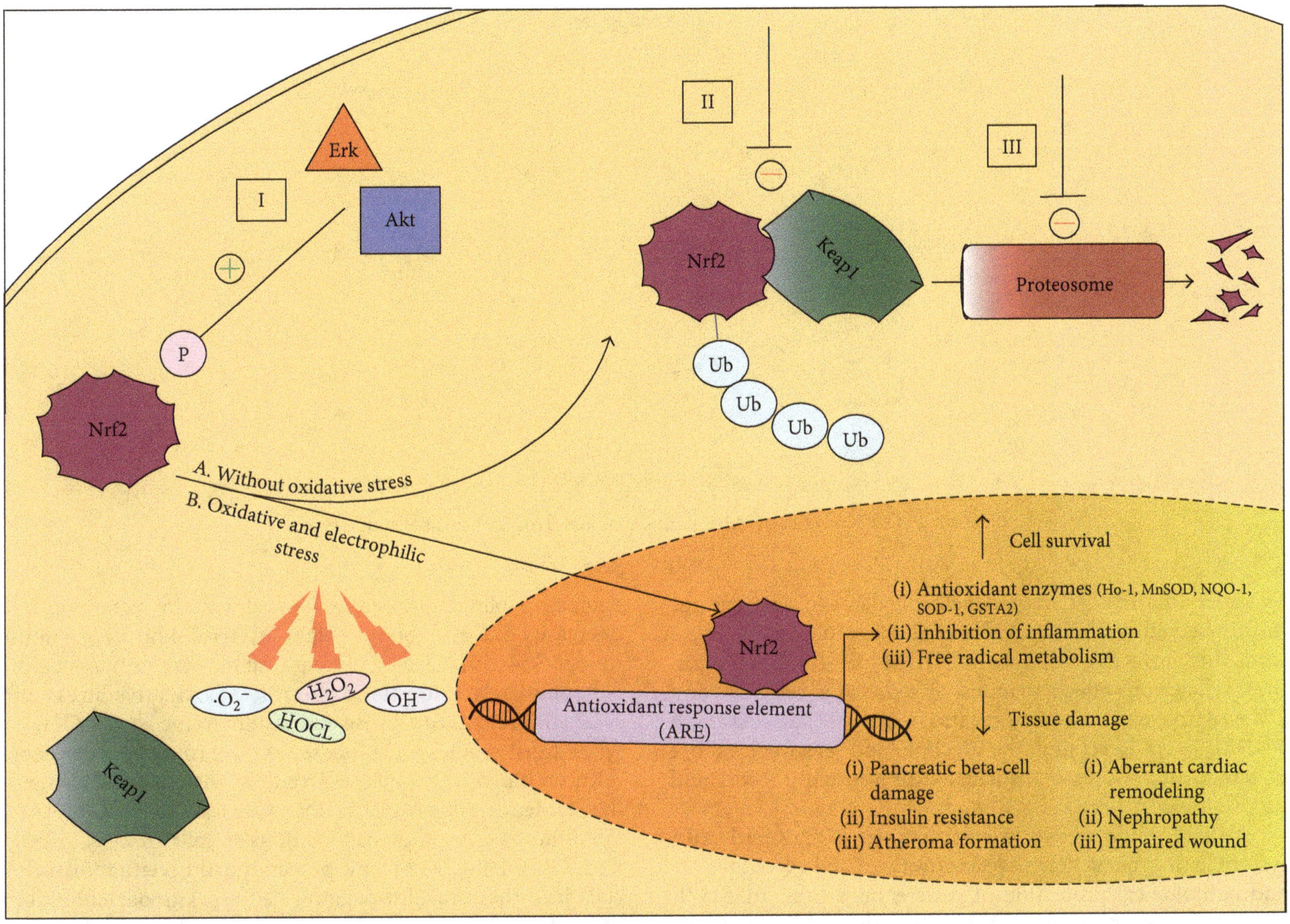

Figure 1: The Nrf2/Keap1/ARE pathway in type II diabetes mellitus. (A) Under nonstressed conditions, the Nrf2 transcription factor is covalently bound to cysteine residues on its native repressor Keap1 in the cytoplasm. This results in the constitutive ubiquitination and degradation of Nrf2 in the proteasome and inhibition of the anti-oxidant response. (B) Under conditions of electrophilic or oxidative stress, cysteine residues on Keap1 are modified, resulting in the stabilization and translocation of Nrf2 into the nucleus, where it can bind to the promoter region of the ARE and initiate the transcription of various cytoprotective enzymes which function to promote cellular survival through a variety of mechanisms, including the upregulation of antioxidant function, inflammatory inhibition, and the transport of toxic metabolites. These cellular adaptations have been shown to improve a wide array of tissue damage underlying the pathogenesis and progression of diabetes. (B) There are three major mechanisms of Nrf2 induction by small molecule activators. (I) Upstream kinases such as Akt and Erk phosphorylate Nrf2 at specific sites, favoring its release by Keap1 and nuclear translocation. (II) Modification of Keap1 cysteine residues disrupts the Nrf2-Keap1 complex, favoring dissociation of Nrf2 and subsequent nuclear translocation. (III) Inhibition of Nrf2 ubiquitination by Keap1 and degradation by the proteasome augments Nrf2 availability, thus favoring nuclear translocation of Nrf2. Ub: ubiquitination; P: phosphorylation.

pathogenesis of diabetic complications has been tied to a singular hyperglycemia-induced event in the mitochondria, overproduction of superoxide by the electron-transport chain [13]. Furthermore, studies have shown that the absence of Nrf2 may exacerbate both type I and type II diabetes [33, 34]. This hyperglycemia-specific increase in ROS overproduction by the mitochondria may explain why classic antioxidants, low molecular-weight compounds that can scavenge reactive oxygen intermediates, have not been proven beneficial in the treatment of diabetic complications. In contrast to these classic or direct antioxidants, the battery of cytoprotective agents that are upregulated by the Nrf2/Keap1/ARE pathway have been termed "ultimate antioxidants," which possess long half-lives, are not depleted throughout the course of their wide range of chemical detoxification reactions, and can even accelerate regeneration of other antioxidants, such as glutathione [35]. Lastly, the ability to target this pathway at a variety of locations, as will be discussed later, grants an incredibly rich degree of flexibility and diversity as the search for rational and clinically relevant therapeutics evolves.

4. Nrf2/Keap1/ARE and the β-Cell

Pancreatic β-cell dysfunction and the resulting impairments in insulin sensitivity and production are a critical component in the development and progression of both type I and type II DM [36], and oxidative stress is one important mechanism whereby this damage occurs [37]. Despite overexpression of Nrf2 downstream endogenous antioxidant genes by the

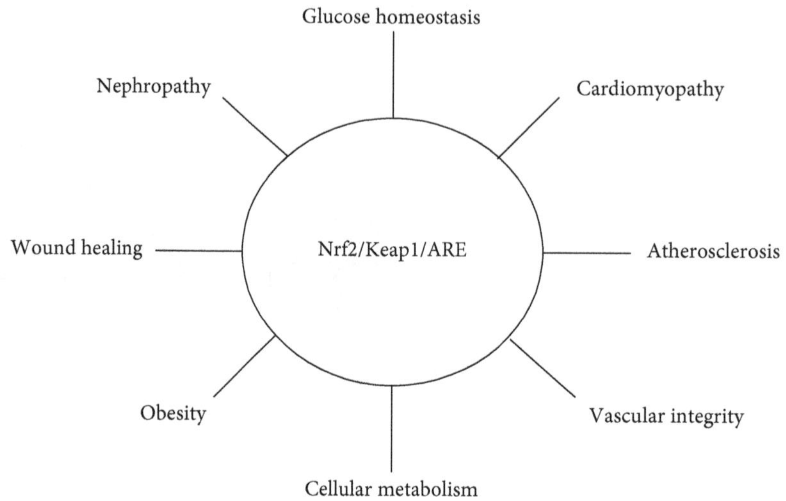

Figure 2: The Nrf2/Keap1/ARE pathway is involved in multiple tissue types.

pancreas in order to curtail cellular damage and salvage insulin-secreting ability, oxidative damage ultimately overloads this protective response in TIIDM [38–40]. In humans, these deleterious effects manifest as reduced β-cell mass and DNA damage in the pancreatic islets of patients with TIIDM [41]. Reversing the decline and eventual failure of pancreatic β-cells is critical for preventing TIIDM and its progression [42].

Animal studies have shown that the Nrf2/Keap1/ARE system is a crucial defensive pathway in the physiological and pathological protection of pancreatic β-cells. In β-cell-specific transgenic mice, Nrf2 depletion depressed the expression of cytoprotective antioxidant genes in pancreatic islets and exacerbated oxidative β-cell damage, while Nrf2 induction suppressed the accumulation of intracellular ROS, the formation of ROS-induced DNA adducts, and pancreatic β-cell apoptosis within the islets [43]. Further studies showed the preservation of β-cell mass and function in diabetic mice with genetically modified upregulation of Nrf2 via Keap1 knockout [44]. Pancreatic β-cell protection by the Nrf2/Keap1/ARE system is not limited to free radical scavenge but includes reduction of inflammation via the NF-kappaB pathway [45] and maintenance of critical cellular degradation systems such as apoptosis, autophagy, and proteosomal degradation [46, 47].

In addition to β-cell injury, oxidative stress also affects pancreatic insulin secretion, although this relationship is less clear. While some studies show that ROS impairs insulin release through mechanisms such as a reduction in ATP production [48] and increased glyceraldehyde 3-phosphate dehydrogenase (GAPDH) activity [49], there is a growing body of evidence indicating that oxidative and electrophilic stress can actually augment, and may even be necessary for, insulin release [50, 51]. The role of the Nrf2/Keap1/ARE pathway in insulin secretion is similarly controversial. While insulin content and secretion are decreased in the pancreatic islets of Nrf2 knockout mice and upregulation of Nrf2 appears to improve the insulin-releasing potential of β-cells [44, 52, 53], Nrf2 deficiency has also been associated with decreased blood glucose, enhanced insulin signaling, and decreased fat and body weight in Nrf2 knockout mouse models [54–57]. Clearly, a great deal of work remains before we completely understand the role of oxidative stress and Nrf2 with regard to glucose and insulin homeostasis. Of note, while most studies have focused on the role of Nrf2/Keap1/ARE on glucose and insulin handling within β-cells, emerging evidence suggests that this pathway may also play a dynamic role in other pancreatic islet cells (α-cells, δ-cells, and PP-cells), possibly by preventing differentiation of β-cells into these insulin-negative cell types under conditions of oxidative stress [58].

5. Nrf2 and Insulin Resistance

In addition to β-cell dysfunction, insulin resistance in a wide range of tissues is a hallmark of TIIDM, resulting in elevated blood glucose levels and exacerbation of pancreatic damage as it attempts to compensate for perceived hypoglycemia. Studies by Uruno et al. in murine models of Nrf2 overexpression via both genetic Keap1 knockdown and pharmacological induction suggest that Nrf2 activation can improve insulin sensitivity in diabetes and abrogate diabetes and obesity in mice [44]. Body weight and blood glucose levels were decreased in diabetic mice with Keap1 knockout. These findings were attributed to Nrf2-mediated stimulation of energy consumption in skeletal muscle and brown adipose tissue. Further studies showed that Nrf2 induction in mice also suppressed gluconeogenesis, owing to transcriptional repression of a variety of enzymes including the gluconeogenic enzyme glucose-6-phosphatase (G-6-P). *In vitro* studies using murine hepatocytes confirmed that Nrf2 attenuates G-6-P expression in these cells, despite stimulation of gluconeogenesis using a cAMP analog. In addition to its inhibitory effect on G-6-P, Nrf2 was shown to decrease expression of other genes related to gluconeogenesis, as well as augment insulin sensitivity in an insulin tolerance test. A more recent study in a murine model suggests that increased Nrf2 signaling may also improve insulin resistance via suppression of oxidative stress

TABLE 1: Nrf2/Keap1/ARE and diabetic complications.

Diabetic complication	Pathogenesis	Nrf2- (or downstream-) mediated effects
Atherosclerosis	(i) oxLDL formation (ii) Proinflammatory response in endothelial cells	(i) Protection from oxLDL transformation of phagocytic cells [77, 78] (ii) Inhibition of proinflammatory response at atherosusceptible sites [71, 79]
Heart failure	(i) Aberrant cardiac and ECM remodeling (ii) Insulin resistance of myocytes (iii) Impaired regulation of intracellular calcium (iv) Accumulation of AGE products	(i) Blood pressure regulation [72] (ii) Protection of myocardium following ischemia (iii) Diminishes ROS and myocardial hypertrophy [99]
Diabetic nephropathy	(i) Renal oxidative and nitrosative stress (ii) Mesangial cell proliferation, inflammation, fibrosis	(i) Improvement of metabolic indices (e.g., polydipsia and polyuria) [110] (ii) Reversal in dysfunction of key growth factors and ECM proteins [111–113]
Wound healing	(i) Keap1 overexpression (ii) Loss of wound redox homeostasis (iii) Chronic inflammatory microenvironment	(i) Impairments in angiogenesis and reepithelialization [120]

in the hypothalamus, a phenomenon that may affect systemic metabolic regulation [59]. Furthermore, obesity is associated with an increased risk of developing insulin resistance and TIIDM, and murine studies have likewise shown that Nrf2 induction can suppress weight gain and increase skeletal muscle oxygen consumption, mitochondrial redox homeostasis, and ATP production, as well as augment cellular glucose uptake [44, 60, 61].

6. Diabetic Complications (Table 1)

6.1. Cardiovascular Disease. The absolute risk of cardiovascular disease (CVD) is 2-fold greater in patients with TIIDM versus those without, and at least 65% of people with DM die of heart disease or stroke [3, 62]. Given this close link between TIIDM and CVD, it is not surprising that oxidative stress has been implicated in the pathogenesis of many CVD disorders, including hypertension [63], heart failure (HF) [64], atherosclerosis [65], and ischemia-reperfusion injury [66]. Free radical-induced endothelial damage is thought to be the initiating step in CVD [67], and hyperglycemia-induced ROS in TIIDM exacerbates impairments in angiogenesis and neovascularization through means such as disruption of endothelial progenitor cell function and vascular homeostasis [68, 69]. The importance of Nrf2 and its downstream elements to vascular integrity has also become increasingly apparent, and studies have illuminated their role in functions such as augmentation of blood vessel branching [70], preservation of endothelial cell function [71], blood pressure regulation [72], and protection of the myocardium following ischemia [73, 74]. In particular, evidence of Ho-1, the Nrf2 downstream enzyme that catalyzes the degradation of heme into biliverdin, ferrous iron, and carbon monoxide, as an important mediator against vascular dysfunction in diabetes has recently emerged. Upregulation of Ho-1 levels was shown to improve left ventricular ejection fraction and inhibit remodeling in diabetic rats with myocardial infarction, and *in vivo* and *in vitro* studies demonstrated that Ho-1 overexpression attenuated angiotensin II-mediated cardiac hypertrophy in these mice [74]. Studies in streptozotocin-induced diabetic mice suggest that these effects are due to reductions in oxidative stress, inflammation, and apoptosis [75]. Therefore, the likely link among ROS and the Nrf2/Keap1/ARE pathway to the plethora of CVD-related complications that afflict diabetic patients has emerged as a subject of intense investigation.

6.2. Atherosclerosis. Nrf2 has been implicated in a variety of processes intrinsic to the formation of atherosclerotic plaque. As an indispensable component of the antioxidant response within macrophages [76], Nrf2 protects these phagocytic cells from oxidized low-density lipoproteins (oxLDL) and foam cell transformation, fundamental steps in atheroma formation [77, 78]. Additionally, Nrf2 appears to inhibit the proinflammatory response in endothelial cells located at atherosusceptible sites, conferring them a protective advantage in response to diabetic hyperglycemia [71, 79]. The significance of these effects is largely attributed to the downstream activation of the Nrf2 downstream antioxidant enzyme HO-1, which has been independently found to play a significant defensive role against atherosclerosis [80]. However, there are also studies suggesting that Nrf2 can promote atheroma formation, possibly due to interactions with a variety of well-described proatherogenic factors such as vascular cell adhesion molecule 1 (VCAM-1) and interleukin-1 (IL-1) [81–83]. For instance, overexpression of Ho-1 was found to be associated with worsening coronary atherosclerosis in an autopsy study of Japanese patients with diabetes mellitus [84]. This seeming contradiction might be explained by a differential response of Nrf2 to laminar versus oscillatory blood flow, as atheroma formation is not uniform throughout the vascular system but rather disposed to bifurcation and branch points [85]. Regardless, mounting evidence of the importance of Nrf2 for vascular integrity and long-term endothelial function suggests that the Nrf2/Keap1/ARE pathway is influential in atherosclerotic resistance and may be a useful target for protection against coronary artery disease (CAD), peripheral vascular disease, and cerebrovascular disease in diabetic populations.

6.3. Heart Failure. Not only is there a well-established association between TIIDM and the development of HF, but this relationship also persists even in the absence of other risk factors such as CAD or hypertension, suggesting that TIIDM may mediate an exclusive form of cardiomyopathy [86]. Multiple mechanisms, such as impaired regulation of intracellular calcium and accumulation of AGE products, have been suggested to underlie this dysfunction, all of which ultimately result in oxidative stress and myocardial toxicity [87]. Not surprisingly, ROS and mitochondrial dysfunction are increased in the diabetic heart [64]. The resulting cardiac cellular necrosis and apoptosis impair contractile and electrical function, two contributing features of HF [88–90]. In addition to causing cellular damage, ROS can modify proteins essential in excitation-contraction coupling [91], activate hypertrophy-signaling kinases [92], and stimulate cardiac extracellular matrix (ECM) remodeling [93]. Furthermore, ROS exacerbates insulin resistance of myocytes, a key element of diabetes-induced cardiac dysfunction [94].

Evidence that aberrant cardiac remodeling is attenuated by a variety of Nrf2 target genes such as SOD [95], HO-1 [96] and glutathione peroxidase (GPx) [97] has motivated investigation into a possible protective role of the Nrf2/Keap1/ARE pathway against cardiomyopathy in DM. In murine models of HF and TIIDM, oxidative stress attenuates the expression of Nrf2 in cardiomyocytes and downregulates glucose utilization, resulting in insulin resistance [98]. Furthermore, Nrf2 overexpression diminishes ROS and myocardial hypertrophy, an effect that was facilitated by extracellular signal-related kinase (Erk), which normally acts to activate Nrf2 during oxidative stress [99]. It has therefore may be that Erk-mediated Nrf2 downregulation may underlie individual susceptibilities to CVD-related diabetic complications.

A number of studies utilizing pharmacologic Nrf2 activators have implicated the antioxidant properties of the Nrf2/Keap1/ARE pathway in cardioprotection [100, 101]. Consequently, there is a great deal of interest in therapeutically targeting this pathway as a means of preventing or reversing pathological cardiac remodeling [102] or delaying ventricular failure, the hemodynamic hallmark of HF in TIIDM [103, 104]. However, chronic overactivation of the Nrf2/Keap1/ARE signaling pathway may actually contribute to cardiomyopathy, which undermines the encouraging results of acute Nrf2 induction [105]. A long-term phase III clinical study in TIID patients with stage 4 chronic kidney disease (CKD) (BEACON trial) was terminated early due to a higher rate of cardiovascular events in the treatment group [106]. It is unclear as to why these adverse events were observed in this study and not in an earlier clinical trial in patients with stage 3 CKD (BEAM trial), but possibilities include significantly longer length of drug exposure or the use of a 20 mg fixed dose as opposed to an adjustable dosage [107]. However, whether this truly reflects a cardiomyopathic tendency of Nrf2 or is alternatively the result of other factors, such as an inherently increased rate of cardiovascular events in patients with more severe CKD, remains unknown.

6.4. Diabetic Nephropathy. Diabetic nephropathy is a well-known microvascular complication of chronic hyperglycemia, and both oxidative stress and an impaired response by the Nrf2/Keap1/ARE system have been implicated in its progression via renal cell apoptosis, fibrosis, and deficiencies in cellular regeneration [11, 108, 109]. In a streptozocin- (STZ-) induced mouse diabetes model, Nrf2 activation with sulforaphane suppressed nephropathy and significantly improved metabolic indices associated with TIIDM, such as hyperglycemia, polydipsia, polyuria, and weight loss [110]. These benefits can be largely attributed to decreases in renal oxidative and nitrosative stress, which act to reverse dysfunction in multiple known mediators of diabetic nephropathy such as transforming growth factor beta (TGF-B), ECM proteins such as fibronectin and collagen IV, and p21, a cell-cycle regulator [111]. Similar findings with other known activators of the Nrf2/Keap1/ARE pathway, such as resveratrol and MG-132, support the therapeutic targeting of this system to ameliorate the oxidative damage and glucose-induced mesangial cell proliferation, inflammation, and fibrosis which underlies diabetic nephropathy [112, 113]. In humans, decreased levels of Nrf2 and expression of target genes in the peripheral blood of patients with CKD further support the contribution of an impaired Nrf2 antioxidant signaling pathway to systemic oxidative overload and inflammation in diabetic nephropathy [114].

6.5. Wound Healing. Impaired wound healing is a well-known and devastating complication of TIIDM and represents the leading cause of chronic wounds and lower extremity amputations in the US [115]. However, despite adherence to tight control of blood glucose levels and advances in synthetic and biologic healing modalities, chronic wounds persist in diabetic patients, suggesting a more fundamental pathology in the diabetic regenerative milieu [116]. As in other diabetic complications, oxidative stress is important for the development of chronic wounds, and AGE in the diabetic wound microenvironment appear to impair wound contraction and remodeling, the inflammatory response, and ECM proliferation. [117] Several natural Nrf2 activators have shown a promise in treating diabetic wounds, and early induction of the Nrf2 pathway through the rhomboid family protein RHBDF2 accelerated cutaneous wound healing in mice [118, 119]. Interestingly, recent work in tissue regeneration models has demonstrated that hyperglycemia in diabetes is associated with Keap1 dysfunction, which prevents nuclear localization of Nrf2 and thus is an appropriate stress response [120]. Utilizing a cutaneous gene therapy model, these studies showed that small-interfering RNA (siRNA) targeted at Keap1 restored wound redox homeostasis, accelerated healing, and counteracted impairments in angiogenesis and reepithelialization, two critical functions of wound healing disrupted in diabetes, by restoring Nrf2 localization. This seems to support the notion that aberrant overexpression of Keap1 and resulting

Nrf2 repression is a possible mechanism of the redox homeostasis dysfunction and impaired wound healing in diabetes. Whether this relationship extends to other aspects of the disease, and the relative contribution of Nrf2 to specific wound healing functions, remains to be seen.

7. The Nrf2/Keap1/ARE Pathway as a Therapeutic Target

Given the broad accountability of oxidative stress for many pathological processes, the Nrf2/Keap1/ARE system has emerged as a logical therapeutic target for the prevention or treatment of disease. This pathway has been studied most intensively in cancer [19] but also in chronic obstructive pulmonary disease (COPD) [121], neurodegenerative disorders [122], and autoimmune diseases such as inflammatory bowel disease (IBD) [123] and rheumatoid arthritis [124]. A multitude of clinical trials has also been pursued in order to assess the efficacy of targeting or modifying elements of the pathway in order to diminish ROS-induced damage in human disease [125–128]. As a critical upstream mediator of the pathway, Nrf2 induction has formed the basis of most of this research. There are three primary mechanisms by which current pharmacological activators increase Nrf2 expression (Figure 2). These consist of (1) activation of upstream kinases such as protein kinase B (Akt) and extracellular signal-regulated kinases (Erk), which phosphorylate specific sites favoring the release of Nrf2 from Keap1; (2) modification of Keap1 cysteine residues, which disrupts the Nrf2-Keap1 complex and favors Nrf2 dissociation; and (3) blockage of ubiquitination and/or proteosomal degradation of Nrf2 [129]. The end result of all of these mechanisms is Nrf2 stabilization and subsequent translocation into the nucleus, where it can exert its transcriptional effects and commence an antioxidant cascade. Of note, Nrf2 activators have already made their way into clinical practice; in 2013, dimethyl fumarate (BG-12, brand name Tecfidera®) was approved by the FDA for the treatment of multiple sclerosis and is thought to exert its therapeutic effects via augmentation of Nrf2's downstream cytoprotective, anti-inflammatory, and antioxidant properties [130, 131]. These achievements represent a promise that the Nrf2 pathway can be effectively used in other diseases in which oxidative stress plays a major role, such as TIIDM.

With regard to TIIDM, knowledge of the pivotal role of oxidative stress in the pathogenesis and progression of the disease originally precipitated investigation into natural antioxidants, such as vitamin E, vitamin C, and coenzyme Q10, as logical initial approaches [132–134]. However, results of these studies have generally been disappointing, and human clinical trials have not shown any benefit of organic molecules as adjunct therapies in preventing or treating diabetic complications [135–137]. Therefore, over the past decade, a significant amount of research, predominantly utilizing high throughput cell-based screening assays, has been devoted to identifying clinically applicable small molecule activators or inducers of endogenous antioxidant mechanisms, such as the Nrf2/Keap1/ARE pathway [138]. These "new mechanism-based antioxidants" have emerged as the new frontier of defense against oxidative stress and inflammation in TIIDM.

An array of Nrf2 small molecule activators, both natural and synthetic, has been identified and studied extensively (Table 2).

These include sulforaphane, curcumin, cinnamaldehyde, pterostilbene, oltipraz, and resveratrol. Some of the most encouraging candidates fall under the category of synthetic triterpenoids; triterpenoid, 2-cyano-3,12-dioxooleane-,1,9(11)-dien-28-oic acid (CDDO), and its derivatives have yielded highly promising results in animal models of heart failure [102], insulin resistance [52], and obesity [155]. Bardoxolone methyl (CDDO-Me), one such derivative originally developed as an anticancer drug, was incidentally found to exhibit renoprotective effects and has made its way into human trials. A phase II clinical trial (BEAM) in adults with TIIDM and advanced CKD showed significant improvements in glomerular filtration rate (GFR) with only mild side effects such as muscle spasms, hypomagnesemia, and gastrointestinal distress [107]. Unfortunately, a subsequent phase III trial (BEACON) in patients with TIIDM and stage IV CKD was terminated early due to serious adverse events [106].

In addition to systemic administration, targeted delivery systems represent a potential approach to treatment of localized diabetes complications. For example, an engineered lipid-protein system (lipoproteoplex) demonstrated safe and efficient delivery of si*Keap1* to diabetic wounds and resulted in accelerated wound healing [156]. Such novel delivery systems could also potentially circumvent the known toxicities resulting from covalent modifications (e.g., alkylation) of Keap1 cysteine residues that form the basis of function for many reported Nrf2 stabilizers [157]. Therefore, Nrf2 pathway modulation via direct, noncovalent inhibition of Nrf2-Keap1 protein-protein complexes is emphasized in current research. Additionally, strategies aimed at adjacent or downstream elements in the Nrf2 pathway have also gained traction as an alternative or combinatorial approaches to treatment. For instance, repression of BTB domain and CNC homolog (Bach1), a nuclear inhibitor of Nrf2, in combination with traditional Nrf2 activators, has shown promising results in neurodegenerative disease models for safely increasing the efficiency and biological activity of these agents [158].

In addition to the pathogenesis of TIIDM and its major complications, treatment of the metabolic alterations in TIIDM has also become a focus of intense investigation. Shin et al. found that Nrf2 regulates fibroblast growth factor 21 (FGF21), a key mediator of glucose and lipid metabolism, in mice [159]. This may have implications in guiding treatment of obesity in TIIDM, which is itself regulated, at least in part, by Nrf2 action on lipogenic gene expression and fatty acid synthesis [156]. Studies have shown that Nrf2/Keap1/ARE activators can exert potent reductions in body weight and hepatic fat accumulation in mice with an excellent safety profile and tolerance, representing potential novel, noninvasive options for managing obesogenesis in TIIDM [156, 160].

As we learn more about the protective aspects of the Nrf2 pathway, we must also appreciate the potential hazards of

TABLE 2: Small molecule activators of Nrf2 in TIIDM.

Molecule	Source	Mechanism of Nrf2 activation	Evidence
Sulforaphane (SFN)	Natural (cruciferous vegetables such as broccoli, brussel sprouts, and cabbage)	Modification of Keap1 cysteine residues	(i) Pancreatic β-cell protection [45] (ii) Prevented cardiac oxidative damage, inflammation, and hyperglycemic-induced fibrosis [139] (iii) Renal protection in db mice [110]
Curcumin (CUR)	Natural (turmeric)	Modification of Keap1 cysteine residues	(i) Reduced number of prediabetic individuals who progressed to type II DM [140] (ii) Activates liver enzymes involved in glycolysis, gluconeogenesis, and lipid metabolism [141]
Bardoxolone methyl (CDDO-Me/RTA 402)	Synthetic (derivative of oleanolic acid)	Modification of Keap1 cysteine residues	(i) Efficacy in short-term clinical trials in patients with type II DM and CKD [107] (ii) Did not reduce risk of end-stage renal disease (ESRD) or death from cardiovascular failure in patients with DM and stage IV CKD and was terminated early due to side effects [106]
Tert-butylhydro-quinone (tBHQ)	Synthetic (preservative in unsaturated vegetable oils and edible animal fats)	Modification of Keap1 cysteine residues/activation of upstream kinases	(i) Prevented glucose-induced impairments in diabetic retinopathy [142]
Cinnamic aldehyde (CA)	Natural (found in bark of cinnamon tree)	Activation of upstream kinases	(i) Lowered blood glucose, total cholesterol, triglycerides, and increased HDL* in diabetic rats and mice [143] (ii) Prevented development of hypertension in conditions of insulin resistance [144] (iii) Improved renal and glomerular function [110]
Resveratrol (RES)	Natural (polyphenol, found in the skin of red grapes, peanuts, and berries)	Activation of upstream kinases	(i) Reduced blood glucose and HbA1c** levels [145] (ii) Restored secretory function of β-cells in response to toxicity [146] (iii) Renoprotective effects in DM [147]
Magnesium lithospermate B (MLB)	Natural (active polyphenol acid of *Radix Salviae miltiorrhizae* herb)	Activation of upstream kinases	(i) Suppressed progression of renal injury in diabetic rats [148] (ii) Protection against DM-related atherosclerosis [149]
MG132	Synthetic peptide aldehyde	Proteosome inhibitor	(i) Renoprotective against DM-induced oxidative damage, inflammation, and fibrosis [113]
Pterostilbene	Natural (blueberries, grapes)	Mechanism unclear	(i) Protective against β-cell apoptosis [150]
Catechins	Natural (flavenols, found in red wine, berries, grapes)	Likely activation of upstream kinases	(i) Reduced hepatic glucose production and enhanced pancreatic function [151, 152] (ii) Decreased cytokine-induced β-cell damage *in vitro* [153] (iii) Prevented reduction in islet mass *in vivo* [154] (iv) Protected against nephrotoxicity [155]

*HDL: high-density lipoprotein; **HbA1c: a marker of chronic hyperglycemia.

targeting Nrf2 as a therapeutic means. Accruing evidence points to a "dark side" of Nrf2, which also regulates cell proliferation [161]. Nrf2 and its downstream genes are overexpressed in many cancer cell lines and human cancer tissues, and ove-activation of this pathway appears to contribute to the evolution of cancer and chemoresistance of cancer cells [162, 163]. Furthermore, mutations in Nrf2 and Keap1 have been found in a large percentage of malignancies [164, 165]. These findings should not impede our pursuit of targeting the Nrf2/Keap1/ARE pathway in the treatment of diabetes but should rather encourage a cautious and vigilant approach.

8. Nrf2 as a Potential Biomarker

Although biomarkers as a means of noninvasive disease prediction or prevention have been a topic of intense investigation for many years, very few have made their way into the clinical setting, and utility is largely limited to ad hoc corroboration of pathologic events, such as myocardial ischemia and heart failure. An increasing number of studies have been published on biomarkers of oxidative stress in a wide array of human disease [166], and AGE [167], nitrotyrosine [168], preoxiredoxin [169], and 8-hydroxy-2′-deoxyguanosine (8-OhdG) [170] levels in the skin, plasma, and urine samples have been investigated for both type I and type II DM. However, lack of validation for these markers remains a major obstacle to clinical utility [171]. The adoption of Nrf2, or elements of the Nrf2/Keap1/ARE pathway, as potential biomarkers has been proposed for prognostic purposes in cancer and neurodegeneration [172, 173]. The pursuit of using the Nrf2 pathway as a biomarker for TIIDM and its complications remains in its infancy, but existing evidence suggests that there may indeed be utility in prediabetic and diabetic patients, and research is likely to accelerate in this field as the medical landscape continues to shift towards a front-end, preventative approach with regard to chronic disease management [31, 174].

9. Conclusion

We have answered many questions regarding the role of the Nrf2/Keap1/ARE pathway and oxidative stress in TIIDM, but more remain before we can capitalize on this relationship to attain widespread, clinical significance in humans. For instance, much of what we know is derived from animal studies, and it is unclear as to what extent the murine antioxidant system reflects that of humans. Additionally, despite clear evidence of dysfunction in the Nrf2/Keap1/ARE antioxidant response across a wide range of tissue types and disease stages in TIIDM, the specific mechanisms underlying Nrf2 dysfunction have yet to be fully elucidated. We must also be cognizant of alternative, potentially confounding effects that independent players within Nrf2/Keap1/ARE pathway may exert. For instance, in addition to its cytoprotective role against oxidative stress as part of the Nrf2/Keap1/ARE pathway, accumulating research indicates that the Nrf2 molecule can also independently control the expression of genes responsible for many aspects of cellular metabolism. These studies, largely dependent on transgenic diabetic and Nrf2 knockout murine models, have implicated this molecule in TIIDM pathogenesis, prevention, and progression, via means that are wholly distinct from its role in oxidative protection. For instance, Nrf2 regulates blood glucose homeostasis and metabolic reprogramming by redirecting anabolic pathways [175], inhibiting lipogenesis [176], and promoting insulin sensitization, thereby ameliorating insulin resistance [177]. A more robust understanding of these varied roles may help explain seeming paradoxes in the role of the Nrf2/Keap1/ARE pathway such as what we see in insulin homeostasis and atheroma formation. These examples highlight not only the pleotropic effects of Nrf2 throughout tissues but also the variety of ways in which it responds and interacts, often contradictorily, with different types of stress.

Looking towards the future, we must continue to validate the Nrf2/Keap1/ARE pathway as a mediator of the oxidative stress underlying TIIDM and further explore this role in less morbid complications such as retinopathy and neuropathy. As we continue to screen for and develop ways to target the Nrf2/Keap1/ARE pathway, the importance of identifying novel delivery systems and nontoxic mechanisms of Nrf2 activation will accelerate translation of these therapeutics into human trials. Finally, encouraging evidence for the use of the Nrf2/Keap1/ARE as a biomarker should catalyze efforts to validate its use in the clinical setting. The intertwining roles of Nrf2, oxidative stress, and TIIDM will continue to provoke interest for a time to come, but it is becoming increasingly clear that further understanding this intimate relationship has preventative, prognostic, and therapeutic value in combatting this devastating disease.

Conflicts of Interest

The authors declare that there is no conflict of interest regarding the publication of this paper.

Acknowledgments

This work was supported by the American Diabetes Association "Pathway to Stop Diabetes" to Daniel J. Ceradini [Grant no. 1-16-ACE-08].

References

[1] G. Roglic, *Global Report on Diabetes*, World Health Organization, 2016.

[2] J. A. O'Brien, A. R. Patrick, and J. Caro, "Estimates of direct medical costs for microvascular and macrovascular complications resulting from type 2 diabetes mellitus in the United States in 2000," *Clinical Therapeutics*, vol. 25, pp. 1017–1038, 2003.

[3] D. Lloyd-Jones, R. J. Adams, T. M. Brown et al., "Heart disease and stroke statistics—2010 update: a report from the American Heart Association," *Circulation*, vol. 121, pp. e46–e215, 2010.

[4] J. L. Dieleman, R. Baral, M. Birger et al., "US spending on personal health care and public health, 1996-2013," *The Journal of the American Medical Association*, vol. 316, pp. 2627–2646, 2016.

[5] American Diabetes Association, "Diagnosis and classification of diabetes mellitus," *Diabetes Care*, vol. 37, Supplement 1, pp. S81–S90, 2014.

[6] W. C. Knowler, E. Barrett-Connor, S. E. Fowler et al., "Reduction in the incidence of type 2 diabetes with lifestyle intervention or metformin," *New England Journal of Medicine*, vol. 346, no. 6, pp. 393–403, 2002.

[7] E. W. Gregg, Y. Li, J. Wang et al., "Changes in diabetes-related complications in the United States, 1990-2010," *The New England Journal of Medicine*, vol. 370, pp. 1514–1523, 2014.

[8] W. R. Rowley, C. Bezold, Y. Arikan, E. Byrne, and S. Krohe, "Diabetes 2030: insights from yesterday, today, and future trends," *Population Health Management*, vol. 20, pp. 6–12, 2017.

[9] S. Reuter, S. C. Gupta, M. M. Chaturvedi, and B. B. Aggarwal, "Oxidative stress, inflammation, and cancer: how are they linked?," *Free Radical Biology and Medicine*, vol. 49, pp. 1603–1616, 2010.

[10] P. Soysal, A. T. Isik, A. F. Carvalho et al., "Oxidative stress and frailty: a systematic review and synthesis of the best evidence," *Maturitas*, vol. 99, pp. 66–72, 2017.

[11] D. M. Small, J. S. Coombes, N. Bennett, D. W. Johnson, and G. C. Gobe, "Oxidative stress, antioxidant therapies and

chronic kidney disease," *Nephrology*, vol. 17, pp. 311–321, 2012.

[12] A. J. McGuinness and E. Sapey, "Oxidative stress in COPD: sources, markers, and potential mechanisms," *Journal of Clinical Medicine*, vol. 6, no. 2, 2017.

[13] M. Brownlee, "Biochemistry and molecular cell biology of diabetic complications," *Nature*, vol. 414, no. 6865, pp. 813–820, 2001.

[14] F. Giacco and M. Brownlee, "Oxidative stress and diabetic complications," *Circulation Research*, vol. 107, pp. 1058–1070, 2010.

[15] P. Dandona, K. Thusu, S. Cook et al., "Oxidative damage to DNA in diabetes mellitus," *Lancet*, vol. 347, pp. 444-445, 1996.

[16] T. Nishikawa, D. Edelstein, X. L. Du et al., "Normalizing mitochondrial superoxide production blocks three pathways of hyperglycaemic damage," *Nature*, vol. 404, pp. 787–790, 2000.

[17] B. Williams, B. Gallacher, H. Patel, and C. Orme, "Glucose-induced protein kinase C activation regulates vascular permeability factor mRNA expression and peptide production by human vascular smooth muscle cells in vitro," *Diabetes*, vol. 46, pp. 1497–1503, 1997.

[18] H. Ishii, M. R. Jirousek, D. Koya et al., "Amelioration of vascular dysfunctions in diabetic rats by an oral PKC beta inhibitor," *Science*, vol. 272, pp. 728–731, 1996.

[19] T. W. Kensler, N. Wakabayashi, and S. Biswal, "Cell survival responses to environmental stresses via the Keap1-Nrf2-ARE pathway," *Annual Review of Pharmacology and Toxicology*, vol. 47, pp. 89–116, 2007.

[20] K. Itoh, T. Chiba, S. Takahashi et al., "An Nrf2/small Maf heterodimer mediates the induction of phase II detoxifying enzyme genes through antioxidant response elements," *Biochemical and Biophysical Research Communications*, vol. 236, pp. 313–322, 1997.

[21] M. McMahon, K. Itoh, M. Yamamoto, and J. D. Hayes, "Keap1-dependent proteasomal degradation of transcription factor Nrf2 contributes to the negative regulation of antioxidant response element-driven gene expression," *The Journal of Biological Chemistry*, vol. 278, pp. 21592–21600, 2003.

[22] P. Moi, K. Chan, I. Asunis, A. Cao, and Y. W. Kan, "Isolation of NF-E2-related factor 2 (Nrf2), a NF-E2-like basic leucine zipper transcriptional activator that binds to the tandem NF-E2/AP1 repeat of the beta-globin locus control region," *Proceedings of the National Academy of Sciences of the United States of America*, vol. 91, pp. 9926–9930, 1994.

[23] R. Venugopal and A. K. Jaiswal, "Nrf1 and Nrf2 positively and c-Fos and Fra1 negatively regulate the human antioxidant response element-mediated expression of NAD(P)H:-quinone oxidoreductase1 gene," *Proceedings of the National Academy of Sciences of the United States of America*, vol. 93, pp. 14960–14965, 1996.

[24] T. Nguyen, P. J. Sherratt, P. Nioi, C. S. Yang, and C. B. Pickett, "Nrf2 controls constitutive and inducible expression of ARE-driven genes through a dynamic pathway involving nucleocytoplasmic shuttling by Keap1," *The Journal of Biological Chemistry*, vol. 280, pp. 32485–32492, 2005.

[25] T. Nguyen, P. Nioi, and C. B. Pickett, "The Nrf2-antioxidant response element signaling pathway and its activation by oxidative stress," *The Journal of Biological Chemistry*, vol. 284, pp. 13291–13295, 2009.

[26] D. D. Zhang and M. Hannink, "Distinct cysteine residues in Keap1 are required for Keap1-dependent ubiquitination of Nrf2 and for stabilization of Nrf2 by chemopreventive agents and oxidative stress," *Molecular and Cellular Biology*, vol. 23, pp. 8137–8151, 2003.

[27] J. Alam, D. Stewart, C. Touchard, S. Boinapally, A. M. Choi, and J. L. Cook, "Nrf2, a Cap'n'Collar transcription factor, regulates induction of the heme oxygenase-1 gene," *The Journal of Biological Chemistry*, vol. 274, pp. 26071–26078, 1999.

[28] L. F. Chasseaud, "The role of glutathione and glutathione S-transferases in the metabolism of chemical carcinogens and other electrophilic agents," *Advances in Cancer Research*, vol. 29, pp. 175–274, 1979.

[29] A. Uruno, Y. Yagishita, and M. Yamamoto, "The Keap1-Nrf2 system and diabetes mellitus," *Archives of Biochemistry and Biophysics*, vol. 566, pp. 76–84, 2015.

[30] M. Long, M. Rojo de la Vega, Q. Wen et al., "An essential role of NRF2 in diabetic wound healing," *Diabetes*, vol. 65, pp. 780–793, 2016.

[31] A. S. Jiménez-Osorio, A. Picazo, S. González-Reyes, D. Barrera-Oviedo, M. E. Rodríguez-Arellano, and J. Pedraza-Chaverri, "Nrf2 and redox status in prediabetic and diabetic patients," *International Journal of Molecular Sciences*, vol. 15, pp. 20290–20305, 2014.

[32] M. C. Lu, J. A. Ji, Z. Y. Jiang, and Q. D. You, "The Keap1-Nrf2-ARE pathway as a potential preventive and therapeutic target: an update," *Medicinal Research Review*, vol. 36, pp. 924–963, 2016.

[33] L. M. Aleksunes, S. A. Reisman, R. L. Yeager, M. J. Goedken, and C. D. Klaassen, "Nuclear factor erythroid 2-related factor 2 deletion impairs glucose tolerance and exacerbates hyperglycemia in type 1 diabetic mice," *The Journal of Pharmacology and Experimental Therapeutics*, vol. 333, no. 1, pp. 140–151, 2010.

[34] M. S. Bitar and F. Al-Mulla, "A defect in Nrf2 signaling constitutes a mechanism for cellular stress hypersensitivity in a genetic rat model of type 2 diabetes," *American Journal of Physiology Endocrinology and Metabolism*, vol. 301, no. 6, pp. 1119–1129, 2011.

[35] A. T. Dinkova-Kostova and P. Talalay, "Direct and indirect antioxidant properties of inducers of cytoprotective proteins," *Molecular Nutrition & Food Research*, vol. 52, no. 1, pp. 128–138, 2008.

[36] M. Cnop, N. Welsh, J. C. Jonas, A. Jörns, S. Lenzen, and D. L. Eizirik, "Mechanisms of pancreatic beta-cell death in type 1 and type 2 diabetes: many differences, few similarities," *Diabetes*, vol. 54, Supplement 2, pp. S97–107, 2005.

[37] S. Fujimoto, E. Mukai, and N. Inagaki, "Role of endogenous ROS production in impaired metabolism-secretion coupling of diabetic pancreatic beta cells," *Progress in Biophysics and Molecular Biology*, vol. 107, pp. 304–310, 2011.

[38] J. S. Harmon, M. Bogdani, S. D. Parazzoli et al., "Beta-cell-specific overexpression of glutathione peroxidase preserves intranuclear MafA and reverses diabetes in db/db mice," *Endocrinology*, vol. 150, pp. 4855–4862, 2009.

[39] H. M. Kubisch, J. Wang, T. M. Bray, and J. P. Phillips, "Targeted overexpression of cu/Zn superoxide dismutase protects pancreatic beta-cells against oxidative stress," *Diabetes*, vol. 46, pp. 1563–1566, 1997.

[40] M. Sasaki, S. Fujimoto, Y. Sato et al., "Reduction of reactive oxygen species ameliorates metabolism-secretion coupling

in islets of diabetic GK rats by suppressing lactate overproduction," *Diabetes*, vol. 62, pp. 1996–2003, 2013.

[41] H. Sakuraba, H. Mizukami, N. Yagihashi, R. Wada, C. Hanyu, and S. Yagihashi, "Reduced beta-cell mass and expression of oxidative stress-related DNA damage in the islet of Japanese type II diabetic patients," *Diabetologia*, vol. 45, pp. 85–96, 2002.

[42] A. Vetere, A. Choudhary, S. M. Burns, and B. K. Wagner, "Targeting the pancreatic beta-cell to treat diabetes," *Nature Reviews. Drug Discovery*, vol. 13, pp. 278–289, 2014.

[43] Y. Yagishita, T. Fukutomi, A. Sugawara et al., "Nrf2 protects pancreatic beta-cells from oxidative and nitrosative stress in diabetic model mice," *Diabetes*, vol. 63, pp. 605–618, 2014.

[44] A. Uruno, Y. Furusawa, Y. Yagishita et al., "The Keap1-Nrf2 system prevents onset of diabetes mellitus," *Molecular and Cellular Biology*, vol. 33, pp. 2996–3010, 2013.

[45] M. Y. Song, E. K. Kim, W. S. Moon et al., "Sulforaphane protects against cytokine- and streptozotocin-induced beta-cell damage by suppressing the NF-kappaB pathway," *Toxicology and Applied Pharmacology*, vol. 235, pp. 57–67, 2009.

[46] W. Li, W. Wu, H. Song et al., "Targeting Nrf2 by dihydro-CDDO-trifluoroethyl amide enhances autophagic clearance and viability of beta-cells in a setting of oxidative stress," *FEBS Letters*, vol. 588, pp. 2115–2124, 2014.

[47] S. Lee, E. G. Hur, I. G. Ryoo, K. A. Jung, J. Kwak, and M. K. Kwak, "Involvement of the Nrf2-proteasome pathway in the endoplasmic reticulum stress response in pancreatic beta-cells," *Toxicology and Applied Pharmacology*, vol. 264, pp. 431–438, 2012.

[48] B. McEvoy, R. Sumayao, C. Slattery, T. McMorrow, and P. Newsholme, "Cystine accumulation attenuates insulin release from the pancreatic beta-cell due to elevated oxidative stress and decreased ATP levels," *The Journal of Physiology*, vol. 593, pp. 5167–5182, 2015.

[49] K. Sakai, K. Matsumoto, T. Nishikawa et al., "Mitochondrial reactive oxygen species reduce insulin secretion by pancreatic beta-cells," *Biochemical and Biophysical Research Communications*, vol. 300, pp. 216–222, 2003.

[50] M. Saadeh, T. C. Ferrante, A. Kane, O. Shirihai, B. E. Corkey, and J. T. Deeney, "Reactive oxygen species stimulate insulin secretion in rat pancreatic islets: studies using mono-oleoyl-glycerol," *PLoS One*, vol. 7, article e30200, 2012.

[51] C. Leloup, C. Tourrel-Cuzin, C. Magnan et al., "Mitochondrial reactive oxygen species are obligatory signals for glucose-induced insulin secretion," *Diabetes*, vol. 58, pp. 673–681, 2009.

[52] P. K. Saha, V. T. Reddy, M. Konopleva, M. Andreeff, and L. Chan, "The triterpenoid 2-cyano-3,12-dioxooleana-1,9-dien-28-oic-acid methyl ester has potent anti-diabetic effects in diet-induced diabetic mice and Lepr(db/db) mice," *The Journal of Biological Chemistry*, vol. 285, pp. 40581–40592, 2010.

[53] Z. Yu, W. Shao, Y. Chiang et al., "Oltipraz upregulates the nuclear factor (erythroid-derived 2)-like 2 (NRF2) antioxidant system and prevents insulin resistance and obesity induced by a high-fat diet in C57BL/6J mice," *Diabetologia*, vol. 54, pp. 922–934, 2011.

[54] Y. K. Zhang, K. C. Wu, J. Liu, and C. D. Klaassen, "Nrf2 deficiency improves glucose tolerance in mice fed a high-fat diet," *Toxicology and Applied Pharmacology*, vol. 264, pp. 305–314, 2012.

[55] P. J. Meakin, S. Chowdhry, R. S. Sharma et al., "Susceptibility of Nrf2-null mice to steatohepatitis and cirrhosis upon consumption of a high-fat diet is associated with oxidative stress, perturbation of the unfolded protein response, and disturbance in the expression of metabolic enzymes but not with insulin resistance," *Molecular and Cellular Biology*, vol. 34, pp. 3305–3320, 2014.

[56] A. K. Meher, P. R. Sharma, V. A. Lira et al., "Nrf2 deficiency in myeloid cells is not sufficient to protect mice from high-fat diet-induced adipose tissue inflammation and insulin resistance," *Free Radical Biology and Medicine*, vol. 52, pp. 1708–1715, 2012.

[57] J. Pi, L. Leung, P. Xue et al., "Deficiency in the nuclear factor E2-related factor-2 transcription factor results in impaired adipogenesis and protects against diet-induced obesity," *The Journal of Biological Chemistry*, vol. 285, pp. 9292–9300, 2010.

[58] C. Talchai, S. Xuan, H. V. Lin, L. Sussel, and D. Accili, "Pancreatic beta cell dedifferentiation as a mechanism of diabetic beta cell failure," *Cell*, vol. 150, pp. 1223–1234, 2012.

[59] Y. Yagishita, A. Uruno, T. Fukutomi et al., "Nrf2 improves leptin and insulin resistance provoked by hypothalamic oxidative stress," *Cell Reports*, vol. 18, no. 8, pp. 2030–2044, 2017.

[60] S. E. Kahn, R. L. Hull, and K. M. Utzschneider, "Mechanisms linking obesity to insulin resistance and type 2 diabetes," *Nature*, vol. 444, pp. 840–846, 2006.

[61] K. M. Holmström, L. Baird, Y. Zhang et al., "Nrf2 impacts cellular bioenergetics by controlling substrate availability for mitochondrial respiration," *Biology Open*, vol. 2, no. 8, pp. 761–770, 2013.

[62] C. S. Fox, S. Coady, P. D. Sorlie et al., "Trends in cardiovascular complications of diabetes," *The Journal of the American Medical Association*, vol. 292, pp. 2495–2499, 2004.

[63] D. G. Harrison, M. C. Gongora, T. J. Guzik, and J. Widder, "Oxidative stress and hypertension," *Journal of the American Society of Hypertension*, vol. 1, pp. 30–44, 2007.

[64] H. Tsutsui, S. Kinugawa, and S. Matsushima, "Oxidative stress and heart failure," *American Journal of Physiology. Heart and Circulatory Physiology*, vol. 301, pp. H2181–H2190, 2011.

[65] D. Harrison, K. K. Griendling, U. Landmesser, B. Hornig, and H. Drexler, "Role of oxidative stress in atherosclerosis," *The American Journal of Cardiology*, vol. 91, pp. 7a–11a, 2003.

[66] J. L. Zweier, "Measurement of superoxide-derived free radicals in the reperfused heart. Evidence for a free radical mechanism of reperfusion injury," *The Journal of Biological Chemistry*, vol. 263, pp. 1353–1357, 1988.

[67] I. M. Fearon and S. P. Faux, "Oxidative stress and cardiovascular disease: novel tools give (free) radical insight," *Journal of Molecular and Cellular Cardiology*, vol. 47, pp. 372–381, 2009.

[68] M. J. Callaghan, D. J. Ceradini, and G. C. Gurtner, "Hyperglycemia-induced reactive oxygen species and impaired endothelial progenitor cell function," *Antioxidants & Redox Signaling*, vol. 7, pp. 1476–1482, 2005.

[69] A. Martin, M. R. Komada, and D. C. Sane, "Abnormal angiogenesis in diabetes mellitus," *Medicinal Research Reviews*, vol. 23, pp. 117–145, 2003.

[70] Y. Wei, J. Gong, R. K. Thimmulappa, B. Kosmider, S. Biswal, and E. J. Duh, "Nrf2 acts cell-autonomously in endothelium

to regulate tip cell formation and vascular branching," *Proceedings of the National Academy of Sciences of the United States of America*, vol. 110, pp. E3910–E3918, 2013.

[71] Z. Ungvari, L. Bailey-Downs, T. Gautam et al., "Adaptive induction of NF-E2-related factor-2-driven antioxidant genes in endothelial cells in response to hyperglycemia," *American Journal of Physiology. Heart and Circulatory Physiology*, vol. 300, pp. H1133–H1140, 2011.

[72] T. M. Chen, J. Li, L. Liu et al., "Effects of heme oxygenase-1 upregulation on blood pressure and cardiac function in an animal model of hypertensive myocardial infarction," *International Journal of Molecular Sciences*, vol. 14, pp. 2684–2706, 2013.

[73] J. L. Zweier, P. Kuppusamy, and G. A. Lutty, "Measurement of endothelial cell free radical generation: evidence for a central mechanism of free radical injury in postischemic tissues," *Proceedings of the National Academy of Sciences of the United States of America*, vol. 85, no. 11, pp. 4046–4050, 1988.

[74] J. Li, T. M. Chen, J. Cao et al., "Long-term effects of heme oxygenase 1 overexpression on post-infarction heart function in diabetic rats," *Chinese Journal of Applied Physiology*, vol. 30, no. 5, pp. 421–426, 2014.

[75] Y. Zhao, L. Zhang, Y. Qiao et al., "Heme oxygenase-1 prevents cardiac dysfunction in streptozotocin-diabetic mice by reducing inflammation, oxidative stress, apoptosis and enhancing autophagy," *PLoS One*, vol. 8, no. 9, article e75927, 2013.

[76] H. Zhu, Z. Jia, L. Zhang et al., "Antioxidants and phase 2 enzymes in macrophages: regulation by Nrf2 signaling and protection against oxidative and electrophilic stress," *Experimental Biology and Medicine*, vol. 233, pp. 463–474, 2008.

[77] H. K. Jyrkkänen, E. Kansanen, M. Inkala et al., "Nrf2 regulates antioxidant gene expression evoked by oxidized phospholipids in endothelial cells and murine arteries in vivo," *Circulation Research*, vol. 103, pp. e1–e9, 2008.

[78] A. K. Ruotsalainen, M. Inkala, M. E. Partanen et al., "The absence of macrophage Nrf2 promotes early atherogenesis," *Cardiovascular Research*, vol. 98, pp. 107–115, 2013.

[79] M. Zakkar, K. HeidenVan der, A. Luong le et al., "Activation of Nrf2 in endothelial cells protects arteries from exhibiting a proinflammatory state," *Arteriosclerosis, Thrombosis, and Vascular Biology*, vol. 29, pp. 1851–1857, 2009.

[80] K. Ishikawa and Y. Maruyama, "Heme oxygenase as an intrinsic defense system in vascular wall: implication against atherogenesis," *Journal of Atherosclerosis and Thrombosis*, vol. 8, pp. 63–70, 2001.

[81] T. E. Sussan, J. Jun, R. Thimmulappa et al., "Disruption of Nrf2, a key inducer of antioxidant defenses, attenuates ApoE-mediated atherosclerosis in mice," *PLoS One*, vol. 3, article e3791, 2008.

[82] X. L. Chen, S. E. Varner, A. S. Rao et al., "Laminar flow induction of antioxidant response element-mediated genes in endothelial cells. A novel anti-inflammatory mechanism," *The Journal of Biological Chemistry*, vol. 278, pp. 703–711, 2003.

[83] S. Freigang, F. Ampenberger, G. Spohn et al., "Nrf2 is essential for cholesterol crystal-induced inflammasome activation and exacerbation of atherosclerosis," *European Journal of Immunology*, vol. 41, pp. 2040–2051, 2011.

[84] J. Song, S. Sumiyoshi, Y. Nakashima et al., "Overexpression of heme oxygenase-1 in coronary atherosclerosis of Japanese autopsies with diabetes mellitus: Hisayama study," *Atherosclerosis*, vol. 202, no. 2, pp. 573–581, 2009.

[85] T. Hosoya, A. Maruyama, M. I. Kang et al., "Differential responses of the Nrf2-Keap1 system to laminar and oscillatory shear stresses in endothelial cells," *The Journal of Biological Chemistry*, vol. 280, pp. 27244–27250, 2005.

[86] W. B. Kannel and D. L. McGee, "Diabetes and cardiovascular disease. The Framingham study," *The Journal of the American Medical Association*, vol. 241, pp. 2035–2038, 1979.

[87] H. Mönkemann, A. S. VrieseDe, H. J. Blom et al., "Early molecular events in the development of the diabetic cardiomyopathy," *Amino Acids*, vol. 23, pp. 331–336, 2002.

[88] A. Chesley, M. S. Lundberg, T. Asai et al., "The β_2-adrenergic receptor delivers an antiapoptotic signal to cardiac myocytes through G_i-dependent coupling to phosphatidylinositol 3′-kinase," *Circulation Research*, vol. 87, pp. 1172–1179, 2000.

[89] R. Bolli, W. X. Zhu, C. J. Hartley et al., "Attenuation of dysfunction in the postischemic 'stunned' myocardium by dimethylthiourea," *Circulation*, vol. 76, pp. 458–468, 1987.

[90] A. C. Kohler, C. M. Sag, and L. S. Maier, "Reactive oxygen species and excitation-contraction coupling in the context of cardiac pathology," *Journal of Molecular and Cellular Cardiology*, vol. 73, pp. 92–102, 2014.

[91] A. Beresewicz and M. Horackova, "Alterations in electrical and contractile behavior of isolated cardiomyocytes by hydrogen peroxide: possible ionic mechanisms," *Journal of Molecular and Cellular Cardiology*, vol. 23, pp. 899–918, 1991.

[92] A. Sabri, H. H. Hughie, and P. A. Lucchesi, "Regulation of hypertrophic and apoptotic signaling pathways by reactive oxygen species in cardiac myocytes," *Antioxidants & Redox Signaling*, vol. 5, pp. 731–740, 2003.

[93] S. Rajagopalan, X. P. Meng, S. Ramasamy, D. G. Harrison, and Z. S. Galis, "Reactive oxygen species produced by macrophage-derived foam cells regulate the activity of vascular matrix metalloproteinases in vitro. Implications for atherosclerotic plaque stability," *The Journal of Clinical Investigation*, vol. 98, pp. 2572–2579, 1996.

[94] E. Ingelsson, J. Sundström, J. Arnlöv, B. Zethelius, and L. Lind, "Insulin resistance and risk of congestive heart failure," *The Journal of the American Medical Association*, vol. 294, pp. 334–341, 2005.

[95] Z. Lu, X. Xu, X. Hu et al., "Extracellular superoxide dismutase deficiency exacerbates pressure overload-induced left ventricular hypertrophy and dysfunction," *Hypertension*, vol. 51, pp. 19–25, 2008.

[96] C. M. Hu, Y. H. Chen, M. T. Chiang, and L. Y. Chau, "Heme oxygenase-1 inhibits angiotensin II-induced cardiac hypertrophy in vitro and in vivo," *Circulation*, vol. 110, pp. 309–316, 2004.

[97] S. Matsushima, S. Kinugawa, T. Ide et al., "Overexpression of glutathione peroxidase attenuates myocardial remodeling and preserves diastolic function in diabetic heart," *American Journal of Physiology. Heart and Circulatory Physiology*, vol. 291, pp. H2237–H2245, 2006.

[98] Y. Tan, T. Ichikawa, J. Li et al., "Diabetic downregulation of Nrf2 activity via ERK contributes to oxidative stress-induced insulin resistance in cardiac cells in vitro and in vivo," *Diabetes*, vol. 60, pp. 625–633, 2011.

[99] J. Li, T. Ichikawa, L. Villacorta et al., "Nrf2 protects against maladaptive cardiac responses to hemodynamic stress,"

Arteriosclerosis, Thrombosis, and Vascular Biology, vol. 29, pp. 1843–1850, 2009.

[100] T. Ichikawa, J. Li, C. J. Meyer, J. S. Janicki, M. Hannink, and T. Cui, "Dihydro-CDDO-trifluoroethyl amide (dh404), a novel Nrf2 activator, suppresses oxidative stress in cardiomyocytes," *PLoS One*, vol. 4, article e8391, 2009.

[101] H. Ashrafian, G. Czibik, M. Bellahcene et al., "Fumarate is cardioprotective via activation of the Nrf2 antioxidant pathway," *Cell Metabolism*, vol. 15, pp. 361–371, 2012.

[102] Y. Xing, T. Niu, W. Wang et al., "Triterpenoid dihydro-CDDO-trifluoroethyl amide protects against maladaptive cardiac remodeling and dysfunction in mice: a critical role of Nrf2," *PLoS One*, vol. 7, article e44899, 2012.

[103] T. E. Sussan, T. Rangasamy, D. J. Blake et al., "Targeting Nrf2 with the triterpenoid CDDO-imidazolide attenuates cigarette smoke-induced emphysema and cardiac dysfunction in mice," *Proceedings of the National Academy of Sciences of the United States of America*, vol. 106, pp. 250–255, 2009.

[104] T. Abe, Y. Ohga, N. Tabayashi et al., "Left ventricular diastolic dysfunction in type 2 diabetes mellitus model rats," *American Journal of Physiology. Heart and Circulatory Physiology*, vol. 282, pp. H138–H148, 2002.

[105] N. S. Rajasekaran, S. Varadharaj, G. D. Khanderao et al., "Sustained activation of nuclear erythroid 2-related factor 2/antioxidant response element signaling promotes reductive stress in the human mutant protein aggregation cardiomyopathy in mice," *Antioxidants & Redox Signaling*, vol. 14, pp. 957–971, 2011.

[106] D. Zeeuwde, T. Akizawa, P. Audhya et al., "Bardoxolone methyl in type 2 diabetes and stage 4 chronic kidney disease," *The New England Journal of Medicine*, vol. 369, pp. 2492–2503, 2013.

[107] P. E. Pergola, P. Raskin, R. D. Toto et al., "Bardoxolone methyl and kidney function in CKD with type 2 diabetes," *The New England Journal of Medicine*, vol. 365, pp. 327–336, 2011.

[108] L. M. Pedruzzi, M. B. Stockler-Pinto, M. Leite Jr., and D. Mafra, "Nrf2-keap1 system versus NF-kappaB: the good and the evil in chronic kidney disease?," *Biochimie*, vol. 94, pp. 2461–2466, 2012.

[109] H. J. Kim and N. D. Vaziri, "Contribution of impaired Nrf2-Keap1 pathway to oxidative stress and inflammation in chronic renal failure," *American Journal of Physiology Renal Physiology*, vol. 298, pp. F662–F671, 2010.

[110] H. Zheng, S. A. Whitman, W. Wu et al., "Therapeutic potential of Nrf2 activators in streptozotocin-induced diabetic nephropathy," *Diabetes*, vol. 60, pp. 3055–3066, 2011.

[111] K. Yoh, A. Hirayama, K. Ishizaki et al., "Hyperglycemia induces oxidative and nitrosative stress and increases renal functional impairment in Nrf2-deficient mice," *Genes to Cells*, vol. 13, pp. 1159–1170, 2008.

[112] B. Jiang, L. Guo, B. Y. Li et al., "Resveratrol attenuates early diabetic nephropathy by down-regulating glutathione S-transferases mu in diabetic rats," *Journal of Medicinal Food*, vol. 16, pp. 481–486, 2013.

[113] W. Cui, B. Li, Y. Bai et al., "Potential role for Nrf2 activation in the therapeutic effect of MG132 on diabetic nephropathy in OVE26 diabetic mice," *American Journal of Physiology. Endocrinology and Metabolism*, vol. 304, pp. E87–E99, 2013.

[114] L. M. Pedruzzi, L. F. Cardozo, J. B. Daleprane et al., "Systemic inflammation and oxidative stress in hemodialysis patients are associated with down-regulation of Nrf2," *Journal of Nephrology*, vol. 28, pp. 495–501, 2015.

[115] American Diabetes Association, "Economic costs of diabetes in the U.S. in 2012," *Diabetes Care*, vol. 36, pp. 1033–1046, 2013.

[116] W. Duckworth, C. Abraira, T. Moritz et al., "Glucose control and vascular complications in veterans with type 2 diabetes," *The New England Journal of Medicine*, vol. 360, pp. 129–139, 2009.

[117] M. Peppa, P. Stavroulakis, and S. A. Raptis, "Advanced glycoxidation products and impaired diabetic wound healing," *Wound Repair and Regeneration*, vol. 17, pp. 461–472, 2009.

[118] D. R. Senger and S. Cao, "Diabetic wound healing and activation of Nrf2 by herbal medicine," *Journal of Nature and Science*, vol. 2, 2016.

[119] V. Hosur, L. M. Burzenski, T. M. Stearns et al., "Early induction of NRF2 antioxidant pathway by RHBDF2 mediates rapid cutaneous wound healing," *Experimental and Molecular Pathology*, vol. 102, no. 2, pp. 337–346, 2017.

[120] M. A. Soares, O. D. Cohen, Y. C. Low et al., "Restoration of Nrf2 signaling normalizes the regenerative niche," *Diabetes*, vol. 65, pp. 633–646, 2016.

[121] A. Boutten, D. Goven, E. Artaud-Macari, J. Boczkowski, and M. Bonay, "NRF2 targeting: a promising therapeutic strategy in chronic obstructive pulmonary disease," *Trends in Molecular Medicine*, vol. 17, pp. 363–371, 2011.

[122] C. P. Ramsey, C. A. Glass, M. B. Montgomery et al., "Expression of Nrf2 in neurodegenerative diseases," *Journal of Neuropathology and Experimental Neurology*, vol. 66, pp. 75–85, 2007.

[123] L. M. Aleksunes and J. E. Manautou, "Emerging role of Nrf2 in protecting against hepatic and gastrointestinal disease," *Toxicologic Pathology*, vol. 35, pp. 459–473, 2007.

[124] C. J. Wruck, A. Fragoulis, A. Gurzynski et al., "Role of oxidative stress in rheumatoid arthritis: insights from the Nrf2-knockout mice," *Annals of the Rheumatic Diseases*, vol. 70, pp. 844–850, 2011.

[125] T. A. Shapiro, J. W. Fahey, A. T. Dinkova-Kostova et al., "Safety, tolerance, and metabolism of broccoli sprout glucosinolates and isothiocyanates: a clinical phase I study," *Nutrition and Cancer*, vol. 55, pp. 53–62, 2006.

[126] B. S. Cornblatt, L. Ye, A. T. Dinkova-Kostova et al., "Preclinical and clinical evaluation of sulforaphane for chemoprevention in the breast," *Carcinogenesis*, vol. 28, pp. 1485–1490, 2007.

[127] H. Hatcher, R. Planalp, J. Cho, F. M. Torti, and S. V. Torti, "Curcumin: from ancient medicine to current clinical trials," *Cellular and Molecular Life Sciences*, vol. 65, pp. 1631–1652, 2008.

[128] Y. Zhang and R. Munday, "Dithiolethiones for cancer chemoprevention: where do we stand?," *Molecular Cancer Therapeutics*, vol. 7, pp. 3470–3479, 2008.

[129] E. Bhakkiyalakshmi, D. Sireesh, P. Rajaguru, R. Paulmurugan, and K. M. Ramkumar, "The emerging role of redox-sensitive Nrf2-Keap1 pathway in diabetes," *Pharmacological Research*, vol. 91, pp. 104–114, 2015.

[130] R. J. Fox, M. Kita, S. L. Cohan et al., "BG-12 (dimethyl fumarate): a review of mechanism of action, efficacy, and safety," *Current Medical Research and Opinion*, vol. 30, pp. 251–262, 2014.

[131] R. J. Fox, D. H. Miller, J. T. Phillips et al., "Placebo-controlled phase 3 study of oral BG-12 or glatiramer in multiple sclerosis," *The New England Journal of Medicine*, vol. 367, pp. 1087–1097, 2012.

[132] H. Kaneto, Y. Kajimoto, J. Miyagawa et al., "Beneficial effects of antioxidants in diabetes: possible protection of pancreatic beta-cells against glucose toxicity," *Diabetes*, vol. 48, pp. 28–2406, 1999.

[133] K. M. Ramkumar, R. S. Vijayakumar, P. Vanitha et al., "Protective effect of gallic acid on alloxan-induced oxidative stress and osmotic fragility in rats," *Human & Experimental Toxicology*, vol. 33, pp. 638–649, 2014.

[134] M. Latha, L. Pari, K. M. Ramkumar et al., "Antidiabetic effects of scoparic acid D isolated from Scoparia dulcis in rats with streptozotocin-induced diabetes," *Natural Product Research*, vol. 23, pp. 1528–1540, 2009.

[135] S. Golbidi, S. A. Ebadi, and I. Laher, "Antioxidants in the treatment of diabetes," *Current Diabetes Reviews*, vol. 7, pp. 106–125, 2011.

[136] E. Lonn, S. Yusuf, B. Hoogwerf et al., "Effects of vitamin E on cardiovascular and microvascular outcomes in high-risk patients with diabetes: results of the HOPE study and MICRO-HOPE substudy," *Diabetes Care*, vol. 25, pp. 1919–1927, 2002.

[137] J. Belch, A. MacCuish, I. Campbell et al., "The prevention of progression of arterial disease and diabetes (POPADAD) trial: factorial randomised placebo controlled trial of aspirin and antioxidants in patients with diabetes and asymptomatic peripheral arterial disease," *BMJ*, vol. 337, article a1840, 2008.

[138] K. C. Wu, P. R. McDonald, J. J. Liu, R. Chaguturu, and C. D. Klaassen, "Implementation of a high-throughput screen for identifying small molecules to activate the Keap1-Nrf2-ARE pathway," *PLoS One*, vol. 7, article e44686, 2012.

[139] Y. Bai, W. Cui, Y. Xin et al., "Prevention by sulforaphane of diabetic cardiomyopathy is associated with up-regulation of Nrf2 expression and transcription activation," *Journal of Molecular and Cellular Cardiology*, vol. 57, pp. 82–95, 2013.

[140] S. Chuengsamarn, S. Rattanamongkolgul, R. Luechapudiporn, C. Phisalaphong, and S. Jirawatnotai, "Curcumin extract for prevention of type 2 diabetes," *Diabetes Care*, vol. 35, pp. 2121–2127, 2012.

[141] K. I. Seo, M. S. Choi, U. J. Jung et al., "Effect of curcumin supplementation on blood glucose, plasma insulin, and glucose homeostasis related enzyme activities in diabetic db/db mice," *Molecular Nutrition & Food Research*, vol. 52, pp. 995–1004, 2008.

[142] Q. Zhong, M. Mishra, and R. A. Kowluru, "Transcription factor Nrf2-mediated antioxidant defense system in the development of diabetic retinopathy," *Investigative Ophthalmology & Visual Science*, vol. 54, pp. 3941–3948, 2013.

[143] P. Subash Babu, S. Prabuseenivasan, and S. Ignacimuthu, "Cinnamaldehyde—a potential antidiabetic agent," *Phytomedicine*, vol. 14, pp. 15–22, 2007.

[144] H. M. El-Bassossy, A. Fahmy, and D. Badawy, "Cinnamaldehyde protects from the hypertension associated with diabetes," *Food and Chemical Toxicology*, vol. 49, pp. 3007–3012, 2011.

[145] A. Movahed, I. Nabipour, X. Lieben Louis et al., "Antihyperglycemic effects of short term resveratrol supplementation in type 2 diabetic patients," *Evidence-Based Complementary and Alternative Medicine*, vol. 2013, Article ID 851267, 11 pages, 2013.

[146] J. H. Lee, M. Y. Song, E. K. Song et al., "Overexpression of SIRT1 protects pancreatic beta-cells against cytokine toxicity by suppressing the nuclear factor-kappaB signaling pathway," *Diabetes*, vol. 58, pp. 344–351, 2009.

[147] P. Palsamy and S. Subramanian, "Resveratrol protects diabetic kidney by attenuating hyperglycemia-mediated oxidative stress and renal inflammatory cytokines via Nrf2-Keap1 signaling," *Biochimica et Biophysica Acta (BBA) - Molecular Basis of Disease*, vol. 1812, pp. 719–731, 2011.

[148] G. T. Lee, H. Ha, M. Jung et al., "Delayed treatment with lithospermate B attenuates experimental diabetic renal injury," *Journal of the American Society of Nephrology*, vol. 14, pp. 709–720, 2003.

[149] K. Y. Hur, S. H. Kim, M. A. Choi et al., "Protective effects of magnesium lithospermate B against diabetic atherosclerosis via Nrf2-ARE-NQO1 transcriptional pathway," *Atherosclerosis*, vol. 211, pp. 69–76, 2010.

[150] E. Bhakkiyalakshmi, D. Shalini, T. V. Sekar, P. Rajaguru, R. Paulmurugan, and K. M. Ramkumar, "Therapeutic potential of pterostilbene against pancreatic beta-cell apoptosis mediated through Nrf2," *British Journal of Pharmacology*, vol. 171, pp. 1747–1757, 2014.

[151] S. Wolfram, D. Raederstorff, M. Preller et al., "Epigallocatechin gallate supplementation alleviates diabetes in rodents," *Journal of Nutrition*, vol. 136, pp. 2512–2518, 2006.

[152] M. E. Waltner-Law, X. L. Wang, B. K. Law, R. K. Hall, M. Nawano, and D. K. Granner, "Epigallocatechin gallate, a constituent of green tea, represses hepatic glucose production," *Journal of Biological Chemistry*, vol. 277, pp. 34933–34940, 2002.

[153] M. K. Han, "Epigallocatechin gallate, a constituent of green tea, suppresses cytokine-induced pancreatic beta-cell damage," *Experimental & Molecular Medicine*, vol. 35, pp. 136–139, 2003.

[154] E. K. Song, H. Hur, and M. K. Han, "Epigallocatechin gallate prevents autoimmune diabetes induced by multiple low doses of streptozotocin in mice," *Archives of Pharmacal Research*, vol. 26, pp. 559–563, 2003.

[155] K. Sahin, M. Tuzcu, H. Gencoglu et al., "Epigallocatechin-3-gallate activates Nrf2/HO-1 signaling pathway in cisplatin-induced nephrotoxicity in rats," *Life Sciences*, vol. 87, pp. 240–245, 2010.

[156] S. Shin, J. Wakabayashi, M. S. Yates et al., "Role of Nrf2 in prevention of high-fat diet-induced obesity by synthetic triterpenoid CDDO-imidazolide," *European Journal of Pharmacology*, vol. 620, pp. 138–144, 2009.

[157] P. S. Rabbani, A. Zhou, Z. M. Borab et al., "Novel lipoproteoplex delivers Keap1 siRNA-based gene therapy to accelerate diabetic wound healing," *Biomaterials*, vol. 132, pp. 1–15, 2017.

[158] I. G. Gazaryan and B. Thomas, "The status of Nrf2-based therapeutics: current perspectives and future prospects," *Neural Regeneration Research*, vol. 11, pp. 1708–1711, 2016.

[159] Y. Furusawa, A. Uruno, Y. Yagishita, C. Higashi, and M. Yamamoto, "Nrf2 induces fibroblast growth factor 21 in diabetic mice," *Genes to Cells*, vol. 19, pp. 864–878, 2014.

[160] M. Chin, C. Y. Lee, J. C. Chuang et al., "Bardoxolone methyl analogs RTA 405 and dh404 are well tolerated and exhibit efficacy in rodent models of type 2 diabetes and obesity,"

American Journal of Physiology. Renal Physiology, vol. 304, pp. F1438–F1446, 2013.

[161] H. M. Leinonen, E. Kansanen, P. Pölönen, M. Heinäniemi, and A. L. Levonen, "Dysregulation of the Keap1-Nrf2 pathway in cancer," *Biochemical Society Transactions*, vol. 43, pp. 645–649, 2015.

[162] A. Lau, N. F. Villeneuve, Z. Sun, P. K. Wong, and D. D. Zhang, "Dual roles of Nrf2 in cancer," *Pharmacology Research*, vol. 58, pp. 262–270, 2008.

[163] J. D. Hayes and M. McMahon, "The double-edged sword of Nrf2: subversion of redox homeostasis during the evolution of cancer," *Molecular Cell*, vol. 21, pp. 732–734, 2006.

[164] T. Shibata, T. Ohta, K. I. Tong et al., "Cancer related mutations in NRF2 impair its recognition by Keap1-Cul3 E3 ligase and promote malignancy," *Proceedings of the National Academy of Sciences of the United States of America*, vol. 105, pp. 13568–13573, 2008.

[165] T. Ohta, K. Iijima, M. Miyamoto et al., "Loss of Keap1 function activates Nrf2 and provides advantages for lung cancer cell growth," *Cancer Research*, vol. 68, pp. 1303–1309, 2008.

[166] J. Frijhoff, P. G. Winyard, N. Zarkovic et al., "Clinical relevance of biomarkers of oxidative stress," *Antioxidants & Redox Signaling*, vol. 23, pp. 1144–1170, 2015.

[167] J. M. Ashraf, M. Y. Arfat, Z. Arif, J. Ahmad, and K. Alam, "A clinical correlation of anti-DNA-AGE autoantibodies in type 2 diabetes mellitus with disease duration," *Cellular Immunology*, vol. 293, pp. 74–79, 2015.

[168] A. Ceriello, F. Mercuri, L. Quagliaro et al., "Detection of nitrotyrosine in the diabetic plasma: evidence of oxidative stress," *Diabetologia*, vol. 44, pp. 834–838, 2001.

[169] A. Abbasi, E. Corpeleijn, R. T. Gansevoort et al., "Circulating peroxiredoxin 4 and type 2 diabetes risk: the Prevention of Renal and Vascular Endstage Disease (PREVEND) study," *Diabetologia*, vol. 57, pp. 1842–1849, 2014.

[170] M. Serdar, E. Sertoglu, M. Uyanik et al., "Comparison of 8-hydroxy-2′-deoxyguanosine (8-OHdG) levels using mass spectrometer and urine albumin creatinine ratio as a predictor of development of diabetic nephropathy," *Free Radical Research*, vol. 46, pp. 1291–1295, 2012.

[171] I. Dalle-Donne, R. Rossi, R. Colombo, D. Giustarini, and A. Milzani, "Biomarkers of oxidative damage in human disease," *Clinical Chemistry*, vol. 52, pp. 601–623, 2006.

[172] W. C. Tsai, D. Y. Hueng, C. R. Lin, T. C. Yang, and H. W. Gao, "Nrf2 expressions correlate with WHO grades in gliomas and meningiomas," *International Journal of Molecular Sciences*, vol. 17, 2016.

[173] J. A. Johnson, D. A. Johnson, A. D. Kraft et al., "The Nrf2-ARE pathway: an indicator and modulator of oxidative stress in neurodegeneration," *Annals of the New York Academy of Sciences*, vol. 1147, pp. 61–69, 2008.

[174] A. S. Jiménez-Osorio, S. González-Reyes, W. R. García-Niño et al., "Association of nuclear factor-erythroid 2-related factor 2, thioredoxin interacting protein, and heme oxygenase-1 gene polymorphisms with diabetes and obesity in Mexican patients," *Oxidative Medicine and Cellular Longevity*, vol. 2016, Article ID 7367641, 8 pages, 2016.

[175] Y. Mitsuishi, K. Taguchi, Y. Kawatani et al., "Nrf2 redirects glucose and glutamine into anabolic pathways in metabolic reprogramming," *Cancer Cell*, vol. 22, pp. 66–79, 2012.

[176] J. D. Hayes and A. T. Dinkova-Kostova, "The Nrf2 regulatory network provides an interface between redox and intermediary metabolism," *Trends in Biochemical Sciences*, vol. 39, pp. 199–218, 2014.

[177] Z. W. Yu, D. Li, W. H. Ling, and T. R. Jin, "Role of nuclear factor (erythroid-derived 2)-like 2 in metabolic homeostasis and insulin action: a novel opportunity for diabetes treatment?," *World Journal of Diabetes*, vol. 3, pp. 19–28, 2012.

10

Acylcarnitine Profiles in Plasma and Tissues of Hyperglycemic NZO Mice Correlate with Metabolite Changes of Human Diabetes

Anna Weiser, Pieter Giesbertz, Hannelore Daniel, and Britta Spanier

Nutrition Physiology, Technische Universität München, Gregor-Mendel-Str. 2, 85350 Freising, Germany

Correspondence should be addressed to Britta Spanier; spanier@tum.de

Academic Editor: Bernard Portha

The New Zealand obese (NZO) mouse is a polygenic model for obesity and diabetes with obese females and obese, diabetes-prone males, used to study traits of the metabolic syndrome like type 2 diabetes mellitus (T2DM), obesity, and dyslipidaemia. By using LC-MS/MS, we here examine the suitability of this model to mirror tissue-specific changes in acylcarnitine (AC) and amino acid (AA) species preceding T2DM which may reflect patterns investigated in human metabolism. We observed high concentrations of fatty acid-derived ACs in 11 female mice, high abundance of branched-chain amino acid- (BCAA-) derived ACs in 6 male mice, and slight increases in BCAA-derived ACs in the remaining 6 males. Principal component analysis (PCA) including all ACs and AAs confirmed our hypothesis especially in plasma samples by clustering females, males with high BCAA-derived ACs, and males with slight increases in BCAA-derived ACs. Concentrations of insulin, blood glucose, NEFAs, and triacylglycerols (TAGs) further supported the hypothesis of high BCAA-derived ACs being able to mirror the onset of diabetic traits in male individuals. In conclusion, alterations in AC and AA profiles overlap with observations from human studies indicating the suitability of NZO mice to study metabolic changes preceding human T2DM.

1. Introduction

With the generation of the first New Zealand obese (NZO) mouse strain in 1948, a polygenic mouse model entered the diabetes research field which in comparison to monogenic db/db and ob/ob mice has been much less studied and for which "omics studies" are rare [1]. Previously, we studied the monogenic db/db and ob/ob mouse models [2] as well as a mouse model of diet-induced obesity (DIO) [3]. These served as comparative models to elicit and evaluate strengths and weaknesses of the inbred NZO mouse strain to study obesity-induced type 2 diabetes mellitus (T2DM). Although these models all develop obesity, they differ in their susceptibility to developing diabetes. Whereas ob/ob mice develop a strong obesity phenotype, they display an only mild and temporal hyperglycemia associated with pancreatic hypertrophy and hyperplasia. In contrast, db/db mice and male NZO mice suffer from brittle β-cells leading to a severe hyperglycemia and the progression of T2DM [2, 4]. Approximately 50% of the male NZO mice exert T2DM accompanied with a mature hyperinsulinemia and a subsequent β-cell destruction while females remain nondiabetic due to protective effects of oestrogen [5–7]. It was shown that oestrogen decreases hyperphagia via hypothalamic stimuli and furthermore leads to enhanced glucose tolerance, higher insulin sensitivity, and an improved β-cell integrity [8].

Differences between the obesity models can be found as well for their metabolite profiles. Whereas both the monogenic ob/ob and db/db mice display elevated concentrations of branched-chain amino acids (BCAA) as well as BCAA-derived metabolites as robust markers for human T2DM [9], DIO mice do not display this characteristic diabetic fingerprint [3]. Investigation of plasma acylcarnitine (AC) and amino acid (AA) profiles in the DIO C57BL/6 mouse model before and 10 weeks after a high-fat feeding imparted weak predictive value of plasma AC and plasma AA as markers to separate obese insulin-sensitive mice from obese mice with impaired insulin homeostasis [10].

So far, a comprehensive metabolite profiling of the NZO mouse model has not been established. Here, we used targeted metabolite profiling and studied the results of 43 ACs and 35 AAs and their derivatives derived from plasma, liver, kidney, heart muscle, skeletal muscle, and adipose tissue to decipher tissue-specific underlying metabolic alterations that precede T2DM in the NZO strain.

2. Material and Methods

2.1. Animals. The inbred mouse line NZO/HIBomDife was kindly provided from DIfE Institute (Nuthetal, Germany). The strain was originally received from Bomholtgard (Ry, Denmark) and kept as a separate mouse line at DIfE since more than 15 years. The mice were bred in our animal facility, and 12 age-matched males and 11 females were obtained for this study. After 3 weeks of weaning, the mice were subjected to a standard chow diet (ssniff V1534-0 R/M-H) for 5 weeks followed by a chemically defined and controlled diet (CCD; ssniff E15000-04 EF R/M Kontrolle) for 12 weeks. All mice had ad libitum access to clean water and food and were kept in an open mouse facility during the entire study. At 20 weeks of age, body weight and blood glucose were measured in a nonfasted state followed by cervical dislocation under anaesthesia using isoflurane (Baxter, Unterschleißheim, Germany). All animal procedures were in accordance with the Principles of Laboratory Care and approved by the Veterinary Inspection Services.

2.2. Plasma and Tissue Collection. Blood samples were obtained via retroorbital puncture and transferred into EDTA-coated tubes prior to centrifugation at 1.200*g* and 4°C for 10 min to extract plasma. Mice were rapidly dissected, and tissues comprising kidney, liver, heart muscle, skeletal muscle, and adipose tissue were transferred into respective tubes. Plasma and tissues were snap-frozen in liquid nitrogen and stored at −80°C until analysis. For subsequent sample preparation, tissues were ground under constant use of liquid nitrogen to ensure intactness of metabolites.

2.3. Metabolite Profiling via LC-MS/MS. AC and AA profiles were obtained from plasma, skeletal muscle, liver, kidney, heart muscle, and adipose tissues, using a triple quadrupole QTRAP 5500 tandem mass spectrometer (AB Sciex, Framingham, MA, USA) coupled to an Agilent 1260 Infinity Binary HPLC system (Agilent Technologies, Waldbronn, Germany) and an HTC PAL autosampler (CTC Analytics, Zwingen, Switzerland). Plasma and tissues were extracted with methanol and extracts were derivatized to their butyl esters as described previously [11, 12]. The butylated samples additionally contained 14 stable isotope-labelled ACs and 16 deuterated AAs as internal standards. Chromatographic separation was achieved on a reversed-phase Zorbax Eclipse XDB-C18 column (Agilent Technologies, Waldbronn, Germany).

2.4. Analysis of NEFA, Urea, Insulin, and TAG. Quantification of plasma insulin concentrations was performed using the ultrasensitive mouse insulin ELISA kit from Crystal Chem (IL, USA). Nonesterified fatty acids (NEFA) were measured by using the NEFA-HR(2) ACS-ACOD Kit from Wako Chemicals (Neuss, Germany). The concentration of plasma triacylglycerols (TAGs) was determined using a Triglyceride LiquiColor Kit from HUMAN Diagnostics (Wiesbaden, Germany), and urea concentrations in the plasma samples were specified with the Urea Liquicolor Kit from HUMAN Diagnostics.

2.5. Data Analysis. Area ratios of the AC peaks in the chromatogram were calculated using the Analyst 1.5.1 software and converted into concentrations in μmol/l. Multivariate and exploratory data analysis as well as statistical testing were accomplished in R. To reveal the optimal number of clusters, a scree plot followed by hierarchical clustering of principle components (HCPC) and a subsequent k-means consolidation were applied on samples from plasma and each tissue using the R-package FactoMineR. Metabolites were used to further describe the dimensions of the HCPC. Significant metabolites for each cluster were listed, and respective category means were compared to the overall means using a Student's t-test. Obtained p values were transformed to a normal quantile using the v-test transformation by Lebart et al. [13, 14].

Differences among gendered groups (female, male, and diabetic male NZO mice) regarding plasma parameters like blood glucose, insulin, TAG, NEFA, and urea were statistically investigated using ANOVA based on a previous data transformation with the negative reciprocals of the data to achieve normal distribution. For differences between the three groups concerning ACs and AAs in plasma and tissues, a Kruskal-Wallis test was applied to detect significant values. Results were considered as significant at an alpha level of 0.05.

3. Results

HCPC derived from plasma samples separated mice into three distinct clusters. One cluster consisted solely of male animals (cluster 3) while the remaining clusters comprised both genders (Figure 1). Significantly differing metabolite concentrations between the clusters were computed and are listed in Supplemental Table A.1. Cluster 1 was marked by elevated even-numbered long-chain fatty acid-(LCFA-) derived ACs like octadecenyl-carnitine (C18:1), octadecadienyl-carnitine (C18:2), hexadecenyl-carnitine (C16:1), and octadecanoyl-carnitine (C18) and very low abundant BCAAs and BCAA-derived ACs. Cluster 2 was most distinct by high concentrations of essential AAs like threonine (Thr), lysine (Lys), tryptophan (Trp), and methionine (Met). Medium-chain fatty acid (MCFA) and LCFA-derived ACs were strongly negatively linked to cluster 2. For cluster 3, especially high amounts of odd-numbered fatty acid-derived ACs like heptanoyl-carnitine (C7) and pentanoyl-carnitine (C5) as well as BCAA-derived ACs like 2-methylbutyryl-carnitine (2-M-C4) and isovaleryl-carnitine (3-M-C4) showed highly significant results while serine, glycine, alpha-aminoadipic acid (AADP), pentadecenoyl-carnitine (C15), and cystine (Cys-Cys) showed negative associations with cluster 3.

From the three clusters that were found based on metabolite profiling in plasma, we examined variations in blood glucose and insulin concentrations for both genders (Figure 2). As to be expected, females did not show diabetic marks due to the protective effect of oestrogen. For that reason, we focused on the diabetes-prone male mice. When

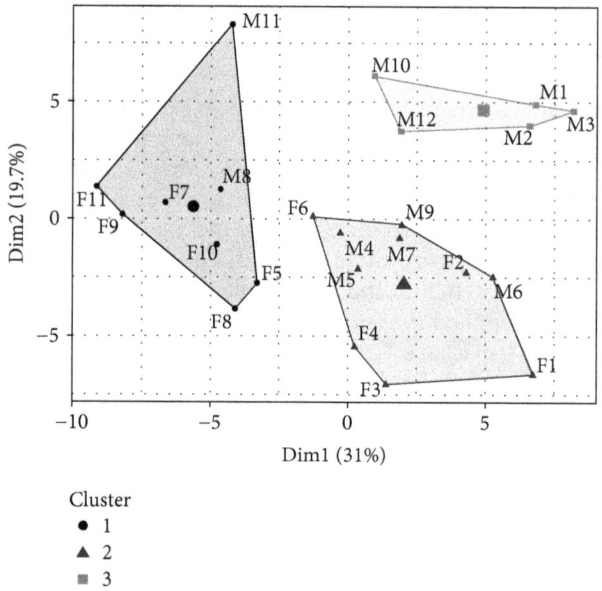

FIGURE 1: Plasma-derived cluster plot of 12 male and 11 female NZO mice to identify groups. HCPC provided three distinct clusters. Clusters 1 and 2 contain female and male NZO mice whereas cluster 3 includes solely male NZO mice. The clustering is based on the input of 78 measured metabolites comprising 43 ACs and 35 AAs. Gender is marked with M (male) and F (female).

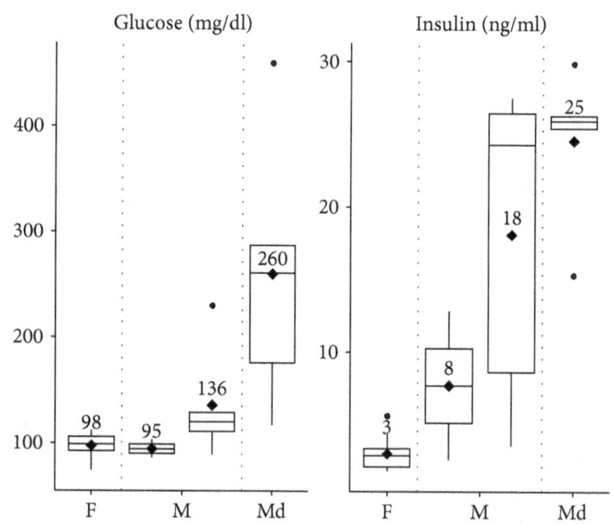

FIGURE 2: Identification of nondiabetic, prediabetic, and diabetic subjects based on blood glucose and plasma insulin concentrations. Plasma glucose and insulin levels were separately analysed based on the HCPC-derived clusters for nondiabetic females (F), non- and prediabetic male mice from clusters 1 and 2 (M), and diabetic male mice from cluster 3 (Md). Rhombuses depict mean values.

considering all male animals in the three clusters, males in cluster 3 showed significantly increased blood glucose values with 260 ± 116 mg/dl (mean ± SD) as well as elevated plasma insulin concentrations with 25 ± 5 ng/ml compared to males in clusters 1 and 2 (Figure 2). Males from cluster 1 showed the lowest blood glucose concentrations with 95 ± 9 mg/dl, comparable to the levels of females in this study with 98 ± 11 mg/dl. However, males from cluster 1 exerted higher insulin concentrations of 8 ± 5 ng/ml compared to females with 3 ± 1 ng/ml. Males from cluster 2 showed intermediate levels of glucose with 136 ± 49 mg/dl and insulin concentrations of 18 ± 10 ng/ml which is consistent with an intermediate condition of hyperglycemia and hyperinsulinemia between nondiabetic and diabetic animals from clusters 1 and 3, respectively.

To reduce the confounding influence of gender specificity, females were kept as one group (F). Males from clusters 1 and 2 were aligned to group M including nondiabetic and prediabetic male mice to increase the number of mice per cluster to gain statistical power as prerequisite for statistical testing. The drawback of increasing group size is the loss of the distinction between healthy and prediabetic male mice which would complete the line-up of dynamic changes in metabolite patterns allowing to characterize nondiabetic, prediabetic, and diabetic mice. Males from cluster 3 consistently exerted diabetic blood glucose concentrations and were denoted as male diabetic (Md).

Plasma- and tissue-specific PCAs showed metabolite-based patterns of similarity among the three mouse groups (Figure 3). In plasma, the metabolite structure of the Md group (Figure 3(a)) is most distinct from M and F compared to the tissue-derived PCAs (Figures 3(b)–3(f)). Next to plasma, adipose tissue is best suited to separate the two male groups (Figures 3(a) and 3(b)). Opposed to this, hepatic and renal tissues depict mainly overlapping features of the M and Md groups (Figures 3(c) and 3(f)).

In the following, only data from the two male groups M and Md will be compared regarding changes in metabolite profiles associated to hyperglycemia. Concentrations that were significantly different between M and Md were depicted as fold changes in Table 1. The derived significant metabolites were coincident with characterizing plasma metabolites for cluster 3 derived from the HCPC (Table A.1). Individuals from groups Md and M were further tested for significant differences in kidney, liver, heart muscle, skeletal muscle, and adipose tissue. Significantly changed hepatic metabolites between Md and M included heptanoyl-carnitine (C7), nonanoyl-carnitine (C9), and 2-methylbutyryl-carnitine (2-M-C4) and appeared to be most akin to those found in plasma opposed to significant metabolites in other tissues (Table 1).

Further phenotypic characteristics of M and Md regarding plasma-derived traits like TAGs, NEFAs, urea, insulin, and blood glucose were examined. However, except for blood glucose concentrations, none of the remaining traits showed a significant difference between M and Md (Table A.2).

Since most significant metabolites were found in plasma and liver, a more detailed analysis of the relations among respective metabolites was performed. For this, relations between plasma and liver metabolites with absolute correlation coefficients of at least 0.6 for group M and Md were depicted (Figure 4).

Squares with highly correlated metabolites between liver and plasma were marked with coloured frames. Metabolites within the purple frame are dominated by plasma BCAAs

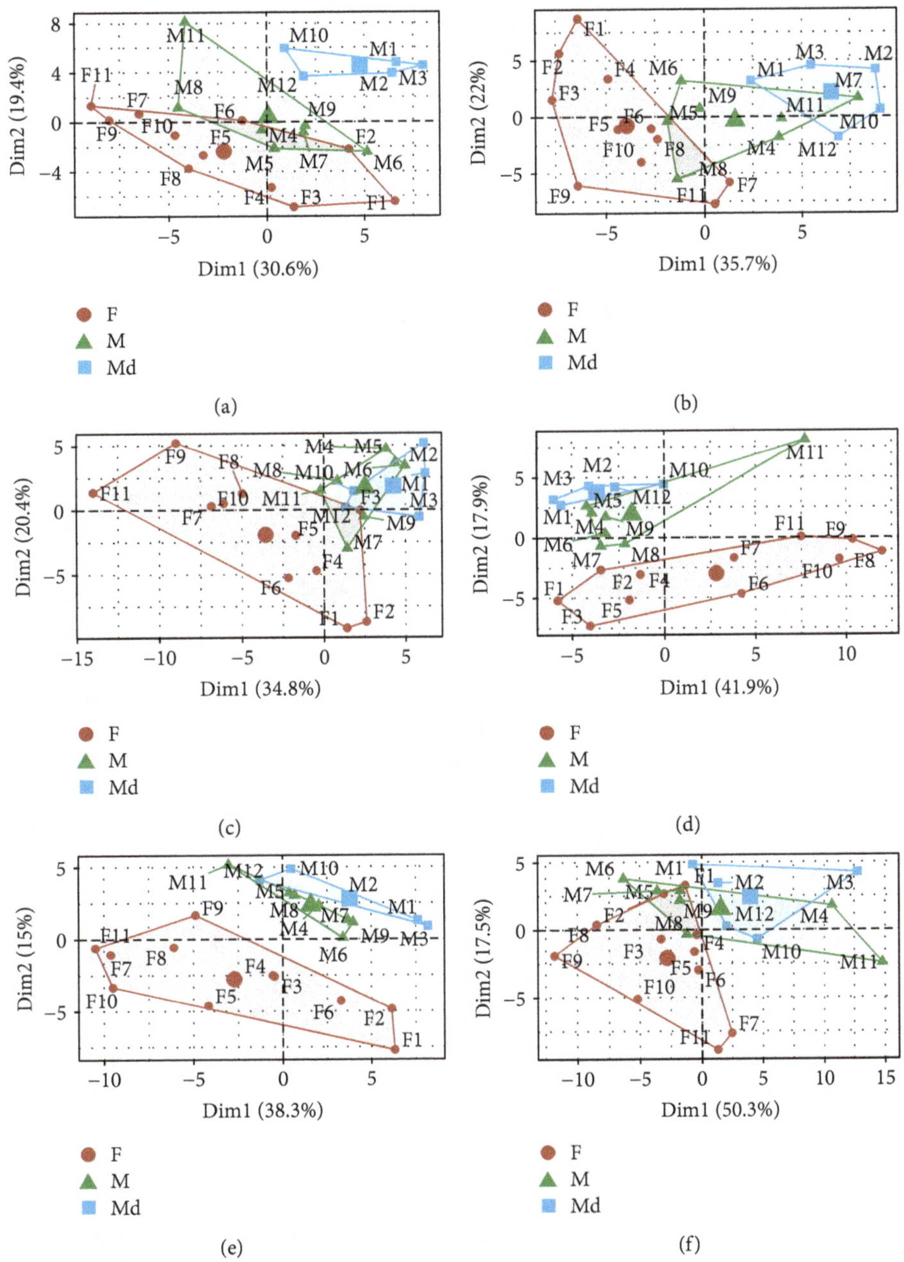

FIGURE 3: PCA to characterize plasma- and tissue-specific metabolite profiles in 12 male and 11 female NZO mice. (a) Plasma; (b) adipose tissue; (c) liver; (d) muscle; (e) heart; (f) kidney. PCAs comprise data of 43 ACs and 35 AAs. Groups are coloured according to female (F), male (M), and male diabetic (Md) mice to examine differences and resemblances among plasma and tissue metabolite profiles. Gender is marked with F (female) and M (male).

and their downstream derived ACs as well as by MCFA-derived ACs which mainly correlated with MCFA-derived ACs in liver tissue. Plasma BCAA-derived and MCFA-derived ACs with significant correlations with hepatic MCFA are 2M-C4, 3M-C4, C4, C4:1, 2M-C3, 2M-C3:1, C3, C5, C6, C7, C8, C9, and C10. Very strong correlations exist between plasma-derived C10 and several LCFA-derived ACs from liver tissue. The yellow frame marks a group of hepatic LCFA-derived ACs which correlate mainly with LCFA-derived ACs from plasma like C18:1, C18:2, C16, C16:1, C16:2, C14, and C15. The correlations do not allow to conclude biochemical relations among liver and plasma; however, it delivers a good overview about plasma metabolites that were previously detected as significant and their closest correlating metabolites from liver tissue and vice versa. This may be useful as a preselection to identify metabolites that dominate the pattern of dysregulated fatty acid oxidation leading to metabolic perturbations like the onset of T2DM.

4. Discussion

4.1. NZO Mice Display Obesity-Induced Insulin Resistance with the Potential to Develop Diabetes. Among the most widely investigated T2DM mouse models are the monogenic

Table 1: Metabolic alterations between the group of diabetic male (Md) and the group of non-/prediabetic male (M) NZO mice in plasma, tissues, and phenotypic traits.

Metabolite	Abbreviation	Fold changes Md : M					
		Plasma	Liver	Adipose tissue	Muscle	Kidney	Heart
Heptanoyl-C	C7	**3.21***	**3.98**†	1.33	1.25	1.18	1.51
Pentanoyl-C	C5	**2.31***	**1.87**‡	1.86	**1.55***	1.40	**1.73**‡
Glucose	Glc	**2.10**†	2.10	2.10	2.10	2.10	2.10
Crotonyl-C	C4:1	**2.07***	0.92	1.56	1.71	3.03	1.29
Hexanoyl-C	C6	**2.04***	1.89	1.10	1.13	0.98	1.52
2-Methylbutyryl-C	2-M-C4	**2.04***	**1.73***	1.28	1.41	1.47	**1.61***
Isobutyryl-C	2-M-C3	**1.99***	0.81	1.25	1.34	0.97	0.65
Isovaleryl-C	3-M-C4	**1.97***	0.64	1.16	1.16	1.52	**1.44**‡
Nonanoyl-C	C9	**1.90**†	5.35†	1.24	0.76	0.99	1.12
Propionyl-C	C3	**1.88***	1.17	1.28	1.05	1.30	1.30
Methacrylyl-C	2-M-C3:1	**1.88**‡	0.90	**1.45***	**2.63**‡	3.03	1.60
Butyryl-C	C4	1.74	0.87	1.16	**1.44**‡	1.14	1.14
3-Methylcrotonyl-C	3-M-C4:1	1.73	0.92	**<LOQ**¶	1.28	1.33	**1.60**‡
Octanoyl-C	C8	1.66	**3.13***	0.95	0.84	0.94	1.15
Tiglyl-C	2-M-C4:1	1.52	1.17	1.42	1.39	1.69	**1.45***
Isoundecanoyl-C	iso-C11:0	1.45	**5.86**†	1.28	0.88	1.44	2.29
α-Aminobutyrate	AAB	1.34	**1.66**‡	1.32	1.15	1.48	1.39
Glutamine	Gln	**1.31***	0.98	**1.21**‡	0.90	1.13	0.99
Hydroxybutyryl-C-b	C4-OH b	1.31	0.75	1.27	**1.77***	1.07	1.46
Isoleucine	Ile	1.30	1.01	**1.38***	1.10	1.11	1.09
Phenylalanine	Phe	**1.27**‡	1.19	1.18	0.97	1.13	1.12
β-Alanine	β-Ala	1.15	**2.07**‡	1.37	0.94	1.29	1.16
γ-Aminobutyric acid	GABA	1.08	1.38	4.02	1.11	**1.54***	1.20
Tryptophan	Trp	1.05	3.83	1.34	1.16	**<LOQ**¶	**1.47**‡
Hydroxybutyryl-C-a	C4-OH a	1.01	0.77	1.29	**1.80**†	0.97	1.00
Arginine	Arg	0.91	0.85	1.04	**0.57**‡	0.84	0.82
3-Methyl-Histidine	3M-His	0.90	**1.29**‡	1.28	0.98	1.23	1.02
Methylglutaryl-C	C5-M-DC	0.62	0.75	**1.34**‡	0.97	0.74	1.12
Cystine	Cys-Cys	**0.46***	**2.44**‡	1.63	1.20	1.48	1.85
Undecanoyl-C	C11	0.19	**3.18**†	1.69	0.91	1.09	0.75
Isotridecanoyl-C	iso-C13:0	0.14	**4.33***	1.01	0.99	1.41	1.18

Differences in plasma- and tissue-derived ACs and AAs between diabetic male NZO mice (Md) and non-/prediabetic male mice (M). Metabolites with p values above 0.05 are shown since the study aims for a holistic approach to define metabolite profiles for diabetic conditions rather than identifying single markers for T2DM. Results were considered as significant at a threshold of $\alpha < 0.05$. LOQ = limit of quantification; C = carnitine. ¶<LOQ; $^{\dagger}0.001 < p < 0.01$; $^{*}0.01 < p < 0.05$; and $^{\ddagger}0.05 < p < 0.1$.

ob/ob and db/db mice as well as models of high-fat DIO and insulin resistance. These models differ in their susceptibility and their speed in which they progress from an obese insulin-resistant towards an insulin-deficient type 2 diabetic state, depending on the stability of their β-cells. Moreover, we and others observed distinct metabolic alterations between the respective models. BCAAs, prominent marker metabolites of human T2DM, were reported as increased in the monogenic ob/ob and db/db mice [2], but these changes could not be confirmed in DIO mice [3]. In the present study, we examined NZO mice as a polygenic model of obesity-induced insulin resistance and T2DM. This model has been used in quantitative trait locus analysis to discover risk alleles for the development of T2DM [15, 16], but is rather scarcely studied within the context of metabolite alterations related to obesity-induced T2DM. Here, we aimed to explore metabolite alterations in the NZO model to determine to what extent these mice can reproduce respective metabolic conditions in human. Using a targeted LC-MS/MS analysis, we explored changes in AA and AC concentrations, which include BCAAs and BCAA-derived metabolites, described as prominent diabetes markers.

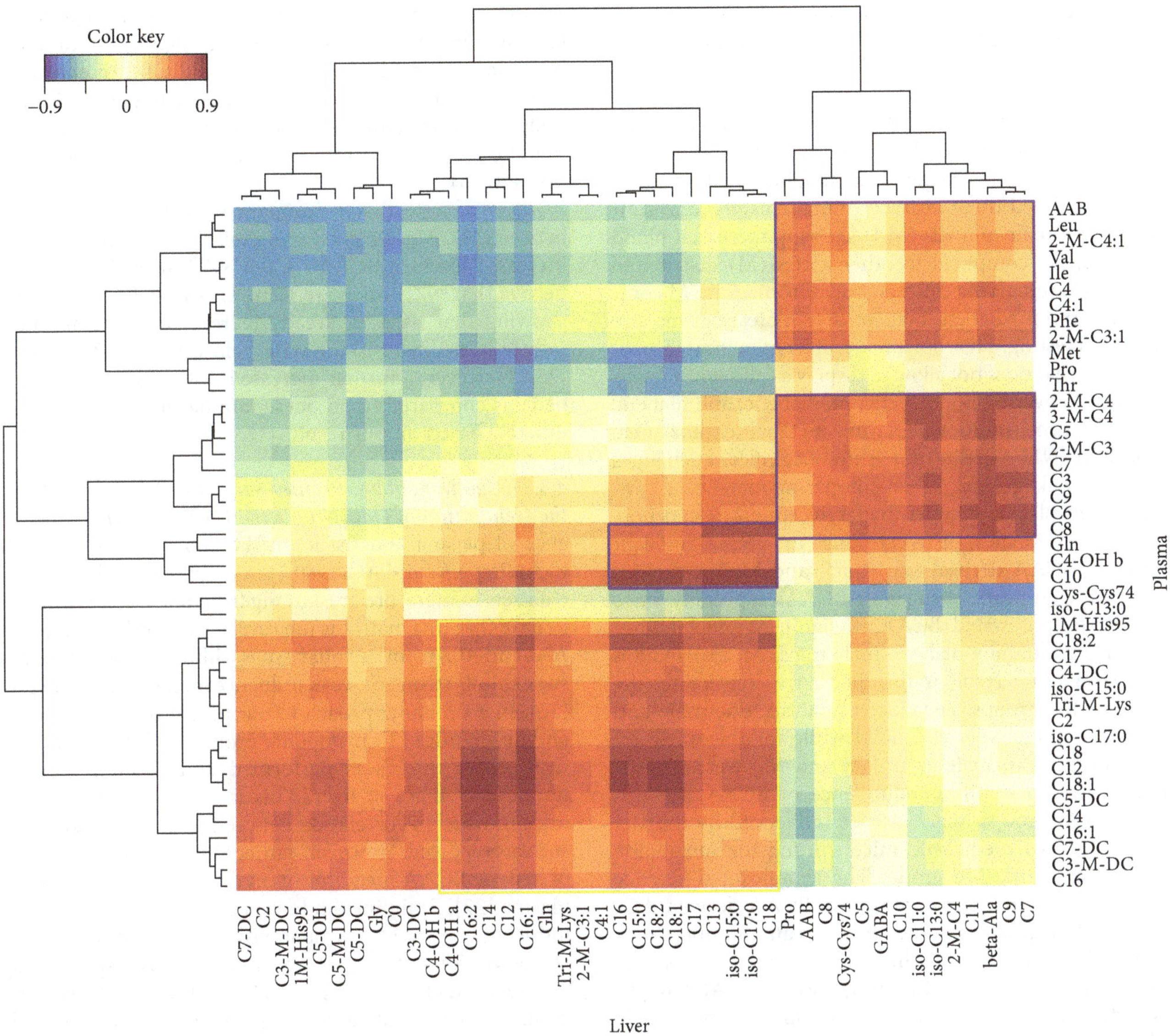

FIGURE 4: Heat map of hierarchical clustering of plasma and liver metabolites from diabetic (Md) and non-/prediabetic (M) male NZO mice. Highly correlating metabolites from plasma and liver are marked with coloured frames, while purple frames comprise mainly BCAA-derived and MCFA-derived ACs while yellow-marked frames comprise mainly LCFA-derived ACs. The threshold for the absolute correlation was set to at least 0.6. The colour scale reflects the distance score between each metabolite pair, with dark red indicating strong positively correlated pairs of metabolites and blue indicating strong negative correlations.

The preceding metabolite profiling in monogenic ob/ob and db/db mice [2] and mice fed a high-fat diet [3] allowed to perform a comparison of metabolite profiles in the NZO mice studied here with our previous measurements.

In our study, female mice remained normoglycemic, which is in line with previous literature stating protective effects of oestrogen [1, 6]. We furthermore observed a large variation in the development and severity of hyperglycemia within the male group since numbers for age and fasted blood glucose concentrations at the onset of T2DM vary among the studies and make it difficult to define the beginning of diabetic perturbations by distinct biomarkers [2, 17, 18]. Previous studies describe that only around 50% of male animals progress to a state of T2DM [1].

One reason for this is the progression of obesity in NZO mice which determines the development of diabetes-like metabolic circumstances [1]. Dependent on the fed diet and the individual progression of gaining weight, overt diabetes-like conditions can appear already in 5-week-old NZO mice with blood glucose levels higher than 300 mg/dl [19]. Besides a large interindividual genetic variation in obesity genes determining the progression speed towards obesity, variation in a large number of other genes determines the progression of individual mice towards obesity-associated diabetes [20]. The comparison of our results derived from db/db and NZO mice showed a more progressive severity of T2DM in db/db opposed to NZO mice when comparing the average blood glucose levels at an age of 20 weeks. However, on an individual basis, it is important to keep in mind that the development of T2DM in NZO is a more dynamic procedure as compared to the db/db model.

4.2. Hyperglycemic Male NZO Mice Show Increased Plasma Levels of BCAA-Derived and MCFA-Derived ACs, but Not of BCAAs. Using the targeted metabolite profiles from plasma, we defined three distinct animal clusters, one consisting only of male animals (Md) showing increased blood glucose levels as compared to other males (M) distributed within the two remaining clusters. Males from group M comprised non- and prediabetic male mice to increase group size for statistical testing. This, however, represents a limitation of our study since it does not allow to display a full set of metabolite patterns covering nondiabetic, prediabetic, and diabetic male NZO mice. Additional plasma metabolites like urea, insulin, and NEFAs did not show significant changes between the male groups. When comparing metabolite concentrations in plasma between hyperglycemic Md and normoglycemic M males, it is striking to find significant increases in BCAA derived and short- and MCFA-derived ACs but no significant changes in BCAAs especially since the HCPC output stated BCAA as significant metabolites for cluster 3 containing diabetic male mice. An explanation for this conflicting result is the difference concerning the structure of the groups. For cluster analysis, one male and two mixed clusters were examined while for the statistical testing only the two male groups M and Md were considered. The lacking significant difference of BCAA between the Md and M groups might also be influenced by the fact that M comprises prediabetic mice shifting the metabolite pattern closer to the Md group. The significant difference among the male groups regarding the BCAA-derived ACs suggests a dysregulation more downstream of mitochondrial BCAA breakdown. A likely involvement of short-chain 3-hydroxyacyl-CoA dehydrogenase (SCHAD) might be expected, as its according gene (Hadh) was previously identified as an obesity gene via quantitative trait locus analysis in NZO mice [21]. Furthermore, SCHAD has been shown to impact thermogenesis and nutrient-dependent insulin secretion, characterizing knockout mice with significantly lowered blood glucose levels and increased insulin concentrations. It is likely that SCHAD exerts an important regulatory impact on the usage of ACs as energy source. In our study, MCFA-derived ACs up to iso-C13 were significantly characteristic for hepatic tissue of Md mice. MCFA-derived ACs are potential indicators to reflect an incomplete fatty acid oxidation imparting a progressive dysregulation of lipid metabolism [22]. At the age of 20 weeks, metabolite profiles of male mice were not dominated by LCFAs; however, MCFAs have been revealed to be characterizing for the progression towards T2DM. For the dynamic NZO model subjected to a CCD, the effects of an impaired β-oxidation are not as distinct as they might evolve under a high-fat diet and therefore are only expected to evolve over time with the progression of obesity-induced T2DM. ACs derived from C12 to C14 fatty acids are associated with the inflammatory transcription factor NFκB triggering a low chronic inflammation that drives obesity-associated insulin resistance [23]. Except for iso-C13 in liver tissue, there were no significant differences between M and Md for C12, C13, and C14. In comparison to female mice, all male mice exerted higher C12 to C14 metabolites in adipose tissue whereas other tissues did not show such a distinct separation between genders (data not shown).

It is of note that a comparison of plasma AA profiles between NZO and New Zealand black (NZB) mice did show increased levels of BCAAs in the NZO mice [24]. Important here is that NZB mice are lean. This is in line with reports showing that BCAAs already increase in an early obesity-induced insulin-resistant state before the onset of diabetes [25]. However, a further increase in BCAAs in an obese diabetic as compared to an obese nondiabetic state thus seems unlikely based on our results.

4.3. Tissue Metabolite Profiles Suggest a Role for the Liver in the Generation of Odd-Numbered Carbon Chains. The influence of plasma and tissue on the allocation of metabolites including AAs and ACs is still poorly understood. While most data sets in literature are coming from plasma, it is important to note that this matrix is the result of the influx and efflux of AAs and ACs from various tissues without knowing which tissue exhibits strong or weak influence on the metabolite profile [26]. In a similar approach to our previous study with ob/ob and db/db mice [2], metabolite profiling of individual tissues from NZO mice was performed and showed most pronounced changes in liver. This is in contrast to the db/db mice in which a correlation between plasma and adipose tissue was reported. However, earlier Shin et al. stated an impact of hepatic BCAA metabolism on the BCAA concentration in plasma [27]. Brain insulin lowers circulating BCAA levels by inducing hepatic BCAA catabolism [27]. Increases in hepatic concentrations of various odd-numbered AC species can be observed, including heptanoyl-carnitine (C7), nonanoyl-carnitine (C9), and undecanoyl-carnitine (C11), as well as isomeric forms of undecanoyl-carnitine (iso-C11) and tridecanoyl-carnitine (iso-C13). The exact origin for these odd-numbered carbon chains remains unknown, and various metabolic routes of formation have been described. Peroxisomal processes of fatty acid alpha oxidation are known to generate odd-numbered carbon chains by chain-shortening fatty acids by one single carbon atom. This is however thought to be a minor process and seems important in catabolic situations [28]. More recently, a study in adipocytes shows that it is principally possible to generate longer odd-numbered acyl chains via elongation of BCAA-derived carbon chains [29].

5. Conclusion

In summary, our study has examined the NZO mouse model by investigating AC and AA species in plasma, liver, kidney, skeletal muscle, heart muscle and adipose tissue to provide detailed and comprehensive fingerprints of different states in the development of T2DM in male mice—from non- to prediabetic to severely diabetic states. Thereby, metabolites derived from BCAAs as well as MCFA derived ACs turned out to be characteristic for diabetic perturbations in male NZO mice. This is coinciding with studies conducted in human trials and highlights the benefits of the polygenic NZO mouse model in mirroring human T2DM conditions for further investigations.

Abbreviations

AA: Amino acid
AADP: Alpha-aminoadipic acid
AC: Acylcarnitine
BCAA: Branched-chain amino acid
C: Carnitine
CCD: Chemically defined and controlled diet
DIO: Diet-induced obesity
EDTA: Ethylenediaminetetraacetic acid
Glc: Glucose
HCPC: Hierarchical clustering of principal components
HOMA-IR: Homeostatic model assessment-insulin resistance
LCFA: Long-chain fatty acid
MCFA: Medium-chain fatty acid
Md: Male diabetic
NEFA: Nonesterified fatty acid
NZB: New Zealand black
NZO: New Zealand obese
PCA: Principal component analysis
SCHAD: Short-chain 3-hydroxyacyl-CoA dehydrogenase
T2DM: Type 2 diabetes mellitus
TAG: Triacylglycerol.

Conflicts of Interest

The authors declare that there is no conflict of interest regarding the publication of this article.

Acknowledgments

The authors thank Hans-Georg Joost and Reinhardt Kluge from the Deutsches Institut für Ernährungsforschung, Nuthetal (DIfE), for the NZO/HiBomDife mice. The authors also thank Ronny Scheundel for animal handling and sample collection. For fruitful discussions and comments on the manuscript, the authors thank their colleagues, especially Kurt Gedrich. This work was supported by the German Research Foundation (DFG) and the Technical University of Munich within the funding program Open Access Publishing.

References

[1] R. Kluge, S. Scherneck, A. Schürmann, and H. G. Joost, "Pathophysiology and genetics of obesity and diabetes in the New Zealand obese mouse: a model of the human metabolic syndrome," in *Animal Models in Diabetes Research*, H.-G. Joost, H. Al-Hasani, and A. Schürmann, Eds., pp. 59–73, Humana Press, Totowa, NJ, USA, 2012.

[2] P. Giesbertz, I. Padberg, D. Rein et al., "Metabolite profiling in plasma and tissues of *ob*/*ob* and *db*/*db* mice identifies novel markers of obesity and type 2 diabetes," *Diabetologia*, vol. 58, no. 9, pp. 2133–2143, 2015.

[3] M. Sailer, C. Dahlhoff, P. Giesbertz et al., "Increased plasma citrulline in mice marks diet-induced obesity and may predict the development of the metabolic syndrome," *PLoS One*, vol. 8, no. 5, article e63950, 2013.

[4] A. J. F. King, "The use of animal models in diabetes research," *British Journal of Pharmacology*, vol. 166, no. 3, pp. 877–894, 2012.

[5] C. Lange, K. Jeruschke, L. Herberg, E. H. Leiter, and E. Junger, "The diabetes-prone NZO/Hl strain. Proliferation capacity of beta cells in hyperinsulinemia and hyperglycemia," *Archives of Physiology and Biochemistry*, vol. 112, no. 1, pp. 49–58, 2006.

[6] M. Lubura, D. Hesse, M. Kraemer et al., "Diabetes prevalence in NZO females depends on estrogen action on liver fat content," *American Journal of Physiology - Endocrinology and Metabolism*, vol. 309, no. 12, pp. E968–E980, 2015.

[7] E. Junger, L. Herberg, K. Jeruschke, and E. H. Leiter, "The diabetes-prone NZO/Hl strain. II. Pancreatic immunopathology," *Laboratory Investigation*, vol. 82, no. 7, pp. 843–853, 2002.

[8] R. W. Schwenk, C. Baumeier, B. Finan et al., "GLP-1–oestrogen attenuates hyperphagia and protects from beta cell failure in diabetes-prone New Zealand obese (NZO) mice," *Diabetologia*, vol. 58, no. 3, pp. 604–614, 2015.

[9] S. E. McCormack, O. Shaham, M. A. McCarthy et al., "Circulating branched-chain amino acid concentrations are associated with obesity and future insulin resistance in children and adolescents," *Pediatric Obesity*, vol. 8, no. 1, pp. 52–61, 2013.

[10] O. Horakova, J. Hansikova, K. Bardova et al., "Plasma acylcarnitines and amino acid levels as an early complex biomarker of propensity to high-fat diet-induced obesity in mice," *PLoS One*, vol. 11, no. 5, article e0155776, 2016.

[11] U. Harder, B. Koletzko, and W. Peissner, "Quantification of 22 plasma amino acids combining derivatization and ion-pair LC–MS/MS," *Journal of Chromatography B*, vol. 879, no. 7-8, pp. 495–504, 2011.

[12] P. Giesbertz, J. Ecker, A. Haag, B. Spanier, and H. Daniel, "An LC-MS/MS method to quantify acylcarnitine species including isomeric and odd-numbered forms in plasma and tissues," *Journal of Lipid Research*, vol. 56, no. 10, pp. 2029–2039, 2015.

[13] D. Grangé and L. Lebart, *Traitements Statistiques des Enquêtes*, ed Jacques Antoine, Dunod, Paris, France, 1993.

[14] S. Le, J. Josse, and F. Husson, "FactoMineR: an R package for multivariate analysis," *Journal of Statistical Software*, vol. 25, no. 1, pp. 1–18, 2008.

[15] R. Kluge, K. Giesen, G. Bahrenberg, L. Plum, J. R. Ortlepp, and H. G. Joost, "Quantitative trait loci for obesity and insulin resistance (Nob1, Nob2) and their interaction with the leptin receptor allele (LeprA720T/T1044I) in New Zealand obese mice," *Diabetologia*, vol. 43, no. 12, pp. 1565–1572, 2000.

[16] H.-J. Pan, Y. Lin, Y. E. Chen, D. E. Vance, and E. H. Leiter, "Adverse hepatic and cardiac responses to rosiglitazone in a new mouse model of type 2 diabetes: relation to dysregulated phosphatidylcholine metabolism," *Vascular Pharmacology*, vol. 45, no. 1, pp. 65–71, 2006.

[17] B. J. Lamont, M. F. Waters, and S. Andrikopoulos, "A low-carbohydrate high-fat diet increases weight gain and does not

improve glucose tolerance, insulin secretion or β-cell mass in NZO mice," *Nutrition & Diabetes*, vol. 6, no. 2, article e194, 2016.

[18] F. Mirhashemi, S. Scherneck, O. Kluth et al., "Diet dependence of diabetes in the New Zealand obese (NZO) mouse: total fat, but not fat quality or sucrose accelerates and aggravates diabetes," *Experimental and Clinical Endocrinology & Diabetes*, vol. 119, no. 3, pp. 167–171, 2011.

[19] C. Baumeier, D. Kaiser, J. Heeren et al., "Caloric restriction and intermittent fasting alter hepatic lipid droplet proteome and diacylglycerol species and prevent diabetes in NZO mice," *Biochimica et Biophysica Acta (BBA) - Molecular and Cell Biology of Lipids*, vol. 1851, no. 5, pp. 566–576, 2015.

[20] H.-G. Joost and A. Schürmann, "The genetic basis of obesity-associated type 2 diabetes (diabesity) in polygenic mouse models," *Mammalian Genome*, vol. 25, no. 9-10, pp. 401–412, 2014.

[21] N. Schulz, H. Himmelbauer, M. Rath et al., "Role of medium- and short-chain L-3-hydroxyacyl-CoA dehydrogenase in the regulation of body weight and thermogenesis," *Endocrinology*, vol. 152, no. 12, pp. 4641–4651, 2011.

[22] S. H. Adams, C. L. Hoppel, K. H. Lok et al., "Plasma acylcarnitine profiles suggest incomplete long-chain fatty acid β-oxidation and altered tricarboxylic acid cycle activity in type 2 diabetic African-American women," *The Journal of Nutrition*, vol. 139, no. 6, pp. 1073–1081, 2009.

[23] J. M. Rutkowsky, T. A. Knotts, K. D. Ono-Moore et al., "Acylcarnitines activate proinflammatory signaling pathways," *American Journal of Physiology. Endocrinology and Metabolism*, vol. 306, no. 12, pp. E1378–E1387, 2014.

[24] A. Maida, J. S. K. Chan, K. A. Sjøberg et al., "Repletion of branched chain amino acids reverses mTORC1 signaling but not improved metabolism during dietary protein dilution," *Molecular Metabolism*, vol. 6, no. 8, pp. 873–881, 2017.

[25] T. J. Wang, M. G. Larson, R. S. Vasan et al., "Metabolite profiles and the risk of developing diabetes," *Nature Medicine*, vol. 17, no. 4, pp. 448–453, 2011.

[26] M. G. Schooneman, N. Achterkamp, C. A. Argmann, M. R. Soeters, and S. M. Houten, "Plasma acylcarnitines inadequately reflect tissue acylcarnitine metabolism," *Biochimica et Biophysica Acta (BBA) – Molecular and Cell Biology of Lipids*, vol. 1841, no. 7, pp. 987–994, 2014.

[27] A. C. Shin, M. Fasshauer, N. Filatova et al., "Brain insulin lowers circulating BCAA levels by inducing hepatic BCAA catabolism," *Cell Metabolism*, vol. 20, no. 5, pp. 898–909, 2014.

[28] T. Takahashi, H. Takahashi, H. Takeda, and M. Shichiri, "Alpha-oxidation of fatty acids in fasted or diabetic rats," *Diabetes Research and Clinical Practice*, vol. 16, no. 2, pp. 103–108, 1992.

[29] C. R. Green, M. Wallace, A. S. Divakaruni et al., "Branched-chain amino acid catabolism fuels adipocyte differentiation and lipogenesis," *Nature Chemical Biology*, vol. 12, no. 1, pp. 15–21, 2016.

11

Suppression of Excessive Histone Deacetylases Activity in Diabetic Hearts Attenuates Myocardial Ischemia/Reperfusion Injury via Mitochondria Apoptosis Pathway

Yang Wu, Yan Leng, Qingtao Meng, Rui Xue, Bo Zhao, Liying Zhan, and Zhongyuan Xia

Department of Anesthesiology, Renmin Hospital of Wuhan University, Wuhan, Hubei Province 430060, China

Correspondence should be addressed to Zhongyuan Xia; xiazhongyuanmz@aliyun.com

Academic Editor: Hiroshi Okamoto

Background. Histone deacetylases (HDACs) play a pivotal role in signaling modification and gene transcriptional regulation that are essential for cardiovascular pathophysiology. Diabetic hearts with higher HDACs activity were more vulnerable to myocardial ischemia/reperfusion (MI/R) injury compared with nondiabetic hearts. We are curious about whether suppression of excessive HDACs activity in diabetic heart protects against MI/R injury. *Methods.* Diabetic rats were subjected to 45 min of ischemia, followed by 3 h of reperfusion. H9C2 cardiomyocytes were exposed to high glucose for 24 h, followed by 4 h of hypoxia and 2 h of reoxygenation (H/R). *Results.* Both MI/R injury and diabetes mellitus elevated myocardium HDACs activity. MI/R induced apoptotic cell death was significantly decreased in diabetic rats treated with HDACs inhibitor trichostatin A (TSA). TSA administration markedly moderated dissipation of mitochondrial membrane potential, protected the integrity of mitochondrial permeability transition pore (mPTP), and decreased cell apoptosis. Notably, cotreatment with Akt inhibitor partly or absolutely inhibited the protective effect of TSA in vivo and in vitro. Furthermore, TSA administration activated Akt/Foxo3a pathway, leading to Foxo3a cytoplasm translocation and attenuation proapoptosis protein Bim expression. *Conclusions.* Both diabetes mellitus and MI/R injury increased cardiac HDACs activity. Suppression of HDACs activity triggered protective effects against MI/R and H/R injury under hyperglycemia conditions through Akt-modulated mitochondrial apoptotic pathways via Foxo3a/Bim.

1. Introduction

Histone deacetylases (HDACs) and the histone acetyl transferases (HATs) regulated global acetylation levels in mammals. They keep a delicate balance and mainly function through acetylation/deacetylation of histone and nonhistone substrates [1]. HDACs family is composed of three distinct groups, nonsirtuin HDACs (class I, II) and longevity protein sirtuin deacetylases (class III) [2]. Previous analyses have grouped nonsirtuin HDACs into two different classes, based on DNA sequence similarity and function [3]. Class I HDACs (1, 2, 3, and 8) display an extensive presence in nucleus and exhibit tissue-specific distributions [4]. Class II HDACs (4, 5, 6, 7, 9, and 10) can shuttle between the nucleus and cytoplasm [5]. Class I HDACs have been extensively studied in their classical role as histone modifiers and transcriptional repressors [6, 7]. Class II HDACs primarily control gene expression by recruiting other proteins; in some cases, these enzymes can also act as transcriptional activators [8]. Many studies indicated that acetylation levels of mammal are linked strongly with cardiovascular diseases, including coronary heart diseases [9], diabetic cardiomyopathy [10], hypertension [11], ventricular remodeling [12, 13], and arrhythmia [14]. Recently, selective inhibition of classes I and II HDACs with an inhibitor, trichostatin A (TSA), showed protective effects against MI/R injury [15]. This is in line with the observations that inhibition of HDACs in cardiac myocytes silences fetal gene activation, attenuates cardiac hypertrophy, and prevents cardiac remodeling [16, 17]. Furthermore, HDACs inhibition was recently reported to improve myocardial function and prevent cardiac remodeling in diabetic mice [18].

Epidemiological surveys indicated that diabetic patients are more likely to develop cardiovascular complications [19]. Despite current optimal therapy, the mortality rate of acute myocardial infarction in diabetic patients is more than double that of nondiabetic patients [20]. Uncontrolled chronic hyperglycemia with mitochondrial bioenergetics deficit and increased oxidative stress led to an inadequate physiological reserve in the myocardium when challenged by MI/R insult [21–24]. Diabetes also attenuates the endogenous antiapoptosis signaling pathways, thus invalidating powerful therapeutic programs, such as ischemic pre- and postconditioning [25–27]. Therefore, mitochondrial dysfunction and signaling events characteristic of apoptosis are responsible for the exacerbated cardiac ischemic injury in diabetic patients [28, 29]. The activation of prosurvival signaling cascades, such as PI3K/Akt, shows cardioprotective effects through recruitment of antiapoptotic proteins during MI/R in nondiabetes animals [30]. Consistent with our previous studies, diabetes mellitus markedly impairs the PI3K/Akt pathway and exacerbates MI/R injury [31, 32].

Many observations showed that HDACs inhibitor promotes an increase in Akt phosphorylation in different type of cells [33, 34]. HDACs inhibitor was found to protect brain white matter injury by activating the PI3K/Akt signaling pathway in neurons [34]. In fact, in Akt deleted mice, protective effects of TSA administration in reducing infarct size were blocked [35].

It has been best characterized that Forkhead box O3 (Foxo3a) plays a crucial role in regulating cell survival, oxidative stress resistance, and apoptosis. Foxo3a has been extensively studied in myocardial I/R injury [36, 37]. Phosphorylation of Foxo3a by serine/threonine kinase Akt results in nucleus exclusion and cytoplasm relocalization [38]. Recent work in mouse tissues demonstrated that the endogenous HDACs inhibitor caused an increased expression of Foxo3a [39]. It is worth noting that Foxo3a has been shown to modulate proapoptotic pathway through binding to consensus sequence of Bim promoter region and induce Bim expression [40].

Trichostatin A (TSA), a class I/II HDACs inhibitor [41], could protect the myocardium from I/R injury in nondiabetic rats [35]. Therefore, we aimed to investigate whether TSA elicits cardioprotective effect in an in vivo model of regional I/R in diabetic rat and in vitro model of hypoxia/reoxygenation (H/R) under hyperglycemia. Furthermore, we also detected whether the activation of Akt by TSA pretreatment could increase phosphorylation of Foxo3a.

2. Materials and Methods

2.1. Animals. Ninety Male Sprague-Dawley (SD) rats (250–280 g) were purchased from HFK bioscience (Beijing, China). Rats were housed in an environment with a maintained temperature of 22°C, relative humidity of 50 ± 15%, and a 12-hour light/12-hour dark cycle. All rats had free access to standard chow and water, ad libitum. All animal procedures received the approval of the Wuhan University Animal Care and Use Committee and followed the Principles of Laboratory Animal Care and are in accordance with the Guide for the Care and Use of Laboratory Animals by the National Institutes of Health (NIH Publication Number 80-23, revised 1996).

2.2. Reagents. Streptozotocin (STZ), triphenyl tetrazolium chloride (TTC), and Evans blue (EB) were obtained from Sigma Chemical Co. (MO, USA). TSA, the Akt inhibitor MK-2206, and the PI3K/Akt inhibitor wortmannin were purchased from Selleck Chemicals Co. (Texas, USA). Dulbecco's modified Eagle's medium (DMEM) and fetal bovine serum (FBS) were purchased from Gibco Laboratories (Grand Island, NY, USA). Antibodies directed against Akt, p-Akt (ser473), Foxo3a, p-Foxo3a (ser253), caspase-3, and GAPDH were obtained from Cell Signaling Technology (CST, Beverly, CA, USA). Primary antibodies against Bim, Bax, Bcl-2, cytochrome C (cytc), Lamin b1, acetyl-histone 3 (Ac-H3), acetyl-histone 4 (Ac-H4), histone 3 (H3), and histone 4 (H4) were obtained from Abcam (Cambridge, MA, USA).

2.3. Diabetes Induction. After 5 days of acclimation to the environment, rats were starved for 12 hours for diabetes induction. Diabetes was induced by single intraperitoneal (ip) injection of STZ (65 mg/kg). STZ was dissolved in 0.1 mol/L sodium citrate buffer (pH = 4.5). Control rats were injected with equal volume of buffer (0.1 mol/L sodium citrate buffer, pH 4.5) after an identical starvation process. Three days after STZ administration, blood samples were obtained from tail vein to evaluate the blood glucose, using Onetouch ultra glucometer (Johnson & Johnson, USA). If the fasting blood glucose was ≥16.7 mmol/L for at least three samples, the rats were considered to have diabetes.

2.4. Groups and Experimental Protocols. For the in vivo study, 8 weeks after STZ injection, diabetic and normal rats were randomized into four groups: (1) sham operated normal rats (NS), (2) normal rats subjected to I/R insult (NIR), (3) sham operated diabetic rats (DS), and (4) diabetic rats subjected to I/R insult (DIR). To gain a deeper insight into the prosurvival effect of HDACs inhibition, different interventions were preformed among diabetic rats: (1) diabetic rats subjected to I/R insult (DIR), (2) DIR rats pretreated with TSA (DIR+TSA), (3) DIR rats copretreated with TSA and MK-2206 (DIR+TSA+MK), and (4) DIR rats copretreated with TSA and wortmannin (DIR+TSA+Wor). TSA (1 mg/kg) or vehicle (DMSO, 1‰) was intraperitoneally given for 5 days before MI/R. MK-2206 (300 μg/kg), wortmannin (15 ug/kg), or vehicle (DMSO, 1‰, 1 mL) was administered intravenously (femoral vein) 20 min before coronary ligation was performed. For the in vitro study, H9C2 cardiomyocytes were randomly assigned to seven groups: (1) low glucose control (LG-Control, 5.5 mM), (2) low glucose culture followed by H/R (LG-HR), (3) high glucose control (HG-control, 33 mM), (4) cells exposed to high glucose followed by H/R (HGHR), (5) HGHR cells pretreated with TSA (HGHR+TSA), (6) HGHR cells copretreated with TSA and Akt inhibitor (HGHR+TSA+MK), and (7) HGHR cells copretreated with TSA and PI3K/Akt inhibitor (HGHR+TSA+Wor). H9C2 cardiomyocytes were cultured in low glucose DMED with 10% FBS at 37°C in a humidified atmosphere of 10% CO_2 and exposed to HG medium for 24 h followed by 4 h of hypoxia (94% N_2 and 5% CO_2) and 2 h reoxygenation. TSA (200 nM) or vehicle was administered 6 h before H/R. MK-2206 (300 nM), wortmannin (100 nM), or vehicle was given

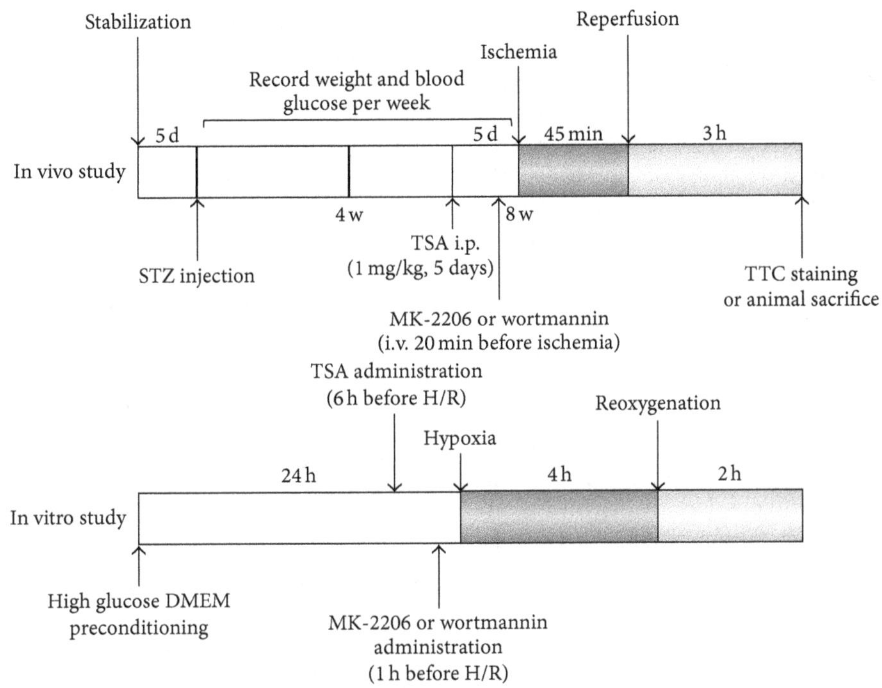

FIGURE 1: Experimental protocols. Diagram showing the experimental procedures including diabetes induction, ischemia/reperfusion model, TSA and MK-2206 administration, and sacrifice end point. Eight weeks after STZ injection, rats were subjected to 45 min of coronary artery occlusion followed by 3 h of reperfusion. TSA or DMSO was administrated at 48, 24, and 1 h before surgery. MK-2206, wortmannin, or vehicle was applied intravenously 20 minutes before ischemia. TSA: HDAC inhibitor; MK-2206: Akt inhibitor.

1 h before hypoxia. The experimental protocol is depicted schematically in Figure 1.

2.5. Myocardial Ischemia and Reperfusion Model. 8 weeks after diabetes induction, rats were anesthetized by pentobarbital sodium (50 mg/kg ip) and subjected to tracheotomy and artificial ventilation. Electrocardiogram and heart rate (HR) were continuously monitored by an electrophysiolograph (BioPAC, MH150, USA). Femoral vein intravenous infusion access had been established for drug or saline administration. The heart was exposed by a fifth-intercostal space thoracotomy and followed by pericardiotomy. A 6-0 silk suture was placed around the left anterior descending artery (LAD) between the first branch of the LAD and the left atrium. A small soft silicon tube was placed between the silk suture and the LAD. The ligature was tightened to occlude the LAD for 45 min. Successful MI/R model was verified by visual inspection of the LV apex for myocardial blanching and ST elevation on the surface electrocardiogram. After 45 min of ischemia, the slipknot was released to perform reperfusion for 3 h. The sham group received the same surgical procedures except for LAD occlusion. The animals were sacrificed after MI/R and part of the cardiac apex was rapidly removed for further analysis. Blood samples were obtained and centrifuged to obtain supernatant for future experiments.

2.6. HDACs Activity Assay. Nuclear extracts from the myocardium or H9C2 cells were suspended in ddH_2O. After HDACs assay buffer addition, a colorimetric substrate comprising an acetylated lysine side chain was added and incubated for 1 h at 37°C. The reaction was stopped by adding lysine developer and then incubated for another 30 min. The lysine developer produces a chromophore that can be analyzed easily by an enzyme linked immunosorbent assay (ELISA) plate reader (Perkin Elmer Co. USA) at 400 nm. Results were expressed as relative OD values/μg (% of sham or control ± SEM.).

2.7. Left Ventricle Function. Invasive hemodynamic measurements were performed to evaluate I/R induced cardiac dysfunction. A saline-filled catheter was inserted into the left ventricle via an incision on the right common carotid artery. The catheter was connected to a pressure transducer (Yixinda, Shenzhen, China). Left ventricular systolic pressure (LVSP) and maximal rates of increase and decrease in LVSP ($\pm dp/dt$max) were continuously monitored by an electrophysiolograph (BioPAC). Statistical analysis was performed by AcqKnowledge 4.0 software.

2.8. Determination of Myocardial Infarct Size. Six rats of each group were sacrificed to assess the sizes of the infarct area (IA), area at risk (AAR), and left ventricle (LV). Rats were administrated with heparin (1 U/g); the left coronary artery ligature was retired and 2 mL of 2% Evans Blue dye (Sigma, USA) was injected into the aorta immediately after 3 hours of reperfusion. Animals were sacrificed, and their hearts were excised and frozen at −70°C after washing with phosphate buffer saline (PBS). Hearts were sliced into 2 mm thick sections, perpendicular to the base-apex, and incubated with freshly prepared 1% TTC solution (pH 7.4) for 10 minutes at 37°C. The viable part was stained red by TTC, while the infarct portion remained pale. The infarct size was determined by an image analysis system (Image-Pro Plus 3.0; Media Cybernetics, MA). Two scientists scored the slides independently to ensure reliability of the results. The percentage of area at risk versus left ventricle (AAR/LV × 100%) and infarct area versus area at risk (IA/AAR × 100%) were calculated.

2.9. Measurement of Lactate Dehydrogenase and Creatine Kinase-MB Activities in Serum. In vivo, arterial blood samples were collected at the end of reperfusion and centrifuged at 2000 rpm for 10 minutes to collect the serum. In vitro, the supernatant was collected to measure the effluent LDH after H/R injury. Levels of cardiovascular biomarkers including creatine kinase-MB (CK-MB) and lactate dehydrogenase (LDH) were detected using a commercially available kit (Jiancheng Bioengineering, China).

2.10. Electron Microscopy. We use transmission electron microscopy to observe sarcomere and mitochondria ultrastructures. Approximately 2 mm^3 tissue from the left ventricle was removed, fixed, and embedded in resin. Thin section slides of 1-2 μm were prepared and oriented for longitudinal sectional views to get a better sight of the mitochondria and sarcomeres. The slides were stained, viewed, and photographed under a transmission electron microscope (HITACHI, HT7700) at ×7,000 (7K) magnification.

2.11. Determination of Apoptosis. In vivo study: the myocardial apoptosis rate was determined using an in situ cardiomyocyte terminal deoxynucleotidyl nick-end labeling assay (TUNEL). Left ventricular apical was quickly removed and incubated with 4% paraformaldehyde overnight at room temperature after reperfusion. Fluorescein-dUTP was added and nuclei were counterstained with 4′,6-diamidino-2-phenylindole (DAPI), according to the manufacturer's protocol (Roche, Indianapolis, USA). Samples were visualized using a laser scanning confocal microscope (Olympus, FV1000). Ten fields were chosen randomly for each sample and the apoptosis index was determined by dividing the number of positive-staining nuclei by the total number of nuclei in a given view field. Caspase-3 is a pivotal mediator of apoptosis; caspase-3 expression was performed to assess myocardial apoptosis specifically. In vitro study: after H/R, cells were collected and resuspended in binding buffer and incubated with fluorescein isothiocyanate- (FITC-) conjugated annexin V and propidium Iodide (PI) for 10 minutes in the dark. Cellular fluorescence was measured using a FACSCalibur instrument (BD Biosciences, USA). The data obtained from the cell population were analyzed using Cell Quest Pro software (BD Biosciences, USA).

2.12. Cell Viability Assay. Cell viability was determined by cell counting kit-8 (Dojindo, Kumamoto, Kyushu, Japan) in 96-well plates. H9C2 cells were cultured in 6-well plates. The CCK-8 solution was add to each well after the treatments and the plates were incubated for 3 h. The absorbance at 450 nm was measured using a microplate reader. The mean optical density (OD) of 6 wells in each group was used to calculate the percentage of cell viability.

2.13. $\Delta\Psi m$ Measurement. JC-1 staining was preformed to measure $\Delta\Psi m$ in H9C2 cells. Cells were incubated with JC-1 for 20 min at 37°C after H/R injury. The red/green fluorescence was detected with a microplate reader (Tecan Infinite 200). The wavelengths of excitation green fluorescence (monomeric form) of JC-1 were 514 nm, and wavelengths of 585 nm were used to detect the aggregated form of JC-1.

2.14. Mitochondrial Permeability Transition Pore (mPTP) in Cardiomyocytes. To examine the mPTP opening, H9C2 cardiomyocytes were measured with the mPTP fluorescence assay kit from Genmed Scientifics Inc. (Arlington, MA, USA). H9C2 cells were loaded with calcein-acetoxymethyl-ester (calcein-AM) (0.25 mM) and 8 mM cobalt chloride at 37°C for 20 min. Fluorescence intensity was observed by fluorescence microscope (Olympus, Bx 50-FLA) at 488 nm excitation and 525 nm emission. Results were represented as relative fluorescence intensity.

2.15. Western Blotting. After reperfusion, hearts were removed rapidly and frozen in liquid nitrogen. Ventricle tissue was sampled (n = 6 rats/group) and homogenized with a mixture of RIPA lysis buffer, PMSF (Beyotime, China), and a protease inhibitor cocktail (Roche, USA). The samples were homogenized and centrifuged at $12 \times 10^3 g$ for 15 minutes at 4°C. Supernatants were collected and total protein concentration was determined by using a BCA kit (Beyotime). Equivalent amounts of proteins (20–50 μg) were separated on a 10% SDS polyacrylamide gel and electrotransferred onto a PVDF membrane. The PVDF membrane was blocked with 5% bovine serum albumin (BSA, Sigma) for 1 hour at room temperature and then incubated with primary antibodies (1:1000) diluted in 5% bovine serum albumin (BSA), respectively, with gentle agitation overnight at 4°C. The membranes were washed three times in Tris Buffered Saline with Tween-20 (TBST) for 7 minutes each and incubated with secondary antibody (1:10000 goat anti-rabbit IgG, Cell Signaling Technology, USA) for 1 hour at room temperature. Signals were detected using a fluorescence imaging scanner (Odyssey, Germany) and optical densities were quantified using the Odyssey Image Analysis Software.

2.16. Statistical Analysis. All data were expressed as means ± SEM. Statistical analyses were performed using one-way or two-way ANOVA, followed by the Tukey HSD test. Statistical analysis was performed using Graphpad Prism 6.0 for Windows (GraphPad Software, USA). Statistical significance was accepted at $p < 0.05$.

3. Results

3.1. Diabetes Per Se and MI/R Injury Both Elevated HDACs Activity and Increased Infarct Size in Rat Hearts. As shown

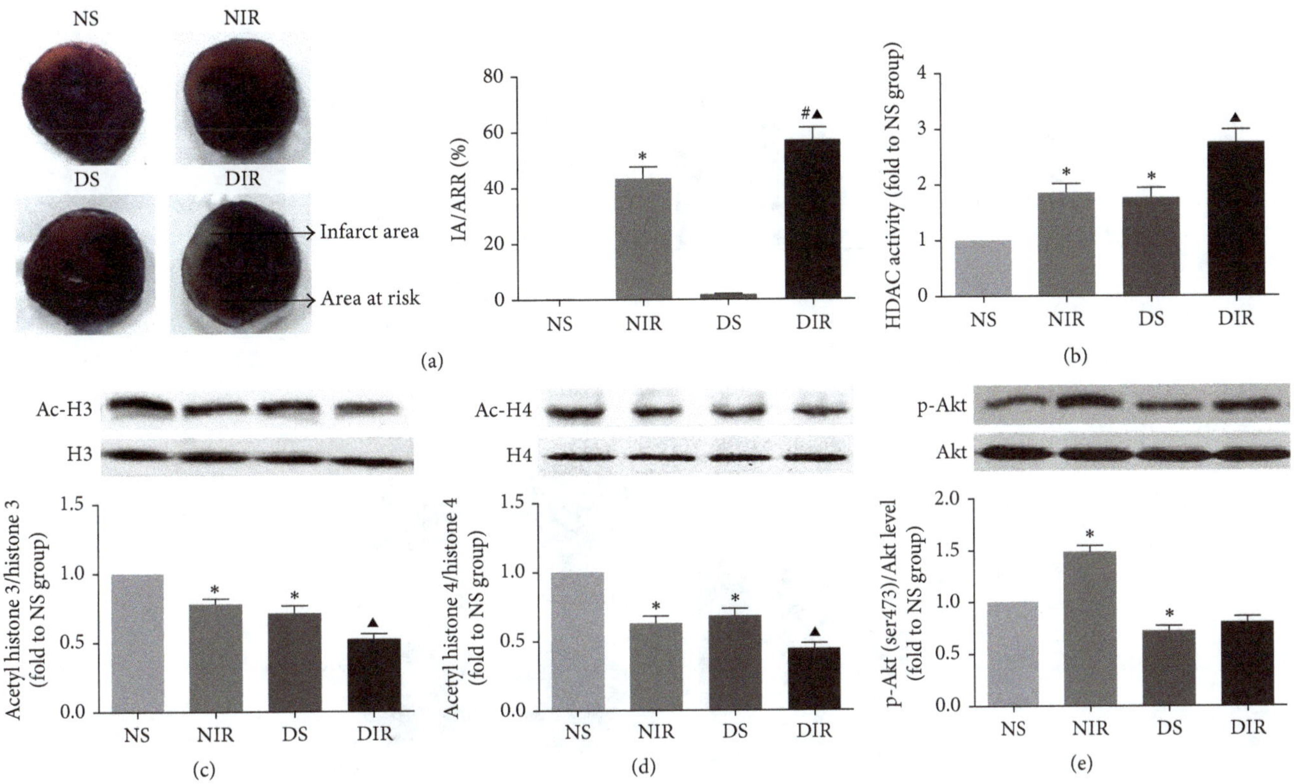

FIGURE 2: Myocardial infarct size and HDAC activity assessment in diabetic and normal rats. (a) Infarct area versus area at risk (IA/AAR × 100%). (b) Effect of MI/R and diabetes per se on total HDAC activity in myocardium. (c, d) Western blot analysis of myocardium acetylated histones H3 and H4 (Ac-H3, Ac-H4), with histones 3 or 4 (H3, H4) serving as the loading control. (e) p-Akt (ser473) and Akt protein expression in myocardium. All the results are presented as mean ± SEM, $n = 6$/group. $^*p < 0.05$ versus NS group. $^▲p < 0.05$ versus DS group. $^\#p < 0.05$ versus NIR group.

in Figure 2(a), the myocardium infarct size of diabetic rats was significantly increased compared with the normal group (NIR versus DIR, $p < 0.05$). Total HDACs activity and specific HDACs substrates (Ac-H3 and Ac-H4) of the myocardium were measured to further investigate the relationship between HDACs activity and myocardial injury (Figure 2(b)). MI/R injury significantly elevated HDACs activity and reduced Ac-H3/H3 and Ac-H4/H4 ratios (Figures 2(c) and 2(d)) in both normal and diabetic rats (NS versus NIR, DS versus DIR, all $p < 0.05$). The total HDACs activity was increased in diabetic rats as compared with the normal rats, which was further confirmed by decreased ratios of Ac-H3/H3 and Ac-H4/H4 (NS versus DS, $p < 0.05$). Next we used immunoblotting to evaluate phosphorylation level of Akt in diabetic and nondiabetic rats, in an attempt to explain why diabetes aggravates MI/R injury. The results showed that MI/R injury elicited a remarkable rise in p-Akt levels in the NIR group compared with NS group; however, this protective reaction was attenuated by diabetes mellitus (DS versus DIR, $p < 0.05$, Figure 2(e)).

3.2. HDACs Inhibition Attenuated Myocardial Injury in Diabetic Rats. We further evaluated the effect of TSA on MI/R injury. Serum CK-MB and LDH levels were significantly increased in diabetic rats compared with age-matched control rats (DS versus DIR, $p < 0.05$, Figures 3(a) and 3(b)). However, TSA pretreatment alleviated MI/R induced cardiomyocyte injury in diabetic rats, as demonstrated by the lower CK-MB and LDH levels (DIR versus DIR+TSA, $p < 0.05$, Figures 3(a) and 3(b)). TSA pretreatment markedly reduced the infract size in diabetic rats (55.9% ± 2.97% versus 38.6% ± 3.45%, $p < 0.05$, Figure 3(c)). Hemodynamic parameters were measured to evaluate the left ventricle function (Table 1). TSA treatment significantly increased $+dp/dt$, $-dp/dt$, and LVSP after 3 h of reperfusion (DIR versus DIR+TSA, $p < 0.05$). Notably, copretreatment with MK-2206 or wortmannin inhibited the TSA-induced protective effects on LV function, infarct size, and release of CK-MB and LDH (DIR+TSA versus DIR+TSA+MK or DIR+TSA+Wor, all $p < 0.05$). TSA was proved to be an effective HDACs inhibitor in present study; pretreatment of TSA for 5 days before surgery in diabetic rats significantly reduced HDACs activity and increased the level of acetylated H3 and H4 (DIR versus DIR+TSA, all $p < 0.05$, Figures 3(d), 3(e), and 3(f)) in myocardium.

3.3. TSA Pretreatment Attenuated I/R Induced Apoptosis. To examine whether TSA pretreatment could alleviate I/R induced myocardial cells apoptosis in diabetic

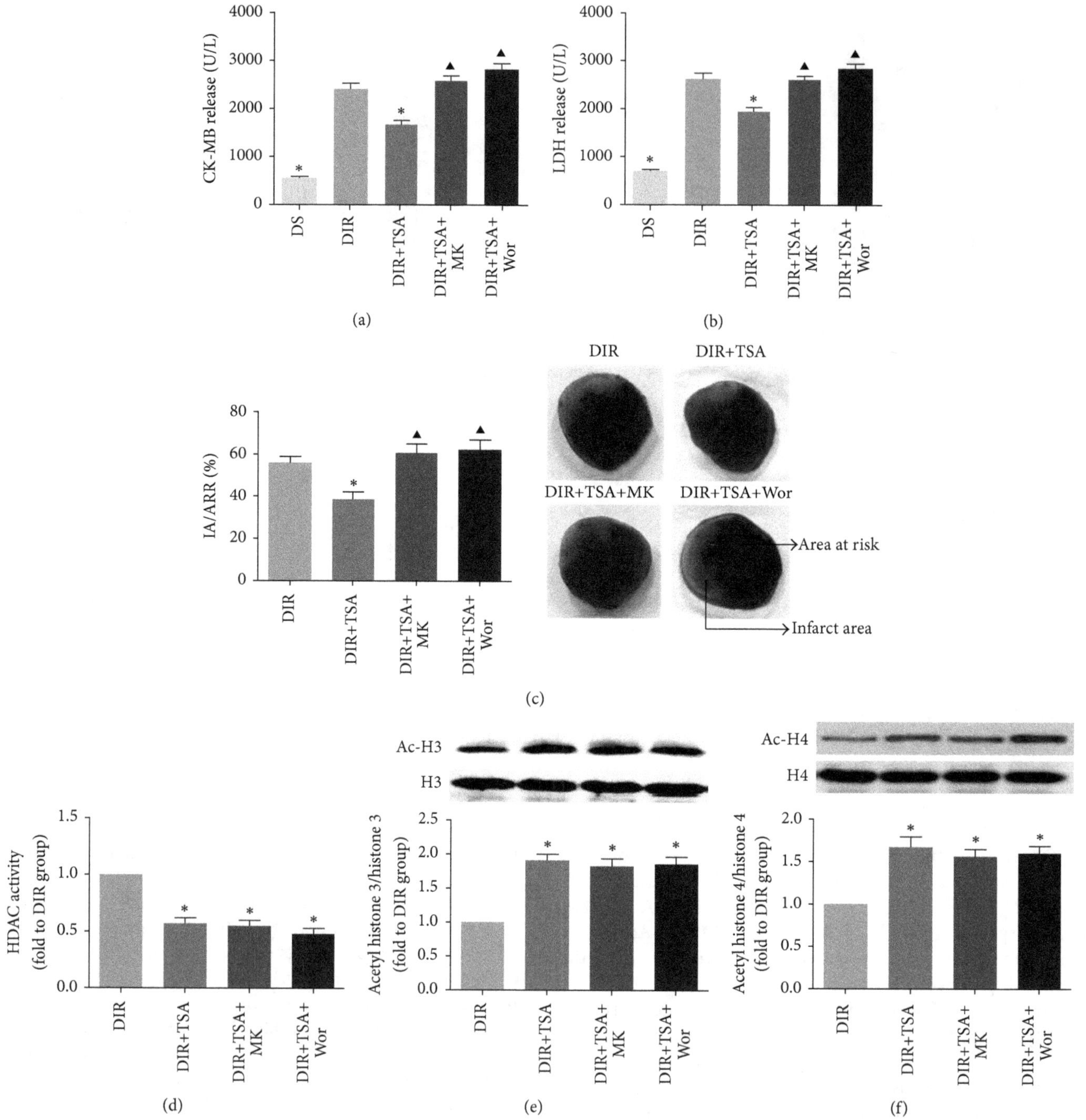

FIGURE 3: The HDAC inhibitor attenuated MI/R injury in diabetic hearts. Serum levels of myocardial injury marker CK-MB (a) and LDH (b). (a) Infarct area versus area at risk (IA/AAR × 100%). Blue-stained areas represent the nonischemic part; red-stained areas represent the area at risk and pale areas indicate myocardial infarction. Area at risk and infarct area were pointed out by arrows. HDACs activity (d) and acetylated level of histone 3 (e) and histone 4 (f). All the results are presented as mean ± SEM, $n = 6$/group. $^*p < 0.05$ versus DIR group. $^▲p < 0.05$ versus DIR+TSA group.

TABLE 1: Effects of TSA on LV hemodynamic parameters after MI/R.

Group/parameters	DIR	DIR+TSA	DIR+TSA+MK	DIR+TSA+Wor
LVDP (mmHg)	52.32 ± 2.78	72.47 ± 4.26*	54.24 ± 3.29▲	48.11 ± 2.96▲
$+dp/dt$max (mmHg/s)	2361 ± 227.5	3582 ± 264.3*	2564 ± 238.7▲	2371 ± 219.8▲
$-dp/dt$max (mmHg/s)	2574 ± 189.1	3672 ± 232.6*	2658 ± 263.4▲	2021 ± 209.8▲

Results represent mean ± SEM. $^*p < 0.05$ versus DIR; $^▲p < 0.05$ versus DIR+TSA; $n = 9$–12/group.

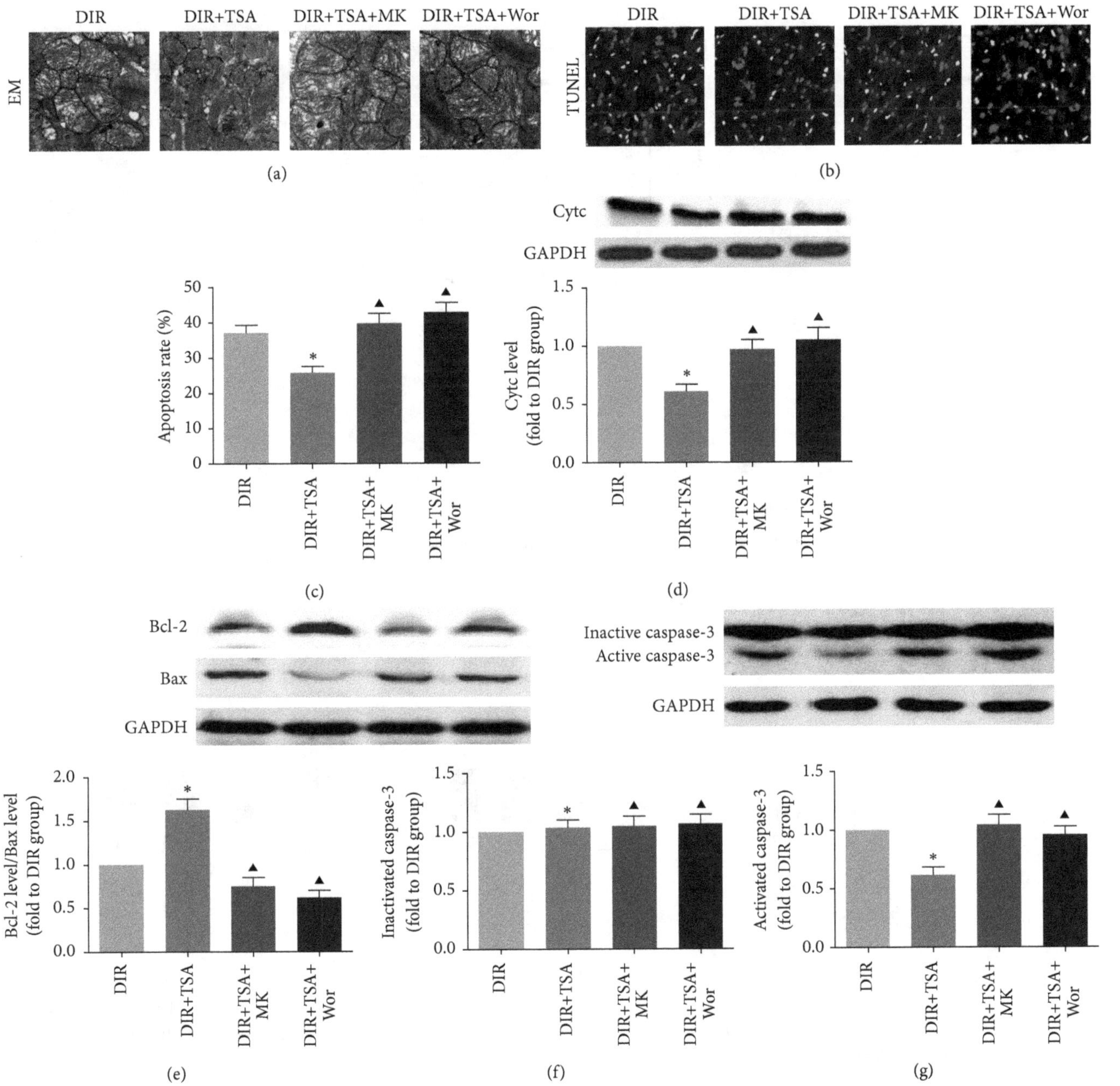

FIGURE 4: HDAC inhibition attenuated mitochondria-associated apoptosis in diabetic rats. (a) Representative electron micrographs of each group (×7000). (b) Representative TUNEL staining images of each group. (c) Quantitative analysis of the apoptosis rate in each group. (d, e) Representative immune blot images and assessment of the cytochrome C (cytc), Bcl-2, and Bax level in each group. (f, g) Representative immune blot images and assessment of activated and inactivated caspase-3 in cardiac tissue. All results are presented as the mean ± SEM, $n = 6$/group. $^{*}p < 0.05$ versus DIR group. $^{\blacktriangle}p < 0.05$ versus DIR+TSA group.

rats, we evaluated the apoptosis rate by a TUNEL assay (Figures 4(b) and 4(c)), further confirmed by the expression of mitochondrial apoptosis-associated proteins caspase-3 (Figures 4(f) and 4(g)), cytc (Figure 4(d)), and Bcl-2/Bax ratio of each group (Figure 4(e)). There were no changes in total (inactivated) caspase-3 levels in the 4 groups. TSA pretreatment significantly decreased the activated caspase-3, the number of TUNEL-positive cells, and cytc expression; however, Bcl-2/Bax ratio was upregulated (DIR+TSA versus DIR, all $p < 0.05$). Copretreatment with MK-2206 or wortmannin in diabetic rats before MI/R significantly elevated expression of activated caspase-3 and increased the number of TUNEL-positive cells compared with that observed in the DIR+TSA group (both $p < 0.05$). Further study found that the effects of TSA on Bcl-2/Bax ratio and cytc expression were reversed by MK-2206 or wortmannin administration (DIR+TSA versus DIR+TSA+MK or DIR+TSA+Wor group, all $p < 0.05$). The ultrastructure changes of myocardium were observed under

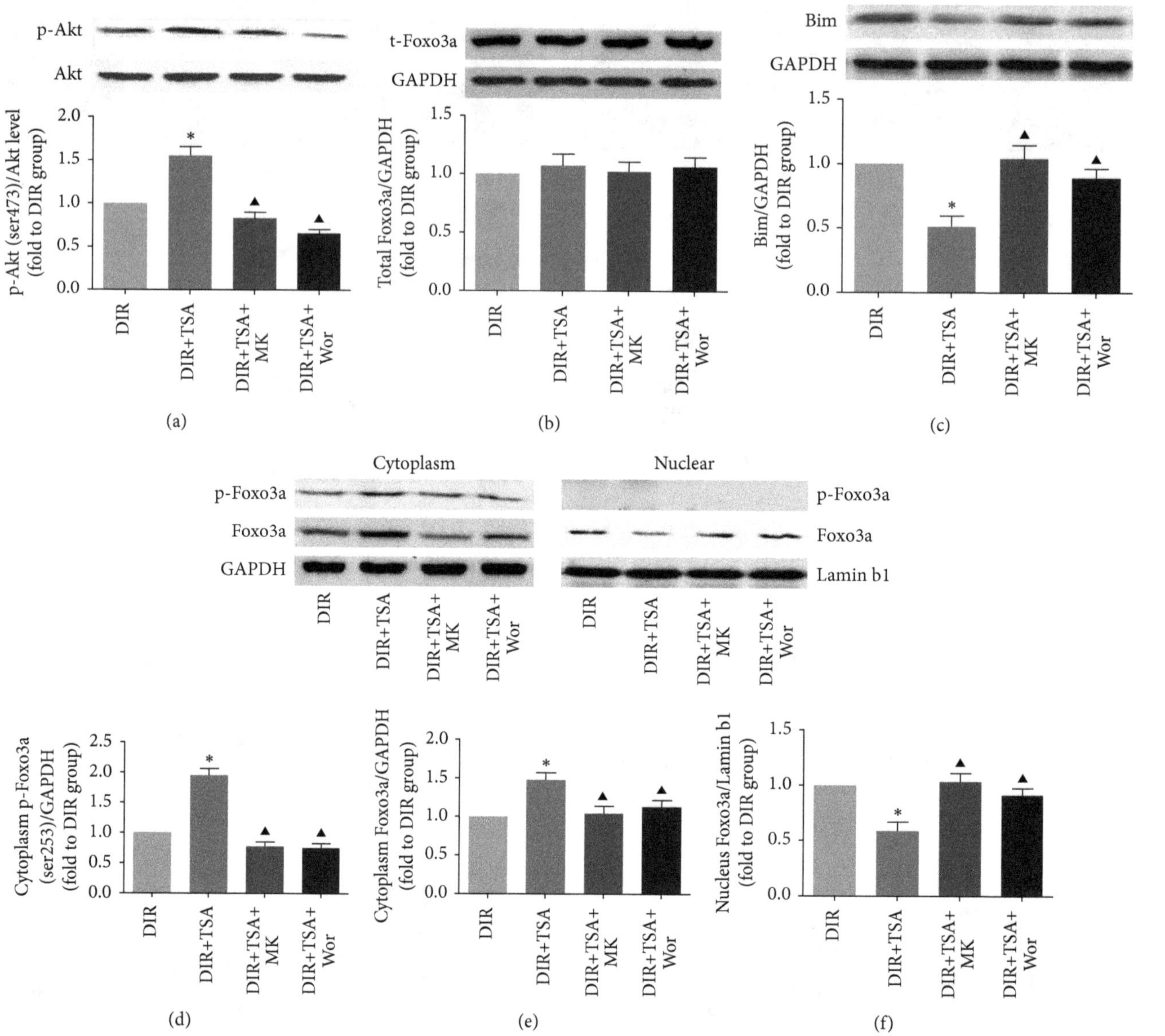

FIGURE 5: Expressions of p-Akt, p-Foxo3a, and Bim. Representative myocardial p-Akt, total-Akt (a), total-Foxo3a (b), Bim (c), cytoplasm p-Foxo3a (d), cytoplasm Foxo3a (e), and nuclear Foxo3a (f) Western blots images and protein levels analysis. GAPDH or Lamin b1 served as the loading control. All values are presented as the mean ± SEM, $n = 6$/group. $^{*}p < 0.05$ versus DIR group. $^{▲}p < 0.05$ versus DIR+TSA group.

an electron microscope. Representative electron micrographs of each group are shown in Figure 4(a). Vacuolar degeneration and cristae fragmentation of myocardial mitochondria caused by MI/R were observed. However, TSA pretreatment mitigated myocardial mitochondrial swelling and attenuated the cellular edema.

3.4. Akt and Foxo3a Play a Crucial Role in the Protective Effect of TSA. The expressions of Akt/p-Akt, Foxo3a/p-Foxo3a, and Bim were determined by Western blotting. Notably, TSA administration increased the expression of p-Akt in diabetic rats when exposed to MI/R insult (DIR versus DIR+TSA, $p < 0.05$), while the p-Akt level was markedly decreased after an Akt inhibitor was applied (DIR+TSA versus DIR+TSA+MK or DIR+TSA+Wor, $p < 0.05$, Figure 5(a)). As total-Foxo3a level remained unchanged in each group (Figure 5(b)), we measured p-Foxo3a and Foxo3a levels in both cytoplasm and nucleus lysate (Figures 5(d), 5(e), and 5(f)). Immunoblotting results showed that TSA administration significantly increased phosphorylation level of p-Foxo3a and Foxo3a in cytoplasm. However, copretreatment with the Akt inhibitor decreased the expression of p-Foxo3a and Foxo3a in cytoplasm (DIR+TSA versus DIR+TSA+MK or DIR+TSA+Wor, all $p < 0.05$). These results suggested that phosphorylation of Foxo3a leads to nuclear exclusion and cytoplasm relocalization. Next, we measured the expression of proapoptosis protein Bim. Researchers have shown that Foxo3a binds to a consensus sequence in the Bim promoter region and

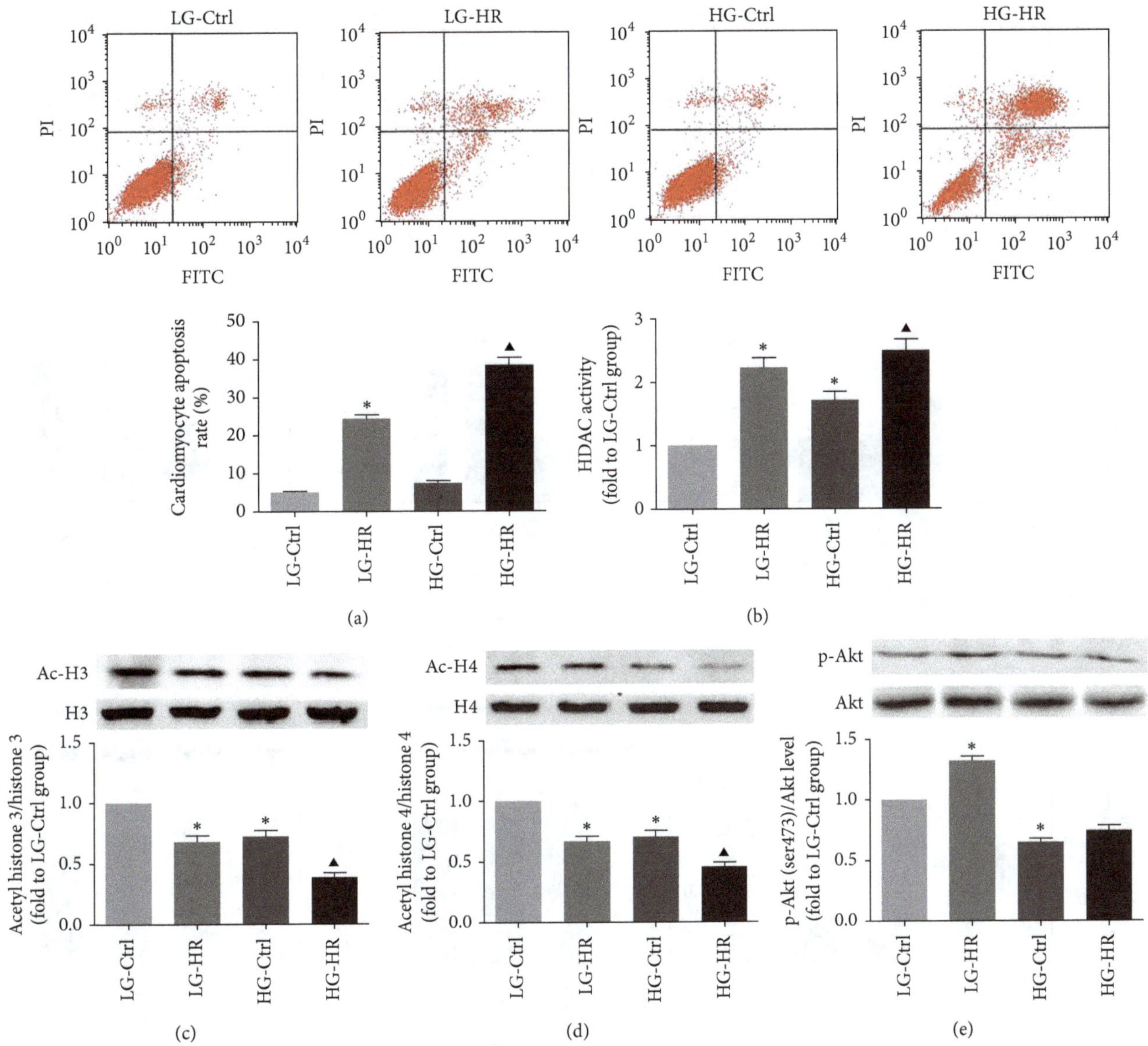

FIGURE 6: Apoptosis rate and HDAC activity assessment in H9C2 cells. Apoptosis of H9C2 cells was assessed by flow cytometry. (b) Total HDAC activity of cardiomyocytes in each group. (c, d) Western blot analysis of cardiomyocyte Ac-H3/H3 and Ac-H4/H4. (e) p-Akt (ser473)/Akt ratio in H9C2 cells. All values are presented as the mean ± SEM, $n = 6$/group. $^{*}p < 0.05$ versus LG-Ctrl group. $^{\blacktriangle}p < 0.05$ versus HG-Ctrl group.

activates Bim transcription [42]. As expected, Bim expression was downregulated by the HDACs inhibitor in diabetic rats (DIR versus DIR+TSA, $p < 0.05$, Figure 5(c)). However, the suppression of Bim by TSA pretreatment was abolished by MK-2206 or wortmannin administration (DIR+TSA versus DIR+TSA+MK or DIR+TSA+Wor, all $p < 0.05$).

3.5. High Glucose Induced Cardiomyocytes Apoptosis and Prosurvival Akt Pathway Deactivation When Exposed to Hypoxia/Reoxygenation Injury. The representative flow cytometry images of LG-Control, LG-HR, HG-Control, and HGHR groups are shown in Figure 6. H9C2 cells exposed to high glucose for 24 h and followed by H/R showed a marked increase in apoptosis compared with the LG-HR group (Figure 6(a)). To further evaluate the relationship between HDACs activity and myocardial injury, total HDACs activity (Figure 6(b)) and the levels of Ac-H3/H3 (Figure 6(c)) and Ac-H4/H4 (Figure 6(d)) in H9C2 cells were measured. HDACs activity of H9C2 cells lysate was elevated after 24 h exposure to high glucose, while Ac-H3/H3 and Ac-H4/H4 ratios were decreased. H/R injury also elevated the total HDACs activity, which was further confirmed by decreased expression of Ac-H3/H4 and Ac-H4/H4 ratios (LG-Ctrl versus LG-HR; HG-Ctrl versus HGHR; all $p < 0.05$). Furthermore, we measured the effect of HG on Akt activation in H9C2 cells. Immunoblotting showed that H/R injury elicited a remarkable increase of p-Akt levels in the LG-HR group (LG-Ctrl versus LG-HR, $p < 0.05$). However,

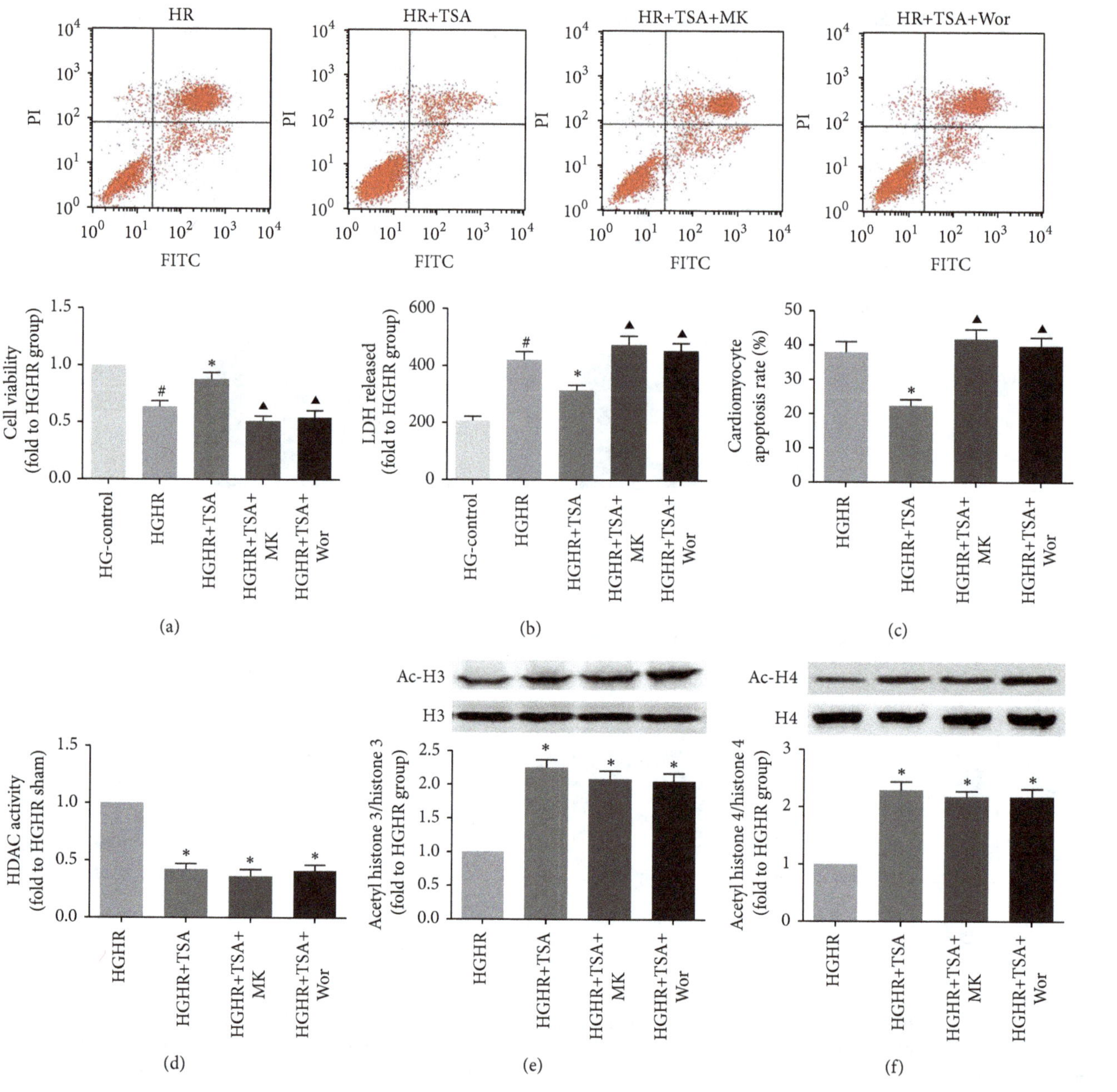

FIGURE 7: TSA administration has a protective effect on cardiomyocytes. Apoptosis in H9C2 cardiomyocytes was assessed by cell viability (a) and LDH leakage (b) and apoptosis rate (c) in each group. Cell lysate HDAC activity of each group was measured (d, e, f). Representative Ac-H3/H3 and Ac-H4/H4 Western blots images and protein levels analysis. GAPDH served as the loading control. All values are presented as the mean ± SEM, $n = 6$/group. $^{\#}p < 0.05$ versus HG-Control group. $^{*}p < 0.05$ versus HGHR group. $^{\blacktriangle}p < 0.05$ versus HGHR+TSA group.

high glucose attenuated this spontaneous protective reaction (HG-Ctrl versus HGHR, $p < 0.05$, Figure 6(e)).

3.6. The HDACs Inhibitor Induced Protection of Cardiomyocytes Exposed to HGHR Injury. The representative flow cytometry images from the HGHR, HGHR+TSA, HGHR+TSA+MK, and HGHR+TSA+Wor groups were shown in Figure 7. H/R injury significantly decreased cell viability and increased LDH leakage (HG-Control versus HGHR, $p < 0.05$, Figures 7(a) and 7(b)), while TSA pretreatment attenuated cellular injury and reduced cell apoptosis, as demonstrated by a decreased cells apoptosis rate, reduced LDH leakage, and increased cell viability (HGHR versus HGHR+TSA, $p < 0.05$, Figures 7(a), 7(b), and 7(c)). Copretreatment with MK-2206 or wortmannin partly blocked the protective effects of the HDACs inhibitor (HGHR+TSA versus HGHR+TSA+MK or HGHR+TSA+Wor, $p < 0.05$). TSA was proved to be an effective HDACs inhibitor in H9C2 cardiomyocytes; administration of TSA 6 h before H/R in H9C2 cells significantly reduced HDACs activity and increased acetylated level of H3 and H4 (HGHR versus HGHR+TSA, all $p < 0.05$, Figures 7(d), 7(e), and 7(f)).

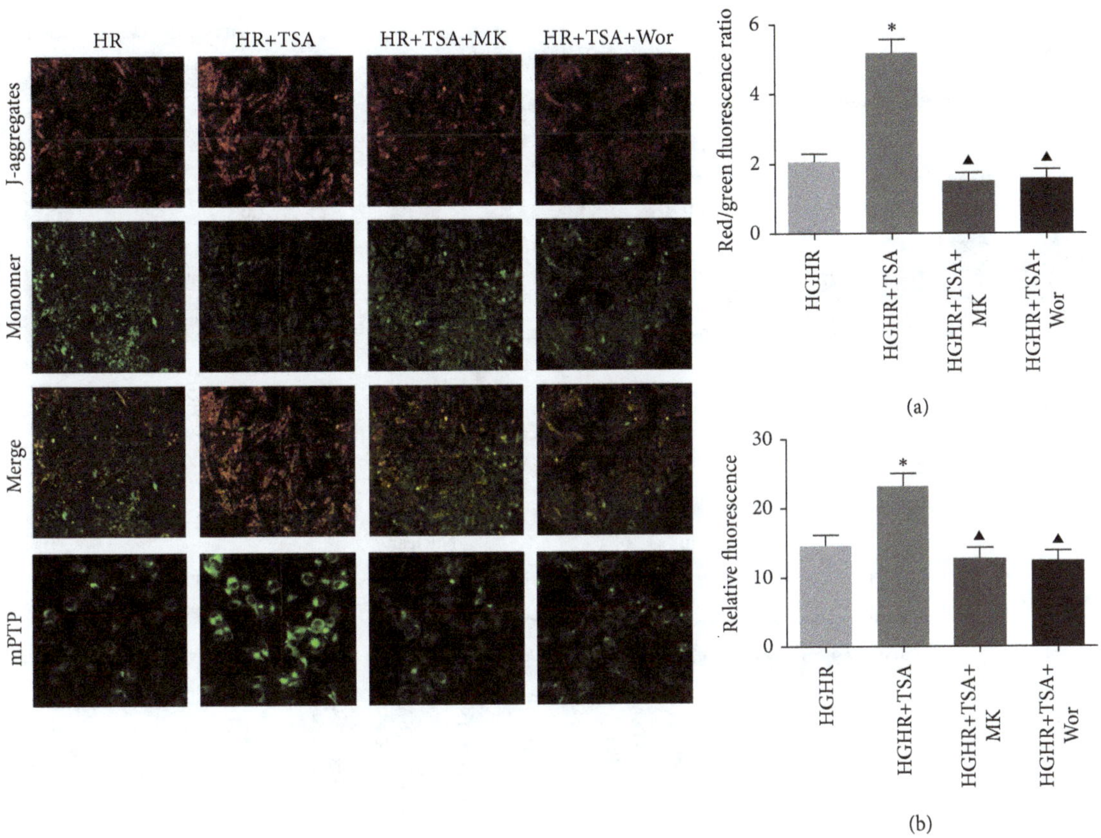

Figure 8: Effect of HDAC inhibition on mitochondrial membrane potential and integrity of mitochondrial permeability transition pore (mPTP). Representative fluorescent images and quantitative analysis in each group. (a) Red fluorescence represented JC-1 aggregation on the mitochondria membrane, reflecting the mitochondrial membrane potential ($\Delta\Psi m$). Green emission of the dye represented the monomeric form of JC-1 after mitochondrial membrane depolarization. (b) Fluorescent images of the cells show the change in integrity of mPTP. Reduced fluorescence in cells indicate opening of mPTP. All values are presented as the mean ± SEM, $n = 6$/group. $^*p < 0.05$ versus HGHR group. $^\blacktriangle p < 0.05$ versus HGHR+TSA group.

3.7. Effects of TSA Administration on mPTP. Due to the property of calcein-AM and cobalt chloride, the fluorescence intensity of calcein-AM following treatment with cobalt chloride can reflect the extent of mPTP opening. Compared with the HGHR, integrity of mPTP was altered significantly in TSA treated cells which was evident from increased calcein fluorescence (Figure 8(b)). However, cotreatment of MK-2206 or wortmannin demonstrated a significant reduced fluorescence level compared with TSA group (Figure 8(b)). These results indicated that TSA decreased the degree of mPTP opening in response to H/R induced injury under high glucose condition.

3.8. TSA Suppressed $\Delta\Psi m$ Dissipation in H9C2 Cells. Mitochondrial membrane potential ($\Delta\Psi m$) was assessed by JC-1 staining (Figure 8(a)). JC-1 aggregates mitochondria and shows red fluorescence under normal conditions. Exposure of H9C2 cells to high glucose for 24 h, followed by H/R resulted in dissipation of $\Delta\Psi m$, which was shown as increased green fluorescence after JC-1 staining. Pretreatment with TSA could moderate the $\Delta\Psi m$ dissipation by HGHR injury, as demonstrated by increased red/green fluorescence ratio, which indicated the protective effect of TSA (HGHR versus HGHR+TSA, $p < 0.05$). Compared with the HGHR+TSA group, cells copretreated with MK-2206 or wortmannin showed aggravated dissipation of $\Delta\Psi m$ (HGHR+TSA+MK or HGHR+TSA+Wor versus HGHR+TSA, $p < 0.05$).

3.9. Inhibition of HDACs Elevated the Phosphorylation Levels of Akt and Its Downstream Effectors in H9C2 Cells Exposed to HG and HR Injury. TSA administration before HGHR injury induced a considerable increase in p-Akt, while Bim expression was suppressed (HGHR versus HGHR+TSA, all $p < 0.05$, Figures 9(a) and 9(c)). As total Foxo3a remained unchanged in each group (Figure 8(b)), we measured p-Foxo3a and Foxo3a levels in both cytoplasm and nuclear lysate (Figures 9(d), 9(e), and 9(f)). Immunoblotting results showed that TSA administration significantly increased phosphorylation level of p-Foxo3a and Foxo3a in cytoplasm. Additionally, copretreatment with the Akt inhibitor decreased the expression of p-Foxo3a/Foxo3a in cytoplasm (DIR+TSA versus DIR+TSA+MK or DIR+TSA+Wor, all $p <$ 0.05, Figure 9(b)). These results showed that phosphorylation

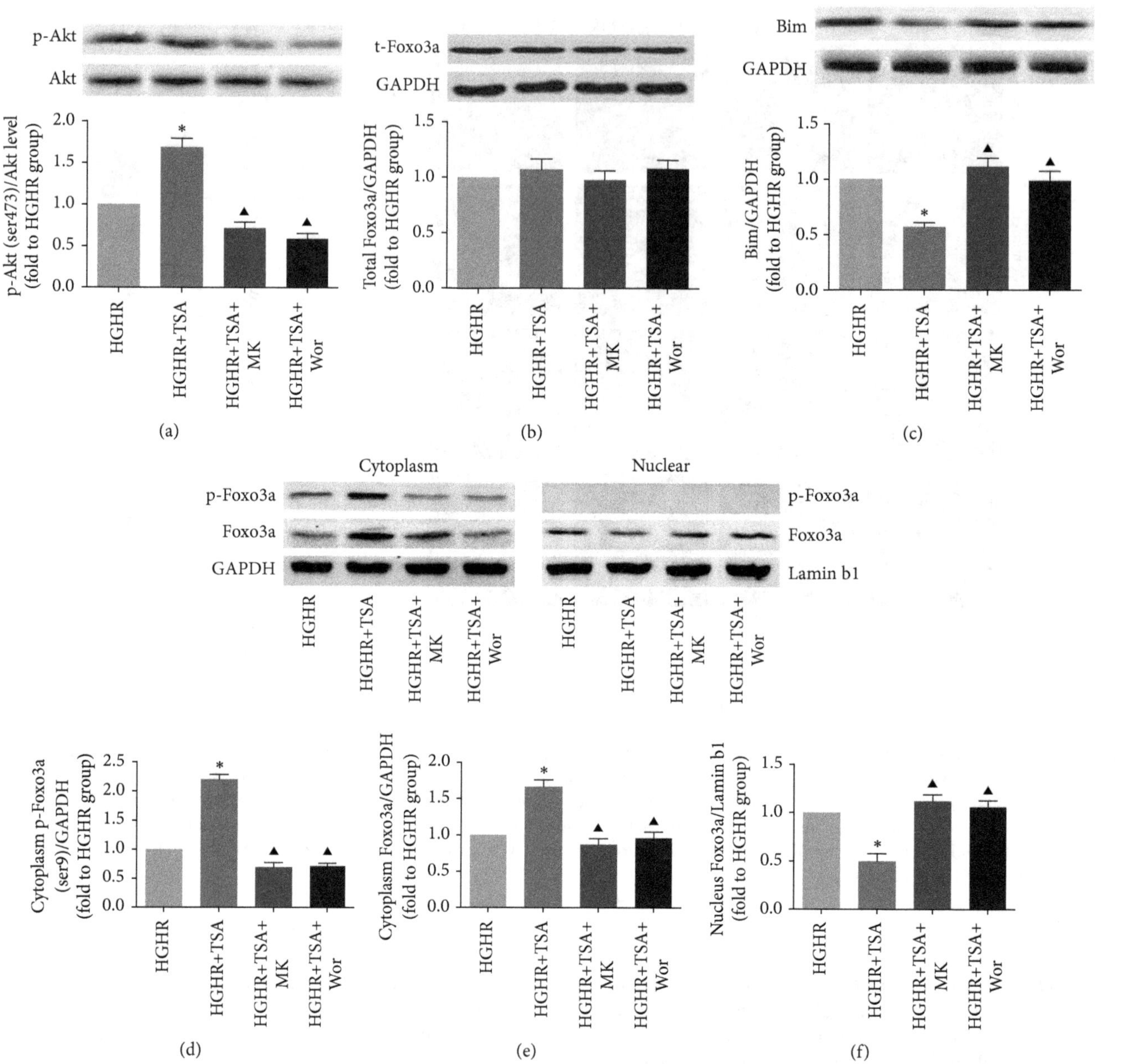

FIGURE 9: Expression of p-Akt/Akt, p-Foxo3a/Foxo3a, and Bim. Cardiomyocyte p-Akt, total-Akt (a), total-Foxo3a (b), Bim (c), cytoplasm p-Foxo3a (d), cytoplasm Foxo3a (e), and nuclear Foxo3a (f) Western blots images and protein levels analysis. GAPDH or Lamin b1 served as the loading control. $^{*}p < 0.05$ versus HGHR group. $^{▲}p < 0.05$ versus HGHR+TSA group.

of Foxo3a may lead to nuclear exclusion and cytoplasm relocalization.

4. Discussion

To the best of our knowledge, this is the first study to demonstrate that the HDACs inhibition confers cardioprotection against MI/R injury in diabetic rats that were more vulnerable to ischemic injury. Reversible acetylation of lysine in histone or nonhistone proteins by HDACs is a key mechanism for signal modification and precise gene transcriptional regulation, which are essential for cardiovascular pathophysiology [43, 44]. Accumulated studies have revealed that diabetes mellitus causes increased HDACs activity in the liver, pancreas [45], and kidney [46]. In line with these researches, our study demonstrated that cardiac HDACs activity is elevated by both the duration of the hyperglycemic state and MI/R injury.

TSA is well established to inhibit class I/II HDACs activity by blocking the active site of HDACs [41]. TSA shows certain cardioprotective effects in nondiabetic heart I/R Injury [47, 48]. In our present study, we found for the first time that both MI/R injury and diabetes per se could increase total HDACs activity in rat heart; furthermore, class I/II HDACs inhibitor TSA triggered protective effects against MI/R and H/R injury under diabetic conditions.

Recent studies indicated that inhibition of histone deacetylases is a promising drug target to confer protection against ischemic or hypoxic injury [13, 35, 49]; the molecule mechanisms that underlie the HDACs inhibition-induced cardioprotection still remain unknown [50]. Accumulated experimental data indicated that TSA activates PI3K/Akt signaling. Wang et al. reported that TSA transiently activated PI3K/Akt cell survival pathway and inhibition of this signaling pathway promoted TSA's effect on cell death and migration in ovarian cancer cells [34]. Furthermore, recent study showed TSA could significantly reduce the cerebral infarct volume during cerebral ischemia/reperfusion injury, which was achieved partly by activation of the PI3K/Akt signaling pathway via upgrading of p-Akt protein. Importantly, our results demonstrated that the selective inhibition of PI3K/Akt signaling pathways by wortmannin could weaken cardioprotective effect induced by TSA treatment dramatically, indicating the essential effect of PI3K/Akt pathways in mediating cardioprotection elicited by HDACs inhibition.

Loss of endogenous reactive Akt activation in the diabetic myocardium may help to explain why diabetic rats are more vulnerable to MI/R injury [51, 52]. We further investigated the role of downstream apoptosis-associated effectors of Akt in the TSA-induced protective effect. We found that TSA treatment caused an increased expression of phosphorylated Foxo3a in cytoplasm but a decreased expression of Foxo3a in nuclear; however these effects were suppressed by Akt inhibitor. Furthermore, we found that the decreased expression of nuclear p-Foxo3a was accompanied by a reduction of Bim expression. We concluded that phosphorylation of Foxo3a by Akt may result in nucleus exclusion and cytoplasm relocalization, thus deactivating the Foxo3a pathway [38, 53]. Notably, Foxo3a modulates proapoptotic pathways by binding to the consensus sequence of the Bim promoter region and inducing Bim expression [40]. In vivo and vitro experiments revealed that TSA administration induced Foxo3a's cytoplasmic relocation and downregulated Bim expression. Bim blocks stress signals transduced from the cytoplasm to mitochondria and triggers the Bax-mediated mitochondria apoptosis pathway [54]. Our result may help explain how TSA protected diabetic rats from the cardiac-damage induced by ischemia or hypoxia.

The survival and antiapoptosis effects of HDACs inhibition were closely associated with the reduction of the apoptosis rate of cardiomyocytes. Signaling events characteristic of apoptosis and mitochondrial dysfunction resulted in the diabetic myocardium being more vulnerable to I/R injury [28, 29]. Ischemic or hypoxic injury renders the mitochondrial membrane permeable and causes dissipation of the proton gradient across the mitochondrial membrane. One of the main events that trigger mitochondrial dysfunction is mPTP opening, with subsequent mitochondrial swelling [55]. Cytochrome C is located within the intermembrane space of mitochondria under normal conditions [56]. I/R injury results in the mPTP opening and cytochrome C release [57]. In the present study, class I/II HDACs inhibition mitigated the effects of MI/R on $\Delta\Psi m$ loss, integrity of mPTP, and cytochrome C release. Pretreatment with a HDACs inhibitor before MI/R or H/R moderated the dissipation of $\Delta\Psi m$ and protected integrity of mPTP by suppressing Bim expression, which mediates the mitochondrial apoptosis process by opening mPTP on the mitochondrial membrane [57].

Our observation shows that HDACs inhibition protects diabetic heart against I/R injury; however the roles of class I HDACs or class II HDACs in myocardial protection is still controversial. The study of Aune et al. demonstrated that class I HDACs inhibition elicits protection of contractile function following I/R, which is associated with increased expression of endogenous antioxidant enzymes [58]. Class II HDACs are abundantly expressed in the heart [59]. Study from Zhao et al. supports that class II serves as a potential target in MI/R injury through TSA inhibition [35]. Further studies need to be done to determine whether the selective inhibition of HDACs exerts cardiac protection from MI/R injury in diabetic heart. Pretreated diabetic rats with a HDACs inhibitor suppressed the excessive HDACs activity in the myocardium and conferred protection against MI/R injury. We believe that high levels of cardiac HDACs activity in diabetes exacerbate ischemic heart injury; however, the underlying mechanisms require further investigation.

5. Conclusions

Both duration of diabetes per se and MI/R injury increased cardiac HDACs activity. Suppression of HDACs activity triggered protective effects against MI/R and H/R injury under hyperglycemia conditions through Akt-modulated mitochondrial apoptotic pathways via Foxo3a/Bim.

Competing Interests

The authors declare that they have no competing interest.

Authors' Contributions

Yang Wu and Yan Leng are equal contributors.

Acknowledgments

This research was supported by a grant from the National Natural Science Foundation of China (nos. 81201458, 81170768, and 81471844).

References

[1] B. Li, M. Carey, and J. L. Workman, "The role of chromatin during transcription," *Cell*, vol. 128, no. 4, pp. 707–719, 2007.

[2] I. V. Gregoretti, Y.-M. Lee, and H. V. Goodson, "Molecular evolution of the histone deacetylase family: functional implications of phylogenetic analysis," *Journal of Molecular Biology*, vol. 338, no. 1, pp. 17–31, 2004.

[3] S. Thiagalingam, K.-H. Cheng, H. J. Lee, N. Mineva, A. Thiagalingam, and J. F. Ponte, "Histone deacetylases: unique players in shaping the epigenetic histone code," *Annals of the New York Academy of Sciences*, vol. 983, pp. 84–100, 2003.

[4] W. S. Xu, R. B. Parmigiani, and P. A. Marks, "Histone deacetylase inhibitors: molecular mechanisms of action," *Oncogene*, vol. 26, no. 37, pp. 5541–5552, 2007.

[5] S. Khochbin, A. Verdel, C. Lemercier, and D. Seigneurin-Berny, "Functional significance of histone deacetylase diversity," *Current Opinion in Genetics and Development*, vol. 11, no. 2, pp. 162–166, 2001.

[6] M. Grunstein, "Histone acetylation in chromatin structure and transcription," *Nature*, vol. 389, no. 6649, pp. 349–352, 1997.

[7] M. A. Moser, A. Hagelkruys, and C. Seiser, "Transcription and beyond: the role of mammalian class I lysine deacetylases," *Chromosoma*, vol. 123, no. 1-2, pp. 67–78, 2014.

[8] M. Martin, R. Kettmann, and F. Dequiedt, "Class IIa histone deacetylases: regulating the regulators," *Oncogene*, vol. 26, no. 37, pp. 5450–5467, 2007.

[9] M. A. Thal, P. Krishnamurthy, A. R. MacKie et al., "Enhanced angiogenic and cardiomyocyte differentiation capacity of epigenetically reprogrammed mouse and human endothelial progenitor cells augments their efficacy for ischemic myocardial repair," *Circulation Research*, vol. 111, no. 2, pp. 180–190, 2012.

[10] S. S. Vadvalkar, C. N. Baily, S. Matsuzaki, M. West, Y. A. Tesiram, and K. M. Humphries, "Metabolic inflexibility and protein lysine acetylation in heart mitochondria of a chronic model of Type 1 diabetes," *Biochemical Journal*, vol. 449, no. 1, pp. 253–261, 2013.

[11] H.-A. Lee, D.-Y. Lee, H.-M. Cho, S.-Y. Kim, Y. Iwasaki, and I. K. Kim, "Histone deacetylase inhibition attenuates transcriptional activity of mineralocorticoid receptor through its acetylation and prevents development of hypertension," *Circulation Research*, vol. 112, no. 7, pp. 1004–1012, 2013.

[12] C. M. Trivedi, Y. Luo, Z. Yin et al., "Hdac2 regulates the cardiac hypertrophic response by modulating Gsk3β activity," *Nature Medicine*, vol. 13, no. 3, pp. 324–331, 2007.

[13] L. Zhang, X. Qin, Y. Zhao et al., "Inhibition of histone deacetylases preserves myocardial performance and prevents cardiac remodeling through stimulation of endogenous angiomyogenesis," *Journal of Pharmacology and Experimental Therapeutics*, vol. 341, no. 1, pp. 285–293, 2012.

[14] Q. Xu, X. Lin, L. Andrews, D. Patel, P. D. Lampe, and R. D. Veenstra, "Histone deacetylase inhibition reduces cardiac connexin43 expression and gap junction communication," *Frontiers in Pharmacology*, vol. 4, article 44, 2013.

[15] T. C. Zhao, G. Cheng, L. X. Zhang, Y. T. Tseng, and J. F. Padbury, "Inhibition of histone deacetylases triggers pharmacologic preconditioning effects against myocardial ischemic injury," *Cardiovascular Research*, vol. 76, no. 3, pp. 473–481, 2007.

[16] Y. Kong, P. Tannous, G. Lu et al., "Suppression of class I and II histone deacetylases blunts pressure-overload cardiac hypertrophy," *Circulation*, vol. 113, no. 22, pp. 2579–2588, 2006.

[17] C. L. Antos, T. A. McKinsey, M. Dreitz et al., "Dose-dependent blockade to cardiomyocyte hypertrophy by histone deacetylase inhibitors," *Journal of Biological Chemistry*, vol. 278, no. 31, pp. 28930–28937, 2003.

[18] Y. Chen, J. Du, Y. T. Zhao et al., "Histone deacetylase (HDAC) inhibition improves myocardial function and prevents cardiac remodeling in diabetic mice," *Cardiovascular Diabetology*, vol. 14, no. 1, article 99, 2015.

[19] A. Lopez-de-andres, R. Jimenez-Garcia, V. Hernandez-Barrera et al., "National trends over one decade in hospitalization for acute myocardial infarction among Spanish adults with type 2 diabetes: cumulative incidence, outcomes and use of percutaneous coronary intervention," *PLoS ONE*, vol. 9, no. 1, Article ID e85697, 2014.

[20] H. Li, Z. Liu, J. Wang et al., "Susceptibility to myocardial ischemia reperfusion injury at early stage of type 1 diabetes in rats," *Cardiovascular Diabetology*, vol. 12, no. 1, p. 133, 2013.

[21] S. Hicks, N. Labinskyy, B. Piteo et al., "Type II diabetes increases mitochondrial DNA mutations in the left ventricle of the Goto-Kakizaki diabetic rat," *American Journal of Physiology—Heart and Circulatory Physiology*, vol. 304, no. 7, pp. H903–H915, 2013.

[22] A. K. Sharma and D. Khanna, "Diabetes mellitus associated cardiovascular signalling alteration: a need for the revisit," *Cellular Signalling*, vol. 25, no. 5, pp. 1149–1155, 2013.

[23] M. Muravyeva, I. Baotic, M. Bienengraeber et al., "Cardioprotection during diabetes: the role of mitochondrial DNA," *Anesthesiology*, vol. 120, no. 4, pp. 870–879, 2014.

[24] S. Koka, A. Das, F. N. Salloum, and R. C. Kukreja, "Phosphodiesterase-5 inhibitor tadalafil attenuates oxidative stress and protects against myocardial ischemia/reperfusion injury in type 2 diabetic mice," *Free Radical Biology and Medicine*, vol. 60, pp. 80–88, 2013.

[25] K. Przyklenk, "Reduction of myocardial infarct size with ischemic 'conditioning' : physiologic and technical considerations," *Anesthesia and Analgesia*, vol. 117, no. 4, pp. 891–901, 2013.

[26] R. Engbersen, N. P. Riksen, M. J. Mol et al., "Improved resistance to ischemia and reperfusion, but impaired protection by ischemic preconditioning in patients with type 1 diabetes mellitus: a pilot study," *Cardiovascular Diabetology*, vol. 11, article 124, 2012.

[27] P. Ferdinandy, R. Schulz, and G. F. Baxter, "Interaction of cardiovascular risk factors with myocardial ischemia/reperfusion injury, preconditioning, and postconditioning," *Pharmacological Reviews*, vol. 59, no. 4, pp. 418–458, 2007.

[28] F. Giacco and M. Brownlee, "Oxidative stress and diabetic complications," *Circulation Research*, vol. 107, no. 9, pp. 1058–1070, 2010.

[29] R. C. Sloan, F. Moukdar, C. R. Frasier et al., "Mitochondrial permeability transition in the diabetic heart: contributions of thiol redox state and mitochondrial calcium to augmented reperfusion injury," *Journal of Molecular and Cellular Cardiology*, vol. 52, no. 5, pp. 1009–1018, 2012.

[30] K. Ban, A. J. Cooper, S. Samuel et al., "Phosphatidylinositol 3-kinase γ is a critical mediator of myocardial ischemic and adenosine-mediated preconditioning," *Circulation Research*, vol. 103, no. 6, pp. 643–653, 2008.

[31] Y. Wu, Z.-Y. Xia, J. Dou et al., "Protective effect of ginsenoside Rb1 against myocardial ischemia/reperfusion injury in streptozotocin-induced diabetic rats," *Molecular Biology Reports*, vol. 38, no. 7, pp. 4327–4335, 2011.

[32] M. Liu, B. Zhou, Z.-Y. Xia et al., "Hyperglycemia-induced inhibition of DJ-1 expression compromised the effectiveness of ischemic postconditioning cardioprotection in rats," *Oxidative Medicine and Cellular Longevity*, vol. 2013, Article ID 564902, 8 pages, 2013.

[33] H. Shi, L. Chen, H. Wang et al., "Synergistic induction of miR-126 by hypoxia and HDAC inhibitors in cardiac myocytes," *Biochemical and Biophysical Research Communications*, vol. 430, no. 2, pp. 827–832, 2013.

[34] G. Wang, Y. Shi, X. Jiang et al., "HDAC inhibition prevents white matter injury by modulating microglia/macrophage polarization through the GSK3β/PTEN/Akt axis," *Proceedings of the National Academy of Sciences of the United States of America*, vol. 112, no. 9, pp. 2853–2858, 2015.

[35] T. C. Zhao, J. Du, S. Zhuang, P. Liu, and L. X. Zhang, "HDAC inhibition elicits myocardial protective effect through modulation of MKK3/Akt-1," *PLoS ONE*, vol. 8, no. 6, Article ID e65474, 2013.

[36] M. Paillard, E. Tubbs, P.-A. Thiebaut et al., "Depressing mitochondria-reticulum interactions protects cardiomyocytes from lethal hypoxia-reoxygenation injury," *Circulation*, vol. 128, no. 14, pp. 1555–1565, 2013.

[37] M. Li and N. K. Fukagawa, "Age-related changes in redox signaling and VSMC function," *Antioxidants and Redox Signaling*, vol. 12, no. 5, pp. 641–655, 2010.

[38] S. Ganesan, B. L. Unger, A. T. Comstock et al., "Aberrantly activated EGFR contributes to enhanced IL-8 expression in COPD airways epithelial cells via regulation of nuclear FoxO3A," *Thorax*, vol. 68, no. 2, pp. 131–141, 2013.

[39] T. Shimazu, M. D. Hirschey, J. Newman et al., "Suppression of oxidative stress by β-hydroxybutyrate, an endogenous histone deacetylase inhibitor," *Science*, vol. 339, no. 6116, pp. 211–214, 2013.

[40] K.-J. Yin, C. Y. Hsu, X.-Y. Hu et al., "Protein phosphatase 2A regulates bim expression via the Akt/FKHRL1 signaling pathway in amyloid-β peptide-induced cerebrovascular endothelial cell death," *Journal of Neuroscience*, vol. 26, no. 8, pp. 2290–2299, 2006.

[41] P. A. Marks, "Histone deacetylase inhibitors: a chemical genetics approach to understanding cellular functions," *Biochimica et Biophysica Acta—Gene Regulatory Mechanisms*, vol. 1799, no. 10-12, pp. 717–725, 2010.

[42] S. Zhu, S. Evans, B. Yan et al., "Transcriptional regulation of Bim by FOXO3a and Akt mediates scleroderma serum-induced apoptosis in endothelial progenitor cells," *Circulation*, vol. 118, no. 21, pp. 2156–2165, 2008.

[43] H. Rafehi, A. Balcerczyk, S. Lunke et al., "Vascular histone deacetylation by pharmacological HDAC inhibition," *Genome Research*, vol. 24, no. 8, pp. 1271–1284, 2014.

[44] L. Zhao, C.-N. Chen, N. Hajji et al., "Histone deacetylation inhibition in pulmonary hypertension: therapeutic potential of valproic acid and suberoylanilide hydroxamic acid," *Circulation*, vol. 126, no. 4, pp. 455–467, 2012.

[45] S. Khan and G. B. Jena, "Protective role of sodium butyrate, a HDAC inhibitor on beta-cell proliferation, function and glucose homeostasis through modulation of p38/ERK MAPK and apoptotic pathways: study in juvenile diabetic rat," *Chemico-Biological Interactions*, vol. 213, pp. 1–12, 2014.

[46] S. Khan and G. Jena, "Sodium butyrate, a HDAC inhibitor ameliorates eNOS, iNOS and TGF-β1-induced fibrogenesis, apoptosis and DNA damage in the kidney of juvenile diabetic rats," *Food and Chemical Toxicology*, vol. 73, pp. 127–139, 2014.

[47] M. Xie, Y. Kong, W. Tan et al., "Histone deacetylase inhibition blunts ischemia/reperfusion injury by inducing cardiomyocyte autophagy," *Circulation*, vol. 129, no. 10, pp. 1139–1151, 2014.

[48] T. A. McKinsey, "Therapeutic potential for HDAC inhibitors in the heart," *Annual Review of Pharmacology and Toxicology*, vol. 52, pp. 303–319, 2012.

[49] L. Yu, M. Lu, P. Wang, and X. Chen, "Trichostatin A ameliorates myocardial ischemia/reperfusion injury through inhibition of endoplasmic reticulum stress-induced apoptosis," *Archives of Medical Research*, vol. 43, no. 3, pp. 190–196, 2012.

[50] C. Zhou, L. Qiu, Y. Sun et al., "Inhibition of EGFR/PI3K/AKT cell survival pathway promotes TSA's effect on cell death and migration in human ovarian cancer cells," *International Journal of Oncology*, vol. 29, no. 1, pp. 269–278, 2006.

[51] B. Huisamen, "Protein kinase B in the diabetic heart," *Molecular and Cellular Biochemistry*, vol. 249, no. 1-2, pp. 31–38, 2003.

[52] A. Tsang, D. J. Hausenloy, M. M. Mocanu, R. D. Carr, and D. M. Yellon, "Preconditioning the diabetic heart: the importance of Akt phosphorylation," *Diabetes*, vol. 54, no. 8, pp. 2360–2364, 2005.

[53] C. Peng, J. Ma, X. Gao, P. Tian, W. Li, and L. Zhang, "High glucose induced oxidative stress and apoptosis in cardiac microvascular endothelial cells are regulated by FoxO3a," *PLoS ONE*, vol. 8, no. 11, Article ID e79739, 2013.

[54] D. Ren, H.-C. Tu, H. Kim et al., "BID, BIM, and PUMA are essential for activation of the BAX- and BAK-dependent cell death program," *Science*, vol. 330, no. 6009, pp. 1390–1393, 2010.

[55] G. Wang, T. Hamid, R. J. Keith et al., "Cardioprotective and antiapoptotic effects of heme oxygenase-1 in the failing heart," *Circulation*, vol. 121, no. 17, pp. 1912–1925, 2010.

[56] P. Korge, H. M. Honda, and J. N. Weiss, "Protection of cardiac mitochondria by diazoxide and protein kinase C: implications for ischemic preconditioning," *Proceedings of the National Academy of Sciences of the United States of America*, vol. 99, no. 5, pp. 3312–3317, 2002.

[57] D. A. Kubli and Å. B. Gustafsson, "Mitochondria and mitophagy: the yin and yang of cell death control," *Circulation Research*, vol. 111, no. 9, pp. 1208–1221, 2012.

[58] S. E. Aune, D. J. Herr, S. K. Mani, and D. R. Menick, "Selective inhibition of class I but not class IIb histone deacetylases exerts cardiac protection from ischemia reperfusion," *Journal of Molecular and Cellular Cardiology*, vol. 72, pp. 138–145, 2014.

[59] M. Yoshida, "Potent and specific inhibition of mammalian histone deacetylase both in vivo and in vitro by trichostatin A," *Tanpakushitsu Kakusan Koso*, vol. 52, supplement 13, pp. 1788–1789, 2007.

12

Transgenerational Glucose Intolerance of Tumor Necrosis Factor with Epigenetic Alteration in Rat Perirenal Adipose Tissue Induced by Intrauterine Hyperglycemia

Rina Su, Jie Yan, and Huixia Yang

Department of Obstetrics and Gynecology, Peking University First Hospital, No. 8, Xishiku Street, Xicheng District, Beijing 100034, China

Correspondence should be addressed to Huixia Yang; yanghuixia@bjmu.edu.cn

Academic Editor: Kimber Stanhope

Changes in DNA methylation may play a role in the genetic mechanism underlying glucose intolerance in the offspring of mothers with diabetes. Here, we established a rat model of moderate intrauterine hyperglycemia induced by streptozotocin to detect glucose and lipid metabolism of first-generation (F1) and second-generation (F2) offspring. Moderate intrauterine hyperglycemia induced high body weight in F1 and F2 offspring of diabetic mothers. F1 offspring had impaired glucose tolerance and abnormal insulin level. Additionally, F1 and F2 offspring that were exposed to intrauterine hyperglycemia had impaired insulin secretion from the islets. The tumor necrosis factor (*Tnf*) gene was upregulated in perirenal adipose tissue from F1 offspring and relatively increased in F2 offspring. Both F1 and F2 offspring showed similar hypomethylation level at the −1952 site of *Tnf*. We confirmed that DNA methylation occurs in offspring exposed to intrauterine hyperglycemia and that the DNA methylation is intergenerational and inherited.

1. Introduction

Gestational diabetes mellitus (GDM) is characterized by intrauterine hyperglycemia and has been reported to affect 17.5% of pregnant women in China [1]. GDM is associated with health issues in offspring. The offspring of mothers with GDM have been shown to have higher birth weights and are reportedly prone to obesity, hypertension, and dyslipidemia compared to offspring of mothers without diabetes [2, 3]. It has been suggested that, apart from genetic influences, the intrauterine environment may also influence the phenotype of the offspring.

"Programming" refers to the process by which a stimulus at a critical window of development has long-term effects. Numerous studies have investigated the effects of adverse intrauterine environment and found that it is correlated with poor fetal growth and increased risk of type 2 diabetes and obesity in adulthood [4]. Some studies have shown that obesity and type 2 diabetes are a global metabolic disorder and systemic inflammation, and the intersection of these phenomena is especially evident in visceral adipose tissue [5, 6]. Nevertheless, the potential mechanism of glucose intolerance induced by intrauterine hyperglycemia remains to be fully understood, and it is yet unknown whether inflammation is related to metabolic disturbances in offspring exposed to intrauterine hyperglycemia.

It has been suggested that epigenetic mechanisms may be the link between environmental and nutritional factors and regulation of gene expression. DNA methylation is one of the major epigenetic modifications. We hypothesized that changes in DNA methylation could participate in the expression of genes related to glucose intolerance in offspring. Furthermore, DNA methylation might also determine the transgenerational disease transmission.

In this study, we established a rat model of streptozotocin-(STZ-) induced moderate intrauterine hyperglycemia. F1 female rats were fed either normal diet or high-fat diets after weaning. The F1 adult female rats obtained from the control and diabetic rats were mated with control male rats, and the phenotypes of F2 female offspring were characterized to study transgenerational influences. Furthermore, we analyzed the methylation status in perirenal adipose tissue to investigate whether intrauterine hyperglycemia affected gene expression of inflammatory cytokines by regulating epigenetic modification.

2. Materials and Methods

2.1. Animals and Tissue Isolation. Twenty-one Wistar rats were used in this study. All the rats were fed in the specific-pathogen-free (SPF) grade animal test room with stable room temperature and humidity. The rats were housed in a 12 : 12 light : dark cycle. All animal protocols were reviewed and approved by the Institutional Animal Care and Use Committee of Peking University First Hospital (J201010). At 12 weeks, female Wistar rats (Vital River Laboratory Animal Technology Co., Ltd., Beijing, China) were mated with male rats. Onset of pregnancy was determined by the presence of a vaginal plug after overnight mating (designated as day 0 [D0] of pregnancy). After the rats were made to fast for a 12 h period, the female rats were randomly divided into two groups: intrauterine hyperglycemia group (F0-D), in which fourteen rats were injected with a single intraperitoneal injection of 25 mg/kg STZ (Sigma) in citrate buffer (pH 4.4) on D0.5, and control group (F0-C), in which the seven pregnant rats received an equal volume of citrate buffer on D0.5. On D4 of pregnancy and every three days thereafter, the blood glucose concentration was measured via the tail vein to check for diabetes. The pregnant rats were allowed to deliver spontaneously. Female offspring were studied and fed either a normal diet (12% kcal fat, 24% kcal protein, and 64% kcal carbohydrates; Beijing KeAoXieLi Feeds Co., Ltd., Beijing, China) or a high-fat diet (45% kcal fat, 20% kcal protein, and 45% kcal carbohydrates; Beijing KeAoXieLi Feeds Co., Ltd., Beijing, China) after weaning: the control group rats were fed a normal diet (F1-CN, $n = 9$) or high-fat diet (F1-CF, $n = 9$), and the diabetic group rats were fed a normal diet (F1-DN, $n = 9$) or high-fat diet (F1-DF, $n = 9$). The F1-CN and F1-DN female adult rats were then mated with control male rats. The phenotypes of F2 female offspring were characterized. F2 female offspring were divided into F2-C and F2-D groups (Figure 1). The F1 and F2 offspring were sacrificed at 28 weeks. Blood from the abdominal aorta was obtained and centrifuged at 3,000 ×g for 10 min to separate the serum and stored at −80°C until analysis. The heart, liver, pancreas, kidney, and fat pads (including mesenteric, perirenal, and ovarian fat) were carefully dissected and weighed. Perirenal adipose tissues were dissected from visible blood vessels and immediately frozen in liquid nitrogen, and the perirenal adipose tissue samples were stored at −80°C before further processing.

2.2. Oral Glucose Tolerance Test. F1 rats from all the four F1 groups (F1-CN, F1-DN, F1-CF, and F1-DF) were fasted overnight and given 2 g/kg glucose by gavage for the oral glucose tolerance test (OGTT) conducted at 16, 20, and 24 weeks. Blood samples were collected from the tail vein before ($t = 0$) and at 30, 60, and 120 min of glucose administration.

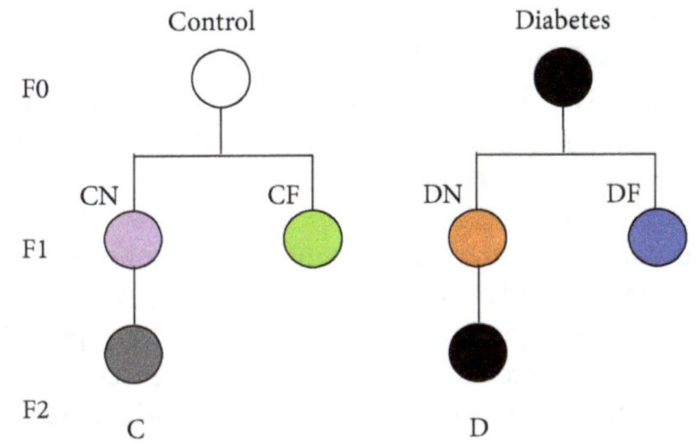

FIGURE 1: GDM rat model with moderate hyperglycemia induced by streptozotocin. Study design: female offspring were fed either normal or high-fat diets after weaning: control groups were fed normal diet (F1-CN) or high-fat diet (F1-CF) and rats in the diabetic group were fed normal diet (F1-DN) or high-fat diet (F1-DF). Adult females of the F1-CN and F1-DN groups were mated with control males to obtain F2 female offspring (F2-C and F2-D). Purple denotes the F1-CN group; green, F1-DN; orange, F1-CF; blue, F1-DF; and grey, F2-C group; and the plain circle denotes the F2-D group.

2.3. Biochemical Test and Analysis. The fasting insulin (FINS) levels were measured in the F1-CN, F1-DN, F2-C, and F2-D groups by enzyme-linked immunosorbent assay (ELISA) at 28 weeks (rat insulin ELISA kit, Cayman Chemical, 589501, USA), according to the manufacturer's instructions. The total triglyceride (TG) and high-density lipoprotein (HDL) levels in the F1-CN, F1-DN, F2-C, and F2-D groups were detected in a fully automatic biochemical analyzer at 28 weeks. The reagents used in the assays were provided by Beijing BHKT Clinical Reagent Co., Ltd., China.

2.4. Histology and Morphometric Analysis. Morphological evaluation was carried out as follows: briefly, pancreases were dissected rapidly, cleaned of connective tissue, weighed, and fixed in 4% paraformaldehyde solution for 48 h. The pancreases were then embedded in wax and serially sliced to obtain 5 μm wide histological sections. The sections were stained with hematoxylin and eosin and then the morphological features were analyzed under a microscope. The areas and diameters of pancreatic islets were measured using Image-Pro Plus 6.0 (Media Cybernetics). Ten different fields were analyzed per rat, and six rats in each of the F1-CN, F1-DN, F2-C, and F2-D groups were analyzed.

2.5. Immunohistochemistry of Pancreatic Islets. Immunolocalization was performed for anti-insulin reaction on 5 μm thick sections, and the sections were subsequently stained with streptavidin biotin peroxidase. Paraffin sections were deparaffinized in xylene and rehydrated in descending grades of alcohol followed by heat-induced epitope retrieval. Endogenous peroxidase and nonspecific antibody binding sites were suppressed by treating the sections with 0.3% hydrogen peroxide for 10 min at room temperature.

The sections were then washed in phosphate-buffered saline and incubated for 1 h with primary antibodies for rat insulin (ZSGB-BIO, Beijing, China). The sections were washed again with phosphate-buffered saline and incubated with biotinylated secondary antibody (PV6000, ZSGB-BIO, Beijing, China) for 40 min. Finally, the nuclei were stained using hematoxylin and eosin and mounted in 3,3′-diaminobenzidine (DAB). Antibody binding was evaluated by high-power light microscopy (cellSens, Olympus DP72, Japan). The pancreatic islet area and fluorescence intensity were measured using Image-Pro Plus 6.0 (Media Cybernetics). Ten different fields were analyzed per rat, and six rats per group were analyzed.

2.6. MeDIP Array. A purified genomic DNA pool was prepared from three perirenal adipose tissue samples from the F1-CN and F1-DN groups and digested overnight with *Mse*I restriction enzyme (NEB, R0525S). Denatured DNA was immunoprecipitated using monoclonal antibodies against 5-methyl cytidine (Abcam, Ab10805). Immunoprecipitated DNA was recovered with proteinase K digestion followed by column-based purification, amplified, and hybridized on a Rat DNA Methylation 3 × 720 K CpG Island Plus RefSeq Promoter Array according to the protocol of Roche NimbleGen. Immunoprecipitated (IP) and input DNA samples were labeled with Cy5 and Cy3, respectively. Hybridization was performed using a NimbleGen Hybridization Kit and NimbleGen Hybridization System 12. Scanning was done using high-resolution NimbleGen MS 200 Microarray Scanner. MeDIP array data were analyzed using NimbleScan software, and the array results could be visualized using SignalMap software. Microarray data reported in the paper were deposited to the Gene Expression Omnibus (GEO) at the National Center for Biotechnology Information (NCBI) under the series accession number GSE65779.

2.7. DNA Methylation ChIP Analysis. MeDIP samples from the F1-CN and F1-DN groups were hybridized to Rat DNA Methylation 3 × 720 K CpG Island Plus RefSeq Promoter Array representing 15,287 putative promoters (−3.88 kb to +0.97 kb to the transcription start site (TSS)) and 15,790 CpG islands. Chromatin immunoprecipitation (ChIP) analysis was carried out by CapitalBio Corporation (Beijing, China). We identified 923 and 2150 promoters as significantly hypermethylated and significantly hypomethylated, respectively. The biological significance of the microarray data was analyzed by the Molecular Annotation System (CB-MAS, CapitalBio Corporation, Beijing, China, http://bioinfo.capitalbio.com/mas3/).

2.8. DNA Methylation Analysis Using Bisulfite Sequencing. Genomic DNA of three perirenal adipose tissue samples from the F1-CN, F1-DN, F2-C, and F2-D groups was treated and purified with the EpiTect bisulfite kit (Qiagen), according to the manufacturer's instructions. The methylation status was evaluated by cloning and sequencing the bisulfite-treated DNA. The following primers were used to amplify region −2012 to −1829 of the *Tnf* promoter: sense 5′-GGT TTT TTT TGG AGA AAG TTG TTT-3′, antisense 5′-AAA AAC ACA ACC CCC TAA TAC ATT A-3′. The following primers were used to amplify region −220 to +26 of the *Tnf* promoter: sense 5′-TTT TGA TGT TTG GGT GTT TTT AAT T-3′, antisense 5′-TTC TCC CTC CTA ACT AAT CCC TTA A-3′. The purified PCR products were cloned using a pEASY-T1 Simple Cloning Vector system (TransGen Biotech, Beijing, China), and ten individual clones in each sample were sequenced. A total of three samples were evaluated in each group. The sequence obtained by cloning was analyzed at Beijing General GeneTest Co., Ltd. (Beijing, China).

2.9. Nucleic Acid Purification and Real-Time PCR. For RNA extraction, perirenal adipose tissues from the F1-CN, F1-DN, F2-C, and F2-D groups were homogenized in 1 mL of TRIzol reagent and RNA was purified according to the manufacturer's recommendations. The RNA was used as a template for synthesis of the same amount of cDNA (2 μg) using First Strand Synthesis Kit (Applied Biosystems, USA). cDNA quantity was measured using real-time PCR with the ABI PRISM 7500 sequence detection system and fluorescence-based SYBR Green technology. The PCR reaction mixture consisted of 2 μg of diluted cDNA sample, 2x SYBR Green PCR Master Mix (Molecular Probes, USA), primers optimized for each target gene, and nuclease-free water to achieve a final volume of 20 μL. All the samples were analyzed in duplicate. Primers were designed using Primer Express 3.0 software. The following primers were used: *Rplp0*, sense 5′-GGC GAC CTG GAA GTC CAA-3′ and antisense 5′-TCT GCT CCC ACA ATG AAG CA-3′; *Tnf*, sense 5′-TGA TCG GTC CCA ACA AGG A-3′ and antisense 5′-GGG CCA TGG AAC TGA TGA GA-3′; *IL-1β*, sense 5′-CCCAAGCACCTTCTTTTCCTT-3′ and antisense 5′-CGTCATCATCCCACGAGTCA-3′; *IL-6*, sense 5′-ACAGAGGATACCACCCACAACAG-3′ and antisense 5′-TCAGAATTGCCATTGCACAAC-3′; *IL-10*, sense 5′-CAGTCAGCCAGACCCACATG-3′ and antisense 5′-TGTTGTCCAGCTGGTCCTTCT-3′; *IFN-γ*, sense 5′-ATCGAATCGCACCTGATCACT-3′ and antisense 5′-GTGCTGGATCTGTGGGTTGTT-3′.

2.10. Western Blot Analysis. Perirenal adipose biopsies from the F1-CN, F1-DN, F2-C, and F2-D groups were homogenized in RIPA lysis buffer (KeyGen Biotech, KGP702, Nanjing, China) and 1 mM phenylmethylsulfonyl fluoride (PMSF; Amresco, M221, USA). The protein content was determined using a bicinchoninic acid (BCA) protein assay kit from KeyGen Biotech (Nanjing, China). Protein samples were placed at equal concentrations on polyacrylamide gel and separated using 12% sodium dodecyl sulfate-polyacrylamide gel electrophoresis (SDS-PAGE). Proteins were transferred to polyvinylidene difluoride (PVDF) membranes (Applygen, P2110, Beijing, China) and subjected to Western blot analysis. After incubation with primary antibodies (Cell Signaling Technology, 11948S, USA) overnight, the PVDF membranes were washed and incubated with horseradish peroxidase-conjugated secondary antibodies (ZSGB-BIO, Beijing, China) for 1 h at room temperature. The results were

Table 1: Body weight (grams) of F1 and F2 females.

	N	Birth	3 weeks	7 weeks	11 weeks	15 weeks	19 weeks	23 weeks	28 weeks
F1-CN	8	6.26 ± 0.13	37.51 ± 1.25	171.88 ± 4.73	242.00 ± 7.70	259.38 ± 7.52	284.25 ± 10.70	301.13 ± 11.02	309.50 ± 12.84
F1-DN	9	6.90 ± 0.14^{a}	41.93 ± 4.08	179.11 ± 7.86	255.56 ± 9.29	284.33 ± 8.57^{a}	305.44 ± 8.92	318.22 ± 10.11	325.44 ± 10.91
F1-CF	8	6.37 ± 0.08	38.01 ± 1.68	169.38 ± 4.38	248.63 ± 6.70	281.50 ± 8.20^{a}	311.50 ± 11.34	328.38 ± 14.23	332.57 ± 15.16
F1-DF	8	7.04 ± 0.09^{b}	42.56 ± 1.91	179.50 ± 4.32	259.50 ± 7.08	292.50 ± 9.43	306.86 ± 10.07	317.43 ± 14.78	318.86 ± 14.85
F2-C	6	7.2 ± 0.4	57.62 ± 1.49	187 ± 3.96	248.66 ± 6.11	274.17 ± 3.7	286.5 ± 7.53	288.66 ± 9.61	300.17 ± 6.63
F2-D	6	7.1 ± 0.8	56.80 ± 1.94	198.83 ± 6.69	256.66 ± 9.59	284 ± 9.08	299.17 ± 6.62	310.83 ± 5.64*	322.33 ± 6.65*

Data are means ± SEM. Significance was determined by ANOVA. $^{a}p < 0.05$ versus F1-CN, $^{b}p < 0.05$ versus F1-CF, and $^{*}p < 0.05$ versus F2-C.

Table 2: Body composition (grams) of F1 and F2 females at 28 weeks.

	N	Mesenteric adipose tissue weight (g)	Perirenal adipose tissue weight (g)	Ovarian adipose tissue weight (g)	Visceral adipose tissue weight (g)	Pancreas weight (g)	Liver weight (g)	Heart weight (g)	Kidney weight (g)
F1-CN	8	4.34 ± 0.79	3.79 ± 0.89	7.69 ± 1.42	15.82 ± 3.03	1.97 ± 0.06	7.68 ± 0.21	0.92 ± 0.04	1.98 ± 0.06
F1-DN	7	3.78 ± 0.44	4.21 ± 0.42	9.57 ± 0.96	17.56 ± 1.72	1.96 ± 0.08	7.67 ± 0.46	0.89 ± 0.04	1.96 ± 0.08
F1-CF	7	5.34 ± 1.18	6.93 ± 1.96	11.88 ± 2.10	24.16 ± 4.99	1.90 ± 0.10	7.13 ± 0.47	0.90 ± 0.05	1.90 ± 0.10
F1-DF	4	3.9 ± 1.01	4.28 ± 0.92	8.87 ± 1.92	17.05 ± 3.81	1.98 ± 0.06	8.49 ± 0.64	0.77 ± 0.03	1.98 ± 0.06
F2-C	8	3.87 ± 0.43	3.56 ± 0.30	9.95 ± 0.44	17.37 ± 0.75	0.91 ± 0.09	9.31 ± 0.33	0.91 ± 0.03	2.38 ± 0.05
F2-D	8	4.18 ± 0.63	4.49 ± 0.27*	8.88 ± 0.69	17.89 ± 1.46	0.89 ± 0.07	8.68 ± 0.44	0.89 ± 0.02	2.11 ± 0.34

Data are means ± SEM. Significance was determined by ANOVA. $^{*}p < 0.05$ versus F2-C.

quantified by densitometry using AlphaEaseFC FluorChem SA software for Windows (Alpha Innotech Corporation, California, USA).

2.11. Statistics. One-way ANOVA was used to determine the comparisons among the four groups. Post hoc comparisons using Tukey's test were performed when a significant F-score was detected. Comparisons between two groups were performed using two-tailed unpaired Student's t-test. All the values are presented as mean ± SEM. Statistically significant differences were defined at $p < 0.05$.

3. Results

3.1. Moderate Intrauterine Hyperglycemia Induced High Body Weight in F1 Females. As previously described [7], we established a moderate intrauterine hyperglycemia rat model by injecting Wistar rats with a single intraperitoneal injection of streptozotocin (STZ). The average glucose level of diabetic mothers during pregnancy was 11.2–15.0 mmol/L. Further morphological studies of the pancreas samples confirmed that rats with GDM had smaller pancreatic islets than rats without GDM.

The birth weight was significantly higher in the F1-DN group than in the F1-CN group (Table 1). The body weight was also significantly higher in the F1-DN group than in the F1-CN group at 15 weeks (Table 1). Furthermore, intrauterine hyperglycemia was found to induce adipopexis in F1 offspring, and the perirenal adipose tissue, ovarian adipose tissue, and whole visceral adipose tissue weighed more in the F1-DN group than in the F1-CN group; however, the tissue weights did not significantly differ between the two groups (Table 2). The pancreas, liver, heart, and kidney weights also showed no significant differences between the F1-DN and F1-CN groups (Table 2).

The body weight was higher in the F1-CF group than in the F1-CN group at 15 weeks (Table 1). The high-fat diet did not further exacerbate the effect of intrauterine hyperglycemia exposure on body weight (F1-DF versus F1-DN, Table 1).

The weights of perirenal adipose tissue and whole visceral adipose tissue were higher in the F1-CF group than in the F1-CN group with borderline significance ($p = 0.065$ and $p = 0.094$, resp.). There were no significant differences in the weights of the pancreas, liver, heart, and kidney in each group (Table 2).

3.2. Moderate Intrauterine Hyperglycemia Induced Glucose Intolerance and Abnormal Insulin and Lipid Levels in F1 Females. At birth, there was no significant difference in the blood glucose level between the F1-CN and F1-DN groups (Figure 2(a)). The fasting glucose levels were monitored in the F1 rats at 16, 20, 24, and 28 weeks. The fasting glucose level was higher in the F1-DN group than in the F1-CN group at 20 weeks (Figure 2(b)). The fasting glucose level was also elevated in the F1-DF group compared to that in the F1-CF group at 24 and 28 weeks (Figure 2(b)). Results of the GTT revealed impaired glucose tolerance (IGT) in the F1-DN group at 20 weeks. In this group, the blood glucose level had significantly increased at 0, 30, 60, and 120 min after glucose load, and the AUC was significantly higher in the F1-DN group than in the F1-CN group (Figures 3(b) and 3(e)). The GTT revealed IGT at 30 and 120 min in the F1-DN group at

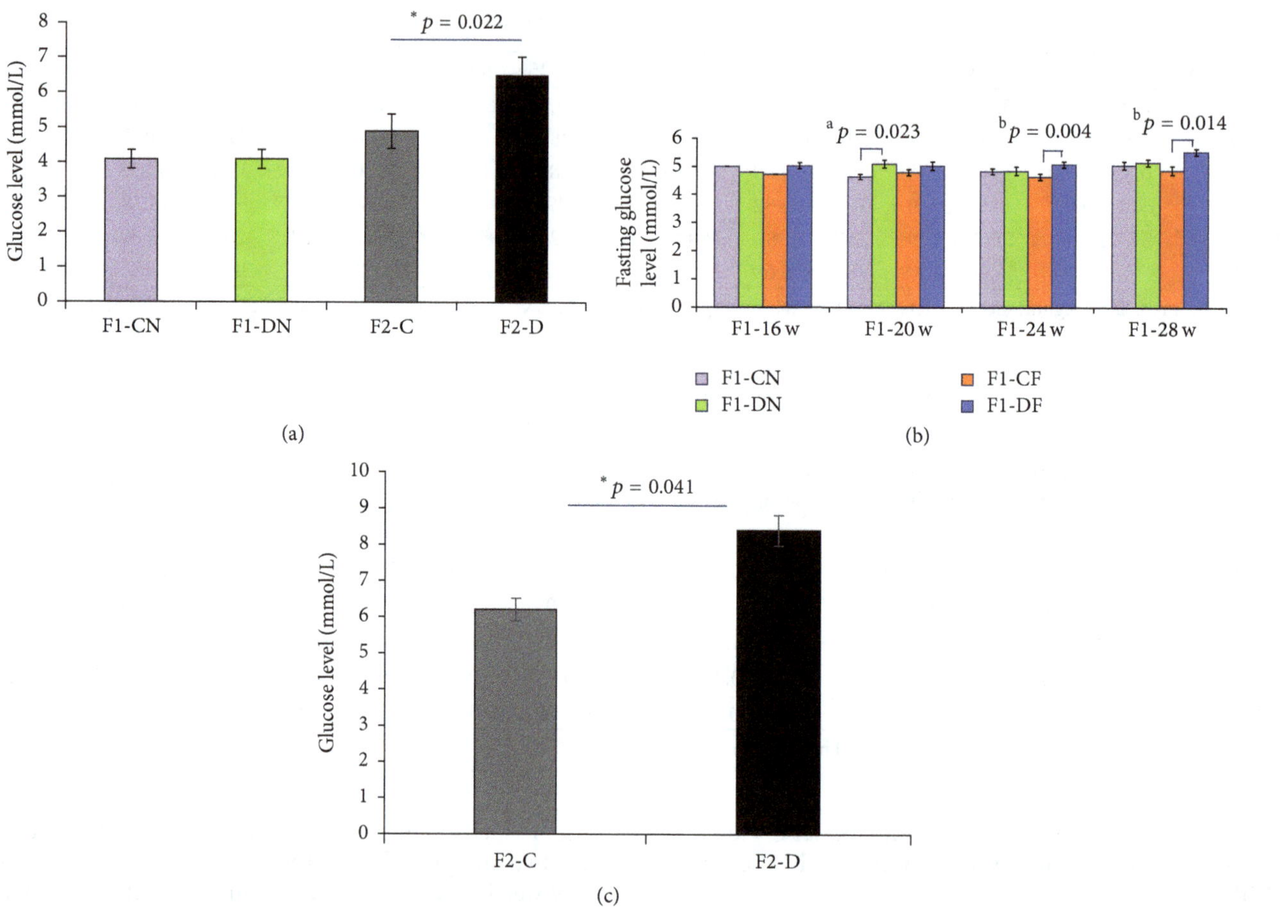

FIGURE 2: Glucose levels in Fl and F2 offspring. (a) The F2 offspring in the F2-D group have a higher glucose level at birth. (b) Rats in the Fl-DN group have a higher fasting glucose level at 20 weeks, and rats in the Fl-DF group have a higher fasting glucose level at 24 and 28 weeks than rats in the Fl-CF group. (c) Rats in the F2-D group have a higher glucose level at 28 weeks. The results are means ± SEM, $N = 8$-9; $^{a}p < 0.05$ versus Fl-CN; $^{b}p < 0.05$ versus Fl-CF; $^{*}p < 0.05$ versus F2-C.

24 weeks, and there were no differences in the AUC between the Fl-DN and Fl-CN groups at 24 weeks (Figures 3(c) and 3(f)). The GTT revealed no difference in the glucose tolerance at 16 weeks (Figures 3(a) and 3(d)).

The high-fat diet also induced glucose intolerance. The blood glucose level significantly increased at 60 min after glucose load at 16 weeks, at 60 and 120 min at 20 weeks, and at 30 min at 24 weeks in the Fl-CF group compared to the Fl-CN group (Figures 3(a)–3(c)). The high-fat diet could exacerbate glucose intolerance of offspring exposed to intrauterine hyperglycemia, as evidenced by the blood glucose level, which was significantly increased at 30 min after glucose load at both 16 and 24 weeks in the Fl-DF group compared to the Fl-DN group, and the AUC was significantly increased at 24 weeks (Figures 3(a), 3(c), and 3(f)). Moreover, IGT was found in the Fl-DF group compared to the Fl-CF group, and the blood glucose level of the former group significantly increased at 30 min at 16 weeks; 30 min at 20 weeks; and 0, 30, and 60 min at 24 weeks. Furthermore, the AUC was significantly higher at 20 and 24 weeks (Figures 3(a), 3(b), 3(c), 3(e), and 3(f)).

The FINS, triglyceride, and HDL levels in the Fl rats were monitored at 28 weeks (Figures 4(a)–4(c)). The FINS and HDL levels were significantly decreased in the Fl-DN group compared to the Fl-CN group (Figures 4(a) and 4(c)).

3.3. Moderate Intrauterine Hyperglycemia Induced High Body Weight and Hyperglycemia in F2 Females. The birth weights of F2 females were similar between the diabetes and control groups, and body weight increased in the F2-D group compared to the controls at 23 and 28 weeks (Table 1). In addition, the blood glucose levels at birth and at 28 weeks were significantly increased in the F2-D group compared to those in the F2-C group (Figures 2(a) and 2(c)). Moreover, the weight of perirenal adipose tissue was significantly higher in the F2-D than that in the F2-C group, whereas the weights of the pancreas, liver, heart, and kidney did not significantly differ between the two groups (Table 2). In addition, the FINS, TG, and HDL levels were similar between the two F2 groups (Figures 4(a)–4(c)).

3.4. Moderate Intrauterine Hyperglycemia Induced Transgenerational Effects on Islet Structure and Impaired Insulin

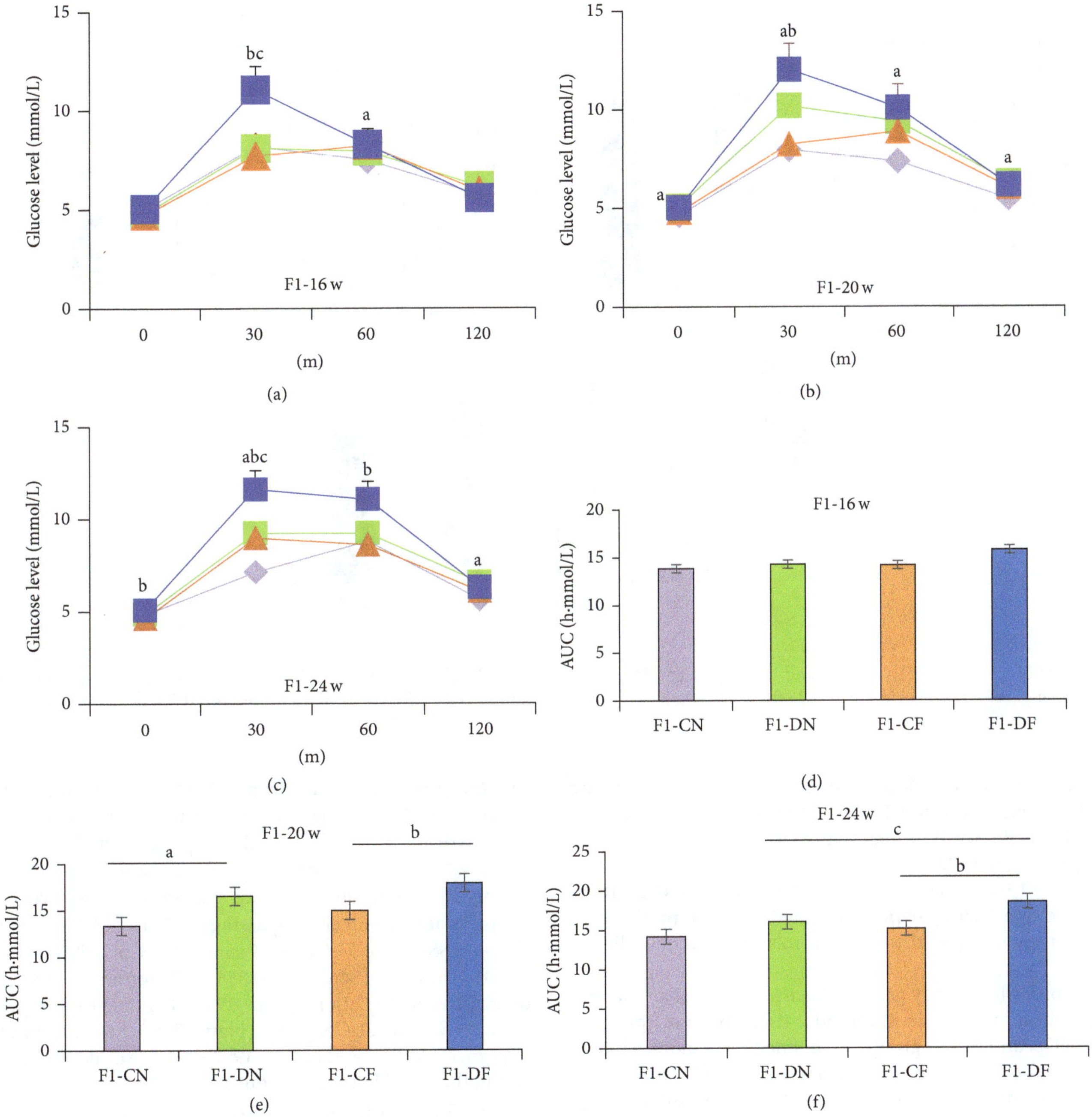

FIGURE 3: Glucose tolerance test. (a–c) Glucose tolerance test (GTT) was performed at 16, 20, and 24 weeks using 2 g glucose/kg body weight given by gavage. (d–f) AUC was performed at 16, 20, and 24 weeks. The results are presented as means ± SEM, $N = 8\text{-}9$; $^{a}p < 0.05$ versus F1-CN; $^{b}p < 0.05$ versus F1-CF; $^{c}p < 0.05$ versus F1-DN.

Secretion. A morphological study of the pancreas samples confirmed that the F1-DN group had obviously smaller pancreatic islets and atrophied β-cell mass compared to the F1-CN group (Figures 5(a) and 5(b)). Pancreatic islets in the F2-D group were similar to those in the control group (Figures 5(a) and 5(b)). To further define the potential secretory defects that may be related to the abnormal structure of islets in offspring exposed to intrauterine hyperglycemia, pancreatic islets were immunohistochemically analyzed. The level of insulin-positive cells in the islets was borderline significantly reduced in F1-DN group compared to F1-CN group (Figures 5(c) and 5(d)); interestingly, the level of insulin-positive cell area of islets was borderline significantly increased in F2-D group compared to that in F2-C group (Figures 5(c) and 5(d)).

3.5. Altered Genome-Wide Methylation Levels in F1 Female Offspring Exposed to Intrauterine Hyperglycemia. We used methylated DNA immunoprecipitation (MeDIP) combined with microarray technology to discover whether changes in DNA methylation are specific to intrauterine hyperglycemia

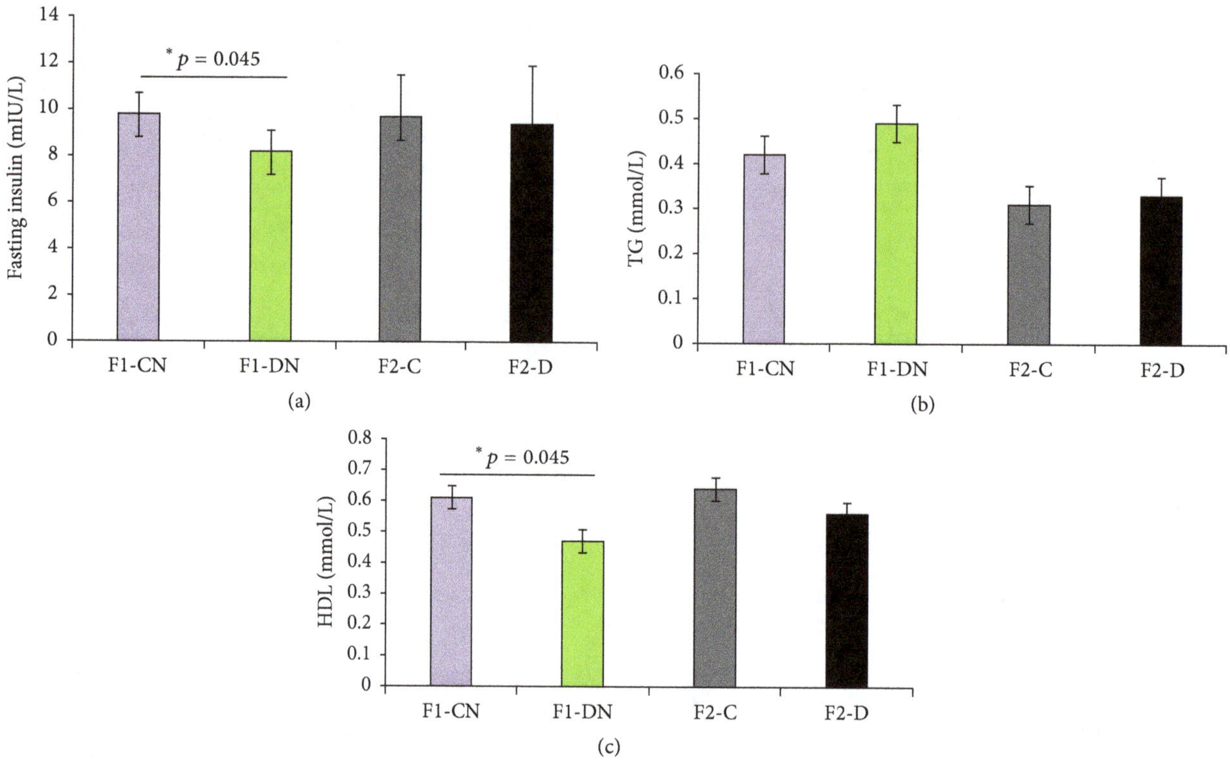

FIGURE 4: Biochemical analysis of F1 and F2 offspring at 28 weeks. (a) Level of fasting insulin in F1 and F2 offspring. (b) TG level in F1 and F2 offspring. (c) HDL level in F1 and F2 offspring. Results are presented as means ± SEM, $N = 6$ per group; $^*p < 0.05$ versus F1-CN.

exposure. We identified differentially methylated genes in the F1-DN group using Rat DNA Methylation 3 × 720 K CpG Island Plus RefSeq Promoter Array representing 15,287 putative promoters (−3.88 kb to +0.97 kb respective to the TSS) and 15,790 CpG islands. A total of 923 and 2150 promoters were significantly hypermethylated and hypomethylated, respectively, compared to the controls in perirenal adipose tissue.

In order to identify groups of genes with similar changes in methylation in perirenal adipose tissue from offspring in the F1-DN and F1-CN groups, we defined the biological processes of the identified genes using a molecular annotation system. Genes were ranked by the level of significance (p values) according to the difference in methylation (Figure 6, Tables S1 and S2 in Supplementary Material available online at http://dx.doi.org/10.1155/2016/4952801). It is noteworthy that some genes associated with adipocytokine signaling pathway were significantly hypomethylated, including *Camkk2*, *Pck1*, *Rxrb*, *Adipoq*, *Tnf*, *Prkag3*, *Nfkbib*, and *Mapk10*. Moreover, the methylation level of genes related to type II diabetes mellitus was also prominently decreased, including *Prkce*, *Prkcz*, *Adipoq*, *Tnf*, *Slc2a2*, *Prkcd*, and *Mapk10* (Figure S1). As a key gene associated with adipocytokine signaling pathway and diabetes, the *Tnf* promoter was hypomethylated in perirenal adipose tissue from F1-DN group compared to controls ($p <$ 0.05).

3.6. Methylation Levels of Tnf Promoter Region in F1 and F2 Offspring. MeDIP data showed that the portion of the *Tnf* promoter region from −2914 to −1717 was hypomethylated. Bisulfite sequencing was used to validate results of MeDIP for *Tnf*. Genomic DNA was extracted from perirenal adipose tissue obtained from F1 and F2 female offspring. Bisulfite sequencing was performed on a portion of the promoter region encompassing −2012 to −1829 relative to the +1 TSS of the *Tnf* gene, including 5 CpG sites (−1952, −1901, −1881, −1866, and −1858). We found a significant decrease in methylation in the −1952 site in the F1-DN group compared to the F1-CN group (Figure 7(a)). Interestingly, the hypomethylation level at the −1952 site was similar in the F2-D and the F1-DN groups (Figure 7(a)).

We further carried out bisulfite sequencing on another portion of the *Tnf* promoter region encompassing −220 to +26 relative to the +1 TSS, which included 8 CpG sites (−178, −138, −91, −89, −66, −35, −20, and −7). The methylation level did not significantly differ between the F1-DN and F1-CN groups, and similar results were obtained for the F2 generation (Figure 7(a)).

3.7. Tnf Methylation May Control the Expression of Tnf. In order to investigate the physiological importance of methylation in gene and protein expression, we measured the *Tnf* gene and protein expression levels using real-time PCR and Western blot analysis, respectively. The *Tnf* gene expression was significantly higher in the F1-DN group than in the F1-CN group ($p < 0.05$), and the *Tnf* gene expression showed an increasing trend in the F2-D group compared to the F2-C

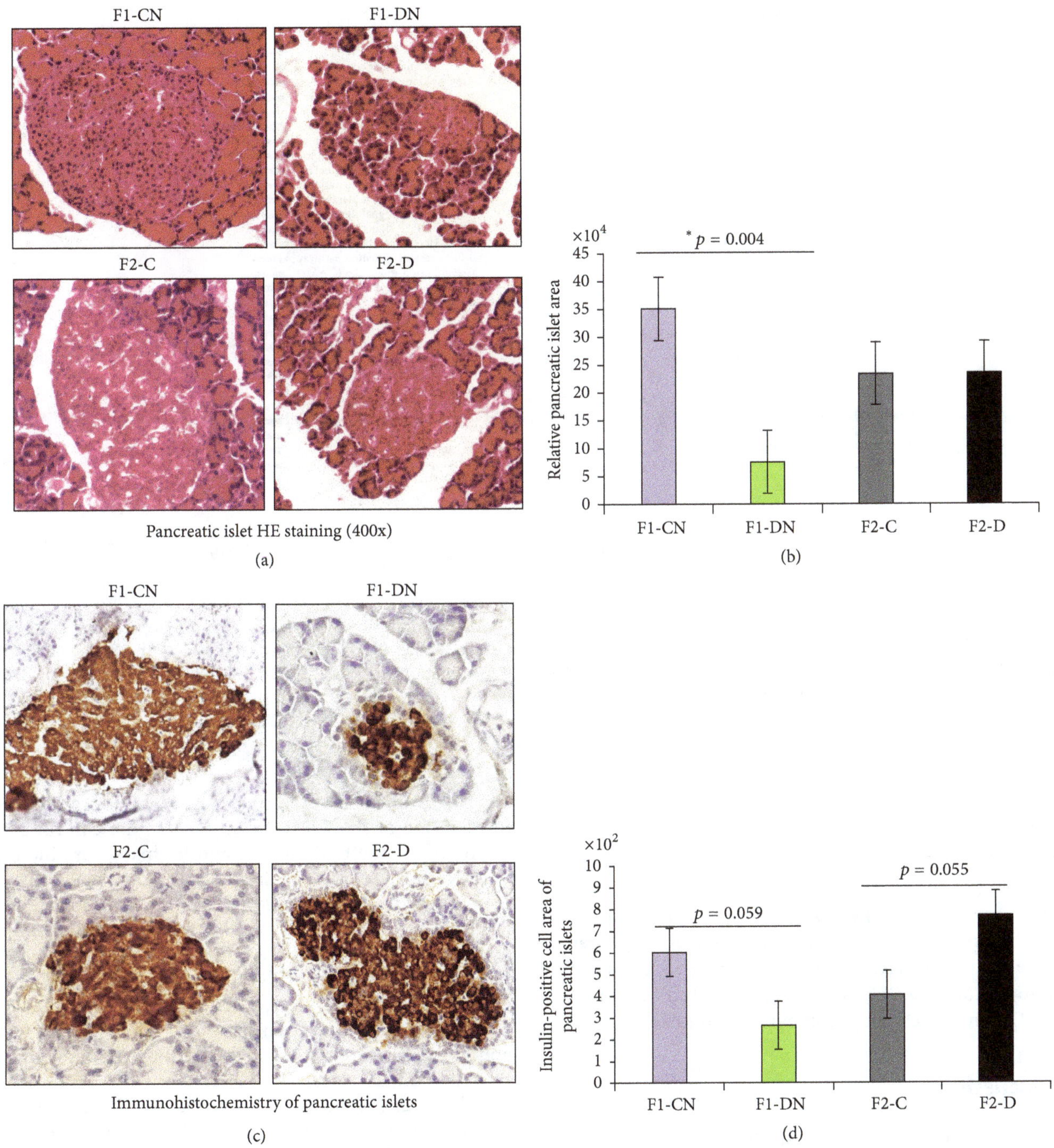

FIGURE 5: Histology and immunohistochemistry of pancreatic islets. (a) HE staining images (400x) of pancreatic islets obtained from F1 and F2 offspring. (b) The area and diameters of pancreatic islets were measured using Image-Pro Plus 6.0, Media Cybernetics. Ten different fields were analyzed for each rat, with a total of six rats per group. (c) Immunohistochemistry of pancreatic islets. (d) Insulin-positive cell area of pancreatic islets was measured using Image-Pro Plus 6.0. Ten different fields were analyzed for each rat; totally six rats in each group were analyzed. Results are presented as means ± SEM, $N = 6$ per group; $^*p < 0.05$ versus F1-CN.

group, but this difference was not statistically significant ($p = 0.09$; Figure 7(b)). The protein expression did not significantly differ in the F1-DN and F2-D groups compared to the corresponding control groups (Figure 7(c)).

Hypomethylation of the *Tnf* promoter region at −1952 site was negatively correlated with the increased gene expression in diabetic offspring ($r = -0.36$). The transcription factors *Tfap2a*, *Tfap2c*, *Ebf1*, *Egr1*, *Rxra*, *c-Rel*, *RelA*, and *Nfic*

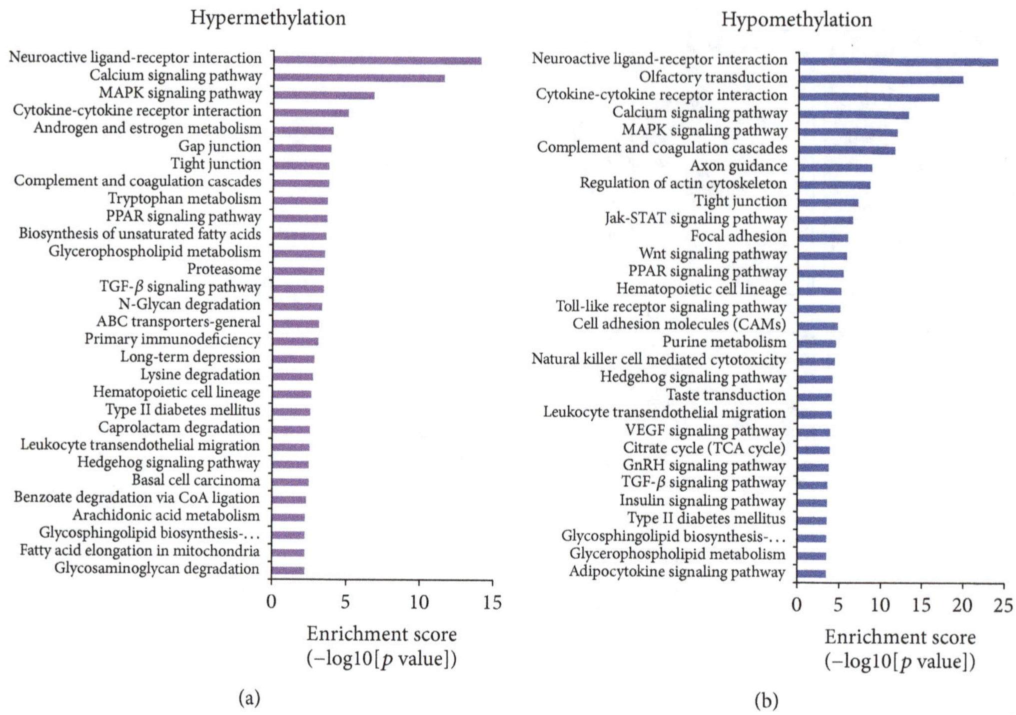

FIGURE 6: The pathways of DNA methylation changes in F1 offspring exposed to intrauterine hyperglycemia. Immunoprecipitated DNA was amplified and hybridized on Rat DNA Methylation 3 × 720 K CpG Island Plus RefSeq Promoter Array according to the Roche NimbleGen protocol. Microarray data was extracted and analyzed by the Molecular Annotation System (CB-MAS, CapitalBio Corporation, Beijing, China, http://bioinfo.capitalbio.com/mas3/).

predicted by the JASPAR database may be involved in the regulation of *Tnf* expression by binding to the specific CpG site in a methylation-sensitive manner.

3.8. Expression of Inflammatory Cytokines in Perirenal Adipose Tissue. Expression of inflammatory cytokines in perirenal adipose tissue was detected, and the expression levels of *IL-1β*, *IL-6*, *IL-10*, and *IFN-γ* did not significantly differ between the F1-DN and F2-D groups compared to controls (Figure 8).

4. Discussion

A GDM rodent model can be established using streptozotocin, which is directly toxic to maternal pancreatic β-cells. A previous study found that small fetuses were delivered following severe intrauterine hyperglycemia induced by a high dose of streptozotocin [8]. Nevertheless, GDM women with moderate hyperglycemia and large babies are more common in the clinical setting. Previous studies have found that administering a low dose of streptozotocin for five consecutive days can also induce moderate intrauterine hyperglycemia [8]. We established a GDM rat model with a single intraperitoneal injection of 25 mg/kg streptozotocin. The resultant moderate glucose level and the large fetus were used to mimic human macrosomia in offspring from mothers with GDM.

The birth weight of F1 offspring was significantly higher in offspring of the GDM group than in the control group; furthermore, the body weight and fat mass were increased in the offspring during adulthood. Although the F1 offspring of mothers in the GDM group had normal blood glucose levels at birth, impaired glucose tolerance and abnormal insulin and HDL levels were displayed in adulthood. The pancreatic islets were smaller in size and disordered and the insulin secretion was affected in F1 offspring of mothers with GDM, indicating that intrauterine hyperglycemia may lead to abnormal structure of fetal islets. The impaired β-cells may be related to the development of IGT.

The birth weights did not significantly differ between F2 offspring of mothers with GDM and controls. Nevertheless, the F2 offspring showed higher body weight and fat mass in adulthood. Furthermore, F2 offspring displayed hyperglycemia at birth and increased insulin secretion from the pancreatic islets in adulthood.

Together, these data contribute to the idea that early-life exposure to hyperglycemia in utero can influence glucose metabolism and induce insulin resistance in offspring up to the F2 generation. In addition, transgenerational offspring will be prone to obesity and hyperlipidemia in adulthood. It is indicated that a certain developmental pattern is programmed in utero. Ding et al. [9] demonstrated that intrauterine hyperglycemia induced IGT and abnormal insulin levels in both F1 and F2 offspring, which are partly due to the deficient islet ultrastructure. Future studies should aim to

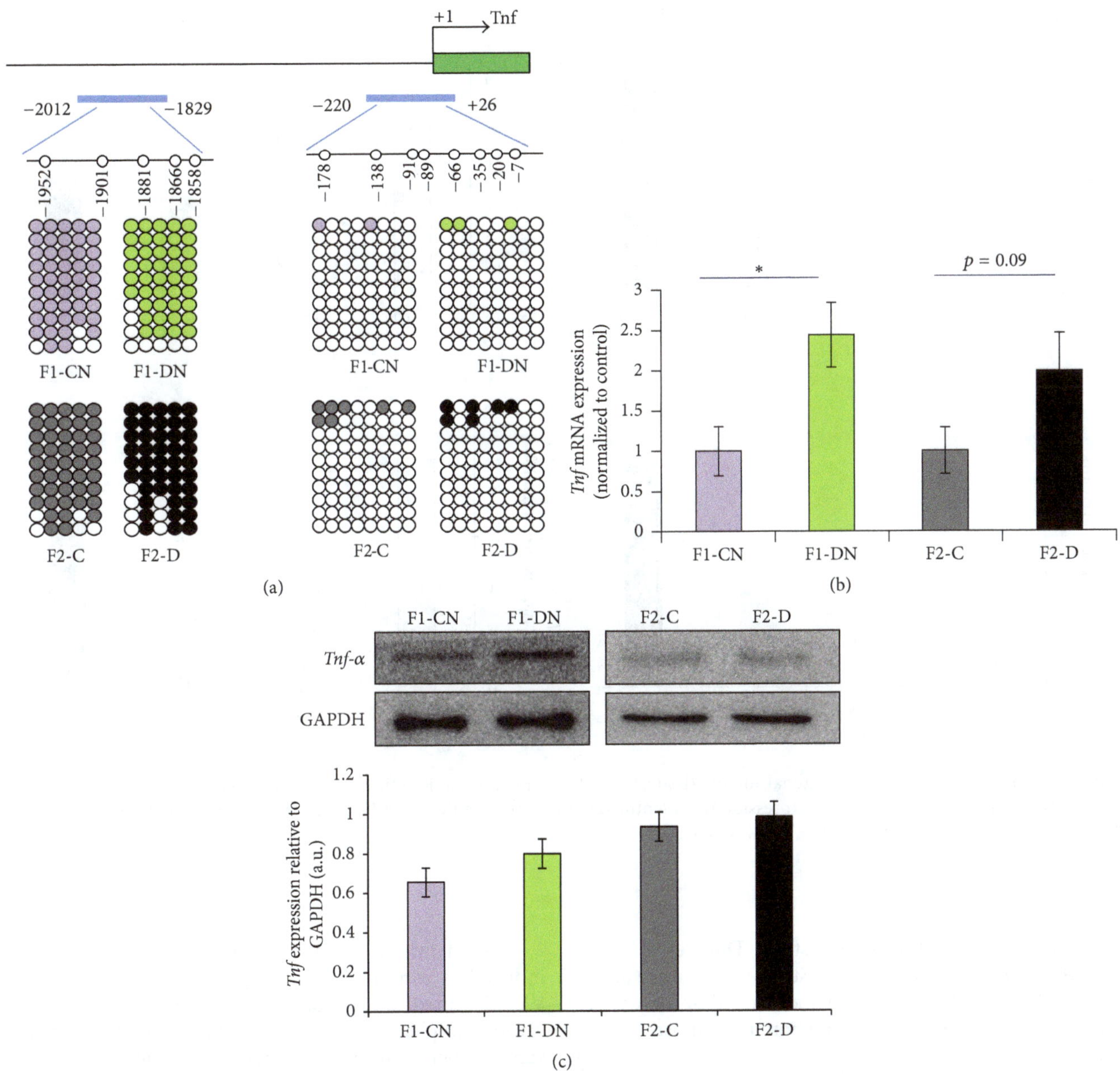

FIGURE 7: Methylation analysis and gene expression of *Tnf*. (a) Bisulfite sequencing was performed on the portion of the promoter regions encompassing −2012 to −1829 relative to the +1 transcription start site of the *Tnf* gene including 5 CpG sites and −220 to +26 including 8 CpG sites. Each line represents the average methylation level of the sequence of all the clones. CpG sites are shown as blank (unmethylated) or filled (methylated) circles ($N = 3$ per group). (b) The expression of *Tnf* was identified using real-time PCR ($N = 8$-9). (c) The protein expression of *Tnf* was identified using Western blotting ($N = 5$ per group). Results are presented as the means ± SEM. $^*p < 0.05$ versus F1-CN. $N = 4$–9.

investigate the potential mechanisms by which environmental factors can influence the expression of genes involved in insulin resistance.

Previous studies have showed that a low-grade inflammation characterized by increased circulating levels of proinflammatory cytokines in adipose tissue, such as *IL-6* and *Tnf*, and chemokines is a common feature of obesity and diabetes [10]. The overexpression of *Tnf* is closely related to insulin resistance, reduced lipoprotein lipase activity, and increased lipase activity. Moreover, *Tnf* is an adipokine involved in systemic inflammation, and inflammatory factors secreted from adipocytes may interfere with the insulin signaling pathway and impair the action of insulin and glucose transport [11–14]. In our study, *Tnf* expression was increased in the F1 generation born from mothers with GDM and relatively increased in F2 offspring. Additionally, chronic inflammation was found in adipose tissue, and the levels of *IL-1β* and *IL-10* tended to increase in both F1 and F2 offspring obtained from F0 mothers with GDM. Transgenerational transmission of inflammatory state may be presented between F1 and

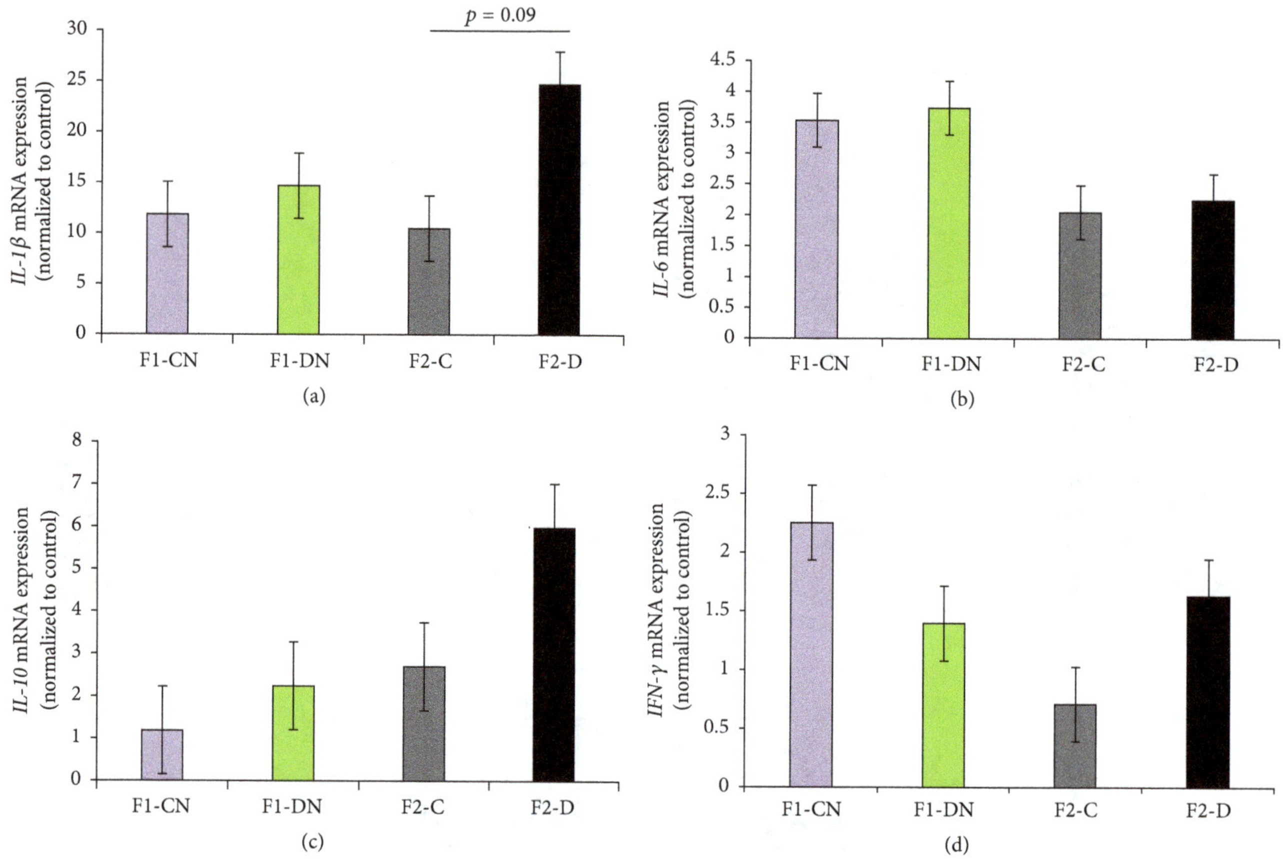

FIGURE 8: Inflammatory cytokines in perirenal adipose tissue. (a) *IL-1β* expression was identified using real-time PCR. (b) *IL-6* expression was identified using real-time PCR. (c) *IL-10* expression was identified using real-time PCR. (d) *IFN-γ* expression was identified using real-time PCR. Results are presented as the means ± SEM. $N = 4$-5.

F2 offspring. Consistent with our study, Ding et al. [15] showed that a feed-forward cycle exists in female mice after continuous high-fat diet stress, as demonstrated by increased adiposity and progressive inflammation in adipose tissue across generations.

Epigenetic mechanisms have been cited as a possible link between environmental and nutritional factors and the regulation of gene expression. DNA methylation is a major epigenetic modification. Evidence suggests that gene expression can be regulated by DNA methylation in diabetic patients, and the differential methylation may be responsible for the progression of type 2 diabetes [16]. Environmental events and nutritional conditions during early pregnancy may induce permanent DNA methylation changes in the fetus in utero. These studies emphasized the effect of early intrauterine exposure on epigenetic changes, which may be "memorized" and last throughout the lifetime of the offspring. Additionally, these epigenetic changes could also be transmitted to the F2 generation and show transgenerational effects [17, 18]. Nevertheless, most studies in this area have only focused on restricted intrauterine nutrition and reported the epigenetic modifications in intrauterine growth restriction (IUGR) models [19–21]. Our study is the first to provide further evidence of intrauterine exposure to excess nutrition.

We identified specific changes in DNA methylation induced by intrauterine hyperglycemia using MeDIP array. We identified a total of 923 and 2150 promoters in the visceral adipose tissue of F1 offspring that had been significantly hypermethylated and hypomethylated, respectively. It is noteworthy that the *Tnf* promoter was hypomethylated in diabetic offspring compared to the controls. Further bisulfite sequencing of the *Tnf* promoter encompassing −220 to +26 revealed that, overall, hypomethylation did not broadly alter the chromatin in diabetic offspring; rather, it was confined to the specific cytosine.

The *Tnf* promoter sequence contains CpG dinucleotides within or next to transcription factor-binding sites. The CpG site at site −1952 of the *Tnf* promoter was distinctly hypomethylated both in F1 and F2 offspring of diabetic mothers and the 1952-bp 5′-flanking region of the promoter may be a *c-Rel-*, *EBF1-*, *NFIC-*, *RelA-*, and *NF-κB*-binding site. Therefore, DNA methylation is proposed to participate in regulating the expression of the *Tnf* gene by interfering with transcription binding sites, playing a role in the progression of insulin resistance. Consistent with our findings, a study by Lou et al. [22] showed that the activation and upregulation of proinflammatory cytokines such as *IL-1β*, *IL-6*, *TNF-α*, and *IFN-γ* mainly occurred in the arterial intima of diabetic rats, and reduced levels of DNA methylation at the specific cytosine-phosphate-guanosine sites of *IL-1β*, *IL-6*, *TNF-α*, and *IFN-γ* may be one of the mechanisms to regulate the expression of these genes. Our results emphasized the effect of early intrauterine exposure on insulin sensitivity via epigenetic changes, which may persist throughout the lifetime as well as get transmitted to the next generation.

Another factor related to insulin resistance is lifestyle, and previous studies have reported that accumulation of intracellular lipid metabolites from incomplete lipid oxidation could inhibit signal transduction to glucose transport [23–25], suggesting the involvement of a high-fat diet in the development of insulin resistance. In the current study, offspring were given high-fat diets, and we found that fat overload could exaggerate the programmed glucose intolerance in offspring exposed to intrauterine hyperglycemia. The underlying mechanism for this phenomenon is not yet fully understood. Barrès et al. reported that elevated free fatty acids might induce insulin resistance through epigenetic mechanisms [16].

5. Conclusions

Overall, our results revealed that intrauterine hyperglycemia can influence the DNA methylation level in the promoter regions of inflammatory factors involved in insulin resistance, such as *TNF-α*, and the DNA methylation is intergenerational and inherited.

Abbreviations

GDM: Gestational diabetes mellitus
MeDIP: Methylated DNA immunoprecipitation
STZ: Streptozotocin
GTT: Glucose tolerance test
IGT: Impaired glucose tolerance
IUGR: Intrauterine growth restriction
OGTT: Oral glucose tolerance test
IP: Immunoprecipitated
TNF: Tumor necrosis factor
IL-1β: Interleukin-1β
IL-6: Interleukin-6
IL-10: Interleukin-10
IFN-γ: Interferon-γ.

Conflict of Interests

No potential conflict of interests relevant to this paper was reported.

Authors' Contribution

Rina Su and Jie Yan contributed equally to this work.

Acknowledgments

This study was supported by the National Natural Science Foundation of China (81370722, 30973212) and the Scientific Research Foundation for the Returned Overseas Chinese Scholars, State Education Ministry ([2014]1685).

References

[1] W. W. Zhu, H. X. Yang, Y. M. Wei et al., "Evaluation of the value of fasting plasma glucose in the first prenatal visit to diagnose gestational diabetes mellitus in China," *Diabetes Care*, vol. 36, no. 3, pp. 586–590, 2013.

[2] P. W. Franks, H. C. Looker, S. Kobes et al., "Gestational glucose tolerance and risk of type 2 diabetes in young Pima Indian offspring," *Diabetes*, vol. 55, no. 2, pp. 460–465, 2006.

[3] J. G. Manderson, B. Mullan, C. C. Patterson, D. R. Hadden, A. I. Traub, and D. McCance, "Cardiovascular and metabolic abnormalities in the offspring of diabetic pregnancy," *Diabetologia*, vol. 45, no. 7, pp. 991–996, 2002.

[4] D. J. P. Barker, "The fetal origins of type 2 diabetes mellitus," *Annals of Internal Medicine*, vol. 130, no. 4, pp. 322–324, 1999.

[5] O. Izaola, D. De Luis, I. Sajoux, J. C. Domingo, and M. Vidal, "Inflammation and obesity (lipoinflammation)," *Nutrición Hospitalaria*, vol. 31, no. 6, pp. 2352–2358, 2015.

[6] E. D. Buras, L. Yang, P. Saha et al., "Proinsulin-producing, hyperglycemia-induced adipose tissue macrophages underlie insulin resistance in high fat-fed diabetic mice," *The FASEB Journal*, vol. 29, no. 8, pp. 3537–3548, 2015.

[7] J. Yan, X. Li, R. Su, K. Zhang, and H. Yang, "Long-term effects of maternal diabetes on blood pressure and renal function in rat male offspring," *PLoS ONE*, vol. 9, no. 2, Article ID e88269, 2014.

[8] F. A. Van Assche, K. Holemans, and L. Aerts, "Long-term consequences for offspring of diabetes during pregnancy," *British Medical Bulletin*, vol. 60, pp. 173–182, 2001.

[9] G.-L. Ding, F.-F. Wang, J. Shu et al., "Transgenerational glucose intolerance with Igf2/H19 epigenetic alterations in mouse islet induced by intrauterine hyperglycemia," *Diabetes*, vol. 61, no. 5, pp. 1133–1142, 2012.

[10] B. D. Kayser, C. M. Toledo-Corral, T. L. Alderete, M. J. Weigensberg, and M. I. Goran, "Temporal relationships between adipocytokines and diabetes risk in Hispanic adolescents with obesity," *Obesity*, vol. 23, no. 7, pp. 1479–1485, 2015.

[11] G. S. Hotamisligil, P. Peraldi, A. Budavari, R. Ellis, M. F. White, and B. M. Spiegelman, "IRS-1-mediated inhibition of insulin receptor tyrosine kinase activity in TNF-α- and obesity-induced insulin resistance," *Science*, vol. 271, no. 5249, pp. 665–668, 1996.

[12] K. T. Uysal, S. M. Wiesbrock, M. W. Marino, and G. S. Hotamisligil, "Protection from obesity-induced insulin resistance in mice lacking TNF-alpha function," *Nature*, vol. 389, no. 6651, pp. 610–614, 1997.

[13] M. Yuan, N. Konstantopoulos, J. Lee et al., "Reversal of obesity- and diet-induced insulin resistance with salicylates or targeted disruption of *Ikkβ*," *Science*, vol. 293, no. 5535, pp. 1673–1677, 2001.

[14] S. N. Vallerie, M. Furuhashi, R. Fucho, and G. S. Hotamisligil, "A predominant role for parenchymal c-Jun amino terminal kinase (JNK) in the regulation of systemic insulin sensitivity," *PLoS ONE*, vol. 3, no. 9, Article ID e3151, 2008.

[15] Y. Ding, J. Li, S. Liu et al., "DNA hypomethylation of inflammation-associated genes in adipose tissue of female mice after multigenerational high fat diet feeding," *International Journal of Obesity*, vol. 38, no. 2, pp. 198–204, 2014.

[16] R. Barrès, M. E. Osler, J. Yan et al., "Non-CpG methylation of the PGC-1α promoter through DNMT3B controls mitochondrial density," *Cell Metabolism*, vol. 10, no. 3, pp. 189–198, 2009.

[17] R. C. Painter, C. Osmond, P. Gluckman, M. Hanson, D. I. W. Phillips, and T. J. Roseboom, "Transgenerational effects of prenatal exposure to the Dutch famine on neonatal adiposity and health in later life," *BJOG: An International Journal of Obstetrics & Gynaecology*, vol. 115, no. 10, pp. 1243–1249, 2008.

[18] G. C. Burdge, J. Slater-Jefferies, C. Torrens, E. S. Phillips, M. A. Hanson, and K. A. Lillycrop, "Dietary protein restriction of pregnant rats in the F0 generation induces altered methylation of hepatic gene promoters in the adult male offspring in the F1 and F2 generations," *British Journal of Nutrition*, vol. 97, no. 3, pp. 435–439, 2007.

[19] J. H. Park, D. A. Stoffers, R. D. Nicholls, and R. A. Simmons, "Development of type 2 diabetes following intrauterine growth retardation in rats is associated with progressive epigenetic silencing of Pdx1," *The Journal of Clinical Investigation*, vol. 118, no. 6, pp. 2316–2324, 2008.

[20] Q. Fu, R. A. McKnight, C. W. Callaway, X. Yu, R. H. Lane, and A. V. Majnik, "Intrauterine growth restriction disrupts developmental epigenetics around distal growth hormone response elements on the rat hepatic IGF-1 gene," *The FASEB Journal*, vol. 29, no. 4, pp. 1176–1184, 2015.

[21] D. Goodspeed, M. D. Seferovic, W. Holland et al., "Essential nutrient supplementation prevents heritable metabolic disease in multigenerational intrauterine growth-restricted rats," *The FASEB Journal*, vol. 29, no. 3, pp. 807–819, 2015.

[22] X. D. Lou, H. D. Wang, S. J. Xia, S. Skog, and J. Sun, "Effects of resveratrol on the expression and DNA methylation of cytokine genes in diabetic rat aortas," *Archivum Immunologiae et Therapia Experimentalis*, vol. 62, pp. 329–340, 2014.

[23] K. F. Petersen, S. Dufour, D. Befroy, R. Garcia, and G. I. Shulman, "Impaired mitochondrial activity in the insulin-resistant offspring of patients with type 2 diabetes," *The New England Journal of Medicine*, vol. 350, no. 7, pp. 664–671, 2004.

[24] V. B. Ritov, E. V. Menshikova, J. He, R. E. Ferrell, B. H. Goodpaster, and D. E. Kelley, "Deficiency of subsarcolemmal mitochondria in obesity and type 2 diabetes," *Diabetes*, vol. 54, no. 1, pp. 8–14, 2005.

[25] J.-Y. Kim, R. C. Hickner, R. L. Cortright, G. L. Dohm, and J. A. Houmard, "Lipid oxidation is reduced in obese human skeletal muscle," *American Journal of Physiology—Endocrinology and Metabolism*, vol. 279, no. 5, pp. E1039–E1044, 2000.

13

High-Salt Intake Ameliorates Hyperglycemia and Insulin Resistance in WBN/Kob-*Lepr*$^{fa/fa}$ Rats: A New Model of Type 2 Diabetes Mellitus

Yoshiichi Takagi, Taichi Sugimoto, Masaya Kobayashi, Mitsuyuki Shirai, and Fumitoshi Asai

Laboratory of Veterinary Pharmacology, School of Veterinary Medicine, Azabu University, Kanagawa, Japan

Correspondence should be addressed to Fumitoshi Asai; asai@azabu-u.ac.jp

Academic Editor: Ed Randell

High-salt intake is a major risk factor for developing hypertension in type 2 diabetes mellitus, but its effects on glucose homeostasis are controversial. We previously found that high-salt intake induces severe hypertension in WBN/Kob diabetic fatty (WBKDF) rats. In the present study, we examined the effects of a high-salt intake on glucose homeostasis in WBKDF rats. Male WBKDF rats and age-matched Wistar rats at 6 weeks of age were each divided into two groups and fed either a normal-sodium (NS, 0.26%) diet or high-sodium (HS, 8%) diet for 7 weeks. Systolic blood pressure and urine volume were increased in WBKDF-HS and Wistar-HS. Body weight gain and food consumption were comparable between NS and HS in both strains. Plasma and urine glucose levels were significantly increased in WBKDF-NS but not in WBKDF-HS. HOMA-IR in WBKDF-HS was significantly lower compared with that in WBKDF-NS. The high plasma adiponectin level in WBKDF-NS compared with that in Wistar-NS was further enhanced in WBKDF-HS. Glycogen deposits and fat droplets in the livers of WBKDF-HS were reduced compared with those of WBKDF-NS. The present study demonstrated that HS intake ameliorated hyperglycemia and insulin resistance in WBKDF rats, which may be due to increased plasma levels of adiponectin.

1. Introduction

Metabolic syndrome is a clustering of several metabolic parameters, including hypertension, diabetes, dyslipidemia, and abdominal obesity. The incidence of metabolic syndrome is increasing rapidly in developed and developing countries [1]. Hypertension is one of the most challenging health problems leading to cardiovascular mortality and morbidity when associated with type 2 diabetes mellitus (T2DM), dyslipidemia, and obesity [2]. Dietary approaches for controlling high blood pressure have historically focused on sodium [3]. Thus, many guidelines recommend that patients with T2DM reduce their sodium intake. However, the connection between sodium intake and glucose homeostasis remains elusive.

Animal models are a useful substitute for humans in studies for both etiology and therapeutic interventions. The WBN/Kob-*Lepr*^{fa} diabetic and fatty (WBKDF), a new rat strain, was developed by introducing the *fa* allele of the leptin receptor from the Zucker fatty rat into the parental WBN/Kob rat genome [4]. Compared with the parental strains, WBKDF rats are characterized by earlier-onset diabetes, more severe pancreatic complications, and endogenous insulin resistance [5–8].

Our previous study demonstrated that WBKDF-HS rats developed salt-sensitive hypertension associated with vascular dysfunction and increased oxidative stress [9]. To further validate WBKDF rats as a metabolic syndrome model, in the present study, we examined the effects of high-salt intake on glucose homeostasis in WBKDF rats in comparison with age-matched Wistar rats.

2. Material and Methods

2.1. Animals. This study was conducted in compliance with the principles of laboratory animal care and was approved by the Committee on the Ethics of Animal Experiments of Azabu University (Sagamihara, Japan). Five-week-old male WBKDF rats and age-matched male Wistar rats were obtained from Japan SLC (Hamamatsu, Japan). Animals were caged alone to allow for individual measurements of food consumption. All rats were maintained under stringent environmental conditions that included strict adherence to temperature (21 ± 1°C), humidity (55 ± 5%), and lighting (illuminated from 07:00 to 19:00).

2.2. Research Protocol. WBKDF rats ($n = 16$) and Wistar rats ($n = 16$) at 6 weeks of age were allocated into one of 2 groups ($n = 8$ in each group) and given either the normal-sodium diet (NS, NaCl content 0.26%) or the high-sodium diet (HS, NaCl content 8%) for 7 weeks: Wistar rats on the NS (Wistar-NS); Wistar rats on the HSD (Wistar-HS); WBKDF rats on the NSD (WBKDF-NS); and WBKDF rats on the HSD (WBKDF-HS). Animals were fed food and tap water ad libitum.

Blood samples using heparin sodium (Mitsubishi Tanabe Pharma, Tokyo, Japan) as an anticoagulant were collected from the tail vein of nonfasted and conscious rats at 6, 10, and 13 weeks of age. Urine was collected for 24 h from rats at 6, 9, and 13 weeks of age, while the animals were kept individually in metabolic cages to measure the urine volume and the urine glucose concentration. Urinary samples were collected by placing the rats at 6, 9, and 13 weeks of age in metabolic cages with their respective diets and water for 24 h. After the urine volume had been measured, the glucose and sodium concentrations in the urine were calculated.

When the rats were 13 weeks old, we performed the intravenous glucose tolerance test (IVGTT), after which the rats were euthanized by exsanguination under anesthesia with pentobarbital sodium (60 mg/kg IP; Kyoritsu Seiyaku, Tokyo, Japan). At the end of the study, the pancreas, liver, mesenteric fat pad, and epididymal fat pad were removed and weighed.

2.3. Measurement of Physiological Parameters. The body weights of the rats and their food intakes were measured once weekly at 6–13 weeks of age between 10:00 and 14:00. Systolic blood pressure (SBP) and heart rate in the conscious nonfasted state were measured at 6, 8, 10, and 12 weeks of ages using a tail-cuff blood pressure analyzer (BP98A-L, Softron, Tokyo, Japan). The rats were prewarmed for 15–20 min at 32°C to improve the detection of pulsation of the tail artery. The arithmetic mean of three successive measurements was used for SBP.

2.4. Intravenous Glucose Tolerance Test (IVGTT). The IVGTT was conducted when the rats were 13 weeks old. After fasting for 18 h, the rats were anesthetized with pentobarbital sodium (50 to 60 mg/kg IP). Glucose (20% *w/v*; Otsuka Pharmaceutical, Tokyo, Japan) was injected into the femoral vein at a dose of 0.5 g/kg. Equivalent volumes (0.2 mL) of blood were sampled from the jugular vein at 0, 2, 5, 10, and 20 min. Heparinized sodium was used as an anticoagulant, and plasma was separated by centrifugation (2000 ×g for 15 min). The plasma levels of glucose and insulin were then analyzed. The area under the curves (AUCs) for plasma glucose and insulin, which represented the total glucose level and total insulin secretion during IVGTT, was calculated according to the trapezoidal rule.

Insulin resistance (IR) was assessed by the homeostasis model assessment of insulin resistance (HOMA-IR), and insulin secretion was evaluated with the β-cell function index of HOMA (HOMA-β), both of which were calculated using the fasting plasma glucose and insulin levels [10].

2.5. Measurement of Blood and Urine Biomarkers. Heparinized plasma was separated from the collected blood by centrifugation at 3000 ×g for 10 min. Plasma concentrations of alanine transaminase (ALT), aspartate aminotransferase (AST), total cholesterol (T-CHO), phospholipid (PL) and triglycerides (TG), and glucose in both the plasma and urine were measured using an automatic analyzer (JCA-BM 2250; JEOL Ltd., Tokyo, Japan). Plasma levels of insulin (Morinaga Institute of Biological Science Inc., Yokohama, Japan) and adiponectin (Otsuka Pharmaceutical Co. Ltd., Tokyo, Japan) were quantitated with ELISA kits.

2.6. Histopathological Examination. The excised pancreas and liver were immediately fixed in 10% phosphate-buffered paraformaldehyde, and the tissues were then paraffin embedded employing standard techniques and thin sectioned (3–5 μm). The sections of the pancreas were immunohistochemically examined for insulin (A0504, Dako Japan, Kyoto, Japan). The sections of the liver were stained with hematoxylin and eosin (HE), periodic acid-Schiff (PAS), and Oil Red O.

2.7. Statistical Analysis. Data are presented as means ± standard error of the mean (SEM). Significant differences between the mean values were tested by two-way ANOVA followed by post hoc Tukey tests. P values less than 0.05 were considered to indicate significance. The data were analyzed using Graph Pad Prism version 7.0. (GraphPad software, San Diego, CA, USA).

3. Results

3.1. Body Weights and Food Consumption. The body weights of WBKDF-NS rats were higher than those of Wistar-NS rats throughout the study (Figure 1(a)). There were no significant differences in body weight or body weight gain among the four groups at the end of the study (Figures 1(a) and 1(b)). At 6 weeks of age, the food intake by the WBKDF rats was two times higher than that by the Wistar rats (Figures 1(c) and 1(d)), confirming that WBKDF rats with the *fa* gene had hyperphagia. During food manipulation, both groups of WBKDF rats consumed more food and calories than Wistar rats (Figures 1(c) and 1(d)), but there was no significant difference between the NS and HS groups.

3.2. Organ Weight. Cardiometabolic parameters in rats from all four groups at the end of the experimental period are shown in Table 1. The weights of the epididymis and mesentery fat pads in WBKDF-NS were significantly higher than those in Wistar-NS. HS loading caused significant reduction

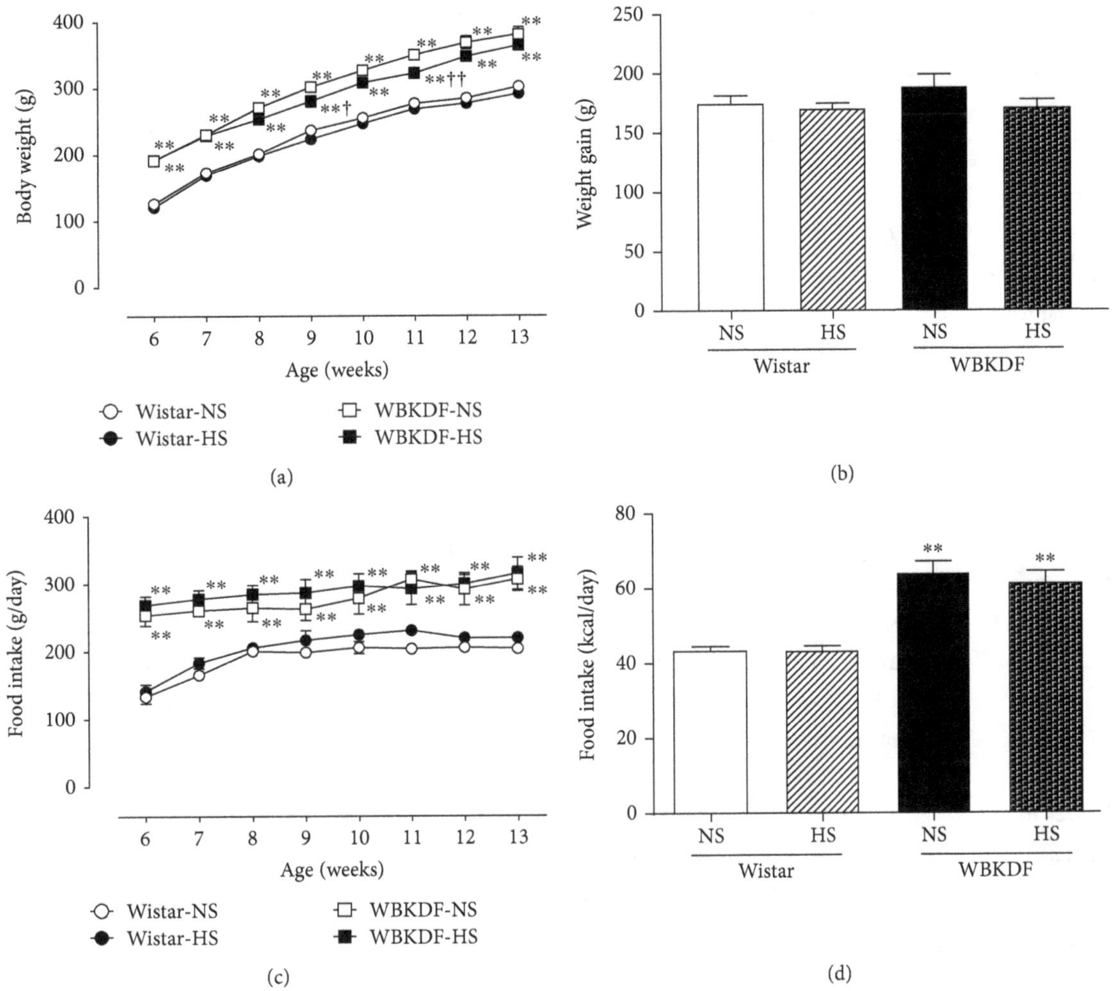

FIGURE 1: Effects of high-salt intake on body weight (a), food intake (g/day) (b), and food intake (kcal/day) (c) in WBKDF and Wistar rats. Data are expressed as mean ± SE ($n = 8$). $^{**}P < 0.01$ versus Wistar rats on the same diet; $^{\dagger}P < 0.05$ versus the same strain of rat on the NS diet; $^{\dagger\dagger}P < 0.01$ versus the same strain of rat on the NS diet.

in the weights of the epididymis ($P < 0.05$) and mesentery ($P < 0.01$) fat tissues in Wistar rats but not in WBKDF rats.

The liver weight in WBKDF-NS was significantly higher than that in Wistar rats. Inversely, the pancreas weight in WBKDF-NS was significantly lower compared with that in Wistar-NS. HS loading caused a significant reduction in the liver weight but not in the pancreas weight in WBKDF rats (Table 1).

3.3. Blood Pressure. Neither Wistar-NS nor WBKDF-NS exhibited significant changes in SBP throughout the experiment, and there were no significant differences in SBP between Wistar-NS and WBKDF-NS (Table 1). In contrast, both WBKDF-HS and Wistar-HS demonstrated significant elevation of SBP, which was more prominent ($P < 0.01$) in WBKDF-HS than in Wistar-HS (Table 1).

3.4. Blood Chemistry. WBKDF-NS rats had significantly higher levels of plasma ALT, TG, T-CHO, and PL compared with Wistar-NS rats. Plasma levels of ALT and AST in WBKDF-HS were significantly lower than those in WBKDF-NS, but there was no difference in plasma levels of TG, T-CHO, or PL between WBKDF-NS and WBKDF-HS (Table 1).

Plasma levels of adiponectin in WBKDF-NS rats were significantly higher than those in Wistar-NS rats at 13 weeks of age ($P < 0.01$). Both HS groups had higher plasma levels of adiponectin compared with NS groups, and only the differences in WBKDF rats were significant ($P < 0.01$, Table 1).

3.5. Nonfasting Plasma Levels of Glucose and Insulin. The nonfasting plasma glucose levels in the Wistar groups remained constant during the experimental period (data not shown). In contrast, WBKDF-NS rats developed hyperglycemia, and their plasma glucose levels at 13 weeks of age were significantly ($P < 0.01$) higher than those in Wistar rats. The HS diet inhibited the increase in plasma glucose level in WBKDF-NS rats (Table 1).

Nonfasting plasma insulin levels in WBKDF-NS rats were significantly higher than those in Wistar-NS rats at 13 weeks of age. However, there was no significant difference in plasma insulin between NS groups and HS groups of both strains (Table 1).

Table 1: Cardio-metabolic parameters in Wistar rats and WBKDF rats fed either the normal sodium (NS) diet or high sodium (HS) diet for 7 weeks.

	Wistar-NS ($N = 8$)	Wistar-HS ($N = 8$)	WBKDF-NS ($N = 8$)	WBKDF-HS ($N = 8$)	ANOVA (Strain)	ANOVA (Treatment)
Organ weight (% body weight)						
Liver weight	2.9 ± 0.1	2.9 ± 0.0	$3.8 \pm 0.1^{**}$	$3.2 \pm 0.1^{\dagger\dagger}$	$P < 0.0001$	$P = 0.0017$
Pancreas weight	0.4 ± 0.0	0.4 ± 0.0	$0.2 \pm 0.0^{**}$	$0.2 \pm 0.0^{**}$	$P < 0.0001$	$P = 0.3124$
Mesenteric fat weight	1.4 ± 0.1	$0.9 \pm 0.1^{\dagger\dagger}$	$2.2 \pm 0.1^{**}$	$1.9 \pm 0.0^{**}$	$P < 0.0001$	$P < 0.0001$
Epididynmal fat weight	1.6 ± 0.1	$1.2 \pm 0.1^{\dagger}$	$2.9 \pm 0.0^{**}$	$2.9 \pm 0.1^{**}$	$P < 0.0001$	$P = 0.0285$
Heart rate (bpm)	390.6 ± 13.3	395.8 ± 17.9	$326.4 \pm 5.1^{**}$	$346.3 \pm 9.6^{*}$	$P < 0.0001$	$P = 0.3203$
SBP (mmHg)	127.9 ± 2.2	$151.2 \pm 3.9^{\dagger}$	120.7 ± 4.1	$192.0 \pm 8.2^{**\dagger\dagger}$	$P = 0.0027$	$P < 0.0001$
Blood						
Glucose (mg/dL)	115.1 ± 3.5	115.0 ± 4.3	$344.8 \pm 44.2^{**}$	$127.0 \pm 8.8^{\dagger\dagger}$	$P < 0.0001$	$P < 0.0001$
Insulin (ng/dL)	2.4 ± 0.3	1.2 ± 0.2	$15.0 \pm 1.5^{**}$	$13.2 \pm 0.9^{**}$	$P < 0.0001$	$P = 0.2161$
AST (U/L)	67.4 ± 4.0	68.8 ± 7.6	74.6 ± 21.4	50.0 ± 2.7	$P = 0.6212$	$P = 0.3262$
ALT (U/L)	36.5 ± 2.7	32.1 ± 2.4	$109.6 \pm 24.3^{**}$	71.6 ± 8.6	$P = 0.0002$	$P = 0.1145$
T-CHO (mg/dL)	56.5 ± 2.6	47.5 ± 3.8	$95.9 \pm 5.7^{**}$	$106.6 \pm 10.6^{**}$	$P < 0.0001$	$P = 0.8960$
TG (mg/dL)	27.1 ± 4.5	26.8 ± 3.1	$304.4 \pm 34.7^{**}$	$315.8 \pm 36.4^{**}$	$P < 0.0001$	$P = 0.8279$
PL (mg/dL)	103.9 ± 2.4	92.9 ± 4.9	$206.0 \pm 7.8^{**}$	$237.6 \pm 13.7^{**}$	$P < 0.0001$	$P = 0.2272$
Adiponectin (ng/mL)	1432 ± 84	1716 ± 105	$2182 \pm 195^{**}$	$2687 \pm 65^{**\dagger}$	$P < 0.0001$	$P = 0.0033$
Urine						
Volume (mL/24 h)	6.3 ± 0.5	$85.1 \pm 1.5^{\dagger\dagger}$	$23.8 \pm 4.7^{*}$	$108.8 \pm 7.5^{**\dagger\dagger}$	$P < 0.0001$	$P < 0.0001$
Glucose (g/24 h)	0.2 ± 0.0	0.0 ± 0.0	$127.9 \pm 39.5^{**}$	$0.0 \pm 0.0^{\dagger\dagger}$	$P = 0.0031$	$P = 0.0031$

Data are expressed as mean ± SE ($n = 8$). Heart rate and SBP are for rats at 12 weeks of ages. Other parameters are for rats at 13 weeks. $^{*}P < 0.05$ versus Wistar rats on the same diet; $^{**}P < 0.01$ versus Wistar rats on the same diet; $^{\dagger}P < 0.05$ versus the same strain of rat on the NS diet; $^{\dagger\dagger}P < 0.01$ versus the same strain of rat on the NS diet. SBP: systolic blood pressure, AST: aspartate aminotransferase, ALT: alanine aminotransferase, T-CHO: total cholesterol, TG: triglyceride, PL: phospholipid.

3.6. Intravenous Glucose Tolerance Test (IVGTT). The IVGTT was performed on anesthetized WBKDF and Wistar rats at 13 weeks of age after 18 h fasting. There was no significant difference in the fasted plasma glucose levels before glucose loading among all groups of rats (Figure 2(a)). Significantly ($P < 0.01$) higher plasma glucose levels in WBKDF-NS rats compared with that in Wistar-NS were observed at 2, 5, 10, and 20 min after glucose loading. Compared with WBKDF-NS, WBKDF-HS exhibited lower plasma glucose levels after glucose loading, but the difference was not significant (Figure 2(a)).

No significant differences in fasted plasma insulin levels were observed among the four groups before glucose loading (Figure 2(b)). The plasma insulin levels in WBKDF-NS rats at 2, 5, and 10 min after glucose loading were significantly ($P < 0.01$, Figure 2(b)) lower than those in Wistar-NS rats. Plasma insulin was lower in HS groups when compared with the respective NS groups, but the difference was only significant for Wistar rats (Figure 2(b)).

The plasma glucose and insulin levels measured periodically during IVGTT were used to calculate AUCs as indexes of glucose intolerance and insulin secretion, respectively. The glucose AUC value for the WBKDF-NS group was significantly higher than that for the Wistar group ($P < 0.01$; Figure 2(c)). The glucose AUC value for WBKDF-HS was lower than that for WBKDF-NS ($P = 0.053$; Figure 2(c)). The insulin AUC value for WBKDF-NS was significantly lower than that for Wistar-NS ($P < 0.01$; Figure 2(d)). The insulin AUC values for the HS groups were lower than those for the NS groups, but only values for Wistar rats were significantly different ($P < 0.05$, Figure 2(d)).

HOMA-IR was significantly ($P < 0.05$) higher in WBKDF-NS compared with that in Wistar-NS (Figure 2(e)). HS had no significant effects on HOMA-IR in Wistar rats, but HS significantly ($P < 0.01$) reduced HOMA-IR in WBKDF rats (Figure 2(e)). In contrast, there were no significant differences in HOMA-β among the four groups (Figure 2(f)).

3.7. Urine Volume and Concentration of Glucose and Sodium. The urine volume in WBKDF-NS rats was significantly higher than that in Wistar-NS rats. Urine volumes in HS groups were significantly higher than those in NS groups in both strains at 6, 9, and 13 weeks of age, whereas the urine volume in WBKDF-HS rats was higher than that in Wistar-HS rats. High urinary glucose excretion was observed in WBKDF-NS rats but not in WBKDF-HS rats (Table 1).

3.8. Histopathological Examination of the Pancreas and Liver. Histopathology of the pancreas in WBKDF-NS rats at 13 weeks of age was characterized by loss of acinar cells, but this was not observed in Wistar-NS (Figures 3(a) and 3(b)). However, there were no morphological differences in the pancreas

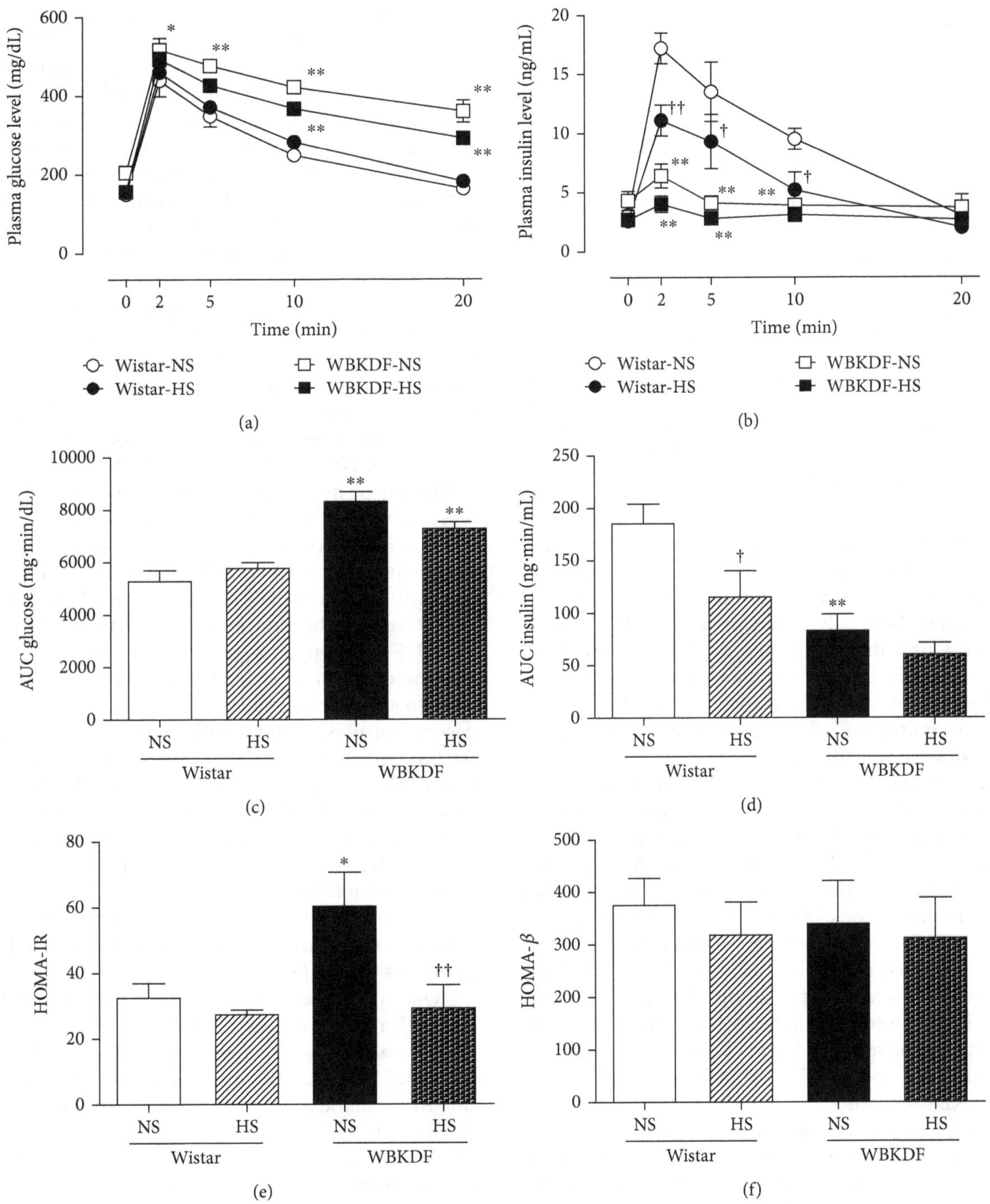

Figure 2: Effects of high-salt intake on plasma glucose concentration (a), plasma insulin concentration (b), AUC-glucose (c), AUC-insulin (d), and HOMA-IR (e) during the intravenous glucose tolerance test (IVGTT) in WBKDF and Wistar rats. Data are expressed as mean ± SE ($n = 8$). $^{*}P < 0.05$ versus Wistar rats on the same diet; $^{**}P < 0.01$ versus Wistar rats on the same diet; $^{\dagger}P < 0.05$ versus the same strain of rat on the NS diet; $^{\dagger\dagger}P < 0.01$ versus the same strain of rat on the NS diet.

between the NS group and HS group in both strains (Figures 3(c) and 3(d)).

The histopathological analysis on the liver is shown in Figure 4. There were no morphological differences in the livers between the NS group and HS group of Wistar rats. In contrast, WBKDF-NS rats had increased hepatic lipid deposits in the peripheral periportal zone compared with WBKDF-HS rats (Figures 4(a) and 4(b)). In addition, the livers of WBKDF-NS rats had less glycogen deposition than those of WBKDF-HS rats (Figure 4(c)).

4. Discussion

T2DM patients are more susceptible to hypertension because of their increased salt sensitivity compared with nondiabetic individuals [11, 12]. The studies on the influence of HS intake

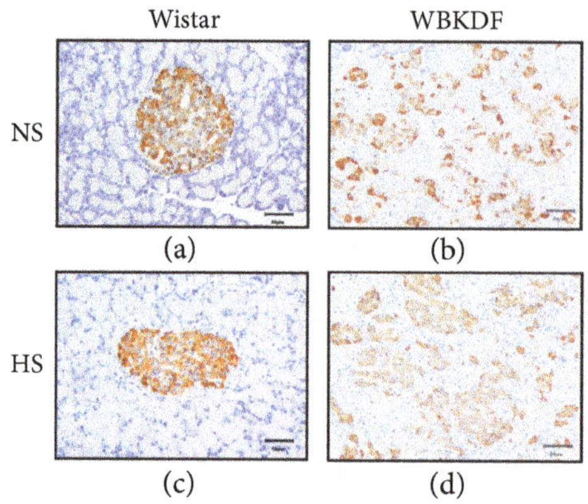

FIGURE 3: Histopathological examination of the pancreas in WBN/Kob-*Lepr*^{fa} (WBKDF) and Wistar rats fed normal-sodium (NS) or high-sodium (HS) diets. Representative immunostaining of insulin in (a) Wistar-NS, (b) WBKDF-NS, (c) Wistar-HS, and (d) WBKDF-HS. Scale bars = 50 μm.

have been limited to hypertensive patients and animals, and little is known about its influence on T2DM. The male WBKDF rat used in this study is a new metabolic syndrome model exhibiting obesity, dyslipidemia, and T2DM [4–6, 8]. Recently, we found that HS intake produces salt-sensitive hypertension in WBKDF rats, suggesting this strain as a useful animal model of metabolic syndrome [9]. This encouraged us to examine the effects of HS intake on T2DM model rats with salt sensitivity.

The main findings of this study are the following: (1) SBP and urine volume increased in WBKDF-HS and Wistar-HS. (2) Body weight gain and food consumption were comparable between NS and HS in both strains. (3) Plasma and urine glucose levels were significantly increased in WBKDF-NS, but not in WBKDF-HS rats. (4) The higher plasma adiponectin level in WBKDF-NS compared with that in Wistar-NS was further increased in WBKDF-HS rats. (5) Reduced glycogen deposits and accumulated fat droplets in the livers of WBKDF-NS rats were ameliorated in WBKDF-HS. (6) Impaired glucose tolerance and high HOMA-IR, a parameter of insulin resistance, observed in WBKDF-NS were ameliorated in WBKDF-HS rats.

According to our previous report [9], the HS diet containing 8% NaCl was demonstrated to be suitable for evaluating the long-term effects of HS in experimental animals [13]. As in the previous study [9], HS significantly increased SBP in WBKDF rats throughout the experiment. However, this salt-sensitive hypertension in WBKDF-HS was associated with the significant inhibition of hyperglycemia evident in WBKDF-NS rats. Although there are few studies examining the relationship between HS intake and hyperglycemia in T2DM model rats, our current data is consistent with reports on SDT-*Lepr*^{fa} rats fed HS diets exhibiting reduction in plasma glucose levels [14].

The WBKDF rat carries the fatty mutation (*fa*) in the leptin receptor gene, and homozygous animals (*fa*/*fa*) exhibit hyperphagia and obesity, in addition to insulin resistance and glucose intolerance [5–8]. Although nonfasting plasma glucose levels in WBKDF-NS rats were significantly higher than those in WBKDF-HS rats, there were no differences in fasting plasma glucose levels between WBKDF-HS and WBKDF-NS rats at 13 weeks of age. Early studies [15] demonstrated that food restriction delayed the development of hyperglycemia in WBKDF rats. These results suggest that hyperglycemia in the WBKDF rat is mainly due to hyperphagia [16]. However, our present and previous studies [9] found no significant differences in food consumption. Thus, inhibition of hyperglycemia by HS intake in WBKDF rats is unlikely due to reduced food and calorie intake.

The renal sodium-glucose cotransporter 2 (SGLT2) plays a crucial role in the regulation of renal glucose transport and sodium reabsorption [17]. SGLT2 inhibitors have been used to treat T2DM through inhibition of glucose reabsorption from the proximal renal tubule [18]. Thus, we examined the urine volume and the concentration of glucose. High urine glucose levels, a typical sign of diabetes, were observed in WBKDF-NS rats but not in WBKDF-HS rats. Thus, the inhibition of hyperglycemia by HS intake in WBKDF rats was due to a different mechanism than SGLT2 inhibition.

The GLP-1 receptor agonist was previously reported to inhibit hyperglycemia via its insulinotropic action in WBKDF rats [16]. In contrast, the normoglycemic WBKDF-HS group had lower insulin concentrations than the hyperglycemic WBKDF-NS group, but there were no significant differences in pancreatic β-cell injury between both groups. HS intake leads to a significant reduction in fasting plasma levels of glucose and insulin in human patients [19]. As the plasma insulin AUCs in the WBKDF-NS group was significantly lower than that in the Wistar-NS group, the reduced insulin secretory function in the WBKDF rats may be due to pancreatic β-cell dysfunction associated with chronic pancreatitis. Furthermore, both plasma insulin levels and HOMA-β were comparable between NS and HS groups in both strains of rats. Thus, the ameliorating effects of HS on hyperglycemia and glucose intolerance in WBKDF rats are unlikely due to the increase in plasma insulin levels.

Our previous and present studies have demonstrated that WBKDF rats have high HOMA-IR values, an indicator of insulin resistance, which are the hallmark of T2DM. Moreover, the IVGTT in the current study revealed that HS intake caused a marked improvement in insulin resistance in WBKDF rats. Obesity and insulin resistance are closely related with fatty liver [20]. Obesity-induced fat accumulation in adipose tissues and the liver, increased fatty acid synthesis in the liver and increased TG level in the plasma are associated with insulin resistance [20]. Indeed, the livers of WBKDF-NS rats had fat accumulation and reduced glycogen due to insulin resistance. The ameliorated histological hepatic changes observed in WBKDF-NS rats due to HS intake may be associated with insulin resistance in the liver. These results suggest that HS intake inhibited hyperglycemia by ameliorating insulin resistance in WBKDF rats.

In contrast to WBKDF rats, there was no obvious change in insulin sensitivity between Wistar-NS and Wistar-HS rats. The connection between sodium intake and insulin resistance has been debated [21]. Our finding on insulin resistance conflicts with the observation that the HS intake led to insulin resistance in rats [22–24]. The reason for this

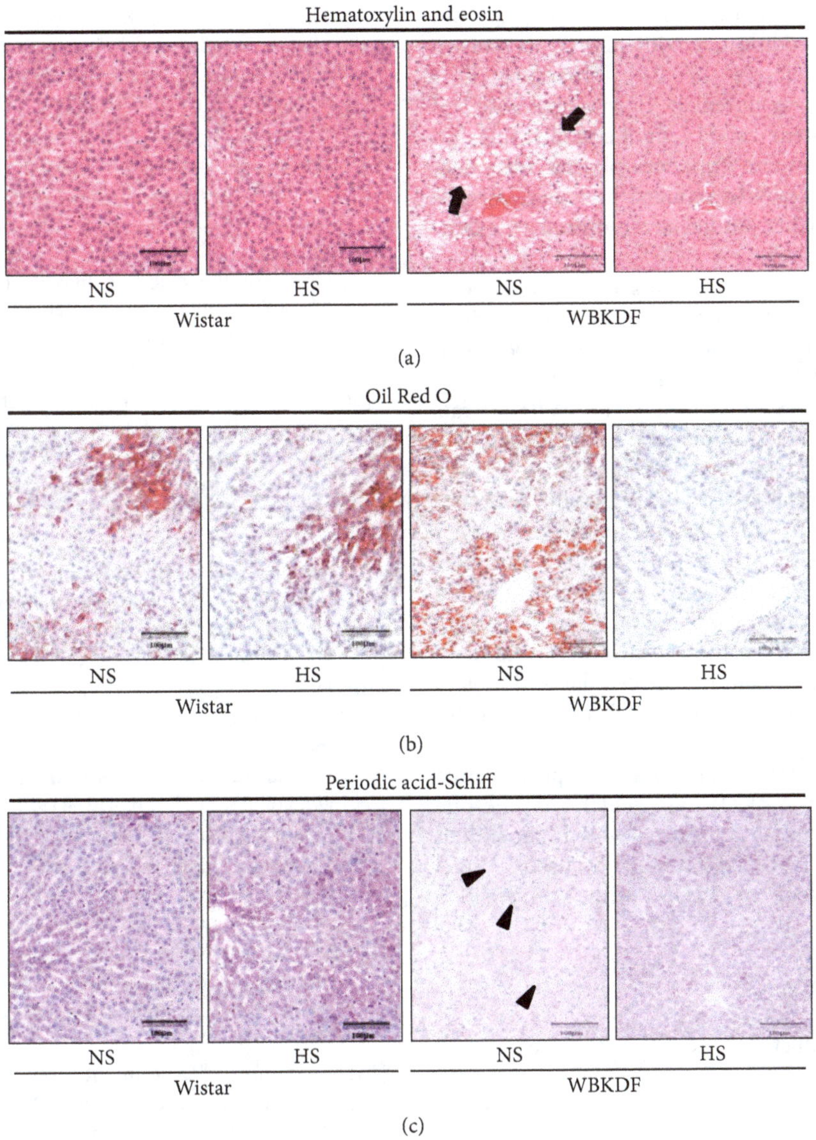

Figure 4: Histopathological examination of the liver in WBN/Kob-*Lepr*^{fa} (WBKDF) and Wistar rats fed normal-sodium (NS) or high-sodium (HS) diets. Representative immunostaining of (a) hematoxylin and eosin (HE), (b) Oil Red O, and (c) periodic acid-Schiff (PAS) in WBKDF and Wistar rats. Scale bars = 50 μm.

apparent discrepancy among the rat studies is unclear, but one possible explanation is that the differences in the rats, such as the rat strain, salt-sensitivity, and insulin-sensitivity, in addition to experimental conditions, including sodium concentration in the diet and duration of HS feeding, may be involved. Indeed, Sprague–Dawley rats, which were used in the aforementioned studies, are generally considered to be salt resistant [25].

The current study demonstrated that the HS diet increased plasma levels of adiponectin, one of the major adipocyte-secreted proteins [26], in WBKDF rats and Wistar rats. These results are in line with early studies reporting that a high-salt intake increased plasma adiponectin levels in normal human volunteers [27] and rodents [28, 29]. Previous studies clarifying and characterizing insulin-sensitizing activities, in vivo tissues, and underlying mechanisms suggested that the liver is a major target tissue of adiponectin, which exerts its insulin-sensitizing effects by binding to its receptors, leading to activation of the AMP-activated protein kinase and other unknown pathways [30]. Our results are consistent with early reports that treatment with recombinant adiponectin markedly alleviated hepatomegaly and fatty liver, as well as significantly attenuated elevated levels of serum ALT in nonalcoholic obese *ob*/*ob* mice [31], which spontaneously develop hyperinsulinemia, insulin resistance, and steatosis due to an inherited leptin deficiency [32]. Taken together, these results suggest that increased adiponectin by HS intake improved hyperglycemia and insulin resistance in WBKDF rats.

Our previous study demonstrated that WBKDF-HS rats developed renal damage and hypertension, which may have been associated with vascular dysfunction and increased oxidative stress [9]. Other groups have reported HS-induced renal tubular damage in spontaneously hypertensive rats [33] and increase in angiotensin II in the proximal tubular system via activation of the intrarenal renin-angiotensin system (RAS) [34]. In addition, angiotensin II is known to increase adiponectin levels [27, 28]. Therefore, it is probable that increased angiotensin II via activation of the intrarenal RAS system by HS intake contributes to salt-sensitive hypertension and enhances plasma adiponectin, which subsequently leads to reduced insulin resistance in WBKDF-HS rats. Further studies are required to examine this hypothesis.

The present study has several limitations. Firstly, disturbed regulation of adipokines, including resistin and visfatin, as well as adiponectin, is implicated in the development of insulin resistance and T2DM [35]. Thus, whether inhibition of hyperglycemia by HS intake observed in WBKDF rats was solely due to adiponectin remains to be elucidated. Secondly, plasma adiponectin levels in WBKDF-NS were higher than those in Wistar-NS rats. This result contrasts with the observation that reduction of adiponectin mainly contributes to T2DM development [26]. A possible explanation for the high adiponectin level in WBKDF-NS is a compensatory mechanism that counteracts high insulin resistance in WBKDF rats. Further studies are needed to clarify this possibility and to examine the cellular and molecular mechanisms that regulate plasma levels of adiponectin in high-salt conditions.

In conclusion, the HS intake ameliorated hyperglycemia and insulin resistance in WBKDF rats, which may be due to enhancement of plasma adiponectin levels independent of the increase in BP. The WBKDF rat may be a useful model for examining the etiology of T2DM with salt-sensitive hypertension.

Conflicts of Interest

The authors have no conflicts of interest to disclose.

Acknowledgments

This study was supported in part by a research project grant awarded by Azabu University. The authors wish to thank Dr. Katsuaki Ito for insightful discussions.

References

[1] K. T. Teng, C. Y. Chang, L. F. Chang, and K. Nesaretnam, "Modulation of obesity-induced inflammation by dietary fats: mechanisms and clinical evidence," *Nutrition Journal*, vol. 13, no. 1, article 12, 2014.

[2] J. Titze and F. C. Luft, "Speculations on salt and the genesis of arterial hypertension," *Kidney International*, vol. 91, no. 6, pp. 1324–1335, 2017.

[3] Z. S. Quader, M. E. Cogswell, J. Fang, S. M. Coleman King, and R. K. Merritt, "Changes in primary healthcare providers' attitudes and counseling behaviors related to dietary sodium reduction, DocStyles 2010 and 2015," *PLoS One*, vol. 12, no. 5, article e0177693, 2017.

[4] T. Akimoto, K. Nakama, Y. Katsuta et al., "Characterization of a novel congenic strain of diabetic fatty (WBN/Kob-*Lepr*^{fa}) rat," *Biochemical and Biophysical Research Communications*, vol. 366, no. 2, pp. 556–562, 2008.

[5] N. Kaji, A. Okuno, K. Ohno-Ichiki et al., "Plasma profiles of glucose, insulin and lipids in the male WBN/Kob-*Lepr*^{fa} rat, a new model of type 2 diabetes with obesity," *The Journal of Veterinary Medical Science*, vol. 74, no. 9, pp. 1185–1189, 2012.

[6] A. Okuno, N. Kaji, A. Takahashi et al., "Role of insulin resistance in the pathogenesis and development of type 2 diabetes in WBN/Kob-*Lepr*^{fa} rats," *The Journal of Veterinary Medical Science*, vol. 75, no. 12, pp. 1557–1561, 2013.

[7] D. Nagakubo, M. Shirai, Y. Nakamura et al., "Prophylactic effects of the glucagon-like Peptide-1 analog liraglutide on hyperglycemia in a rat model of type 2 diabetes mellitus associated with chronic pancreatitis and obesity," *Comparative Medicine*, vol. 64, no. 2, pp. 121–127, 2014.

[8] J. Namekawa, Y. Takagi, K. Wakabayashi et al., "Effects of high-fat diet and fructose-rich diet on obesity, dyslipidemia and hyperglycemia in the WBN/Kob-*Lepr*^{fa} rat, a new model of type 2 diabetes mellitus," *The Journal of Veterinary Medical Science*, vol. 79, no. 6, pp. 988–991, 2017.

[9] Y. Takagi, H. Kadowaki, I. Kobayashi et al., "Effects of high-sodium intake on systemic blood pressure and vascular responses in spontaneously diabetic WBN/Kob-*Lepr*$^{fa/fa}$ rats," *Clinical and Experimental Pharmacology and Physiology*, vol. 44, no. 2, pp. 305–312, 2017.

[10] D. R. Matthews, J. P. Hosker, A. S. Rudenski, B. A. Naylor, D. F. Treacher, and R. C. Turner, "Homeostasis model assessment: insulin resistance and β-cell function from fasting plasma glucose and insulin concentrations in man," *Diabetologia*, vol. 28, no. 7, pp. 412–419, 1985.

[11] J. A. O'Hare, J. B. Ferriss, D. Brady, B. Twomey, and D. J. O'Sullivan, "Exchangeable sodium and renin in hypertensive diabetic patients with and without nephropathy," *Hypertension*, vol. 7, no. 6, Part 2, pp. II43–II48, 1985.

[12] M. Imanishi, K. Yoshioka, M. Okumura et al., "Sodium sensitivity related to albuminuria appearing before hypertension in type 2 diabetic patients," *Diabetes Care*, vol. 24, no. 1, pp. 111–116, 2001.

[13] G. Simon, "Experimental evidence for blood pressure-independent vascular effects of high sodium diet," *American Journal of Hypertension*, vol. 16, no. 12, pp. 1074–1078, 2003.

[14] Y. Katsuda, Y. Kemmochi, M. Maki et al., "Physiological changes induced by salt intake in female Spontaneously Diabetic Torii-*Lepr*^{fa} (SDT fatty) rat, a novel obese type 2 diabetic model," *Animal Science Journal*, vol. 85, no. 5, pp. 588–594, 2014.

[15] T. Akimoto, M. Terada, A. Shimizu, N. Sawai, and H. Ozawa, "The influence of dietary restriction on the development of diabetes and pancreatitis in female WBN/Kob-fatty rats," *Experimental Animals*, vol. 59, no. 5, pp. 623–630, 2010.

[16] D. Nagakubo, M. Shirai, K. Wakabayashi, Y. Nakamura, N. Kaji, and F. Asai, "Therapeutic effects of liraglutide, a glucagon-like peptide-1 analog, in diabetic WBN/Kob-Lepr^{fa} rats with obesity and chronic pancreatitis," *Integrative Obesity and Diabetes*, vol. 2, no. 5, pp. 265–270, 2016.

[17] A. Mather and C. Pollock, "Glucose handling by the kidney," *Kidney International*, vol. 79, Supplement 120, pp. S1–S6, 2011.

[18] S. G. Chrysant, "Promising cardiovascular and blood pressure effects of the SGLT2 inhibitors: a new class of antidiabetic drugs," *Drugs Today*, vol. 53, no. 3, pp. 191–202, 2017.

[19] O. Melander, L. Groop, and U. L. Hulthén, "Effect of salt on insulin sensitivity differs according to gender and degree of salt sensitivity," *Hypertension*, vol. 35, no. 3, pp. 827–831, 2000.

[20] P. Dongiovanni and L. Valenti, "A nutrigenomic approach to non-alcoholic fatty liver disease," *The International Journal of Molecular Sciences*, vol. 18, no. 7, article 1534, 2017.

[21] J. J. DiNicolantonio, A. K. Niazi, R. Sadaf et al., "Dietary sodium restriction: take it with a grain of salt," *The American Journal of Medicine*, vol. 126, no. 11, pp. 951–955, 2013.

[22] D. S. Donovan, C. G. Solomon, E. W. Seely, G. H. Williams, and D. C. Simonson, "Effect of sodium intake on insulin sensitivity," *The American Journal of Physiology-Endocrinology and Metabolism*, vol. 264, no. 5, pp. E730–E734, 1993.

[23] T. Ogihara, T. Asano, K. Ando et al., "Insulin resistance with enhanced insulin signaling in high-salt diet–fed rats," *Diabetes*, vol. 50, no. 3, pp. 573–583, 2001.

[24] D. Premilovac, S. M. Richards, S. Rattigan, and M. A. Keske, "A vascular mechanism for high-sodium-induced insulin resistance in rats," *Diabetologia*, vol. 57, no. 12, pp. 2586–2595, 2014.

[25] R. D. Wainford and D. R. Kapusta, "Hypothalamic paraventricular nucleus Gαq subunit protein pathways mediate vasopressin dysregulation and fluid retention in salt-sensitive rats," *Endocrinology*, vol. 151, no. 11, pp. 5403–5414, 2010.

[26] A. E. Achari and S. K. Jain, "Adiponectin, a therapeutic target for obesity, diabetes, and endothelial dysfunction," *The International Journal of Molecular Sciences*, vol. 18, no. 6, article 1321, 2017.

[27] A. T. Lely, J. A. Krikken, S. J. Bakker et al., "Low dietary sodium and exogenous angiotensin II infusion decrease plasma adiponectin concentrations in healthy men," *The Journal of Clinical Endocrinology & Metabolism*, vol. 92, no. 5, pp. 1821–1826, 2007.

[28] Y. Kamari, N. Shimoni, F. Koren, E. Peleg, Y. Sharabi, and E. Grossman, "High-salt diet increases plasma adiponectin levels independent of blood pressure in hypertensive rats: the role of the renin–angiotensin–aldosterone system," *Journal of Hypertension*, vol. 28, no. 1, pp. 95–101, 2010.

[29] Y. Zhao, P. Gao, F. Sun et al., "Sodium intake regulates glucose homeostasis through the PPARδ/adiponectin-mediated SGLT2 pathway," *Cell Metabolism*, vol. 23, no. 4, pp. 699–711, 2016.

[30] H. Ruan and L. Q. Dong, "Adiponectin signaling and function in insulin target tissues," *Journal of Molecular and Cellular Biology*, vol. 8, no. 2, pp. 101–109, 2016.

[31] A. Xu, Y. Wang, H. Keshaw, L. Y. Xu, K. S. Lam, and G. J. Cooper, "The fat-derived hormone adiponectin alleviates alcoholic and nonalcoholic fatty liver diseases in mice," *The Journal of Clinical Investigation*, vol. 112, no. 1, pp. 91–100, 2003.

[32] L. A. Campfield, F. J. Smith, and P. Burn, "The OB protein (leptin) pathway - a link between adipose tissue mass and central neural networks," *Hormone and Metabolic Research*, vol. 28, no. 12, pp. 619–632, 1996.

[33] K. Hosohata, D. Yoshioka, A. Tanaka, H. Ando, and A. Fujimura, "Early urinary biomarkers for renal tubular damage in spontaneously hypertensive rats on a high salt intake," *Hypertension Research*, vol. 39, no. 1, pp. 19–26, 2016.

[34] K. A. Nath, "Tubulointerstitial changes as a major determinant in the progression of renal damage," *American Journal of Kidney Diseases*, vol. 20, no. 1, pp. 1–17, 1992.

[35] O. O. Elekofehinti, O. C. Ejelonu, J. P. Kamdem, O. B. Akinlosotu, and I. G. Adanlawo, "Saponins as adipokines modulator: a possible therapeutic intervention for type 2 diabetes," *The World Journal of Diabetes*, vol. 8, no. 7, pp. 337–345, 2017.

14

Effects of Type 2 Diabetic Serum on Proliferation and Osteogenic Differentiation of Mesenchymal Stem Cells

Xiangqun Deng,[1] Min Xu,[2] Moyu Shen,[2] and Jinluo Cheng[2]

[1]*Department of Endocrinology, Wuhan Third Hospital, Wuhan University, Wuhan 430062, China*
[2]*Department of Endocrinology, Changzhou No. 2 People's Hospital, Nanjing Medical University, Changzhou 213003, China*

Correspondence should be addressed to Xiangqun Deng; dengxiangqun@hotmail.com

Academic Editor: Paolo Fiorina

Diabetic patients have an increased risk of osteoporosis-associated fractures. However, the results of most studies of the effects of diabetes on bone mass in patients with type 2 diabetes (T_2DM) have been contradictory. To clarify these conflicting findings, we investigated the effects of diabetic serum on the proliferation and osteogenic differentiation of mesenchymal stem cells (MSCs). We used human sera from subjects with different levels of glycemic control to culture the MSCs and induce osteogenic differentiation. The rate of MSC proliferation differed when MSCs were cultured with sera from diabetic subjects with different levels of hyperglycemia. Hyperglycemic sera promoted MSC proliferation to some extent, but all the diabetic sera inhibited the differentiation of MSCs to osteoblasts. The effects of type 2 diabetic sera on the proliferation and osteogenic differentiation of MSCs are closely related to glycemic control. Our data demonstrate the importance of stratifying the study population according to glycemic control in clinical research into diabetic osteoporosis.

1. Introduction

Diabetes mellitus (DM) is a pandemic chronic metabolic disorder, with substantial morbidity and mortality, which is increasing in tandem with industrial development and an aging population. Growing evidence corroborates the notion that DM influences the skeletal metabolism, and patients with diabetes have an increased risk of osteoporosis-associated fractures. Many studies have demonstrated that patients with type 1 diabetes mellitus have reduced bone mineral density (BMD) and an increased risk of fracture [1–6]. However, although the relationship between type 2 diabetes mellitus (T_2DM) and osteoporosis has been widely investigated, it remains controversial. A systematic review that analyzed 47 studies from the United States, Japan, China, Europe, and Africa [7] showed that all the studies reported conflicting effects of T_2DM on bone mass. The majority of articles (26) showed increased BMD in T_2DM, whereas 13 articles reported reduced BMD, and eight articles reported normal or no difference in bone mass. Several authors have reported elevated BMD among patients with T_2DM in China [8], whereas other studies have reported reduced BMD [9–11]. These conflicting results regarding the influence of T_2DM on BMD are probably partly attributable to differences in the sex, age, ethnicity, glycemic control, and body mass indices of the study subjects, but the specific mechanisms at the cellular and molecular levels require clarification.

The balance of osteoblasts and osteoclasts is an important factor in maintaining a normal bone mass. A reduction in osteoblast activity or an increase in osteoclast activity can influence the deposition and resorption of bone, inducing osteoporosis. Mesenchymal stem cells (MSCs) from the bone marrow are multipotent cells that can differentiate into multiple cell lineages, including osteoblasts, adipocytes, fibroblasts, myoblasts, and chondrocytes [12, 13]. Therefore, the quantity of MSCs and the proportion of MSCs that differentiate into osteoblast cells directly control the production of osteoblasts and, therefore, influence bone formation. Many studies have suggested that the differentiation of MSCs into a specific cell type should simultaneously inhibit their differentiation into other cell types [14–17]. The thiazolidinediones, peroxisome proliferator-activated receptor gamma agonists that are generally used in the treatment of T_2DM, prevent osteoblast differentiation, thus increasing the differentiation of MSCs into adipocytes [18]. Consequently, an increase in the onset of osteoporosis is observed in diabetic patients treated with a thiazolidinedione, such as rosiglitazone. Osteoporosis is often accompanied by a histologically detectable increase in adipose tissue in the bone marrow, indicating the gradual replacement of the bone marrow by adipose tissue [19]. Therefore, a dysfunction in the proliferation and osteogenic differentiation of MSCs may be an important mechanism of osteoporosis in patients with T_2DM.

In this study, to clarify the conflicting results regarding the influence of T_2DM on BMD, we investigated the effects of T_2DM on the proliferation and osteogenic differentiation of MSCs.

2. Materials and Methods

2.1. Instruments and Biochemical Reagents. A BD FACSCanto™ II flow cytometer (Becton Dickinson, Franklin Lakes, NJ, USA) was used to identify MSCs. The TC10™ Automated Cell Counter, iMark™ Microplate Absorbance Reader, CFX96™ Real-Time PCR System, PowerPac™ Electrophoresis System, and Gel DOC™ XR+ Imaging System were from Bio-Rad Laboratories, Inc. (Carlsbad, CA, USA). Percoll® cell-separating solution, used for gradient centrifugation, was from Santa Cruz Biotechnology, Inc. (Dallas, TX, USA). Gibco® cell culture reagents, such as penicillin, streptomycin, trypsin–EDTA (0.25%) with phenol red, fetal bovine serum (FBS), phosphate-buffered saline (PBS), minimum essential medium α (α-MEM), and Dulbecco's modified Eagle's medium (DMEM), were purchased from Thermo Fisher Scientific Inc. (Carlsbad,CA, USA). TRIzol Reagent and dimethyl sulfoxide (DMSO) were purchased from Invitrogen (Carlsbad, CA, USA). The RNA primers were synthesized by Shanghai Sangon Biotechnology Company Ltd (Shanghai, China). The iScript™ cDNA Synthesis Kit and SsoFast™ EvaGreen® Supermix for Quantitative Real-Time PCR were from Bio-Rad Laboratories, Inc. 3-(4,5-Dimethylthiazol-2-yl)-2,5-diphenyltetrazolium bromide (MTT), L-ascorbic acid 2-phosphate, L-glutamine, dexamethasone, β-glycerophosphate, and Alizarin red were purchased from Sigma (St. Louis, MO, USA).

Fluorescein isothiocyanate- (FITC-) conjugated mouse anti-human STRO-1 IgM antibody and the isotype control, FITC-conjugated mouse anti-human IgM antibody, were from Santa Cruz Biotechnology, Inc. RabMAbs® rabbit monoclonal antibodies directed against human RUNX2, osteopontin (OPN), osteocalcin (OCN), and glyceraldehyde 3-phosphate dehydrogenase (GAPDH) and a horseradish peroxidase- (HRP-) conjugated goat polyclonal secondary antibody directed against rabbit IgG H&L were purchased from Abcam (Hong Kong) Ltd. (New Territories, Hong Kong, China). Prestained marker, an SDS–polyacrylamide gel preparation kit, RIPA lysis buffer for western blotting, a BCA protein assay kit, and an enhanced chemiluminescence kit were supplied by Beyotime Biotechnology Company (Jiangsu, China). Other biochemical reagents were purchased from Shanghai Sangon Biotechnology Company Ltd.

2.2. Isolation, Culture, and Identification of Bone Marrow-Derived MSCs. All the protocols involving serum and cells that originated from humans, used either for experimentation or maintenance, were approved by the Ethics Committee of Changzhou Second People's Hospital Affiliated to Nanjing Medical University, Nanjing, China, and were performed in accordance with the Laboratory Guidelines of China. All the subjects gave their written informed consent in accordance with the Declaration of Helsinki.

Bone marrow aspirates (3–5 mL) were collected in heparin from four healthy volunteers and washed twice with PBS. The bone marrow cells were suspended and mixed with 5 mL of α-MEM containing 10% FBS. Each cell suspension was then added to an equal volume of 1.073 g/mL Percoll cell-separating solution for gradient centrifugation. After the bone marrow mononuclear cells were separated, they were placed in a 25 cm^2 culture bottle and cultured (37°C, 5% CO_2, saturated humidity) in α-MEM supplemented with 10% FBS, 10,000 units/mL penicillin, 10,000 μg/mL streptomycin, and 0.2 mmol/L glutamine. The medium was changed every 3 days. The nonadherent cells were removed, and fresh general medium was added to allow further growth. After the adherent cells reached 80%–90% confluence, the culture medium was removed and the cells were washed three times with PBS. The adherent cells were detached with preheated 0.25% trypsin–EDTA and then subcultured in two new 75 cm^2 culture bottles at a concentration of 8×10^3 cells/cm^2. The subcultured amplified cells were collected in the third generation and frozen for storage in cell-freezing medium, which contained α-MEM, 10% FBS, 10,000 units/mL penicillin, 10,000 μg/mL streptomycin, and 10% DMSO. All the experiments were performed with cells from passage 4. The MSCs in the fourth generation were analyzed with flow cytometry for the expressions of the surface molecular marker STRO-1, as previously described [20].

2.3. Preparation of Human Blood Serum. To harvest the human blood sera, we collected blood samples from healthy and diabetic volunteers and classified them according to the level of glycosylated hemoglobin A1c (HbA1c), after each subject had given their written informed consent in accordance with the Declaration of Helsinki. The four human blood serum groups were divided according to HbA1c: <6.5%, 6.5%–8.0%, 8.0%–10%, and >10% HbA1c. 90 diabetic volunteers were enrolled in the study to supply their blood samples according to HbA1c level. Each subgroup included 30 diabetic volunteers, which their clinical parameters were matched for age, gender, and duration of T_2DM. All diabetic volunteers received insulin therapy, and some were combined with metformin and/or acarbose in recent one year (Table 1). To avoid the influences of medicine on osteogenic differentiation of MSCs, all diabetic volunteers who received thiazolidinedione (rosiglitazone or pioglitazone) therapy were excluded. In addition, the diabetic patients with osteoporotic fracture were not enrolled in the study. 30 healthy volunteers with normal glycometabolic parameters were matched for age and gender to supply their blood samples with HbA1c < 6.5%. They were not being administered any medication. After the blood samples were collected, the sera

Table 1: Clinical characteristics of diabetic volunteers.

Variable	HbA1c 6.5%–8.0%	HbA1c 8.0%–10%	HbA1c above 10%	*P* value
Number of diabetic patients	30	30	30	
Sex				0.87
Male	18 (60)	17 (57)	18 (60)	
Female	12 (40)	13 (43)	12 (40)	
Age (years)	48.2 ± 8	48.6 ± 9	48.4 ± 10	0.92
Duration of diabetes (years)	12.1 ± 5	12.6 ± 7	13.2 ± 5	0.68
Diabetes therapy				
Insulin alone	20 (67)	18 (60)	18 (60)	0.92
Insulin and metformin	2 (7)	2 (7)	2 (7)	>0.99
Insulin and acarbose	1 (3)	1 (3)	2 (7)	0.94
Insulin and metformin and acarbose	7 (23)	9 (30)	8 (26)	0.25

Data were presented as means ± SD or *n* (%).

were separated and mixed well according to HbA1c group. The serum mixtures were heated to 56°C in a water bath for about 30 min to inactivate the complement and then filter sterilized through a 0.22 μm membrane. Each treated serum sample was split into aliquots for cryopreservation at −20°C.

2.4. MTT Cell Proliferation Assay of MSCs. Exponentially growing MSCs from passage 4 were collected for an MTT assay. The MSCs were seeded in 96-well plates at 10^3 cells/well and cultured in 200 μL of α-MEM supplemented with different blood sera for 2, 4, 5, 6, or 7 days. The medium was changed every 3 days. The 96-well plates were removed from the incubator at different time points, and 20 μL of 0.5 mg/mL MTT solution was added to each well containing MSCs. The plate was centrifuged at low velocity for 5 min and incubated continuously for 4 h, and the medium removed. The plates were dried on paper towel, and 150 μL of DMSO was added to each well to dissolve the cellular staining products. The optical density at a wavelength of 490 nm (OD_{490}) was measured with a Bio-Rad iMark Microplate Absorbance Reader. The data derived from four healthy volunteers are shown as the mean ± SD of three independent wells. To determine the effects of T_2DM on the proliferation of MSCs, we used cell culture solution α-MEM supplemented with different blood sera: 10% FBS, 5% FBS + 5% human blood serum or 10% human blood serum.

2.5. Induced Osteogenic Differentiation of MSCs. To induce the osteogenic differentiation of MSCs, MSCs (5000 cells/well) were plated in six-well plates. The osteoblast differentiation medium was high-glucose DMEM supplemented with 10% FBS, 50 mg/L ascorbic acid, 100 nM dexamethasone, and 10 mM β-glycerophosphate. The cells were cultured for 3 weeks and then stained with Alizarin red to detect the calcium phosphate deposits. To clarify the effects of diabetic serum on the osteogenic differentiation of MSCs, human sera with different concentrations of HbA1c were used to replace FBS in the MSC culture medium.

2.6. Quantitative Real-Time PCR. Total RNA was extracted from the cultured MSCs with TRIzol Reagent (Invitrogen), according to the manufacturer's instructions. The first-strand cDNA was synthesized from 1 μg of total RNA in a 20 μL reaction mixture using the iScript cDNA synthesis kit and then used as the template for PCR. Quantitative real-time PCR was performed with the Bio-Rad CFX96 Real-Time PCR System, with SsoFast EvaGreen Supermix, according to the manufacturer's instructions. GAPDH was used as the internal control. The PCR primers used in this study are listed in Table 2. The relative expression levels of the osteogenesis-associated genes were quantified with the comparative Ct($2^{-\Delta\Delta Ct}$) method [21].

Table 2: Primer sequences and product lengths for real-time PCR.

Gene	Primer sequences	Product (bp)
GAPDH-F	CTCTGCTCCTCCTGTTCGACA	112
GAPDH-R	ACGACCAAATCCGTTGACTC	
RUNX2-F	CCGGAATGCCTCTGCTGTTATGA	238
RUNX2-R	ACTGAGGCGGTCAGAGAACAAACT	
OPN-F	ACAGCCACAAGCAGTCCAGATT	109
OPN-R	TGGAATTCACGGCTGACTTTG	
OCN-F	GACTGTGACGAGTTGGCTGA	119
OCN-R	CTGGAGAGGAGCAGAACTGG	

2.7. Western Blotting Analysis. After osteogenic differentiation was induced in MSCs cultured for 21 days, the expression of osteogenesis-associated proteins RUNX2, OPN, and OCN, was analyzed with Western blotting. RabMAbs rabbit monoclonal antibodies directed against human RUNX2, OPN, OCN, and GAPDH were used to detect the corresponding proteins. The Western blotting analysis was performed as described previously [22]. Briefly, the MSCs were lysed in cold RIPA lysis buffer, and the lysed cell solutions were centrifuged at 12,000 ×g for 20 min at 4°C. The protein concentrations in the supernatants were determined with a BCA protein assay kit. Equivalent amounts of proteins were then separated with sodium dodecyl sulfate–polyacrylamide gel electrophoresis in a 10% acrylamide resolving gel. The separated proteins were electrotransferred onto

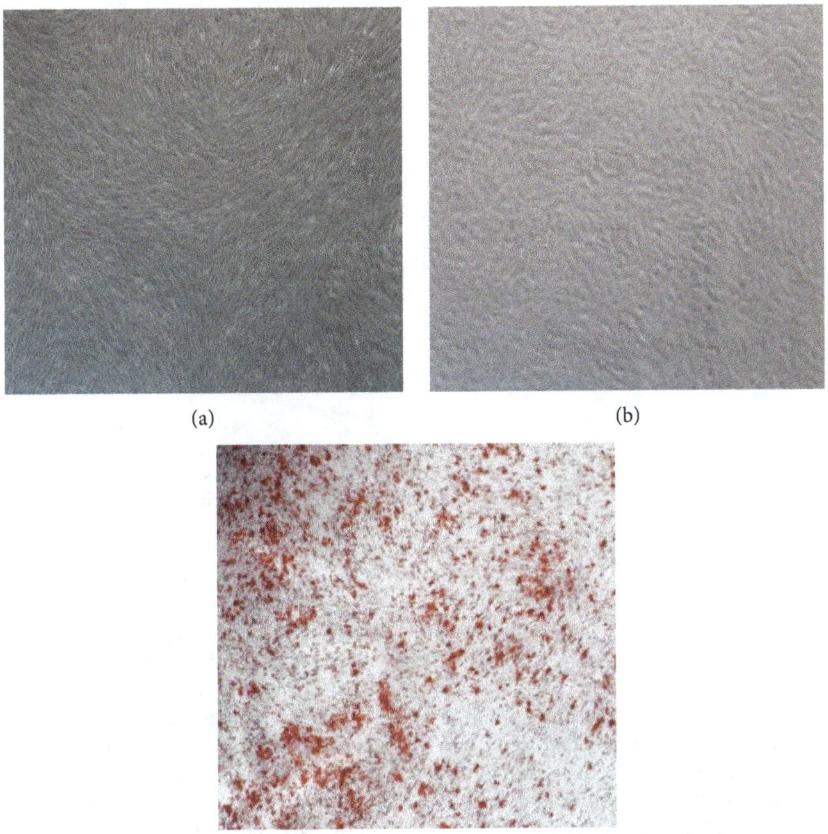

(a) (b) (c)

Figure 1: Morphology of primary and osteogenically differentiated MSCs (×40). (a) Primary cultured MSCs, slender, spindle-shaped, fibroblast-like cells with the typical spiral distribution. (b) MSCs after the induction of osteogenic differentiation; cells became round, with a cobble stone distribution. (c) After 21 days of osteogenic differentiation, large quantities of calcium nodules appeared in the MSCs. Alizarin red stained the calcium nodules scarlet.

polyvinylidene difluoride (PVDF) membrane, which were then blocked in TBS-T (1 × TBS, 0.1% Tween 20) containing 5% nonfat milk for 1 h at room temperature. The membrane was incubated at 4°C overnight with the RUNX2 antibody (1 : 1000), OPN antibody (1 : 1000), OCN antibody (1 : 1000), and GAPDH antibody (1 : 1000) as the internal reference. The PVDF membrane was then incubated with mouse anti-rabbit secondary antibody (1 : 20,000) for 2 h at room temperature and visualized with enhanced chemiluminescence reagent. After the membranes were exposed to Kodak film for 5–10 min, and the resulting images were quantitated with densitometry. The intensity of the bands was analyzed with the Image Lab™ software version 4.0 (Bio-Rad). The results were normalized to the density of the GAPDH bands.

2.8. Statistical Analysis. All the results were presented as me an ± SD and were analyzed with one-way ANOVA. The Student–Newman–Keuls multiple-range test was used to compare the results for two groups. $P < 0.05$ was considered statistically significant. To compare baseline and clinical characteristics of diabetic volunteers, we used Kruskal-Wallis tests for continuous variables and Fisher exact tests for discrete variables. All statistical analyses were performed with the SAS 8.1 software.

3. Results

3.1. MSC Morphology, Identification, and Osteogenic Differentiation. After the bone marrow mononuclear cells were separated from the bone marrow with gradient centrifugation, they were seeded in a 25 cm^2 culture flask. The primary MSCs had adhered to the culture flask wall 2 days after seeding. Several rounds of medium replacements and washing with PBS removed the nonadherent cells. The morphology of the adherent cells gradually changed, and they became slender, spindle-shaped, fibroblast-like cells from day 3 in culture. The cells proliferated rapidly and displayed clustering growth. The primary MSCs required culture for 2 weeks to reach 80%–90% confluence. However, the growth rate of the MSCs clearly increased after passaging, and the cells reached 100% confluence after only 1 week in culture. The typical spiral distribution of the MSCs is shown in Figure 1. The expression of STRO-1 is the best-known phenotypic characteristic of MSCs, and 99.6% of the cells tested positive for STRO-1. After osteogenic differentiation, the cell morphology of the MSCs changed markedly as they gradually became round, with a cobble stone distribution. Calcium nodules stained scarlet with Alizarin red, which are characteristic of osteogenic differentiation, were observed

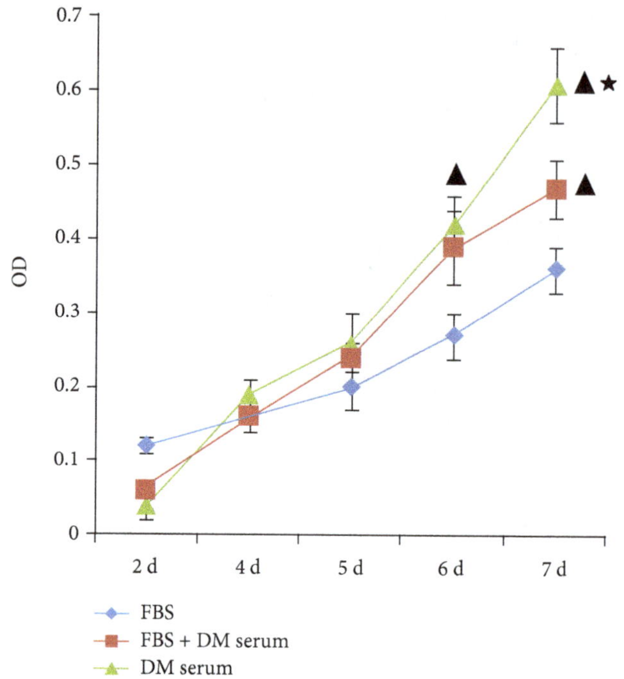

Figure 2: Proliferation of MSCs cultured with different amounts of serum, detected with an MTT assay. MCSs were divided into three groups: one group was cultured with 10% FBS; in one group, 10% FBS was replaced with 5% FBS + 5% diabetic serum; and in one group, 10% FBS was replaced with 10% diabetic serum. After 6 days in culture, the proliferation of the MSCs in the three groups differed significantly. All results were expressed as the mean ± SD and analyzed using one-way ANOVA. Student–Newman–Keuls multiple-range test was used to compare results between two groups: versus group FBS, $^{\blacktriangle}P < 0.01$; versus group FBS + DM serum, $^{\bigstar}P < 0.01$. $n = 4$.

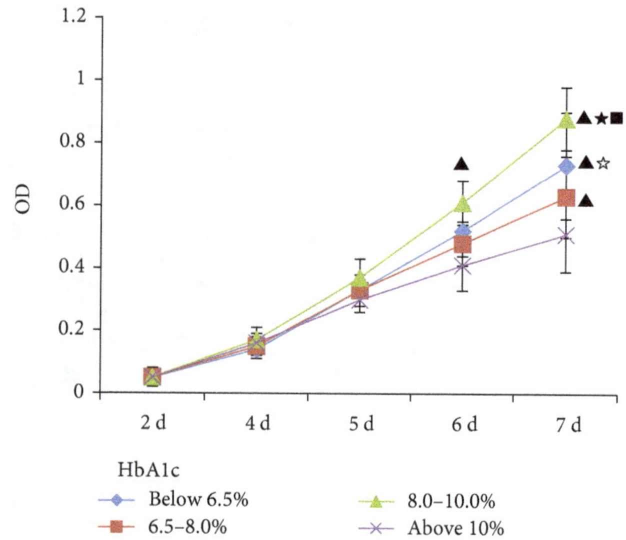

Figure 3: Proliferation of MSCs cultured with serum containing different levels of HbA1c, detected with an MTT assay. MCSs were divided into four groups, to which were added human blood sera with different levels of HbA1c: <6.5%, 6.5%–8.0%, 8.0%–10%, and >10%. After 6 days in culture, the proliferation of the MSCs differed significantly. Diabetic serum containing 8%–10% HbA1c stimulated cell proliferation most effectively. All results were expressed as the mean ± SD and analyzed using one-way ANOVA. Student–Newman–Keuls multiple-range test was used to compare results between two groups: versus group above 10%, $^{\blacktriangle}P < 0.01$; versus group 6.5–8.0%, $^{\bigstar}P < 0.01$, $^{\star}P < 0.05$; versus group below 6.5%, $^{\blacksquare}P < 0.01$. $n = 4$.

in the MSCs after osteogenic differentiation for 21 days (Figure 1). However, when we stained the cells with Alizarin red in different subgroups, we did not find the differences of staining images.

3.2. Effects of T_2DM Sera on MSC Proliferation, Detected with an MTT Assay. To analyze the proliferation of the MSCs, they were seeded in 96-well plates at 10^3 cells/well, the optimal density for the MTT assay. When cultured with FBS for about 7 days, the cells in the 96-well plates reached 100% confluence. The 10% FBS was then replaced partly or fully with T_2DM serum: either 5% FBS + 5% diabetic serum or 10% diabetic serum. Surprisingly, the diabetic serum significantly increased the proliferation of the MSCs (Figure 2). The diabetic sera were divided into different grades with different concentrations of HbA1c and then added to the culture medium for MSCs. Compared with FBS treatment alone, human serum (including normal and diabetic serum) clearly increased cell proliferation. The sera from diabetic patients in which HbA1c was 8%–10% stimulated cell proliferation more effectively than normal serum (<6.5% HbA1c). In contrast, serum from diabetic patients in which HbA1c was >10% stimulated cell proliferation less effectively than normal serum (<6.5% HbA1c) (Figure 3).

3.3. Effects of Diabetic Serum on mRNA Expression of Osteogenic Differentiation-Associated Genes. First, we induced the osteogenic differentiation of MSCs in FBS-supplemented culture medium. The mRNA expression of the osteogenic differentiation factors RUNX2, OPN, and OCN increased gradually as the culture time increased. When MSCs had been cultured for about 21 days, calcium nodules were observed and the mRNA expression of the osteogenic differentiation-associated genes had increased significantly, suggesting that the MSCs had differentiated into osteoblasts (Figure 4(a)). The serum used to induce osteogenic differentiation was then replaced with human serum. All the diabetic sera inhibited the mRNA expression of the osteogenic differentiation-associated genes relative to their expression in MSCs treated with normal human serum. Sera with higher concentrations HbA1c more effectively reduced the expression of these genes after the MSCs had been cultured for about 21 days (Figure 4(b)).

3.4. Expression of Osteogenic Differentiation-Associated Proteins. We investigated the expression of osteogenic differentiation-associated proteins when MSCs were cultured with human serum containing different levels of HbA1c to induce the osteogenic differentiation of MSCs. Protein expression was detected after 21 days in culture. Compared with normal serum (<6.5% HbA1c), the expression of proteins RUNX2, OPN, and OCN clearly decreased as the HbA1c concentration increased (Figure 5).

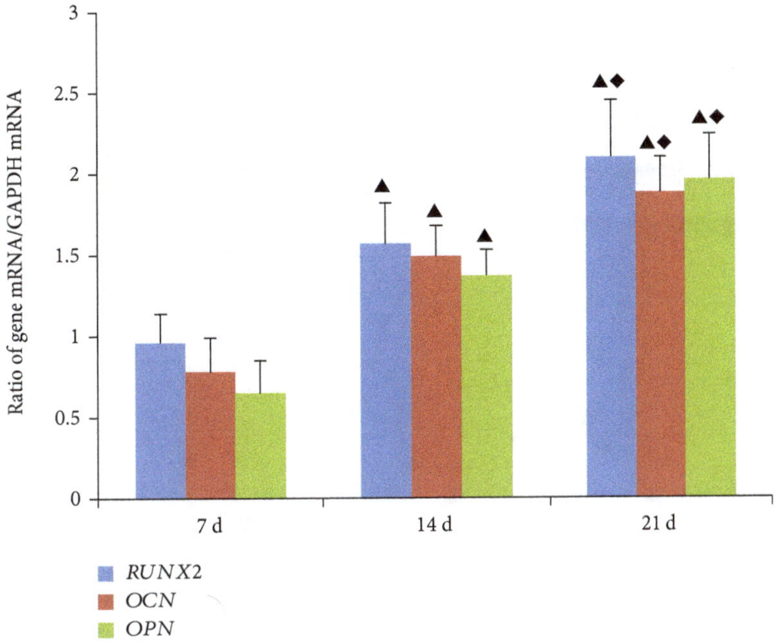

(a)

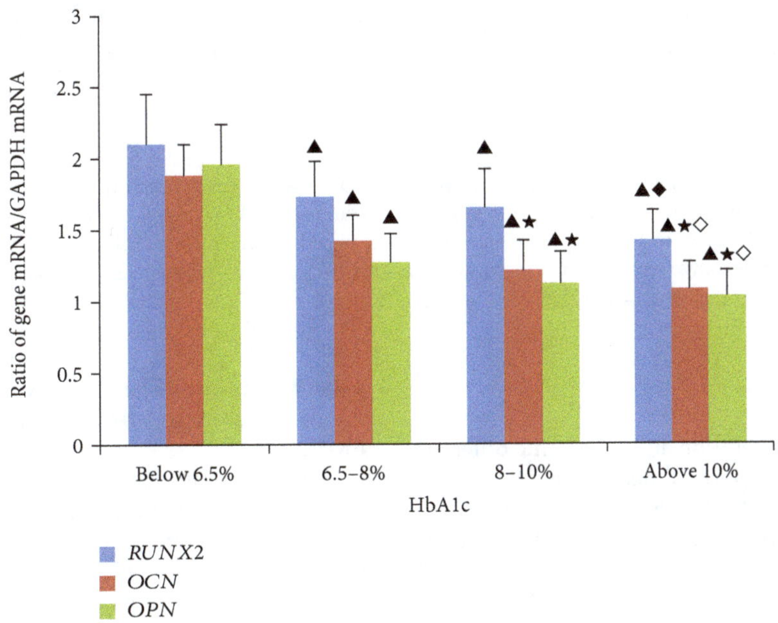

(b)

FIGURE 4: (a) mRNA expression of osteogenic differentiation-associated genes in different periods of culture, detected with quantitative real-time PCR. Osteogenic differentiation-related genes *RUNX2*, *OPN*, and *OCN* were detected after MSCs were cultured for different periods. mRNA expression increased gradually as the culture time increased. All results were expressed as the mean ± SD and analyzed using one-way ANOVA. Student–Newman–Keuls multiple-range test was used to compare results between two groups: versus culture 7 d, ▲$P < 0.01$; versus culture 14 d, ◆$P < 0.01$. $n = 4$. (b) mRNA expression of osteogenic differentiation-associated genes in MSCs cultured with human sera. Osteogenic differentiation of MSCs was induced by culture with human serum. Cells were cultured in sera containing different concentrations of HbA1c: <6.5%, 6.5%–8.0%, 8.0%–10%, or >10%. mRNA expression was detected when the MSCs had been cultured for about 21 days. Diabetic sera inhibited the expression of osteogenic differentiation-associated genes. All results were expressed as the mean ± SD and analyzed using one-way ANOVA. Student–Newman–Keuls multiple-range test was used to compare results between two groups: versus group below 6.5%, ▲$P < 0.01$; versus group 6.5–8%, ★$P < 0.01$; versus group 8–10%, ◆$P < 0.01$, ◇$P < 0.05$. $n = 4$.

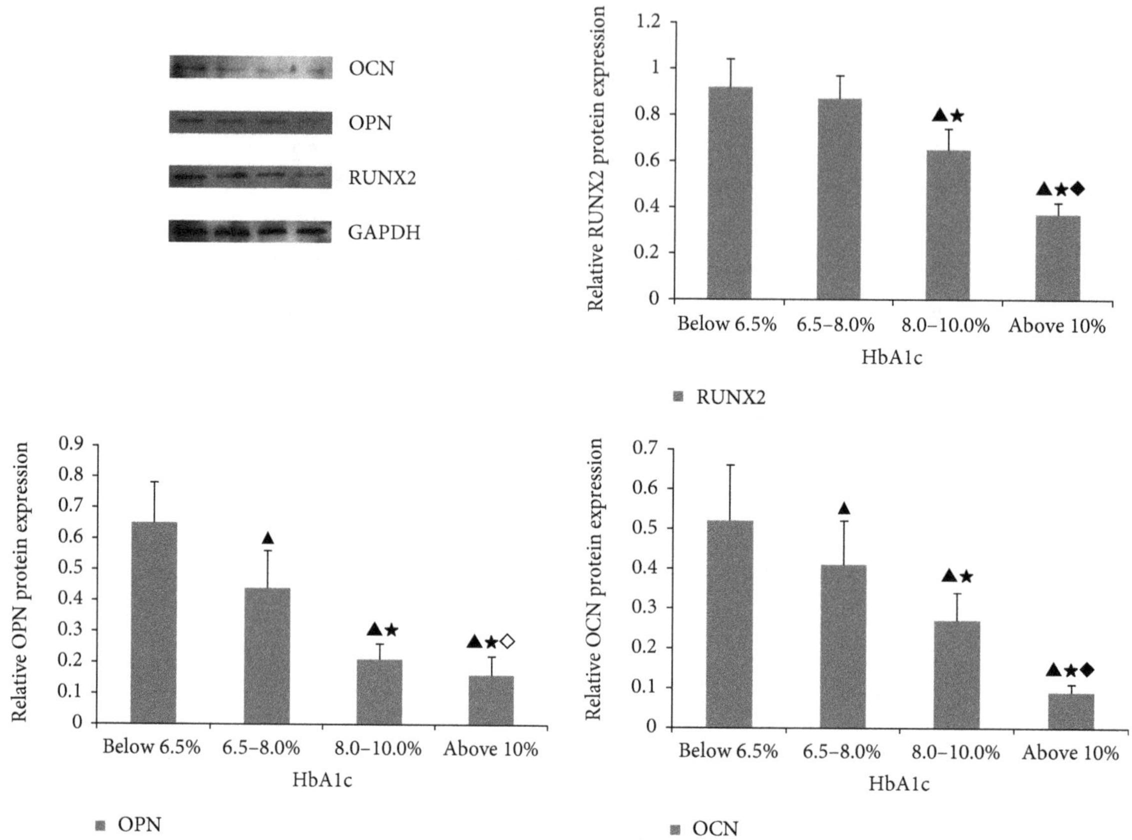

Figure 5: Expression of osteogenic differentiation-associated proteins. Osteogenic differentiation of MSCs was induced by culture with human serum. Human diabetic sera were divided into four groups according to HbA1c: <6.5%, 6.5%–8.0%, 8.0%–10%, and >10%. Protein expression was detected after 21 days in culture. All results were expressed as the mean ± SD and analyzed using one-way ANOVA. Student–Newman–Keuls multiple-range test was used to compare results between two groups: versus group below 6.5%, ▲$P < 0.01$; versus group 6.5–8.0%, ★$P < 0.01$; versus group 8.0–10%, ◆$P < 0.01$, ◊$P < 0.05$. $n = 4$.

4. Discussion

The dysfunction in the proliferation and osteogenic differentiation of MSCs may be an important mechanism of osteoporosis in patients with T_2DM. We used human sera from subjects with different levels of glycemic control to culture the MSCs and induce osteogenic differentiation. We found that the rate of MSC proliferation differed when MSCs were cultured with sera from diabetic subjects with different levels of hyperglycemia, but all the diabetic sera inhibited the differentiation of MSCs to osteoblasts. The effects of type 2 diabetic sera on the proliferation and osteogenic differentiation of MSCs are closely related to glycemic control.

At present, the development of osteoporosis is considered to be associated with factors such as endocrine levels, genes, nutrition, vitamins, and lifestyle [23–29]. However, the specific causes of osteoporosis are not yet completely understood. The diabetic population is a high-risk group for osteoporosis, but even in developed countries, there have been few systematic studies of diabetes-induced osteoporosis [30]. Among the many causes of osteoporosis, the suppression of MSC differentiation to osteoblasts may be the most basic and direct mechanism. Therefore, studying the proliferation and osteogenic differentiation of MSCs in diabetic patients may be an effective way to clarify at the cellular level the so far discrepant findings on the influence of T_2DM on BMD.

Several studies [31, 32] have suggested that FBS plays an important role in the culture of MSCs. The equal quantity MSCs can generate greater quantitative difference colony-forming units of fibroblasts (CFU-Fs) and different quantity cells in each CFU-Fs when different levels of FBS were used to culture the MSCs. In the present study, we examined the effects of human diabetic serum on MSC proliferation and osteogenic differentiation. First, we isolated MSCs from the bone marrow of healthy volunteers and grew them in primary culture. We then used diabetic sera to partly or completely replace FBS in the MSC culture medium. The diabetic serum stimulated MSC proliferation significantly more effectively than FBS. Because the diabetic serum we used was a mixture of sera from different T_2DM patients, it did not reflect the effects of diabetic sera from patients with different degrees of glycemic control. Because HbA1c is the gold standard for assessing glycemic control [33, 34], we mixed the human blood sera according to their HbA1c concentrations: <6.5%, 6.5%–8.0%, 8.0%–10%, or >10%. The MSC proliferation rate differed when the MSCs were cultured with human blood sera containing different levels of HbA1c.

The MSC proliferation rate in the 8%–10% HbA1c group was significantly higher that than in the normal control group (<6.5% HbA1c), whereas the MSC proliferation rate in the >10% HbA1c group was significantly reduced. These results suggest that a certain degree of hyperglycemia promotes MSC proliferation, whereas high HbA1c levels (>10%), which reflect poor glycemic control, significantly inhibit MSC proliferation.

The osteogenic differentiation of MSCs, which differs from their proliferation, displayed consistent results when cultured with different levels of HbA1c. During the induction of MSC differentiation to osteoblasts, all the diabetic sera inhibited the expression of osteogenic differentiation-associated genes at the mRNA and protein levels, suggesting that diabetic serum inhibits the differentiation of MSCs to osteoblasts. Furthermore, higher levels of HbA1c more effectively inhibited the osteogenic differentiation of the MSCs. This suggests that poor glycemic control has a large negative effect on the differentiation of MSCs to osteoblasts.

At the cellular level, the abnormal proliferation and osteogenic differentiation of MSCs induce osteoporosis, and osteoporosis is the combined effect of defects in the proliferation and osteogenic differentiation of MSCs [35, 36]. The present study may partly explain previous conflicting results regarding the influence of T_2DM on BMD. In diabetic patients, a moderate increase in hyperglycemia significantly promotes MSC proliferation, but slightly inhibits their differentiation to osteoblasts, and these combined effects on MSC proliferation and osteogenic differentiation may increase BMD. However, with poorly controlled hyperglycemia, when HbA1c exceeds 10%, for example, BMD is reduced because both the proliferation and osteogenic differentiation of MSCs are inhibited. Our results show that the BMD of patients with T_2DM is closely related to their long-term glycemic control and demonstrate the importance of stratifying study subjects according to their glycemic control in clinical investigations of diabetic osteoporosis.

However, we only investigated the effects of T_2DM sera on the proliferation and osteogenic differentiation of MSCs in this study. Diabetic serum is a very complex mixture, and the key factors in the serum that affect MSCs are not yet clear. Nevertheless, the use of human serum for in vitro assays used by D'Addio et al. [37] is still a valuable tool to test the effect of unknown circulating factors. Furthermore, diabetic T_2DM MSCs themselves may be abnormal in their capacities for proliferation and osteogenic differentiation. Therefore, further studies are required to clarify these issues.

5. Conclusions

This study demonstrates that a moderate increase in hyperglycemia promotes the proliferation of MSCs, whereas poorly controlled hyperglycemia inhibits them. Hyperglycemia also inhibits the osteogenic differentiation of MSCs and the extent of this inhibition is also closely related to glycemic control. Our findings demonstrate the importance of stratifying study subjects according to their glycemic control in clinical research into diabetic osteoporosis. This study partly clarifies the previous conflicting findings regarding the influence of T_2DM on BMD.

Conflicts of Interest

There is no conflict of interest to be reported for this manuscript.

Acknowledgments

This work was supported by a grant from the National Natural Science Foundation of China (81070694) and the Research Project of Wuhan Health and Family Planning Commission (WX16B10).

References

[1] J. Auwerx, J. Dequeker, R. Bouillon, P. Geusens, and J. Nijs, "Mineral metabolism and bone mass at peripheral and axial skeleton in diabetes mellitus," *Diabetes*, vol. 37, no. 1, pp. 8–12, 1988.

[2] P. Gunczler, R. Lanes, V. Paz-Martinez et al., "Decreased lumbar spine bone mass and low bone turnover in children and adolescents with insulin dependent diabetes mellitus followed longitudinally," *Journal of Pediatric Endocrinology & Metabolism*, vol. 11, no. 3, pp. 413–419, 1998.

[3] B. Lettgen, B. Hauffa, C. Möhlmann, C. Jeken, and C. Reiners, "Bone mineral density in children and adolescents with juvenile diabetes: selective measurement of bone mineral density of trabecular and cortical bone using peripheral quantitative computed tomography," *Hormone Research*, vol. 43, no. 5, pp. 173–175, 1995.

[4] M. Leon, L. Larrodera, G. Lledo, and F. Hawkins, "Study of bone loss in diabetes mellitus type 1," *Diabetes Research and Clinical Practice*, vol. 6, no. 3, pp. 237–242, 1989.

[5] T. Forst, A. Pfützner, P. Kann et al., "Peripheral osteopenia in adult patients with insulin-dependent diabetes mellitus," *Diabetic Medicine*, vol. 12, no. 10, pp. 874–879, 1995.

[6] L. D. Mastrandrea, J. Wactawski-Wende, R. P. Donahue, K. M. Hovey, A. Clark, and T. Quattrin, "Young women with type 1 diabetes have lower bone mineral density that persists over time," *Diabetes Care*, vol. 31, no. 9, pp. 1729–1735, 2008.

[7] S. A. Abdulameer, S. A. Sulaiman, M. A. Hassali, K. Subramaniam, and M. N. Sahib, "Osteoporosis and type 2 diabetes mellitus: what do we know, and what we can do?," *Patient Preference and Adherence*, vol. 6, pp. 435–448, 2012.

[8] P. F. Shan, X. P. Wu, H. Zhang et al., "Bone mineral density and its relationship with body mass index in postmenopausal women with type 2 diabetes mellitus in mainland China," *Journal of Bone and Mineral Metabolism*, vol. 27, no. 2, pp. 190–197, 2009.

[9] Y. Hsu, C. Chen, and F. Feng, "Major determinants of bone mineral density (BMD) at multiple skeletal sites in Chinese," *Journal of Bone and Mineral Research*, vol. 19, p. S421, 2004.

[10] L. Xu, M. Cheng, X. Liu, P. Shan, and H. Gao, "Bone mineral density and its related factors in elderly male Chinese patients with type 2 diabetes," *Archives of Medical Research*, vol. 38, no. 2, pp. 259–264, 2007.

[11] Y. Zhou, Y. Li, D. Zhang, J. Wang, and H. Yang, "Prevalence and predictors of osteopenia and osteoporosis in postmenopausal Chinese women with type 2 diabetes," *Diabetes*

Research and Clinical Practice, vol. 90, no. 3, pp. 261–269, 2010.

[12] K. A. Kilian, B. Bugarija, B. T. Lahn, and M. Mrksich, "Geometric cues for directing the differentiation of mesenchymal stem cells," *Proceedings of the National Academy of Sciences of the United States of America*, vol. 107, no. 11, pp. 4872–4877, 2010.

[13] M. Valtieri and A. Sorrentino, "The mesenchymal stromal cell contribution to homeostasis," *Journal of Cellular Physiology*, vol. 217, no. 2, pp. 296–300, 2008.

[14] M. L. Knothe Tate, T. D. Falls, S. H. McBride, R. Atit, and U. R. Knothe, "Mechanical modulation of osteochondroprogenitor cell fate," *The International Journal of Biochemistry & Cell Biology*, vol. 40, no. 12, pp. 2720–2738, 2008.

[15] T. J. Heino and T. A. Hentunen, "Differentiation of osteblasts and osteocytes from mesenchymal stem cells," *Current Stem Cell Research & Therapy*, vol. 3, no. 2, pp. 131–145, 2008.

[16] L. Zhao and B. M. Hantash, "Chapter seven—TGF-β1 regulates differentiation of bone marrow mesenchymal stem cells," *Vitamins & Hormones*, vol. 87, pp. 127–141, 2011.

[17] J. Li, N. Zhang, X. Huang et al., "Dexamethasone shifts bone marrow stromal cells from osteoblasts to adipocytes by C/EBPalpha promoter methylation," *Cell Death & Disease*, vol. 4, no. 10, article e832, 2013.

[18] M. J. Jeon, J. A. Kim, S. H. Kwon et al., "Activation of peroxisome proliferator-activated receptor-gamma inhibits the Runx2-mediated transcription of osteocalcin in osteoblasts," *Journal of Biological Chemistry*, vol. 278, no. 26, pp. 23270–23277, 2003.

[19] M. Kawai, F. J. A. de Paula, and C. J. Rosen, "New insights into osteoporosis: the bone–fat connection," *Journal of Internal Medicine*, vol. 272, no. 4, pp. 317–329, 2012.

[20] Y. Shen, W. Wang, X. Li, Z. Liu, D. C. Markel, and W. Ren, "Impacts of age and gender on bone marrow profiles of BMP7, BMPRs and Stro-1^+ cells in patients with total hip replacement," *International Orthopaedics*, vol. 36, no. 4, pp. 879–886, 2012.

[21] M. W. Pfaffl, "A new mathematical model for relative quantification in real-time RT–PCR," *Nucleic Acids Research*, vol. 29, no. 9, article e45, 2001.

[22] J. G. Mabley, V. Belin, N. John, and I. C. Green, "Insulin-like growth factor I reverses interleukin-1β inhibition of insulin secretion, induction of nitric oxide synthase and cytokine-mediated apoptosis in rat islets of Langerhans," *FEBS Letters*, vol. 417, no. 2, pp. 235–238, 1997.

[23] L. G. Raisz, "Pathogenesis of osteoporosis: concepts, conflicts, and prospects," *The Journal of Clinical Investigation*, vol. 115, no. 12, pp. 3318–3325, 2005.

[24] N. O. Kuchuk, N. M. van Schoor, S. M. Pluijm, J. H. Smit, W. de Ronde, and P. Lips, "The association of sex hormone levels with quantitative ultrasound, bone mineral density, bone turnover and osteoporotic fractures in older men and women," *Clinical Endocrinology*, vol. 67, no. 2, pp. 295–303, 2007.

[25] W. F. Li, S. X. Hou, B. Yu, M. M. Li, C. Férec, and J. M. Chen, "Genetics of osteoporosis: accelerating pace in gene identification and validation," *Human Genetics*, vol. 127, no. 3, pp. 249–285, 2010.

[26] S. Ferrari, "Human genetics of osteoporosis," *Best Practice & Research Clinical Endocrinology & Metabolism*, vol. 22, no. 5, pp. 723–735, 2008.

[27] P. G. Masse, J. L. Jougleux, C. Tranchant, J. Dosy, M. Caissie, and S. P. Coburn, "Enhancement of calcium/vitamin d supplement efficacy by administering concomitantly three key nutrients essential to bone collagen matrix for the treatment of osteopenia in middle-aged women: a one-year follow-up," *Journal of Clinical Biochemistry and Nutrition*, vol. 46, no. 1, pp. 20–29, 2010.

[28] K. L. Tucker, "Osteoporosis prevention and nutrition," *Current Osteoporosis Reports*, vol. 7, no. 4, pp. 111–117, 2009.

[29] N. S. Ali, C. Shonk, and M. S. El-Sayed, "Bone health in men: influencing factors," *American Journal of Health Behavior*, vol. 33, no. 2, pp. 213–222, 2009.

[30] D. L. Chau, S. V. Edelman, and M. Chandran, "Osteoporosis and diabetes," *Current Diabetes Reports*, vol. 3, no. 1, pp. 37–42, 2003.

[31] D. P. Lennon, S. E. Haynesworth, S. P. Bruder, N. Jaiswal, and A. I. Caplan, "Human and animal mesenchymal progenitor cells from bone marrow: identification of serum for optimal selection and proliferation," *In Vitro Cellular & Developmental Biology - Animal*, vol. 32, no. 10, pp. 602–611, 1996.

[32] S. A. Kuznetsov, M. H. Mankani, P. Bianco, and P. G. Robey, "Enumeration of the colony-forming units–fibroblast from mouse and human bone marrow in normal and pathological conditions," *Stem Cell Research*, vol. 2, no. 1, pp. 83–94, 2009.

[33] D. B. Sacks, "Measurement of hemoglobin A_{1c}: a new twist on the path to harmony," *Diabetes Care*, vol. 35, no. 12, pp. 2674–2680, 2012.

[34] S. I. Sherwani, H. A. Khan, A. Ekhzaimy, A. Masood, and M. K. Sakharkar, "Significance of HbA1c test in diagnosis and prognosis of diabetic patients," *Biomarker Insights*, vol. 11, no. 11, pp. 95–104, 2016.

[35] Y. K. Luu, E. Capilla, C. J. Rosen et al., "Mechanical stimulation of mesenchymal stem cell proliferation and differentiation promotes osteogenesis while preventing dietary-induced obesity," *Journal of Bone and Mineral Research*, vol. 24, no. 1, pp. 50–61, 2009.

[36] N. Sun, L. Yang, Y. Li et al., "Effect of advanced oxidation protein products on the proliferation and osteogenic differentiation of rat mesenchymal stem cells," *International Journal of Molecular Medicine*, vol. 32, no. 2, pp. 485–491, 2013.

[37] F. D'Addio, S. La Rosa, A. Maestroni et al., "Circulating IGF-I and IGFBP3 levels control human colonic stem cell function and are disrupted in diabetic enteropathy," *Cell Stem Cell*, vol. 17, no. 4, pp. 486–498, 2015.

15

L-Carnitine: An Antioxidant Remedy for the Survival of Cardiomyocytes under Hyperglycemic Condition

Fernanda Vacante,[1] Pamela Senesi,[1] Anna Montesano,[2] Alice Frigerio,[1] Livio Luzi,[1,2] and Ileana Terruzzi[2]

[1]*Metabolism Research Center, IRCCS Policlinico San Donato, San Donato Milanese, Milan, Italy*
[2]*Department of Biomedical Sciences for Health, Università degli Studi di Milano, Milan, Italy*

Correspondence should be addressed to Ileana Terruzzi; terruzzi.ileana@hsr.it

Guest Editor: Gaetano Santulli

Background. Metabolic alterations as hyperglycemia and inflammation induce myocardial molecular events enhancing oxidative stress and mitochondrial dysfunction. Those alterations are responsible for a progressive loss of cardiomyocytes, cardiac stem cells, and consequent cardiovascular complications. Currently, there are no effective pharmacological measures to protect the heart from these metabolic modifications, and the development of new therapeutic approaches, focused on improvement of the oxidative stress condition, is pivotal. The protective effects of levocarnitine (LC) in patients with ischemic heart disease are related to the attenuation of oxidative stress, but LC mechanisms have yet to be fully understood. *Objective.* The aim of this work was to investigate LC's role in oxidative stress condition, on ROS production and mitochondrial detoxifying function in H9c2 rat cardiomyocytes during hyperglycemia. *Methods.* H9c2 cells in the hyperglycemic state (25 mmol/L glucose) were exposed to 0.5 or 5 mM LC for 48 and 72 h: LC effects on signaling pathways involved in oxidative stress condition were studied by Western blot and immunofluorescence analysis. To evaluate ROS production, H9c2 cells were exposed to H_2O_2 after LC pretreatment. *Results.* Our *in vitro* study indicates how LC supplementation might protect cardiomyocytes from oxidative stress-related damage, preventing ROS formation and activating antioxidant signaling pathways in hyperglycemic conditions. In particular, LC promotes STAT3 activation and significantly increases the expression of antioxidant protein SOD2. Hyperglycemic cardiac cells are characterized by impairment in mitochondrial dysfunction and the CaMKII signal: LC promotes CaMKII expression and activation and enhancement of AMPK protein synthesis. Our results suggest that LC might ameliorate metabolic aspects of hyperglycemic cardiac cells. Finally, LC doses herein used did not modify H9c2 growth rate and viability. *Conclusions.* Our novel study demonstrates that LC improves the microenvironment damaged by oxidative stress (induced by hyperglycemia), thus proposing this nutraceutical compound as an adjuvant in diabetic cardiac regenerative medicine.

1. Introduction

Cardiovascular complications are recognized as the primary cause of mortality in subjects with diabetes mellitus (DM) [1, 2], characterized by hyperglycemia which is determined by a defect of insulin secretion, insulin action, or both [3]. Moreover, DM is associated with inflammation condition.

Chronic hyperglycemia, characterizing overt diabetes, or fluctuant hyperglycemia, present in the prediabetic condition, are responsible for the activation of numerous signaling pathways that exacerbate the systemic inflammation and lead to the development of diabetic complications [4, 5]. Recent evidence establishes how hyperglycemia is involved in the regulation of sirtuin (SIRT) transcription factors. The deregulation of SIRT expression is strictly correlated with the progression of inflammation and atherosclerotic disease. In particular, Balestrieri et al. demonstrated that SIRT6 protein expression is downregulated in atherosclerotic plaques of diabetics, and this defect is linked to the chronic oxidative stress condition [6]. Those evidences indicate that chronic inflammation, oxidative stress condition and predisposition to ischemic heart disease are higher in patients with DM than in nondiabetics [7, 8].

Traditional therapeutic approaches as well as innovative promising strategies [7] (i.e., stem/progenitor cell therapy, existing cardiomyocyte proliferation, and reprogramming noncardiac cells) are limited in patients with DM [8–11]. Periprocedural intensive glycemic control, during early percutaneous coronary intervention in diabetic patients, was shown to improve myocardial protection by increasing SIRT1 expression, endothelial progenitor cell number, and their capability to differentiate in mature cardiomyocytes [12]. Hyperglycemia in diabetic subjects is the major factor responsible for the failure of regenerative myocardial therapeutic strategies. Recent data indicate that the overproduction of reactive oxygen species (ROS) and the oxidative stress condition are the main causes involved in diabetic cardiac injury and in the lack of success in cardiac regenerative therapies [13–17]. Hyperglycemia enhances ROS production impairing cardiac microenvironment and regeneration capacity [16, 17]. In particular, several publications showed that the hyperglycemic and oxidative microenvironment induces mitochondrial abnormalities and cellular damage, eventually leading to senescence and apoptosis of cardiac progenitors [18, 19].

Thus, to optimize regenerative strategies for diabetic patients, the development of new therapeutic approaches focused on the reduction of oxidative stress condition is fundamental.

Noteworthy, in recent years, L-carnitine (LC) has been proposed as a nutraceutical integrator in the treatment of numerous cardiac syndromes, including coronary disease, atherosclerosis, and toxic myocardial injury [20–22]. It is well established that LC, facilitating transport of long-chain fatty acids into the mitochondrial matrix, plays an important role in supporting cardiac energy homeostasis [23–25]. Most importantly, some studies successfully showed LC's ability to reduce oxidative stress, hypoxic cellular damage, and apoptosis of cardiac cells in normal glycemic condition [26, 27]. In particular, Mao et al. have recently demonstrated that LC pretreatment ameliorated cellular damage induced by H_2O_2 in H9c2 rat cardiomyocytes, enhancing mitochondrial function [28].

LC effects on cardiac metabolism and function have been demonstrated under a variety of clinical conditions [29, 30], while LC antioxidative effects in hyperglycemic cardiomyocites were not investigated, yet.

The aim of this study is to investigate *in vitro* LC ability to counteract oxidative stress condition, modifying ROS production and promoting mitochondrial detoxifying function in H9c2 rat cardiomyocytes under hyperglycemic condition (25 mmol/L glucose). The goal is to identify in LC a novel adjuvant agent in cell therapy able to ameliorate the microenvironment of the hyperglycemic heart, thereby supporting cardiac progenitor cell proliferation and differentiation.

2. Materials and Methods

2.1. Chemicals and Reagents. All utilized reagents were obtained from Sigma Chemical Co. (St. Louis, MO, USA).

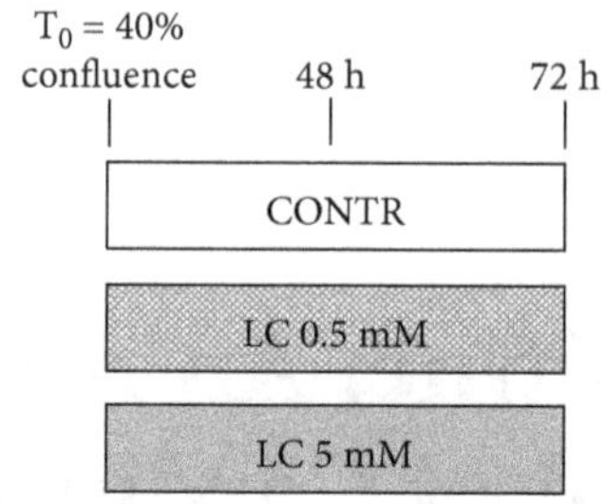

Figure 1: Scheme of treatment. Upon reaching 40% confluence, H9c2 cells were treated for 48 and 72 h with 0.5 or 5 mM LC.

Primary antibodies against GAPDH (FL-335), p-CaMKII α (22B1), CaMKII (M-176), AMPK $\alpha 1/2$ (H-300), SOD2 (FL-222), p21 (C-19), peroxidase-conjugated secondary antibodies for Western blot analysis, and FITC-conjugated antibodies for immunofluorescence study were purchased from Santa Cruz Biotechnology (Santa Cruz, CA, USA). STAT3 (124H6) and p-STAT3 (Ser727) were purchased from Cell Signaling Technology (Danvers, MA, USA).

The CellROX® Oxidative Stress Reagent kit (C10443) was purchased from Thermo Fisher Scientific, Life Technologies Italia (Monza, Italy).

2.2. Cell Line and Culture Conditions. The American Type Culture Collection (ATCC, Manassas, VA, USA) offered the cardiomyoblast H9c2 cell line of rat embryo. The H9c2 cell line was regularly cultured in Dulbecco's modified Eagle's medium (DMEM, Gibco, Grand Island, NY, USA) containing 25 mmol/L glucose, 100 μg/mL streptomycin (Sigma-Aldrich, St. Louis, MO, USA), 100 U/mL penicillin, and 10% fetal bovine serum (FBS, Gibco, Grand Island, NY, USA) in 75 cm^2 tissue culture flasks and then incubated at 37°C by adopting 5% CO_2. H9c2 cells exposed to high glucose (25 mmol/L) represent a validated *in vitro* model in order to mimic cardiac hyperglycemic/diabetic condition [31, 32]. Cells were fed every day; following literature indications, H9c2 cells were split when reaching 70–80% confluence in order to prevent the loss of the differentiation potential [28, 32]. Preliminarily, we evaluated the effective concentration of LC based on our previous work performed on skeletal myoblasts and literature evidence (data not shown) [28, 33]. We identified the correct LC concentrations as the lower concentrations that activated STAT3 signaling. Then, H9c2 cells in the active proliferation phase were treated with 0.5 or 5 mM LC as indicated in Figure 1.

2.3. Growth Curve and Cell Viability Test. H9c2 cells were plated on 60 mm × 15 mm culture dishes at 20% confluence and grown in DMEM. After an overnight phase, the cells were treated or not with 0.5 or 5 mM LC. At 24, 48, and 72 h after treatments, cells were trypsinized and stained with trypan blue and were counted using hemocytometer. The average values for each single day were used to plot a growth curve. Cell viability was calculated by dividing the unstained viable cell count by the total cell count. In addition, morphological changes were observed daily by phase contrast microscopy.

2.4. Western Blot Analysis. Western blot analysis was performed as described previously [34]. Cell lysates were prepared using RIPA buffer implemented with protease inhibitors. 30 μg of proteins was separated by SDS-polyacrylamide gel electrophoreses (SDS-PAGE) and electrophoretically transferred to nitrocellulose membranes (Protran®, Whatman® Schleicher & Schuell). The blots were then blocked and incubated with specific primary antibodies, followed by incubation with anti-species-specific secondary antibodies. To confirm equal protein loading per sample, we used GAPDH protein as housekeeping protein. Finally, detection of specific proteins was performed by enhanced chemoluminescence reagent (Western Lightning ECL Pro, Perkin Elmer). Quantitative measurement of immunoreactive band intensities was performed by densitometric analysis using the Scion Image software (Scion Corporation, Frederick, MD, USA). Data were then converted into fold changes (FC) of the control.

2.5. Immunofluorescence Studies. H9c2 cells were grown on coverslips with or without LC 0.5 or 5 mM LC. After 48 and 72 h of treatment, cells were washed 3 times with PBS, then fixed in prepared 4% paraformaldehyde for 20 minutes. The cells on the coverslips were washed with PBS and incubated for 30 minutes at room temperature with 1% bovine serum albumin in PBS with 0.2% Triton X-100. At that point, H9c2 cells were incubated with primary antibodies for 120 minutes. To detect the primary antibody, binding site cells were washed three times in PBS and followed by incubation with specific antibodies FITC-conjugated for 90 minutes. Nuclei were revealed with DAPI staining. Coverslips with cells were mounted and observed using Nikon Eclipse 50I microscopy. The images were captured using Nis-Elements D 4.00 software. Immunofluorescence signals were estimated using the ImageJ program (http://imagej.nih.gov/ij/). Data were displayed and analyzed using Adobe Photoshop CS4®.

Automated quantification on the immunofluorescence signal was performed by using the ImageJ program (http://imagej.nih.gov/ij/) [34]. For each analyzed protein, the quantified signal was normalized for the total nuclei number.

2.6. Intracellular ROS Determination in H9c2 Cells after H_2O_2 Injury. Intracellular ROS levels were valued using the CellROX® Oxidative Stress Reagent kit. Briefly, H9c2 cells were pretreated with 0.5 or 5 mM LC for 48 h, and then they were exposed to 500 μM H_2O_2 for 30 min. At the end of the H_20_2 injury, the fluorogenic probe of the kit was added (Figure 2(a)). CellROX® Oxidative Stress Reagents are fluorogenic probes designed to reliably measure ROS in live cells. The cell-permeable reagents are nonfluorescent or very faintly fluorescent while in a reduced state and during oxidation exhibit a strong fluorogenic signal. The CellROX® Orange Reagent signal is localized in the cytoplasm.

The images were captured using Nis-Elements D 4.00 software. Data were displayed and analyzed using Adobe Photoshop CS4®.

Automated quantification on the immunofluorescence signal was performed by using the ImageJ program (http://imagej.nih.gov/ij/) [35]. For each analyzed protein, the quantified signal was normalized for the total nuclei number.

2.7. Statistical Analysis. All experiments were performed three times. The data are expressed as the means ± standard deviation, and statistical comparisons were performed with specific statistical packages (Prism v 7.00 GraphPad Software, San Diego, CA, USA). Differences were analyzed by one- or two-way analysis of variance (ANOVA) followed by Tukey's multiple comparison post hoc test. $p < 0.05$ was considered statistically significant.

3. Results

3.1. Attenuation of ROS Production Induced by H_2O_2 in LC Pretreated H9c2 Cells. The diabetic heart usually has ROS levels that exceed normal quantities, and ROS overproduction likely contributes to cardiomyopathy [15, 36, 37]. After stimulus with 500 μM H_2O_2, 48 h pretreatment with 0.5 or 5 mM LC markedly reduced ROS levels with respect to the CONTR condition (Figures 2(b) and 2(c)). Furthermore, DAPI images showed that pretreated H9c2 cells with LC, in particular with 5 mM LC, showed a higher number of nuclei than the control condition (Figures 2(b) and 2(d)): These results suggested that LC pretreatment improved cellular survival after H_2O_2 injury.

3.2. LC Improves Antioxidant Response in H9c2 Cells under Hyperglycemic Condition. Signal transducer and activator of transcription 3 (STAT3) activation thought phosphorylation on Ser^{727} is an important protective mechanism to prevent ROS generation in the setting of oxidative stress [38–40]. Under normoxic conditions, the treatment with 0.5 or 5 mM LC for 48 and 72 h significantly enhanced myocardial STAT3 phosphorylation on Ser^{727} (Figure 3(a)).

Moreover, after 48 and 72 h of treatment, exposure of cells to 0.5 mM LC caused rapid increase of SOD2, a well-known antioxidant enzyme [41]. This effect was significantly augmented with the 5 mM LC dose (Figure 3(b)).

3.3. LC Downregulation of CaMKII Pathway. Ca^{2+}/calmodulin-dependent protein kinase II (CaMKII), a multifunctional serine/threonine protein kinase, is implicated in the pathogenesis of cardiac diseases [42, 43] promoting ROS overproduction [44, 45]. As shown by immunofluorescence analysis (Figure 4(a)), compared with untreated H9c2 cells, LC treatments decreased CaMKII and pCaMKII-positive cell numbers after 72 h of stimuli: immunofluorescence quantification shows a greater effect with the 5 mM LC dose. Furthermore, after 72 h, either 0.5 or 5 mM doses of LC significantly decreased the phosphorylation of CaMKII α isoform, as shown by Western blot analysis (Figure 4(b)).

3.4. LC Action on AMPK Protein Expression. 5′-AMP-activated kinase (AMPK) has become a strategic cellular target for the cure of cardiovascular disease correlated

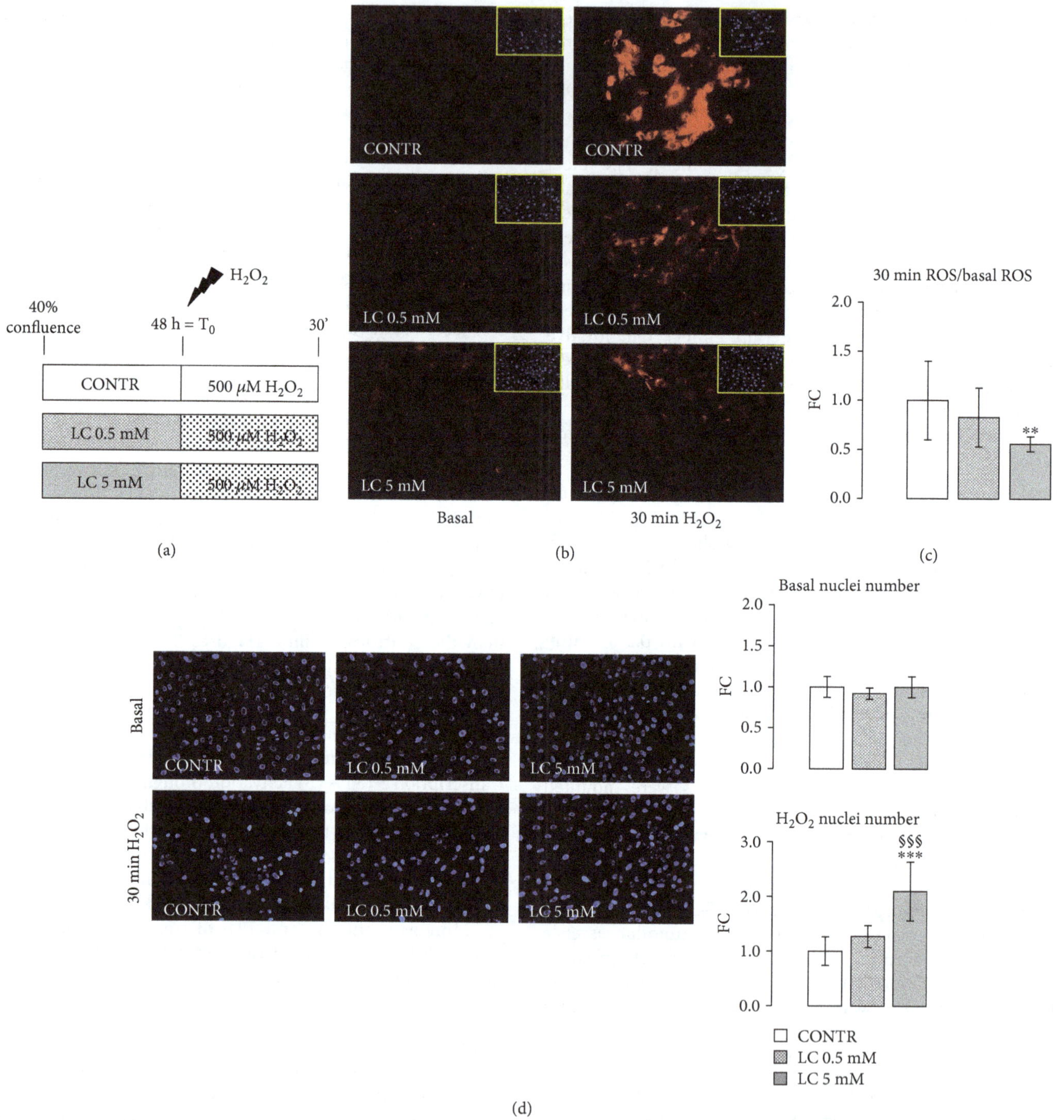

FIGURE 2: Attenuation of ROS production induced by H_2O_2 in LC-pretreated H9c2 cells. (a) Scheme of treatment: H9c2 cardiomyocytes were exposed to a stressful insult with 500 μM of H_2O_2 after pretreatment for 48 h with 0.5 or 5 mM LC. (b) Using the CellROX reagent assay, LC action was evaluated under oxidative stress conditions. The pretreatment with 0.5 or 5 mM LC causes a reduction in ROS production after stimulus with 500 μM of H_2O_2. (c) Quantification of ROS production. The quantified signal was normalized for the total nuclei number. From the DAPI images, it was possible to observe that the cells pretreated with both doses of LC show higher survival compared to the control cells. (d) Quantification of nuclei number pre- and after H_2O_2 injury in LC-pretreated H9c2 cells. Data are expressed as fold changes (FC) of mean ± SD. Significance: $^{**}p \leq 0.01$ vs. CONTR.

with DM [46–48]: it is likely that AMPK activity in the diabetic heart may ameliorate cardiac function. After LC stimuli, immunofluorescence for AMPK showed an increase in AMPK-positive cells in a dose- and time-dependent manner (Figure 5).

3.5. LC Action on Cardiomyocyte Viability. An uncontrolled consequence of sustained hyperglycemia is the induction of cardiomyocyte death that causes a loss of contractile units, which declines organ function and provokes hypertrophy of vital cardiomyocytes [49–51]. We

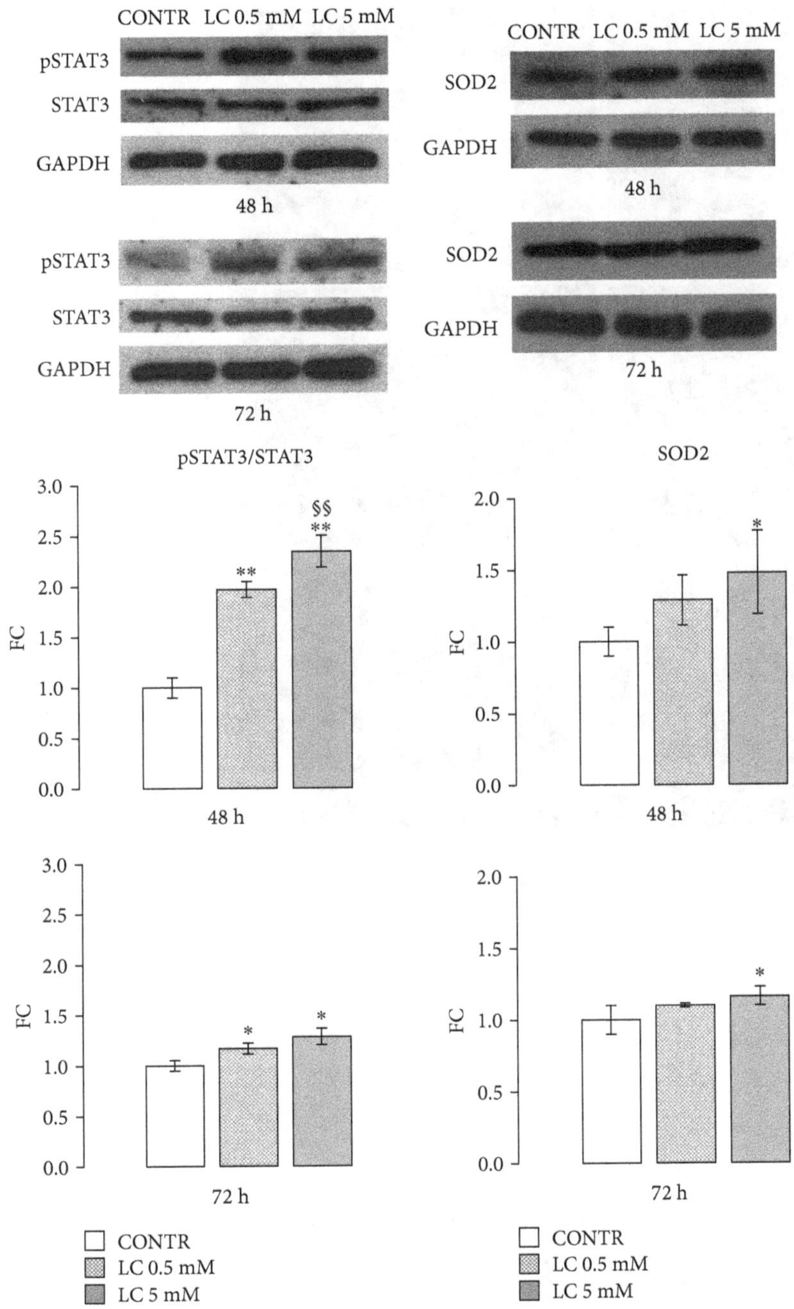

(a) (b)

Figure 3: LC improves antioxidant response in H9c2 cells under hyperglycemic condition. (a) Representative Western blot and relevant quantification: LC stimuli for 48 and 72 h significantly enhanced STAT3 activation (ratio pSTAT3/STAT3). (b) Western blot analysis and relevant quantification: 5 mM LC improved SOD2 protein content in H9c2 cells after 48 and 72 h of treatment with respect to control cells. Data are expressed as fold changes (FC) of mean ± SD. Significance: $^{*}p \leq 0.05$ vs. CONTR; $^{**}p \leq 0.01$ vs. CONTR; $^{\S\S}p \leq 0.01$ vs. LC 0.5 mM.

investigated viability and morphologic features of H9c2 cells after exposure to 0.5 or 5 mM LC (Figure 6(a)). The growth curve showed that LC treatments did not induce a change of cellular proliferation with respect to untreated control cells (Figure 6(b)). Moreover, the viability graph showed the absence of cell mortality in all treatment conditions (Figure 6(b)). To support these data, phase contrast images, collected at day 3 of the growth curve, confirmed the absence of morphological changes in cells treated with 0.5 or 5 mM LC respect to control (Figure 6(c)).

In opposition to its antiproliferative functions, p21 can also play proproliferative and survival roles when it is localized in the cytosol [51]. Figure 6(c) shows that the protein content of p21 in cardiomyocytes treated with 0.5 or 5 mM LC was superimposable to control cells, and this result highlights that there is not p21 translocation from cytoplasm to nuclei.

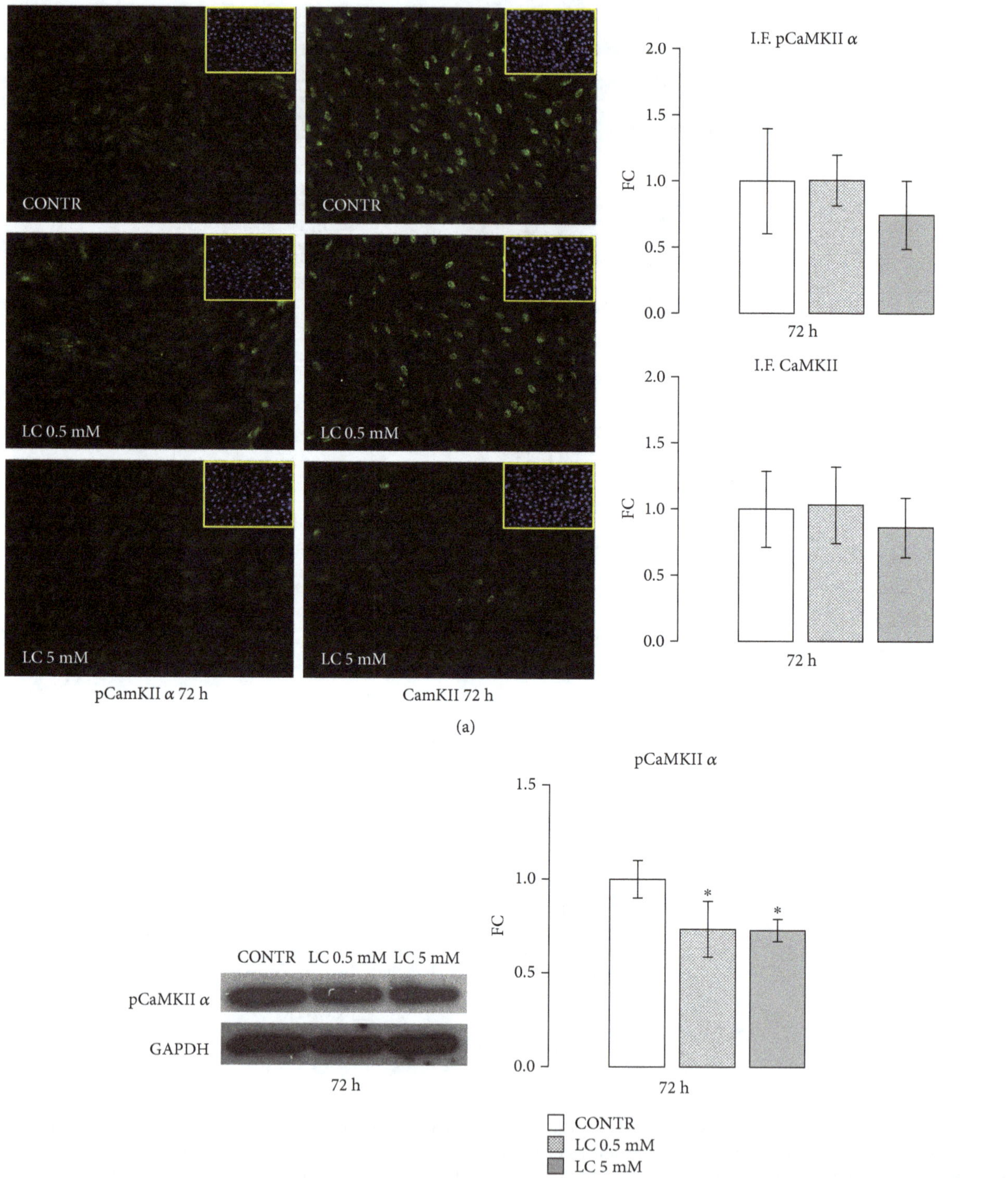

(b)

FIGURE 4: LC downregulation of CaMKII pathway. (a) LC treatments decreased CaMKII-positive cell number and its α phosphorylated form after 72 h of stimuli: this effect was more marked for the 5 mM LC dose. The quantified signal was normalized for the total nuclei number. (b) Representative Western blot and relevant quantification: LC stimuli for 72 h promote CaMKII α isoform activation. Data are expressed as fold changes (FC) of mean ± SD. Significance: $^*p \leq 0.05$ vs. CONTR.

4. Discussion

In the present study, we demonstrated that LC supplementation significantly decreases ROS production in cardiomyocytes during hyperglycemia (Figure 2). ROS generation induced by high glucose causes apoptosis of cardiac cells and important decrease in growth factor secretion [15, 16, 52–55]. In the heart microenvironment, the oxidative stress induced by hyperglycemia can lead to stem cell senescence which is characterized by the production and secretion of

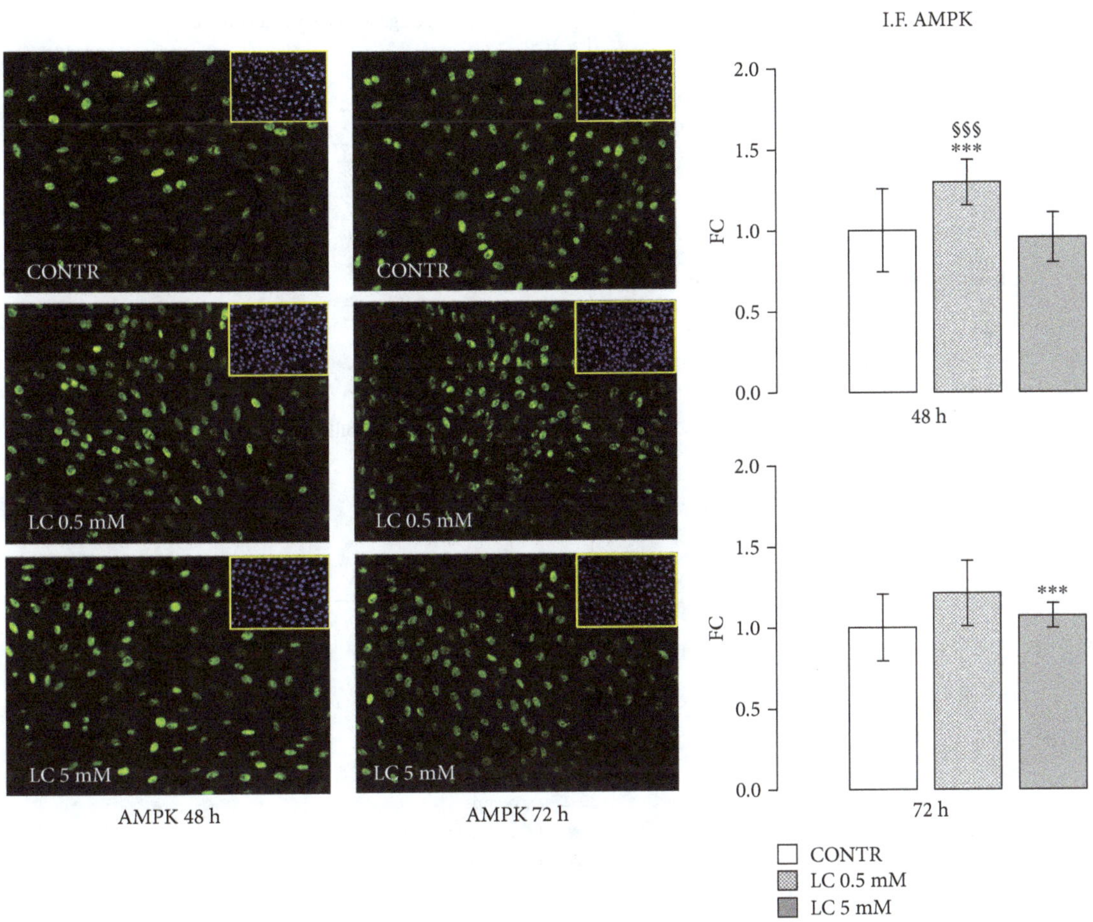

FIGURE 5: LC action on AMPK protein expression. Immunofluorescence assay and relevant quantification showed an increase in the number of AMPK-positive cells in LC condition at 48 and 72 h. The quantified signal was normalized for the total nuclei number. Data are expressed as fold changes (FC) of mean ± SD. Significance: $^{***}p \leq 0.001$ vs. CONTR; $^{\S\S\S}p \leq 0.001$ vs. LC 5 mM.

soluble factor SASP (senescence-associated secretory phenotype). Those factors, responsible for the onset of chronic inflammation and oxidative stress, are considered the pathophysiological link between aging and diabetes in cardiovascular diseases [56].

The association hyperglycemia/ROS/cellular senescence represents a major cause of inefficiency of regenerative medicine [9, 10, 56, 57]. Further, clinical trials established that an altered glycemic control is equal to therapeutic failure [13, 14]. Our data point out that LC could counteract oxidative stress in the hyperglycemic condition. Those observations are consistent with several previous works that reported that LC stimuli decrease ROS generation in the skeletal muscle, bone and cardiac cells grown under normoglycemic condition [26, 27, 58, 59]. Furthermore, as shown in Figure 6, both doses of LC did not modify the H9c2 growth rate and did not induce cellular damages.

Studying the mechanism by which LC may modulate ROS formation, we observed an increase in the serine 727 (Ser^{727}) phosphorylation of STAT3, after 48 and 72 hours of treatment (Figure 3(a)). Recent evidence stresses the critical role of STAT3 in modulating mitochondrial respiratory chain function and ROS production [39, 40]. Serine 727 (Ser^{727}) phosphorylation has a primary part in STAT3 influence on mitochondria: its decrement is associated with the development of cardiac hypertrophy and dilated cardiomyopathy [60]. Moreover, several data showed that STAT3 conserves complex I activity in ischemic condition enhancing cell viability and plays an important role in heart protection from chronic stress induced by hyperglycemia [61]. STAT3 activation promotes the expression of SOD2, the principal enzyme effective in reducing mitochondrial oxidative species [41, 62]. LC treatment significantly increased SOD2 expression in *in vitro* cardiomyocytes, confirming LC capability to counteract oxidative stress in the hyperglycemic condition (Figure 3(b)).

Interestingly, a number of studies have indicated that CaMKII enhances mitochondrial dysfunction, ROS formation, and apoptosis [63], eventually causing cardiomyocyte death both following hyperglycemia [64, 65] and oxidative stress conditions [43, 45, 66].

Hyperglycemic cardiac cells are characterized by a vicious circle between ROS/mitochondrial dysfunction/CaMKII that triggers cellular damages and apoptosis phenomena [42–44]. Taking into consideration that literature evidence, we investigated LC action on CaMKII protein content. As reported in Figure 4, LC treatments reduce CaMKII activation. Remarkably, recent experiments hypothesized

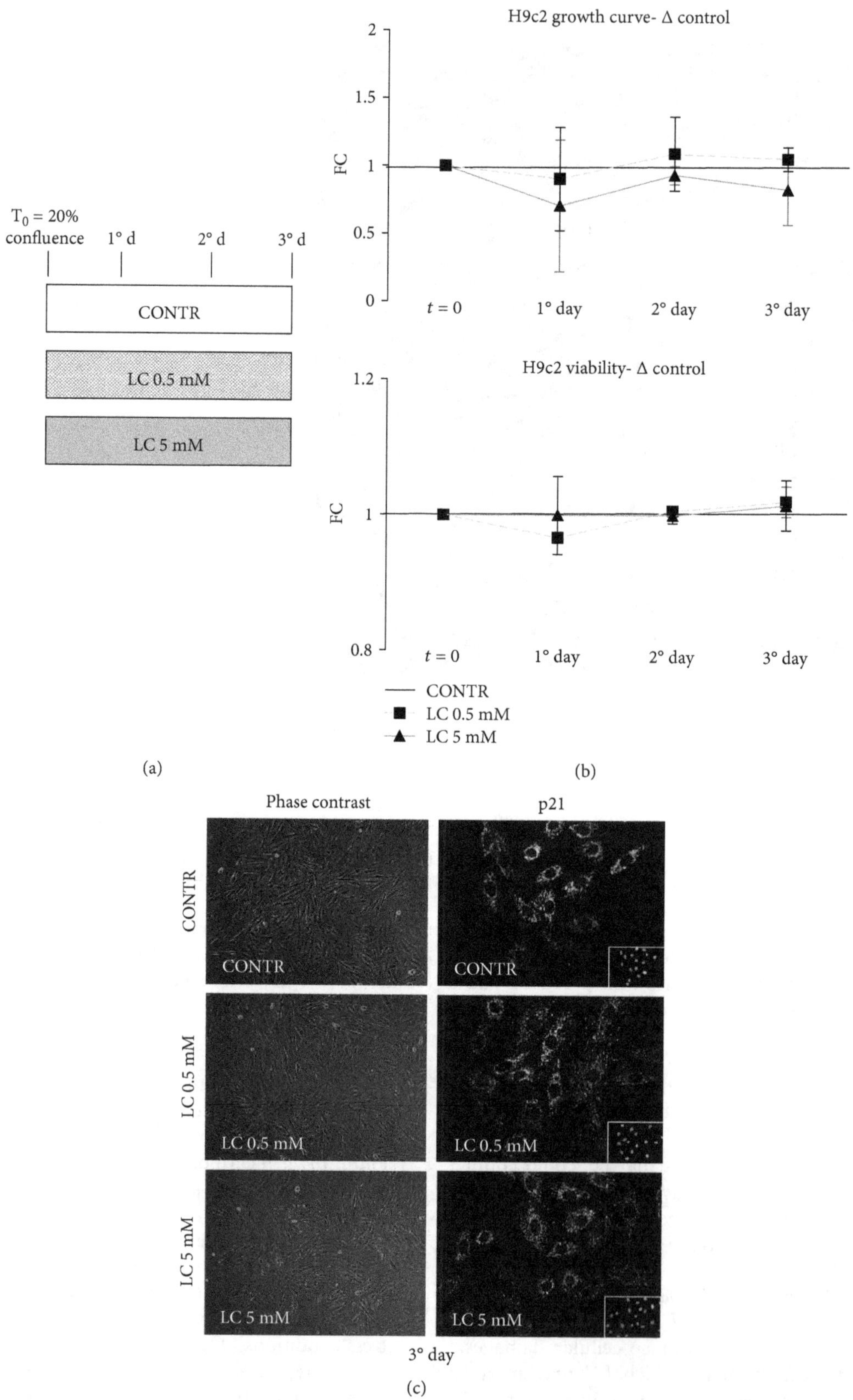

Figure 6: LC action on cardiomyocyte viability. (a) Experimental scheme for growth curve and viability determination. (b) 0.5 or 5 mM LC did not alter the H9c2 proliferative potential. Viability graph shows the absence of cell mortality in all treatment conditions. (c) Phase contrast images show how treatment with 0.5 or 5 mM LC do not modify the morphology of H9c2 cells. Furthermore, there is no p21 translocation from cytoplasm to nuclei following treatment with both doses of LC. Data are expressed as fold changes (FC) of mean ± SD.

TABLE 1: Summary of LC action on hyperglycemic cardiomyocytes (H9c2).

Hyperglycemic cardiomyocites (H9c2)	ROS	STAT3	CaMKII	AMPK	Cellular growth and vitality
L-Carnitine treatment	⇩	⇧	⇩	⇧	=

that CaMKII activation is related to Ca^{2+} movement from the endoplasmic reticulum to mitochondria.

Recently, LC was shown to promote Ca^{2+} availability which is needed for proliferation and differentiation of human osteoblast-like cells, via a depolarization of L-type calcium channels [59]. Despite the Ca^{2+} supply via the L-type channels being essential to ensure appropriate cardiac cell contraction, an excessive Ca^{2+} influx increases mitochondrial ROS production in cardiomyocytes under oxidative stress. Various authors suggested that cardiac damage, induced by CaMKII activation, is caused by an increase in L-type Ca^{2+} current [67].

LC capability of modulating CaMKII in cardiac cells could make LC a molecule appropriate for impeding the cross-talk between L-type Ca^{2+} channels and ROS production and restoring normal mitochondrial function in cardiac cells. Further investigations are necessary to unravel LC action on cardiac calcium channels.

AMPK represents a strategic target in cardiovascular alterations associated with DM. It is well known that impairment of AMPK activation characterizes hyperglycemic cardiomyocytes. In particular, during hypoxia/reoxygenation (H/R) injury in diabetic patients, AMPK deficiency is associated with an increase in ROS production and apoptosis [46, 47]. As shown in Figure 5, LC stimuli enhanced AMPK protein synthesis, suggesting that LC not only could ameliorate the oxidative microenvironment but also could improve metabolic functions of cardiac cells. With this in mind, future studies could investigate LC's possible action on the protein kinase C (PKC) signaling pathway, implicated in diabetic damage. As known, in hyperglycemic condition, the decrease in AMPK activity is associated with an increase of diacylglycerol (DAG) production that activates PKC and NADPH-oxidase causing an abnormal production of ROS [68, 69]. Then, LC ability to stimulate AMPK activation and to regulate the production of acyl-CoA could counteract hyperinsulinemia-correlated oxidative stress.

Whereas the higher risk of developing atrial fibrillation (AF) in diabetic subjects compared to healthy ones is associated with mitochondrial ROS overproduction, ATP depletion, and abnormal calcium homeostasis [70, 71], the key modulator role shown by LC suggests the potential use of this micronutrient as adjuvant therapy in different cardiac pathologies associated with DM.

In conclusion, LC described effects could be useful in association with other cardioactive drugs. Ranolazine is an antianginal drug with hypoglycemic action used in AF treatment, which was shown to enhance skeletal muscle differentiation [35]. In cardiac regenerative medicine, antioxidative LC action, in association with ranolazine, might lead to the improvement of the hyperglycemic-oxidative microenvironment, prevention of apoptosis, and preservation of cell viability. Equally interesting could be the synergistic effect of LC with allopurinol [72] or the α-lipoic acid antioxidant [73] in the prevention and treatment of AF. Remarkable therapeutic perspectives could arise from the association of LC with new hypoglycemic drugs, such as incretins, whose effects on the hyperglycemia control, inflammation, and atherosclerotic plaque progression have recently been demonstrated [74, 75].

Taken together, our results argue that the use of LC as a coadjuvant in therapeutic treatments is very promising, although extensive studies focused on the determination of the effective LC dose and route of administration in humans should be undertaken. Anyway, LC doses used in our study (0.5–5 mM) are compatible with ranges used in humans receiving LC therapy [76, 77].

5. Conclusion

The results of this work (Table 1) provide, for the first time, fundamental *in vitro* cellular evidence that treatment with LC could be a potential strategy to improve the cardiac oxidative microenvironment caused by hyperglycemia.

According to the findings of the present study, demonstrating the LC ability to decrease production of ROS, activate STAT3 and AMPK, and downregulate CaMKII, LC could represent a potential adjuvant therapeutic strategy in diabetic cardiac regenerative medicine.

This adjuvant therapy might be recommended for diabetic patients with high risk of cardiac injury as it exerts a cardioprotective effect by restoring the microenvironmental equilibrium by strengthening cardiomyocytes' defense mechanisms through the stimulation of endogenous antioxidants (SOD2).

Further, *in vitro* and *in vivo* studies on this topic are essential to improve the knowledge on the effects of LC in cardiac diseases associated with diabetes and on its potential synergic action with other antioxidative and hypoglycemic agents.

Conflicts of Interest

The authors declare that there is no conflict of interest regarding the publication of this paper.

Authors' Contributions

FV, PS, and AM are coauthors and contributed equally to this work.

Acknowledgments

This study was partially supported by the Ricerca Corrente funding from the Italian Ministry of Health to IRCCS Policlinico San Donato.

References

[1] M. J. Garcia, P. M. McNamara, T. Gordon, and W. B. Kannell, "Morbidity and mortality in diabetics in the Framingham population: sixteen year follow-up study," *Diabetes*, vol. 23, no. 2, pp. 105–111, 1974.

[2] G. Jia, A. Whaley-Connell, and J. R. Sowers, "Diabetic cardiomyopathy: a hyperglycaemia- and insulin-resistance-induced heart disease," *Diabetologia*, vol. 61, no. 1, pp. 21–28, 2018.

[3] American Diabetes Association, "Diagnosis and classification of diabetes mellitus," *Diabetes Care*, vol. 33, Supplement 1, pp. S62–S69, 2010.

[4] R. J. Pickering, C. J. Rosado, A. Sharma, S. Buksh, M. Tate, and J. B. de Haan, "Recent novel approaches to limit oxidative stress and inflammation in diabetic complications," *Clinical & Translational Immunology*, vol. 7, no. 4, article e1016, 2018.

[5] M. Brownlee, "The pathobiology of diabetic complications: a unifying mechanism," *Diabetes*, vol. 54, no. 6, pp. 1615–1625, 2005.

[6] M. L. Balestrieri, M. R. Rizzo, M. Barbieri et al., "Sirtuin 6 expression and inflammatory activity in diabetic atherosclerotic plaques: effects of incretin treatment," *Diabetes*, vol. 64, no. 4, pp. 1395–1406, 2015.

[7] A. A. Tajik, D. Dobre, D. Aguilar et al., "A history of diabetes predicts outcomes following myocardial infarction: an analysis of the 28 771 patients in the high-risk MI database," *European Journal of Heart Failure*, vol. 19, no. 5, pp. 635–642, 2017.

[8] A. Jorsal, H. Wiggers, and J. J. V. McMurray, "Heart failure: epidemiology, pathophysiology, and management of heart failure in diabetes mellitus," *Endocrinology and Metabolism Clinics of North America*, vol. 47, no. 1, pp. 117–135, 2018.

[9] Z. Lin and W. T. Pu, "Strategies for cardiac regeneration and repair," *Science Translational Medicine*, vol. 6, no. 239, article 239rv1, 2014.

[10] V. R. Satthenapalli, R. R. Lamberts, and R. G. Katare, "Concise review: challenges in regenerating the diabetic heart: a comprehensive review," *Stem Cells*, vol. 35, no. 9, pp. 2009–2026, 2017.

[11] S. K. Sanganalmath and R. Bolli, "Cell therapy for heart failure: a comprehensive overview of experimental and clinical studies, current challenges, and future directions," *Circulation Research*, vol. 113, no. 6, pp. 810–834, 2013.

[12] R. Marfella, M. R. Rizzo, M. Siniscalchi et al., "Peri-procedural tight glycemic control during early percutaneous coronary intervention up-regulates endothelial progenitor cell level and differentiation during acute ST-elevation myocardial infarction: effects on myocardial salvage," *International Journal of Cardiology*, vol. 168, no. 4, pp. 3954–3962, 2013.

[13] L. Cai and B. B. Keller, "Cardiac regeneration and diabetes," *Regenerative Medicine Research*, vol. 2, no. 1, p. 1, 2014.

[14] A. P. Ofstad, D. Atar, L. Gullestad, G. Langslet, and O. E. Johansen, "The heart failure burden of type 2 diabetes mellitus—a review of pathophysiology and interventions," *Heart Failure Reviews*, vol. 23, no. 3, pp. 303–323, 2018.

[15] C. M. O. Volpe, P. H. Villar-Delfino, P. M. F. dos Anjos, and J. A. Nogueira-Machado, "Cellular death, reactive oxygen species (ROS) and diabetic complications," *Cell Death & Disease*, vol. 9, no. 2, p. 119, 2018.

[16] A. Faria and S. J. Persaud, "Cardiac oxidative stress in diabetes: mechanisms and therapeutic potential," *Pharmacology & Therapeutics*, vol. 172, pp. 50–62, 2017.

[17] M. S. Shah and M. Brownlee, "Molecular and cellular mechanisms of cardiovascular disorders in diabetes," *Circulation Research*, vol. 118, no. 11, pp. 1808–1829, 2016.

[18] C. V. Diogo, J. M. Suski, M. Lebiedzinska et al., "Cardiac mitochondrial dysfunction during hyperglycemia–the role of oxidative stress and p66Shc signaling," *The International Journal of Biochemistry & Cell Biology*, vol. 45, no. 1, pp. 114–122, 2013.

[19] K. D. Salpea, C. G. Maubaret, A. Kathagen, G. Ken-Dror, D. W. Gilroy, and S. E. Humphries, "The effect of pro-inflammatory conditioning and/or high glucose on telomere shortening of aging fibroblasts," *PLoS One*, vol. 8, no. 9, article e73756, 2013.

[20] Z. Y. Wang, Y. Y. Liu, G. H. Liu, H. B. Lu, and C. Y. Mao, "L-Carnitine and heart disease," *Life Sciences*, vol. 194, pp. 88–97, 2018.

[21] J. J. Dinicolantonio, A. K. Niazi, M. McCarty, C. J. Lavie, E. Liberopoulos, and J. H. O'Keefe, "L-Carnitine for the treatment of acute myocardial infarction," *Reviews in Cardiovascular Medicine*, vol. 15, no. 1, pp. 52–62, 2014.

[22] J. J. DiNicolantonio, C. J. Lavie, H. Fares, A. R. Menezes, and J. H. O'Keefe, "L-Carnitine in the secondary prevention of cardiovascular disease: systematic review and meta-analysis," *Mayo Clinic Proceedings*, vol. 88, no. 6, pp. 544–551, 2013.

[23] T. V. Fiorentino, A. Prioletta, P. Zuo, and F. Folli, "Hyperglycemia-induced oxidative stress and its role in diabetes mellitus related cardiovascular diseases," *Current Pharmaceutical Design*, vol. 19, no. 32, pp. 5695–5703, 2013.

[24] S. da Silva Guimarães, W. de Souza Cruz, L. da Silva et al., "Effect of L-carnitine supplementation on reverse remodeling in patients with ischemic heart disease undergoing coronary artery bypass grafting: a randomized, placebo-controlled trial," *Annals of Nutrition & Metabolism*, vol. 70, no. 2, pp. 106–110, 2017.

[25] A. P. Wong, A. Niedzwiecki, and M. Rath, "Myocardial energetics and the role of micronutrients in heart failure: a critical review," *American Journal of Cardiovascular Disease*, vol. 6, no. 3, pp. 81–92, 2016.

[26] M. Xue, X. Chen, Z. Guo et al., "L-Carnitine attenuates cardiac dysfunction by ischemic insults through Akt signaling pathway," *Toxicological Sciences*, vol. 160, no. 2, pp. 341–350, 2017.

[27] A. J. Blanca, M. V. Ruiz-Armenta, S. Zambrano et al., "Inflammatory and fibrotic processes are involved in the cardiotoxic effect of sunitinib: protective role of L-carnitine," *Toxicology Letters*, vol. 241, pp. 9–18, 2016.

[28] C. Y. Mao, H. B. Lu, N. Kong et al., "Levocarnitine protects H9c2 rat cardiomyocytes from H_2O_2-induced mitochondrial dysfunction and apoptosis," *International Journal of Medical Sciences*, vol. 11, no. 11, pp. 1107–1115, 2014.

[29] R. Ferrari, E. Merli, G. Cicchitelli, D. Mele, A. Fucili, and C. Ceconi, "Therapeutic effects of L-carnitine and propionyl-L-carnitine on cardiovascular diseases: a review," *Annals of the New York Academy of Sciences*, vol. 1033, no. 1, pp. 79–91, 2004.

[30] R. Lango, R. T. Smolenski, M. Narkiewicz, J. Suchorzewska, and W. Lysiak-Szydlowska, "Influence of L-carnitine and its derivatives on myocardial metabolism and function in ischemic heart disease and during cardiopulmonary bypass," *Cardiovascular Research*, vol. 51, no. 1, pp. 21–29, 2001.

[31] C. Zhang, L. Zhang, S. Chen et al., "The prevention of diabetic cardiomyopathy by non-mitogenic acidic fibroblast growth factor is probably mediated by the suppression of oxidative stress and damage," *PLoS One*, vol. 8, no. 12, article e82287, 2013.

[32] S. Sun, S. Yang, M. Dai et al., "The effect of Astragalus polysaccharides on attenuation of diabetic cardiomyopathy through inhibiting the extrinsic and intrinsic apoptotic pathways in high glucose-stimulated H9C2 cells," *BMC Complementary and Alternative Medicine*, vol. 17, no. 1, p. 310, 2017.

[33] A. Montesano, P. Senesi, L. Luzi, S. Benedini, and I. Terruzzi, "Potential therapeutic role of L-carnitine in skeletal muscle oxidative stress and atrophy conditions," *Oxidative Medicine and Cellular Longevity*, vol. 2015, Article ID 646171, 13 pages, 2015.

[34] I. Villa, P. Senesi, A. Montesano et al., "Betaine promotes cell differentiation of human osteoblasts in primary culture," *Journal of Translational Medicine*, vol. 15, no. 1, p. 132, 2017.

[35] I. Terruzzi, A. Montesano, P. Senesi, F. Vacante, S. Benedini, and L. Luzi, "Erratum to: Ranolazine promotes muscle differentiation and reduces oxidative stress in C2C12 skeletal muscle cells," *Endocrine*, vol. 58, no. 1, p. 46, 2017.

[36] E. Shen, Y. Li, Y. Li et al., "Rac1 is required for cardiomyocyte apoptosis during hyperglycemia," *Diabetes*, vol. 58, no. 10, pp. 2386–2395, 2009.

[37] A. Modesti, I. Bertolozzi, T. Gamberi et al., "Hyperglycemia activates JAK2 signaling pathway in human failing myocytes via angiotensin II-mediated oxidative stress," *Diabetes*, vol. 54, no. 2, pp. 394–401, 2005.

[38] J. A. Meier and A. C. Larner, "Toward a new STATe: the role of STATs in mitochondrial function," *Seminars in Immunology*, vol. 26, no. 1, pp. 20–28, 2014.

[39] K. Szczepanek, Q. Chen, M. Derecka et al., "Mitochondrial-targeted signal transducer and activator of transcription 3 (STAT3) protects against ischemia-induced changes in the electron transport chain and the generation of reactive oxygen species," *The Journal of Biological Chemistry*, vol. 286, no. 34, pp. 29610–29620, 2011.

[40] J. A. Meier, M. Hyun, M. Cantwell et al., "Stress-induced dynamic regulation of mitochondrial STAT3 and its association with cyclophilin D reduce mitochondrial ROS production," *Science Signaling*, vol. 10, no. 472, article eaag2588, 2017.

[41] X. Shen, S. Zheng, N. S. Metreveli, and P. N. Epstein, "Protection of cardiac mitochondria by overexpression of MnSOD reduces diabetic cardiomyopathy," *Diabetes*, vol. 55, no. 3, pp. 798–805, 2006.

[42] L. F. Couchonnal and M. E. Anderson, "The role of calmodulin kinase II in myocardial physiology and disease," *Physiology*, vol. 23, no. 3, pp. 151–159, 2008.

[43] E. D. Luczak and M. E. Anderson, "CaMKII oxidative activation and the pathogenesis of cardiac disease," *Journal of Molecular and Cellular Cardiology*, vol. 73, pp. 112–116, 2014.

[44] K. Odagiri, H. Katoh, H. Kawashima et al., "Local control of mitochondrial membrane potential, permeability transition pore and reactive oxygen species by calcium and calmodulin in rat ventricular myocytes," *Journal of Molecular and Cellular Cardiology*, vol. 46, no. 6, pp. 989–997, 2009.

[45] M. V. Singh, A. Kapoun, L. Higgins et al., "Ca^{2+}/calmodulin-dependent kinase II triggers cell membrane injury by inducing complement factor B gene expression in the mouse heart," *The Journal of Clinical Investigation*, vol. 119, no. 4, pp. 986–996, 2009.

[46] N. B. Ruderman, D. Carling, M. Prentki, and J. M. Cacicedo, "AMPK, insulin resistance, and the metabolic syndrome," *The Journal of Clinical Investigation*, vol. 123, no. 7, pp. 2764–2772, 2013.

[47] C. Beauloye, L. Bertrand, S. Horman, and L. Hue, "AMPK activation, a preventive therapeutic target in the transition from cardiac injury to heart failure," *Cardiovascular Research*, vol. 90, no. 2, pp. 224–233, 2011.

[48] W. Chang, M. Zhang, J. Li et al., "Berberine improves insulin resistance in cardiomyocytes via activation of 5′-adenosine monophosphate-activated protein kinase," *Metabolism*, vol. 62, no. 8, pp. 1159–1167, 2013.

[49] A. Leonardini and A. Avogaro, "Abnormalities of the cardiac stem and progenitor cell compartment in experimental and human diabetes," *Archives of Physiology and Biochemistry*, vol. 119, no. 4, pp. 179–187, 2013.

[50] L. Cai and Y. J. Kang, "Cell death and diabetic cardiomyopathy," *Cardiovascular Toxicology*, vol. 3, no. 3, pp. 219–228, 2003.

[51] E. S. Child and D. J. Mann, "The intricacies of p21 phosphorylation: protein/protein interactions, subcellular localization and stability," *Cell Cycle*, vol. 5, no. 12, pp. 1313–1319, 2006.

[52] H. Wu, L. Cai, J. B. de Haan, and R. Giacconi, "Targeting oxidative stress in diabetic complications: new insights," *Journal of Diabetes Research*, vol. 2018, Article ID 1909675, 2 pages, 2018.

[53] S. Masi, F. D'Aiuto, J. Cooper et al., "Telomere length, antioxidant status and incidence of ischaemic heart disease in type 2 diabetes," *International Journal of Cardiology*, vol. 216, pp. 159–164, 2016.

[54] N. Lal, A. P. L. Chiu, F. Wang et al., "Loss of VEGFB and its signaling in the diabetic heart is associated with increased cell death signaling," *American Journal of Physiology-Heart and Circulatory Physiology*, vol. 312, no. 6, pp. H1163–H1175, 2017.

[55] T. Aliwarga, E. Evangelista, N. Sotoodehnia, R. Lemaitre, and R. Totah, "Regulation of CYP2J2 and EET levels in cardiac disease and diabetes," *International Journal of Molecular Sciences*, vol. 19, no. 7, article 1916, 2018.

[56] H. Shakeri, K. Lemmens, A. B. Gevaert, G. R. Y. de Meyer, and V. F. M. Segers, "Cellular senescence links aging and diabetes in cardiovascular disease," *American Journal of Physiology-Heart and Circulatory Physiology*, vol. 315, no. 3, pp. H448–H462, 2018.

[57] A. S. D. Molgat, E. L. Tilokee, G. Rafatian et al., "Hyperglycemia inhibits cardiac stem cell-mediated cardiac repair and angiogenic capacity," *Circulation*, vol. 130, 11_Supplement_1, pp. S70–S76, 2014.

[58] F. Le Borgne, G. Ravaut, A. Bernard, and J. Demarquoy, "L-Carnitine protects C2C12 cells against mitochondrial superoxide overproduction and cell death," *World Journal of Biological Chemistry*, vol. 8, no. 1, pp. 86–94, 2017.

[59] A. Ferraretto, M. Bottani, I. Villa et al., "L-Carnitine activates calcium signaling in human osteoblasts," *Journal of Functional Foods*, vol. 47, pp. 270–278, 2018.

[60] A. Camporeale, F. Marino, A. Papageorgiou et al., "STAT3 activity is necessary and sufficient for the development of immune-mediated myocarditis in mice and promotes progression to dilated cardiomyopathy," *EMBO Molecular Medicine*, vol. 5, no. 4, pp. 572–590, 2013.

[61] H. Li, W. Yao, Z. Liu et al., "Hyperglycemia abrogates ischemic postconditioning cardioprotection by impairing AdipoR1/Caveolin-3/STAT3 signaling in diabetic rats," *Diabetes*, vol. 65, no. 4, pp. 942–955, 2016.

[62] S. Luo, X. Gu, F. Ma et al., "ZYZ451 protects cardiomyocytes from hypoxia-induced apoptosis via enhancing MnSOD and STAT3 interaction," *Free Radical Biology & Medicine*, vol. 92, pp. 1–14, 2016.

[63] N. Feng and M. E. Anderson, "CaMKII is a nodal signal for multiple programmed cell death pathways in heart," *Journal of Molecular and Cellular Cardiology*, vol. 103, pp. 102–109, 2017.

[64] W. Zhu, S. Tsang, D. M. Browe et al., "Interaction of β1-adrenoceptor with RAGE mediates cardiomyopathy via CaMKII signaling," *JCI Insight*, vol. 1, no. 1, article e84969, 2016.

[65] M. Luo, X. Guan, E. D. Luczak et al., "Diabetes increases mortality after myocardial infarction by oxidizing CaMKII," *The Journal of Clinical Investigation*, vol. 123, no. 3, pp. 1262–1274, 2013.

[66] J. M. Timmins, L. Ozcan, T. A. Seimon et al., "Calcium/calmodulin-dependent protein kinase II links ER stress with Fas and mitochondrial apoptosis pathways," *The Journal of Clinical Investigation*, vol. 119, no. 10, pp. 2925–2941, 2009.

[67] K. Tonegawa, W. Otsuka, S. Kumagai et al., "Caveolae-specific activation loop between CaMKII and L-type Ca^{2+} channel aggravates cardiac hypertrophy in α1-adrenergic stimulation," *American Journal of Physiology. Heart and Circulatory Physiology*, vol. 312, no. 3, pp. H501–H514, 2017.

[68] E. W. Kraegen, A. K. Saha, E. Preston et al., "Increased malonyl-CoA and diacylglycerol content and reduced AMPK activity accompany insulin resistance induced by glucose infusion in muscle and liver of rats," *American Journal of Physiology. Endocrinology and Metabolism*, vol. 290, no. 3, pp. E471–E479, 2006.

[69] S. I. Itani, N. B. Ruderman, F. Schmieder, and G. Boden, "Lipid-induced insulin resistance in human muscle is associated with changes in diacylglycerol, protein kinase C, and IκB-α," *Diabetes*, vol. 51, no. 7, pp. 2005–2011, 2002.

[70] W. Xie, G. Santulli, S. R. Reiken et al., "Mitochondrial oxidative stress promotes atrial fibrillation," *Scientific Reports*, vol. 5, no. 1, article 11427, 2015.

[71] J. Gambardella, D. Sorriento, M. Ciccarelli et al., "Functional role of mitochondria in arrhythmogenesis," *Advances in Experimental Medicine and Biology*, vol. 982, pp. 191–202, 2017.

[72] Y. Yang, J. Zhao, J. Qiu et al., "Xanthine oxidase inhibitor allopurinol prevents oxidative stress-mediated atrial remodeling in alloxan-induced diabetes mellitus rabbits," *Journal of the American Heart Association*, vol. 7, no. 10, 2018.

[73] C. Sardu, G. Santulli, M. Santamaria et al., "Effects of alpha lipoic acid on multiple cytokines and biomarkers and recurrence of atrial fibrillation within 1 year of catheter ablation," *The American Journal of Cardiology*, vol. 119, no. 9, pp. 1382–1386, 2017.

[74] R. Marfella, C. Sardu, M. L. Balestrieri et al., "Effects of incretin treatment on cardiovascular outcomes in diabetic STEMI-patients with culprit obstructive and multivessel non obstructive-coronary-stenosis," *Diabetology and Metabolic Syndrome*, vol. 10, no. 1, p. 1, 2018.

[75] R. Marfella, C. Sardu, P. Calabrò et al., "Non-ST-elevation myocardial infarction outcomes in patients with type 2 diabetes with non-obstructive coronary artery stenosis: effects of incretin treatment," *Diabetes, Obesity and Metabolism*, vol. 20, no. 3, pp. 723–729, 2018.

[76] R. Fielding, L. Riede, J. Lugo, and A. Bellamine, "l-Carnitine supplementation in recovery after exercise," *Nutrients*, vol. 10, no. 3, p. 349, 2018.

[77] A. Sawicka, D. Hartmane, P. Lipinska, E. Wojtowicz, W. Lysiak-Szydlowska, and R. Olek, "l-Carnitine supplementation in older women. A pilot study on aging skeletal muscle mass and function," *Nutrients*, vol. 10, no. 2, p. 255, 2018.

16

Diabetes-Induced Reactive Oxygen Species: Mechanism of Their Generation and Role in Renal Injury

Selim Fakhruddin, Wael Alanazi, and Keith E. Jackson

Department of Basic Pharmaceutical Sciences, School of Pharmacy, University of Louisiana at Monroe (ULM), Pharmacy Building, 1800 Bienville Dr., Monroe, LA 71201, USA

Correspondence should be addressed to Keith E. Jackson; kjackson@ulm.edu

Academic Editor: Carlos Martinez Salgado

Diabetes induces the onset and progression of renal injury through causing hemodynamic dysregulation along with abnormal morphological and functional nephron changes. The most important event that precedes renal injury is an increase in permeability of plasma proteins such as albumin through a damaged glomerular filtration barrier resulting in excessive urinary albumin excretion (UAE). Moreover, once enhanced UAE begins, it may advance renal injury from progression of abnormal renal hemodynamics, increased glomerular basement membrane (GBM) thickness, mesangial expansion, extracellular matrix accumulation, and glomerulosclerosis to eventual end-stage renal damage. Interestingly, all these pathological changes are predominantly driven by diabetes-induced reactive oxygen species (ROS) and abnormal downstream signaling molecules. In diabetic kidney, NADPH oxidase (enzymatic) and mitochondrial electron transport chain (nonenzymatic) are the prominent sources of ROS, which are believed to cause the onset of albuminuria followed by progression to renal damage through podocyte depletion. Chronic hyperglycemia and consequent ROS production can trigger abnormal signaling pathways involving diverse signaling mediators such as transcription factors, inflammatory cytokines, chemokines, and vasoactive substances. Persistently, increased expression and activation of these signaling molecules contribute to the irreversible functional and structural changes in the kidney resulting in critically decreased glomerular filtration rate leading to eventual renal failure.

1. Introduction

Diabetes is a group of chronic metabolic diseases marked by high plasma glucose levels (usually fasting plasma glucose (FPG) is ≥126 mg/dL) resulting from defects in insulin secretion or insulin action or both. The chronic hyperglycemia of diabetes induces several pathophysiological complications including cardiovascular abnormalities to renal failure. According to the American Diabetes Association [1], there are two main classes of diabetes: type 1 or insulin-dependent diabetes mellitus (IDDM) and type 2 or non-insulin-dependent diabetes mellitus (NIDDM). Type 1 diabetes is primarily caused by a cellular-mediated autoimmune destruction of β-cells of the pancreas and accounts for only 5–10% of diabetic cases. Conversely, type 2 diabetes is characterized by insulin resistance with relative insulin deficiency (i.e., patients secrete insulin but not enough to overcome the insulin resistance) and accounts for 90–95% of diagnosed diabetes cases.

The prevalence and incidence of diabetes and diabetic kidney diseases have alarmingly increased during recent decades. According to a 2014 national diabetes statistics report, 29.1 million United States citizens have diabetes which is 9.3% of the U.S. population. Every year, 1.4 million Americans are diagnosed with diabetes [2]. According to the 2014 World Health Organization (WHO) report, worldwide prevalence of diabetes was estimated to be 9% among adults of 18 years of age or older. In 2012, an estimated 1.5 million deaths were directly caused by diabetes [3]. WHO projects that diabetes will be the 7th leading cause of death by 2030 [4].

In line with the increasing incidence of diabetes, cases of chronic kidney disease (CKD) or end-stage renal damage (ESRD) have been growing significantly, since CKD is directly related to diabetes and/or hypertension. Approximately 1 of 3 adults with diabetes and 1 of 5 adults with high blood pressure have CKD. According to the 2014 National Chronic Kidney Disease Fact Sheet, more than 20 million adults (10% of all adults) have CKD in the United States. CKD is more prevalent in older people and most common among adults older than 70 years of age. It has also been observed that diabetes and hypertension are the leading causes of ESRD. In 2011, diabetes and hypertension were identified as the primary cause for 7 of 10 new United States cases of ESRD [5].

Diabetes-mediated chronic hyperglycemia evokes the onset and progression of renal injury because of its role in causing hemodynamic dysregulation along with abnormal morphological and functional nephron changes. The most important event that precedes renal injury is an increase in permeability of plasma proteins such as albumin through a damaged glomerular filtration barrier. This results in excessive urinary albumin excretion (UAE) through the nephron. Excess albumin excretion into urine is used as a prominent marker for diabetic kidney disease. Increased albumin leakage results from the impaired integrity of the glomerular filtration barrier (GFB), which is primarily responsible for retention of all plasma proteins. It is noted that GFB consists of three layers, where the visceral epithelial cells (podocytes) layer is highly vulnerable to ROS because of its nonproliferative nature even in response to injury [6, 7]. This results in early podocyte loss at the onset of diabetes and initiates increased protein excretion in urine.

Reactive oxygen species promote renal injury which eventually develops into chronic kidney disease. Diabetes-mediated ROS could be generated in both enzymatic and nonenzymatic pathways. Among many, NADPH oxidase (Nox) (enzymatic) and mitochondrial electron transport chain (mETC) (nonenzymatic) pathways are the prominent sources of ROS generation in the diabetic kidney and play a critical role in promoting pathophysiological events in kidney disease. In addition to NADPH oxidase (Nox) and mETC, other sources of ROS such as advanced glycation end products (AGEs) and uncoupled nitric oxide synthase (NOS) have been discussed in the current manuscript.

Hyperglycemia-induced ROS, particularly of Nox and mETC origin, are believed to cause the onset of albuminuria followed by progression of renal damage through podocyte depletion. ROS play a significant role in the onset of microalbuminuria through damaging the integrity of all the layers of the GFB. Once microalbuminuria occurs, ROS along with increased protein levels in the tubular ultrafiltrate can activate diverse aberrant signaling pathways to facilitate renal damage from the progressive stage to eventual end-stage renal damage (ESRD). Increased activation and/or production of various signaling mediators such as transcription factors, inflammatory agents, growth factors, cytokines, chemokines, and vasoactive molecules produce deleterious structural and functional glomerular alternations. These abnormal signaling cascades advance renal injury from progression of abnormal renal hemodynamics, increased glomerular basement membrane (GBM) thickness, mesangial expansion, extracellular matrix accumulation, interstitial fibrosis, and glomerulosclerosis to eventual end-stage renal damage. Though, at the outset, hyperglycemia-induced renal damage exhibits moderate structural and functional glomerular changes, such as hyperfiltration, untreated kidney develops most abnormal structural (Kimmelstiel-Wilson syndrome, nodular form of mesangial matrix) and functional (critically decreased filtration rate, <15–29 mL/min/1.73 m^2) condition that warrants kidney dialysis. Albeit the role of glomerulus in progressive renal damage is substantial, tubular segment is not less important at all. Renal tubules rather increasingly contribute to the development of advanced stage of kidney damage which is beyond the scope of this review.

2. Basic Filtration Mechanism

Both kidneys receive about 22 percent of cardiac output that is equal to 1100 mL of blood in an adult. Blood flow into the glomerulus of the kidney is controlled by the afferent and efferent arterioles. The afferent arteriole drives the blood into the glomerulus, whereas efferent arteriole helps the blood flow out of the glomerulus into peritubular capillaries. Both of these arterioles can contribute to the filtration process by either facilitating blood flow to the glomerulus (via afferent arteriolar vasodilation) or increasing intraglomerular pressure (via efferent arteriolar vasoconstriction). Moreover, other physical factors play an important role in maintaining the net intraglomerular filtration pressure. Three critical pressures govern the filtration through the glomerular capillaries. They are (1) hydrostatic pressure inside the glomerular capillaries, also known as glomerular hydrostatic pressure (P_G), which exerts 60 mmHg in favor of filtration, (2) hydrostatic pressure in Bowman's capsule (P_B) that equals about 18 mmHg opposing the filtration, and (3) colloid osmotic pressure of the glomerular capillary plasma proteins, also known as glomerular oncotic pressure (π_G), which shows 32 mmHg acting against the filtration. Hence, mathematically, the net filtration pressure can be calculated from $P_G - P_B - \pi_G$ {(60–18–32) mmHg} which is equivalent to 10 mmHg. This net filtration pressure is maintained in the glomerulus at normal physiologic condition to promote filtration. Filtration of plasma fluid (45% of the total blood coming to the glomerular capillaries) results in easy permeation of relatively low molecular weight plasma components including electrolytes (Na^+, K^+, and Cl^-), organic molecules (e.g., glucose, amino acids, and peptides), HCO_3^-, HPO_4^-, and all waste products such as urea, uric acid, and creatinine along with water into Bowman's space. The filtrate then flows along the renal tubule through which almost all essential components are reabsorbed except the waste products. In addition, it is very interesting to note that glomerular capillary wall is very efficient to retain larger molecules including plasma proteins during filtration, albeit a significant amount of protein can be permeated into the urinary space. The proteins that escape glomerular capillary barriers usually include β-2 microglobulin, immunoglobulin light chains, and small amounts of albumin. Most of these escaped proteins are reabsorbed and catabolized by the proximal tubular epithelium, thus further minimizing urinary excretion of protein content. For a normal adult, urinary protein excretion does not exceed 200 mg/day, of which very little (10–20 mg/day) is albumin [8–10]. However, structural and functional aberration of glomerular capillary barriers can lead to excess urinary excretion of proteins, abundantly albumin in different disease conditions including diabetes [11, 12], hypertension [13], and hyperlipidemia [14]. Excretion of proteins and excretion of albumin into urine are termed as "proteinuria" and "albuminuria," respectively. Proteinuria and albuminuria are synonymously used in clinical practice, since albumin is usually the most abundant urinary protein in different renal diseases. Urinary albumin excretion over 24 hours is used as the "gold standard" to define different albuminuric conditions such as (1) normoalbuminuria that exhibits urinary albumin excretion (UAE) of <30 mg/day, (2) microalbuminuria (UAE range is 30–300 mg/day), and (3) macro/overt albuminuria (UAE > 300 mg/day). Urine collection over 24 hours is a cumbersome job which may lead to inaccurate measurement of truly excreted albumin. That is why clinicians now use albumin/creatinine ratio (mg/mmoL) in a spot urine sample to accurately and conveniently measure albumin that can literally represent albumin concentration in 24 h urine volume [15–17]. In medical literature, microalbuminuria is increasingly recognized as an important marker to characterize acute to chronic renal diseases [18]. Diabetic patients exhibit early microalbuminuria as a sign of onset of renal injury, progression of which can lead to macroalbuminuria with advanced pathological events ranging from decreased glomerular filtration rate (GFR) and glomerulosclerosis to eventual end-stage renal damage (ESRD). Before we review diabetes-induced pathological changes of glomerulus in detail, we will give an account on the contributory role of glomerular filtration barrier in fluid filtration and protein retention underscoring their structural and functional features.

3. Glomerular Filtration Barrier: Structural and Functional Role in Filtration

The glomerular filtration barrier (GFB) is recognized as a highly specialized ultrafiltration device that is capable of filtering large volumes of plasma fluids with a high permeability to water and small and midsized solutes in plasma, while efficiently retaining relatively larger macromolecules within the circulation. The barrier is composed of three layers: the innermost fenestrated vascular endothelium, the glomerular basement membrane, and the outermost podocyte layer (also called the glomerular visceral epithelial cells) [19]. All the layers, more or less, can provide the charge and size selectivity for macromolecules, usually plasma proteins, to prevent their easy passage into the urinary space [20, 21]. However, the exact locations for various selective functions of the barrier are still debatable.

3.1. The Endothelium. The endothelial layer is composed of unusually flattened endothelial cells with a height around the capillary loops of approximately 50–150 nm. Remarkably, endothelial cell bodies are completely perforated by open holes or fenestrae which constitute 20–50% of the entire endothelial surface. The fenestrae are usually round having a diameter of 40–100 nm which is similar in size to that found by Bearer et al. [22] in a study using quick-freeze and deep-etch method in rat kidneys. The abundantly fenestrated endothelium renders high permeability to water and small solutes in the glomeruli. Though larger fenestrae apparently seem to allow free passage of relatively smaller albumin (3.6 nm in diameter), it may not happen due to negatively charged endothelial surface layer (ESL). ESL mainly consists of plasma membrane-bound "glycocalyx" and a larger endothelial cell coat containing proteoglycans, glycoproteins, and plasma proteins [19, 22–24]. The glycocalyx is also composed of proteoglycans and glycoproteins (e.g., selectins, integrin, and members of the immunoglobulin superfamily) which can act as its backbone molecules. The glycoproteins contain acidic oligosaccharides and terminal sialic acids (SAs). Of note, various endothelial cell adhesion molecules which play an important role in cell recruitment during pathogenic condition are good examples of glycoproteins. The glycocalyx includes three families of cell adhesion molecules as glycoproteins: selectin, integrin, and immunoglobulin superfamily. Intercellular cell adhesion molecules (ICAM) and vascular cell adhesion molecules (VCAM) are the members of the immunoglobulin family. On the other hand, the proteoglycans exhibit a complex network of many proteins including glycosaminoglycan (GAG) chains, syndecans, glypicans, mimecan, perlecan, and biglycan. Syndecan is rich in heparan sulfate and chondroitin sulfate chains. Moreover, the glycosaminoglycan contains five chains, namely, heparan sulfate, chondroitin sulfate, dermatan sulfate, keratan sulfate, and hyaluronan (or hyaluronic acid). These highly sulfated chains together with sialic acids of glycoprotein give the glycocalyx a net negatively charged luminal surface [25, 26].

This negatively charged layer can selectively restrict access of negatively charged plasma proteins such as albumin to the endothelial cell membrane leading to limited filtration of albumin. This is manifested by a recent study, where the investigators infused hyaluronidase (ESL degrading enzyme) solution into right jugular vein of mice for 4 weeks and found significant decrease in ESL thickness resulting in increased albumin filtration [27]. Besides hyaluronidase, other high-molecular-weight enzymes, namely, heparinase and chondroitinase, are reported to decrease ESL thickness and charge density with subsequent increment in albumin clearance [28–30].

3.2. The Glomerular Basement Membrane (GBM). Glomerular basement membrane is a gel-like layer interwoven between endothelium and epithelial layer. Electron microscopic study demonstrates that GBM is composed of inner, middle, and outer sublayers designated as lamina rara externa, lamina densa, and lamina rara interna, respectively [31]. All the layers form a tight fibrous meshwork comprising of collagen IV, laminin, and nidogen/entactin along with proteoglycan (i.e., agrin and perlecan) and glycoproteins. Collagen IV is a major skeletal component of GBM and plays an important role in maintaining its integrity. Mutation or loss of collagen IV may lead to progressive renal diseases including basement membrane thinning, podocyte foot process effacement, and Alport syndrome; the latter is manifested by increased ferritin permeability. However, mild proteinuria in patients with Alport syndrome indicates a minor role of this collagen in permselectivity of proteins. Laminin is also an important structural component that can maintain ultrastructure of podocytes by interacting with integrin of basal podocyte membrane. Additionally, laminin is thought to prevent easy permeation of plasma proteins, since its loss or mutation can cause excessive proteinuria [32–34]. Like glomerular endothelium, GBM contributes to charge selective restriction to the passage of polyanionic macromolecules due to its net negative charge imparted by sulfated chains of proteoglycans and sialyl as well as carboxyl groups of glycoproteins. Heparan sulfate proteoglycans are abundantly found in GBM, whereas others (chondroitin, keratan, and dermatan) are rare, but hyaluronic acid is present. On the other hand, agrin proteoglycan predominantly contributes to the total heparan sulfates of GBM, though perlecan may have a part [35, 36]. Based on these observations, it seems that GBM is critical for limited protein leakage as supported by the findings that removal of heparan sulfate by heparanase infusion or anti-heparan sulfate antibody treatment showed massive proteinuria and high GBM permeability. Moreover, heparan sulfate level of GBM was reported to be reduced in patients with both type 1 and type 2 diabetes showing remarkable proteinuria [37]. However, its restrictive protein filtration role has been debated as many studies found insignificant leakage of protein even after reduction of the heparan sulfate components through downregulation of their contributing proteoglycans agrin/perlecan [38–40].

3.3. The Podocytes. The podocytes are terminally differentiated visceral epithelial cells covering the outer surface of the glomerular capillaries and maintain the integrity of the kidney filter. They consist of a voluminous cell body, primary processes (arm-like projections coming from the cell body), and foot processes (numerous slender feet projected from primary processes). The cell body faces urinary space and gives rise to primary processes. Both processes are enriched in microtubules and intermediate filaments such as desmin and vimentin. The primary processes further elongate toward the capillary to make secondary/foot processes that contain an actin-based cytoskeleton. Besides actin, foot processes (FP) also contain other contractile proteins such as myosin, α-actinin, vinculin, and talin, which together help the podocytes get anchored to the basement membrane via mainly $\alpha 3\beta 1$ integrin, whereas α- and β-dystroglycans linked with utrophin also assist in the attachment. The foot processes of podocytes form fine filtration slit by interdigitating with the foot processes of neighboring podocytes. The filtration slits are 30–40 nm in width and are bridged by a thin diaphragm, known as the slit diaphragm (SD). In addition to SD, foot processes can also contain two more membrane domains called apical/luminal and basal membrane domains. All the three membrane domains are structurally and functionally connected to FP actin cytoskeleton, thus giving a pivotal role to actin for podocyte function and dysfunction. Interference in any of these domains causes active reorganization of the actin filament from its parallel and contractile bundles into a dense network resulting in foot processes effacement [41, 42].

On the other hand, slit diaphragm plays a remarkable role in filtration by providing charge and size selective barrier to the macromolecules because of its architectural nature (physical sieve having pore size of ~3.8 nm, the same diameter of an albumin molecule [43, 44]) and various functional proteins. Slit diaphragm (also apical membrane) is lined with a thick coat composed of sialoglycoproteins, including podocalyxin and podoendin, imparting the net surface negative charges to the podocytes. These proteins can charge-selectively prevent filtration of plasma proteins. Additionally, the slit diaphragm consists of many proteins arranged one upon another along a vertical bar conforming to a zipper like structure. Studies of molecular genetics of the slit diaphragm have so far identified many proteins as its integral components, though the list is still growing. Several proteins such as ZO-1 (zonula occludens-1), nephrin, CD2AP (CD2-associated protein), FAT, P-cadherin, NEPH1 (nephrin-like protein-1), and podocin are expressed within the slit diaphragm. Synaptopodin, a novel podocyte marker, is an actin-associated protein, expressed in the foot process, and plays a role in the motility of the foot processes. All these proteins have important structural and functional roles as an integral part of the kidney filter. Though in-depth discussion on each of the podocyte proteins is beyond the scope of our review, the readers are referred to some exciting reviews for more understanding of the podocyte proteins and functions [42, 45, 46] However, we will later discuss injurious effect of reactive oxygen species on these proteins that trigger different pathological events during early to advanced renal damage in both type 1 and type 2 diabetes.

3.4. The Glomerular Mesangial Cells (GMCs). Mesangial cells are smooth muscle-like pericytes located in the intercapillary regions of the glomerulus. Though the mesangial cells are not an integrated structural part of the glomerular capillary barrier in the kidney filter, their contribution to the fluid filtration cannot be underestimated. They, along with the capillary barrier, form a coordinated biochemical unit and control the filtration rate as they have the capacities of regulating filtration surface area, intraglomerular blood volume and filtration pressure, and hormone as well as growth factor secretion. Contracting (e.g., Ang II and vasopressin) and relaxing (i.e., ANP and NO) hormones secreted by GMC can control blood flow to the capillary loops via preferential constriction and dilation of efferent and afferent arterioles, respectively, thus maintaining constant glomerular filtration rate (GFR) [47]. GMC-secreting growth factors such as PDGF, FGF, EGF, and CTGF influence mesangial cell proliferation and matrix production. PDGF is very important for the generation and maintenance of the capillary loops. In addition, GMCs can also cleanse GBM to maintain its permeability feature and take up macromolecules entering into the matrix of the mesangium. In nutshell, GMCs and glomerular layers interplay to maintain the integrity and homeostasis of the glomerulus which has been supported by the evidence that mesangiolysis using toxin or antibodies against mesangial cell antigen results in proteinuria and glomerular abnormalities [48, 49].

4. Hyperglycemia-Induced ROS and Mechanisms of Their Generation

The term reactive oxygen species (ROS) can be defined as highly reactive oxygen-centered chemical species containing one or two unpaired electrons, where an unpaired electron is one that exists in an atomic or molecular orbital alone. The unpaired electron containing chemical species can also be called "free radicals." In medical literature, the term "ROS" is used as a "collective term" to include both radicals and nonradicals, the latter being devoid of unpaired electron. So, ROS are classified into two categories: (1) oxygen-centered radicals and (2) oxygen-centered nonradicals. Oxygen-centered radicals include superoxide anion ($^{\bullet}O_2^-$), hydroxyl radical ($^{\bullet}OH$), alkoxyl radical ($RO^{\bullet}$), and peroxyl radical ($ROO^{\bullet}$). Oxygen-centered nonradicals are hydrogen peroxide (H_2O_2), singlet oxygen ($^1O_2$), and hypochlorous acids (HOCl). Unlike ROS, reactive nitrogen species (RNS) are nitrogen-centered radicals and nitrogen-centered nonradicals. The nitrogen-centered radicals include nitric oxide ($NO^{\bullet}$) and nitrogen dioxide ($NO_2^{\bullet}$), whereas nitrogen-centered nonradicals are peroxynitrite ($ONOO^-$), alkyl peroxynitrite (ROONO), nitroxyl anion (NO^-), nitrous acid (HNO_2), and so on [50].

High glucose-induced ROS can be generated by both enzymatic and nonenzymatic pathways. The enzymatic pathways include nicotinamide adenine dinucleotide phosphate oxidase (NADPH oxidase), uncoupling of nitric oxide synthase (NOS), cytochrome P-450 (CYTP450), cyclooxygenase (COX), lipoxygenase (LOX), xanthine oxidase, and myeloperoxidase (MPO). Conversely, the nonenzymatic pathways include mitochondrial electron transport chain (mETC) deficiencies, advanced glycation end products (AGEs), glucose autooxidation, transition-metal catalyzed Fenton reactions, and polyol (sorbitol) pathway [51–53]. Among these, we will discuss below the major ROS generating pathways, such as NADPH oxidase, uncoupled NOS, mETC, and AGEs that are increasingly involved in the pathogenesis of diabetic kidney diseases as demonstrated by many studies (Figure 2) [54–60].

4.1. NADPH Oxidase. NADPH oxidase is one of the principal sources of ROS production in hyperglycemic conditions of different organs including the kidney. NADPH oxidase is a respiratory burst enzyme that was initially identified in phagocytes in 1933. The enzyme is responsible for production of millimolar amounts of superoxide using cytosolic NADPH as substrate, and the superoxide or its downstream metabolite H_2O_2 can kill microorganisms in burst-dependent manner of phagocytes. Since its early detection in phagocytes, a growing body of scientific studies identified and cloned five major subunits constituting the enzyme, NADPH oxidase. They are membrane-bound flavocytochrome b_{558} forming subunits such as gp91^{phox} (also known as Nox2), p22^{phox}, and cytosolic subunits that include p47^{phox}, p67^{phox}, and p40^{phox}. Membrane-bound and cytosolic subunits are called catalytic and regulatory subunits, respectively. In addition, a small GTP-binding protein called Racl (in nonphagocytes) or Rac2 (in phagocytes) has been recognized as an essential cytosolic component for NADPH oxidase activation. Phagocytic gp91^{phox} (Nox2) subunit does have six different homologs including Noxl, Nox3, Nox4, Nox5, DUOX1, and DUOX2 to make a NOX family of 7 members [61]. In addition to phagocyte, NADPH oxidase has also been identified in other nonphagocytic cell types including fibroblasts, vascular smooth muscle cells, renal cells (podocyte and mesangial and proximal tubular cells), and endothelial cells [62–64]. However, the rate of superoxide production in these nonphagocytic cells by phagocyte-type NADPH oxidase is lower than that of neutrophils, implying the intrinsic functional difference of the enzyme in phagocytic and nonphagocytic cells. Additionally, above-mentioned phagocytic gp91^{phox} (Nox2) homologs can also be expressed in different tissues other than phagocytes with a variation in their abundance from tissue to tissue. For example, Nox4 is highly expressed in renal cells, whereas Noxl is in the colon epithelium and vascular smooth muscle cells (VSMCs) [61, 65]. Though one homolog can be predominantly expressed in a particular cell type, other homologs of the Nox subunit may be expressed as well. NADPH oxidase can be activated in response to different stimuli, namely, pathogens, receptor agonists, and shear stress. Typical activation of the enzyme in phagocyte involves translocation of the cytosolic subunits to the plasma membrane to bind with the cytochrome b_{558}. In doing so, p47^{phox} is first phosphorylated to get released from its autoinhibitory conformation and then recruits other cytosolic subunits (p67^{phox}, p40^{phox}, and Rac2) to make a cytosolic complex. This complex is then translocated to the membrane, where it binds with flavocytochrome b_{558} subunits to trigger transfer of electron from NADPH substrate to molecular O_2, resulting in superoxide formation. p47^{phox} can be phosphorylated by different mediators including Ang II and c-Src. It is notable that p40^{phox} may not be essential for the enzyme activation, while other components paly crucial role in the enzyme activity with a variation in membrane-bound Nox homologs from tissue to tissue. For example, Nox2 is exclusively involved in phagocytic enzyme activation, where Noxl is more upregulated in VSMC and Nox4 is expressed more in renal cells. Noxl-4 isoforms require p22^{phox} subunit for the enzyme activation while Nox5 and DUOX do not [66, 67]. Recently, Paclet et al. in a landmark study by isolating active forms of NADPH oxidase complex showed that translocation of cytosolic p47^{phox} and p67^{phox} subunits and GTPase Rac to plasma membrane and their subsequent binding with cytochrome b_{558} (gp91^{phox} and p22^{phox}) are required to promote ROS generation by NADPH oxidase [68].

4.2. Mitochondrial ETC. Mitochondria are another potential source of ROS production in diabetic condition. However, there is a controversy as to which source of NADPH oxidase and mitochondria is predominantly contributing to ROS generation in diabetic condition, since some scientists identify the first [69, 70] to be more potential source, while others are in favor of the latter [71, 72]. Mitochondria play a pivotal role in maintaining intracellular energy homeostasis by producing ATP from ADP and inorganic phosphate molecule in oxidative phosphorylation pathway. Production of ATP results from two phases: oxidation of NADH (or $FADH_2$) to donate electrons to mitochondrial electron transport chain (ETC) and phosphorylation of ADP to ATP, so named oxidative phosphorylation. It should be noted that the electron donating NADH and $FADH_2$ come from two pathways: (1) glycolytic pathway which produces NADH and pyruvate from oxidation of intracellular glucose by the action of a series of enzymes and (2) mitochondrial Krebs cycle which oxidizes pyruvate derived from glycolysis to further produce NADH and $FADH_2$. Both NADH and $FADH_2$ act as high reducing equivalents for mitochondrial ETC. Mitochondrial ETC is located at the inner membrane and is mainly composed of four stationary enzyme complexes along with two mobile carriers of electrons such as ubiquinone (also known as coenzyme Q_{10}, abbreviated as CoQ_{10}) and cytochrome c. The complexes are complex I (NADH : ubiquinone oxidoreductase), complex II (succinate : ubiquinone oxidoreductase), complex III (ubiquinol : cytochrome c oxidoreductase), and complex IV (cytochrome c oxidase). In addition, an ATP synthesizing complex V (also known as ATP synthase) is located on the inner membrane. Electrons donated by NADH to complex I are transported by mobile ubiquinone to complex III. Ubiquinone can also receive electrons from succinate-derived $FADH_2$ through complex II. Once the electrons reach complex III, its mobile cytochrome c carries the electrons to complex IV, which ultimately sends the electrons to O_2 to reduce it and the reduced oxygen is combined with matrix H^+ to form water. Each NADH or $FADH_2$ donate two electrons to CoQ_{10} at a time and two electrons finally reduce half of molecular oxygen ($1/2O_2$) to give H_2O. During the transport of electrons along the chain, protons from mitochondrial matrix are pumped into inter membrane space using the free energy of the electron transfer. This increases H^+ concentration in the intermembrane space, resulting in increased proton gradient across the inner membrane. The intermembrane protons can again enter into the matrix through ATP synthase which uses the potential energy derived from downward flow of protons for ATP synthesis and the entered protons may either combine with reduced oxygen at complex IV to form water or get pumped into outer space [73].

Any dysregulation in the coordinated transfer of the electrons by the enzyme complexes results in the leakage of electrons. The leaked electrons in turn reduce O_2 to form superoxide ($^{\bullet}O_2^-$) which undergoes dismutation by manganese superoxide dismutase (MnSOD) in the matrix and Cu, Zn-SOD in the inter membrane space to form H_2O_2. Though the major sites for electron leakage in mitochondrial ETC have been controversial, growing scientific evidence showed that complex I and complex III are the prominent sources of electron escape and ROS generation [72, 74–76].

Complex I generates superoxide ($^{\bullet}O_2^-$) from ubiquinone-mediated electron leakage when large electrochemical proton gradient promotes reverse flow of electrons to complex I from downstream ETC sites. In this condition, uncoupling proteins (UCPs) can decrease proton gradient by leaking protons into the matrix, thereby arresting ROS generation [77]. Moreover, iron-sulfur clusters and reduced FMN of complex I may also act as important sources for $^{\bullet}O_2^-$ generation. On the other hand, complex III mediates $^{\bullet}O_2^-$ formation through an electron leakage mechanism arising from autooxidation of ubisemiquinone and reduced cytochrome b [53]. The formation of superoxide may further increase when complex I and complex III are inhibited by rotenone and antimycin, respectively. Inhibition of complex I by rotenone that binds to CoQ_{10} site of the complex can block electron flow from FMN that is fully reduced by high $NADH/NAD^+$ ratio, leading to interaction between reduced FMN and O_2 to form ROS [78]. However, inhibition of the complex by rotenone sometimes shows conflicting results as it can both increase or decrease superoxide formation. For example, increases in superoxide were observed in the human dopaminergic SH-SY5Y cells, mesencephalic neurons, human skin fibroblasts, 3T3-L1 adipocytes, and bovine heart, whereas decreases were found in rat liver mitochondria, mitochondria of rat heart muscle, monocytes and macrophages, and MIN6 cells [79–83]. The exact reason for such discriminating results is unknown. However, it may be possible that substrate-specificity, species- and tissue-specific variation, and surrounding environment (in vivo *or* in vitro) can cause such conflicts. For example, with regard to substrate specificity, rotenone can increase ROS generation in presence of glutamate, whereas it inhibits ROS with succinate [84, 85].

More ROS production occurs when antimycin is used. Because antimycin stabilizes the ubisemiquinone at ubiquinol binding site Q_o (outer site) of complex III by preventing electron transfer from $Q_o \rightarrow Q_i$ (inner antimycin binding site) $\rightarrow$ cytochrome c_1, this in turn causes the ubisemiquinone radical to undergo autooxidation by releasing a singlet electron to be attacked by molecular oxygen leading to $^{\bullet}O_2^-$ formation [53]. Moreover, myxothiazol can bind to Q_o site to prevent electron transfer from QH_2 at Q_o site to Fe-S center, resulting in either increased (probably via reverse electron flow) or decreased (via suppression of mitochondrial inner membrane potential, $\Delta\psi_m$) $^{\bullet}O_2^-$ formation [86, 87].

On the other hand, ROS generation by complex II should not be underestimated, albeit it is considered to have limited role in ROS release. Complex II appears to produce ROS in a condition of high succinate concentration and membrane potential ($\Delta\psi_m$) when the electrons donated by succinate flow back to complex I via ubiquinone that is associated with increased ROS generation. Complex II can also drive electron flow to complex III at higher succinate level, where leakage of electrons occurs from Q_o site of the complex if electron transfer from Q_o to Q_i is slowed down by antimycin leading to ROS generation [88]. In addition, complex II itself can generate superoxide even at lower concentration of succinate at its flavin site. This is demonstrated by the inhibition of complex II with TTFA that binds to the Q-site of the complex to prevent flavin-mediated ubiquinone reduction. Recently,

Anderson et al. showed that TTFA and 3NP (complex II inhibitors) have significantly increased ROS production in comparison to ROS generated by different human skin cells upon exposure to UVA (ultraviolet rays in sunlight), a known ROS stimulator [89]. This supports the notion that complex II inhibitors produce ROS by preventing ubiquinone reduction at Q-site of the complex.

In diabetic milieu, certain factors such as excess reducing equivalents NADH/$FADH_2$ [90], increased proton gradient, and membrane potential ($\Delta\psi_m$) [91] reverse electron transport to complex I [92], and increased ATP synthesis resulting from increased electrochemical proton gradient induces mitochondrial ETC to produce ROS. In addition, intracellular glucose homeostasis is impaired in diabetes due to excess uptake of glucose resulting in its increased flux through glycolytic pathway. This causes excessive production of pyruvate and NADH which shuttle into the mitochondrial matrix, where pyruvate is oxidized to produce more NADH and $FADH_2$ resulting in excess oxidizing substrates for complex I and complex II. Excessive substrates increase electron donations to ETC, thereby producing high proton gradient, increased membrane potential (reduced negativity in the matrix), and increased ATP synthesis. The excess electron transfer by CoQ_{10} oversaturates complex III where, at a point, electron transport can be blocked resulting in either reverse flow of electron to complex I or electron leakage to O_2 forming ROS. It is noted that increased ATP synthesis can be stopped by sustained depletion of ADP. This depleted ADP accompanied by attenuated ATP synthesis can eventually lead to ROS production as high electrochemical proton gradient still exists. This observation is substantiated by the study that rat liver mitochondria stimulate ROS generation when incubated with different mitochondrial complex I substrates such as malate, glutamate, and succinate. This stimulated ROS production is attenuated when ADP is added to the incubation medium containing the substrates [93]. Regarding reverse electron flow, Raza et al. demonstrated that electron back flow from complex III/complex IV occurs due to increased substrate-dependent activity of complex I and complex II with decreased activity of complex III and complex IV which facilitates ROS generation. However, inhibition of complex I by rotenone does not necessarily show significant elevation of ROS due to blockade of electron back flow to complex I [94].

4.3. Advanced Glycation End Products (AGEs). AGEs are a group of heterogeneous compounds produced from the nonenzymatic reaction of reducing sugars with the amino groups of proteins, lipids, and nucleic acids. Their generation involves few steps. The first step is "Maillard reaction" which involves the attachment of the carbonyl group (aldehyde or ketone) of reducing sugars with nucleophilic lysine or N-terminal amino groups of a variety of proteins, lipids, and nucleic acids to form Schiff base. In second step, the Schiff bases undergo reorganization to form more stable ketoamines called Amadori products. Amadori products are highly reactive intermediates that include α-dicarbonyls or oxoaldehydes. Examples of α-dicarbonyls are methylglyoxal, glyoxal, and 3-deoxyglucosone which are also known as precursors of AGEs. In final step, Amadori products undergo further rearrangements through oxidation, dehydration, and degradation to generate highly stable AGEs compounds [95, 96]. AGEs are categorized into 3 classes. These are (1) fluorescent cross-linking AGEs (e.g., pentosidine), (2) nonfluorescent cross-linking AGEs (e.g., imidazolium dilysine cross-links), and (3) non-cross-linking AGEs such as carboxymethyllysine (CML) which arises from the reaction of α-dicarbonyls with lysine and arginine [95]. Diabetes increases risk of forming AGEs due to high plasma glucose which plays a primary role in glycation of proteins, lipids, and nucleic acids [97].

AGEs evoke diverse physiological and pathological effects through interaction with their receptors called receptor for AGEs (RAGE). RAGE is multiligand member of immunoglobulin superfamily, usually located on the cell surface of different cells such as macrophages, adipocytes, endothelial cells, vascular endothelial muscle cells, podocytes, and mesangial cells [96, 98, 99]. RAGE comprises an extracellular VC1 ligand-binding domain [97], a single hydrophobic transmembrane domain, and a highly charged $-COOH^-$ terminal cytosolic tail that mediates intracellular signaling transduction to evoke diverse cellular effects including altered gene expression [100]. However, AGEs can also induce some receptor-independent pathological effects such as modification of structural integrity of basement membrane by cross-linking with long-lived extracellular matrix (ECM) proteins (e.g., collagen) leading to impaired matrix-matrix or matrix-cell interaction [101].

In addition to many receptor-dependent signaling effects of AGEs, ROS generation resulting from AGE-RAGE-mediated activation of NADPH oxidase and mitochondrial ETC is also prominent. For example, evidence from a study showed that interaction of AGE with its receptor RAGE in INS-1 cells caused early phase of ROS production from mitochondria. Moreover, this AGE-mediated early mitochondrial ROS in turn induce NADPH oxidase to produce more ROS, supporting the notion that AGE-RAGE interaction stimulates ROS generation via mitochondrial or NADPH oxidase pathway [102]. Consistent with this finding, Chuang et al. [103] showed that AGE-RAGE-mediated ROS generation in podocytes had been diminished when podocytes cultured in AGE-enriched medium were transfected with a RAGE-specific siRNA. In another study conducted by Wautier et al., they demonstrated that carboxymethyllysine- (CML-) RAGE-mediated activation of NADPH oxidase in human umbilical vein endothelial cells (HUVECs) significantly increased H_2O_2 production, which was diminished upon coincubation of HUVECs with sRAGE and diphenyleneiodonium (DPI), inhibitors of RAGE and NADPH oxidase respectively, suggesting the obvious role of both RAGE and NADPH oxidase in ROS generation [104].

4.4. Uncoupled NOS. Uncoupling nitric oxide synthase (NOS) is also another important enzymatic source for superoxide generation. Three quite distinct isoforms of NOS have been identified with their different location, regulation, catalytic properties, and inhibitor sensitivity. They are (1) nNOS isoform which is first (also predominantly) found in the neuronal tissue, (2) iNOS isoform which is induced in diverse cells and tissues, and (3) eNOS isoform which is first identified and usually located in vascular endothelial cells. Of these, nNOS and eNOS isoforms are constitutively expressed, whereas iNOS is inducible [105]. Physiologically, all the isoforms are responsible for the production of nitric oxide (NO) or arguably first nitroxyl anion (NO^-) followed by NO [106], which plays a pivotal role in vasodilation, anti-inflammation, and antiatherosclerosis. Nitric oxide synthase catalyzes the oxidation of its substrate L-arginine in presence of an essential cofactor called tetrahydrobiopterin (BH_4) to produce NO and L-citrulline. Absence or low levels of arginine and/or BH_4 can lead to superoxide production instead of NO and this phenomenon is known as NOS uncoupling. Moreover, the catalytic function of NOS also requires the dimerization (e.g., forms homodimers) of the enzyme, impairment of which results in $^\bullet O_2^-$ formation. During NO formation, electron is transferred from C-terminally bound NADPH (in reductase domain) to heme on the N-terminal oxygenase domain of the enzyme (via flavin centers (e.g., FDN and FMN). Reduction of NOS ferric (Fe^{3+}) heme by flavin centers enables it to bind with O_2 and subsequently form ferrous (Fe^{2+})-dioxy species as represented by $Fe^{3+} = O_2^{\bullet -} \leftrightarrow Fe^{2+} = O_2^-$. This oxygen bound ferrous heme of NOS can preferentially receive one more electron from BH_4, enabling NOS to hydroxylate L-arginine to initially form N^{ω}-hydroxyl-l-arginine that is ultimately oxidized to NO and L-citrulline. Any aberration in electron flow within NOS can dissociate ferrous-dioxy complex resulting in generation of $O_2^{\bullet -}$ instead of NO from oxygenase domain. Furthermore, in course of catalytic function of the enzyme, BH_4 is converted to $BH_3^\bullet$ or dihydrobiopterin (BH_2) which are no longer capable of reducing heme if they are not either reduced back to BH_4 or replenished by BH_4 [105, 107]. It appears that $BH_3^\bullet$ and BH_2 can be reduced back to BH_4 by flavoprotein of NOS or cellular ascorbates [107] and dihydrofolate reductase or dihydropteridine reductase [108], respectively. Additionally, BH_4 can also be synthesized from GTP by the catalytic action of GTP cyclohydrolase I (GTPCH), 6-pyruvoyl-tetrahydropterin synthase (PTPS), and sepiapterin reductase (SR) to replenish the depleted cellular levels of BH_4 [109]. Lack of any of these enzymes impairs tetrahydrobiopterin biosynthesis leading to increased superoxide and/or H_2O_2 formation by NOS (Figure 1).

All isoforms of NOS can generate superoxide in absence of L-arginine and/or cofactor tetrahydrobiopterin. For example, saphenous veins and internal mammary arteries collected from diabetic patients showed significantly elevated levels of superoxide production especially in the endothelium as demonstrated by fluorescent microtopography. In addition, either denudation of endothelium or inhibition of NOS by N-methyl-l-arginine in diabetic mammary arteries significantly reduced superoxide production suggesting the involvement of eNOS as the mediator of superoxide generation which is reversed in presence of sepiapterin, a BH_4 precursor [110]. In consistency with this study, Satoh et al. found that glomeruli isolated from streptozotocin-induced diabetic rats increased ROS levels, whereas cofactor BH_4 and eNOS dimer formation reduced significantly implicating the importance of BH_4 and eNOS dimerization in the enzyme function. However, addition of BH_4 or inhibition of eNOS by N^G-nitro-L-arginine methyl ester (L-NAME) decreased ROS generation significantly, confirming the existence of uncoupled NOS in diabetic glomeruli [55]. On the other hand, inducible NOS has also been reported to produce superoxide which is inhibited in presence of L-arginine as demonstrated by spin trapping of superoxide [111]. Likewise, neuronal NOS purified from brain also increased superoxide levels quantified by spin trapping technique which was also reduced by addition of L-arginine and NOS inhibitor L-NAME [112, 113]. However, data related to iNOS- and nNOS-mediated superoxide production in diabetic condition is still meager. It is notable that superoxide generated by either uncoupled NOS or NADPH oxidase can further react with NO generated by still existing functional NOS, leading to peroxynitrite ($ONOO^-$) formation. Peroxynitrite is a potent oxidant which not only damages cellular proteins, lipids, and nucleic acid but also oxidizes BH_4 resulting in its depletion which in turn leads to NOS uncoupling and dysfunction.

5. Fate of ROS

As per above discussion, it is clear that superoxide may produce in both physiological and pathological conditions. Once produced, superoxide is immediately neutralized by cellular superoxide dismutase (SOD) to limit its damaging effects on cellular components. Three isozymes of SOD are found in the cell. They are Cu, Zn-SOD, Mn-SOD, and EC-SOD. Among these, Cu, Zn-SOD is believed to be located in cytosol, whereas Mn-SOD and EC-SOD are thought to be localized in mitochondrial matrix and on the outer surface of cell membranes, respectively [114]. All of these isozymes are capable of dismutating superoxide to form hydrogen peroxide. Hydrogen peroxide is further converted to H_2O and O_2 by the action of catalase or glutathione peroxidase (GPx) [52]. Any imbalance between the rates of reactive oxygen species production and their neutralization may lead to accumulation of ROS resulting in oxidative stress. Chronic exposure of tissues to oxidative stress is sufficient to induce a wide range of pathophysiological events leading to eventual cell death.

6. Mechanisms of ROS-Mediated Glomerular Renal Injury in Diabetes: Onset, Progression, and End-Stage Damage

Hyperglycemia-induced onset of renal injury is marked by microalbuminuria, glomerular hemodynamic abnormalities, increased kidney and glomerular size, and hyperfiltration. Once these conditions are set in, diverse pathological events are induced due to aberrant signaling cascades with the progress of time. Impaired signaling functions cause a variety of structural and functional changes ranging from increased glomerular basement membrane (GBM) thickness, mesangial expansion, extracellular matrix deposition, glomerulosclerosis, overt proteinuria, and decreased

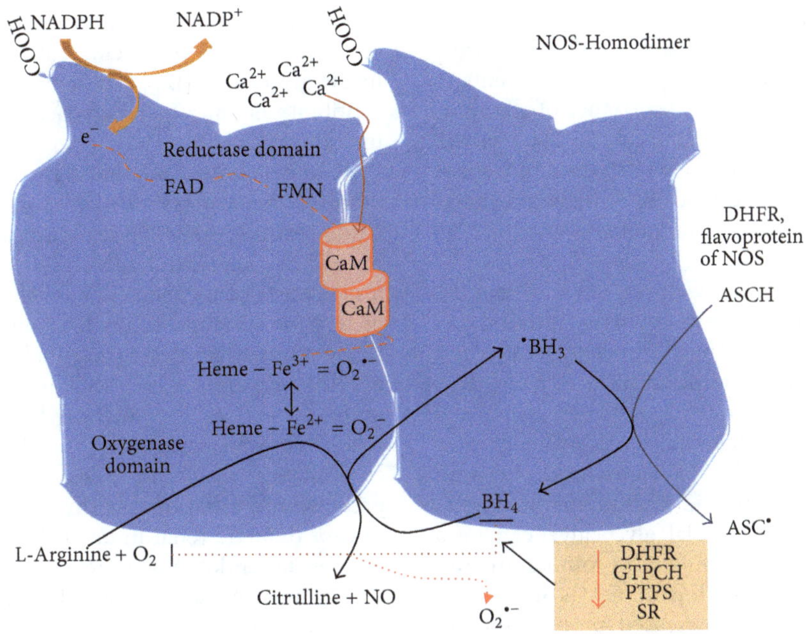

FIGURE 1: *Pictorial presentation of NO production from arginine by nitric oxide synthase (NOS).* FAD: flavin adenine dinucleotide; FMN: flavin mononucleotide; NADPH: nicotinamide-adenine-dinucleotide phosphate; CaM: calmodulin; BH_4: tetrahydrobiopterin; ASCH: ascorbic acid; DHFR: dihydrofolate reductase; GTPCH: GTP cyclohydrolase I; PTPS: 6-pyruvoyl-tetrahydropterin synthase; SR: sepiapterin reductase.

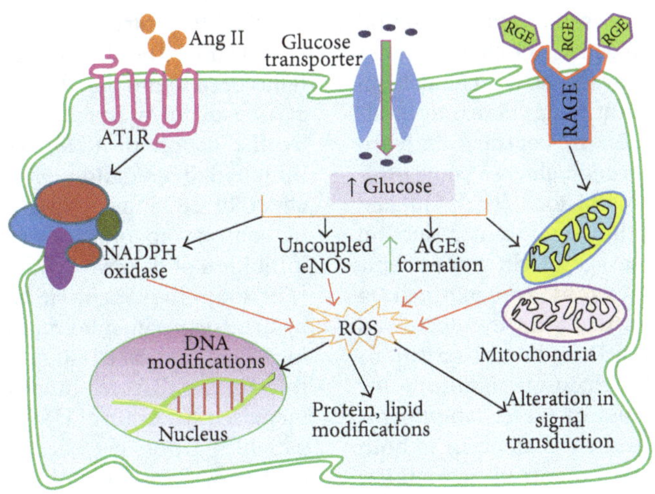

FIGURE 2: Sources of ROS generation and their impact on cellular components and signaling pathways.

glomerular function and filtration rate to eventual end-stage renal damage. Since diabetic renal injury advances through different stages of structural and functional changes in the glomerulus, we will discuss ROS-mediated renal damage in three steps: onset of injury, progression of injury, and end-stage renal damage.

6.1. Onset of Renal Injury through Microalbuminuria. There is an established notion that passage of macromolecules including albumin is highly restricted through normal glomerular capillary wall. However, increased ROS levels in diabetic milieu cause aberration in signaling pathways of different glomerular capillary layers leading to their structural or functional abnormalities which compromise on the glomerular ability of retention of macromolecules. This in turn results in increased leakage of proteins. As all the barriers constitute the capillary wall, it is assumed that each layer's damage by ROS might have a contributory role in protein leakage. Moreover, each layer is likely to communicate with other layer(s) through release of different mediators for the development and the maintenance of functional as well as structural integrity of the glomerular filtration barrier as a composite layer. For example, endothelial layer can communicate with podocytes through secretion of cytokines and growth factors and vice versa [115, 116]. Similarly, podocytes and endothelial cells can also cross-talk through the secretion of various mediators (e.g., type IV collagen) to develop the glomerular basement membrane [117]. This indicates that damage to any of the glomerular layers may induce pathological events to others resulting in excessive fractional clearance of albumin.

Earlier we have discussed microalbuminuria. Here we will focus on how microalbuminuria and hyperfiltration occur at the early phase of renal injury due to ROS-mediated effects inflicted on different glomerular filtration barriers.

6.1.1. ROS-Mediated Damage in Endothelial Layer. From the previous discussion, we have already known that luminal surface of the endothelium is covered by a layer of glycocalyx and endothelial cell coat forming endothelial surface layer (ESL). The glycocalyx is a dynamic hydrated layer largely composed of proteoglycans and glycoproteins of which proteoglycans such as glycosaminoglycans (GAGs) are enriched in heparan sulphate (HS) which gives anionic charge characteristics to the ESL. Interestingly, endothelial glycocalyx can be a major site of action of ROS and different proinflammatory cytokines, which causes degradation of GAGs leading to decreased anionic charges and increased permeability to macromolecules [118, 119]. A study conducted by Singh et al. showed that exposure of glomerular endothelial cell (GEnC) monolayer to ROS such as H_2O_2 significantly reduced heparan sulfate (HS) components of GAG and increased albumin passage across GEnC monolayers [120]. The study also found that H_2O_2 exposure does not actually inhibit biosynthesis of either total or sulfated GAG chains; rather the exposure causes increased cleavage of HS chain from GAG which was confirmed by quantifying increased levels of HS in GEnC supernatant [120]. In contrary, in vitro culture of GEnC monolayers under high glucose concentration showed decreased biosynthesis of total (both sulfated and nonsulfated) GAG chains with a significant reduction of HS biosynthesis. Moreover, cleavage of HS components from cell-associated GAG was reduced as quantified in GEnC supernatant, which is consistent with the decreased biosynthesis of GAG [121]. Taken together, these observations suggest that GAG, especially its HS chains, is significant for GEnC barrier function and the loss of these components indeed leads to leakage of proteins such as albumin in both high glucose and ROS levels. Though these are in vitro studies that might have some inherent limitations, earlier we have also discussed in vivo studies that have demonstrated similar roles of glomerular endothelial surface layer in preventing free passage of plasma proteins [28, 29]. Besides ROS, other radicals such as reactive nitrogen species (RNS) and carbon centered free radicals can also cause oxidation of core proteoglycan proteins and GAG components such as hyaluronic acid (HA), chondroitin sulfate (CS), and heparan sulfate (HS) leading to their fragmentation and the fragmentation in turn generates more free radicals resulting in aggravated condition of glycocalyx of ESL. In addition, ROS/RNS may also increase the rate of proteolysis of glycocalyx through the activation of matrix metalloproteinases (MMPs) and inhibition of endogenous protease inhibitors [122]. ROS mediated glycocalyx degradation can also be supported by ischemia/reperfusion study, where ROS resulting from ischemia-reperfusion remove endothelial glycocalyx which can be reversed by inhibition of xanthine oxidoreductase, an endogenous ROS producing enzyme bound to HS domains in the glycocalyx [123]. These observations confirm the susceptibility of endothelial glycocalyx layer to diverse radicals including ROS.

Glomerular endothelial cells have also been reported to increase the expression of dysfunctional endothelial nitric oxide synthase (eNOS) due to increased monomeric isoforms instead of dimeric in hyperglycemic condition. Either eNOS impairment or its deficiency results in increased superoxide generation as opposed to NO and the superoxide in turn can scavenge NO decreasing its bioavailability. Attenuation of NO levels impairs endothelium-dependent capillary relaxation as well as vasodilation by enhancing formation of vasoconstrictors and alters renal autoregulation which in combination results in increased glomerular intracapillary pressure and filtration rate (hyperfiltration) which is an early sign of diabetic renal injury [124–126]. Moreover, impaired glomerular endothelial functions along with defective eNOS are involved in many other pathological events that have been discussed later.

6.1.2. ROS-Mediated Damage in Glomerular Basement Membrane. Like endothelium, glomerular basement membrane is also considered to have charge- and size-selective properties because of its anionic heparan sulfate (HS) side chains attached to proteoglycan core proteins (e.g., agrin and perlecan) and extracellular matrix (ECM) network, respectively. It has been found that the heparan sulfate component of GBM can be depolymerized from its core proteoglycan proteins by the action of ROS, whereas uses of ROS scavengers inhibited degradation of HS [127]. However, there is no effect of ROS on proteoglycan core proteins [127, 128], in contrary to other studies which found ROS-mediated inhibition of de novo synthesis of core proteoglycan proteins [129, 130]. The loss of HS from GBM can also be confirmed by using experimental rat model of adriamycin nephropathy in which increased ROS levels are considered to play a role in the disease. Interestingly, this model also showed increased secession of HS from its core proteoglycan proteins, which is a possible effect of ROS [127]. Growing body of evidences showed that the loss of HS components from GBM is the prominent reason for increased permeability of GBM resulting in proteinuria [127–129] except some contradictions [38–40]. Furthermore, HS is thought to interact with other extracellular matrix proteins of GBM including collagen IV and laminin, thereby maintaining the integrity and stability of the basement membrane. Therefore, it is assumed that HS not only confers charge selectivity but also does impart size selectivity indirectly by maintaining ECM networks [127, 131]. In short, it can be said that ROS-mediated damage to HS [127] or proteoglycan core proteins [129] or ECM proteins such as laminin and collagen IV [132] is predominantly involved in increased protein leakage in a variety of human and experimental glomerular disease models.

6.1.3. ROS-Mediated Damage to Podocytes. Podocytes, also known as visceral epithelial cells, are the most restrictive barrier to macromolecules, since podocytes form slit diaphragm with very smaller pores by interdigitating neighboring foot processes that ultimately provide efficient size-based permselectivity. However, its charge selectivity for plasma proteins should not be overlooked as apical membrane domain of podocytes contains anionic surface proteins such as podocalyxin (rich in sialic acid) [133], podoplanin [134], and podoendin [135] which repel against anionic albumin to prevent their easy passage. Therefore, structural and functional integrity of podocytes and its slit diaphragm is critical to maintain restrictive fluid filtration through glomerular filtration barrier. In addition, podocytes can also contribute to the structural and functional development of other glomerular parts including GBM, GEnC, and mesangial cells by establishing a cross-talk with them through secreting various mediators. So, damage to the podocytes not only impairs glomerular permeability but also collapses the whole glomerular architecture leading to advanced renal injury. Damage to the podocytes can be reflected by the reduction of their number which is the balance between podocyte loss and proliferation where increased loss and decreased proliferation result in increased depletion of podocytes.

Hyperglycemia-induced ROS can trigger early loss of podocytes by inducing a variety of pathological events which include apoptosis, detachment of podocytes, foot process effacement, reorganization of cytoskeleton, and dysregulation of any single or a group of podocyte proteins. Due to impaired DNA synthesis and hypertrophy podocyte proliferation may be reduced during cell division [136, 137]. Moreover, cells usually may undergo programed cell death through about a dozen mechanisms that might suggest a broader mechanistic platform for podocyte loss. Some of these mechanisms may include autophagy (starvation-induced cell death), aberrant cell cycle progression (e.g., mitotic catastrophe), abnormal proliferation, anoikis (cell death due to absence of cell-matrix interactions), antosis (cell-in-cell death, cannibalism), and necrosis (upregulated lysis of the cell membrane) [138]. Though extensive discussion on all mechanisms is beyond the scope of our current review, we will briefly discuss apoptosis, detachment of podocytes, foot process effacement, autophagy, and cell cycle abnormalities as potential mechanisms of podocyte death and loss.

(1) Apoptosis. Podocytes can be a target of ROS-mediated damage, since many ROS generating pathways are activated in podocytes in high glucose ambience. Several studies have reported that multicomponent complexes of NADPH oxidase [139, 140], mitochondrial respiratory chain [141], and AGEs [142] are the major sources of ROS in podocytes. Moreover, NADPH oxidase [136, 143, 144] and mitochondrial ETC [136] are reported to be activated in podocytes cultured in high glucose, resulting in increased ROS production.

Reactive oxygen species induce dysregulation of different redox signaling cascades in the podocytes causing their apoptosis or detachment. In doing so, high glucose or ROS can upregulate and activate diverse proinflammatory cytokines and transcription factors, proapoptotic molecules, and growth factors. Recently, using type 1 and type 2 diabetic models of mice, Susztak et al. [136] demonstrated that

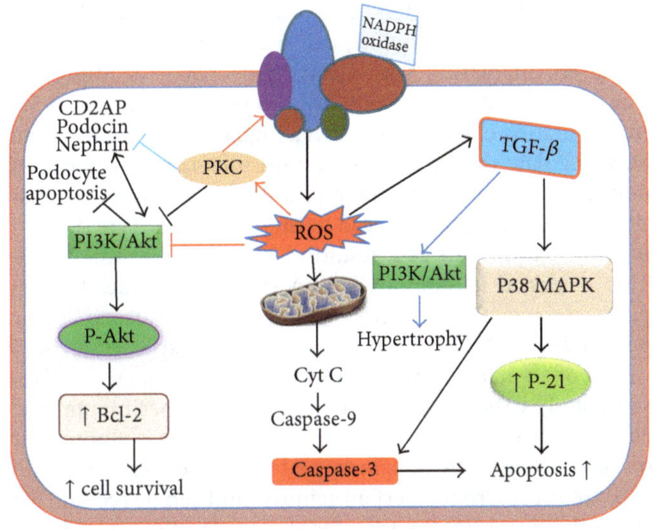

FIGURE 3: Major signaling pathways for induction of apoptosis and hypertrophy of podocyte and mesangial cells.

ROS generated from NADPH oxidase and mitochondrial pathways have significantly increased apoptosis of podocytes with the onset of diabetes through increased activation of proapoptotic mediator p38-MAPK (p38-Mitogen activated protein kinase) and caspase-3. The podocyte apoptosis precedes its depletion which leads to increased urinary albumin excretion. p38-MAPK and caspase-3 are downstream proapoptotic mediators that are required by TGF-β which is highly expressed and activated in podocytes, resulting in their increased apoptosis [145]. However, SMAD7 can independently induce podocyte apoptosis without requiring any of p38-MAPK and caspase-3 or TGF-β. Moreover, TGF-β can enhance synthesis of SMAD7 that can amplify TGF-β-induced p38-MAPK and caspase-dependent apoptosis. TGF-β can also increase Bcl2-associated X protein (Bax) expression through induction of Bax gene transcription and mitochondrial translocation of Bax protein that results in cytochrome c release from mitochondria and subsequent activation of caspase-3 (Figure 3) [146]. In consistency with these findings, Lee et al. reported that both Bax and activated caspase-3 have been significantly overexpressed in the glomeruli isolated from diabetic rats and podocytes cultured in high glucose levels with resultant apoptosis [147]. Interestingly, both high glucose and ROS levels can increasingly induce TGF-β expression in various tissues including the glomerulus [148–150]. Once TGF-β is upregulated, it can further enhance ROS generation via activation of NADPH oxidase complexes [151] and mitochondrial respiratory function [152] leading to exacerbation of TGF-β-induced apoptosis and detachment of podocytes. In addition to induction of podocyte apoptosis and detachment, TGF-β indeed activates diverse signal transduction pathways to elicit pathological changes to the architecture and function of the glomerulus which has been discussed in greater detail later.

(2) Detachment. Podocyte detachment is also promoted by ROS through activation of different signaling pathways.

Podocytes are attached to the GBM via cell surface adhesion proteins such as $\alpha3\beta1$ integrin and dystroglycans (DGs). Impaired interaction with GBM or decreased synthesis of these proteins can apparently lead to podocyte detachment. Accumulating evidences show that high glucose and ROS can downregulate the expression of $\alpha3\beta1$ integrin, an important podocyte anchoring receptor [153–155]. Decreased expression of $\alpha3\beta1$ integrin can lead to increased podocyte detachment due to loss of FPs, resulting in enhanced proteinuria. This evidence is supported by a study where deletion of podocyte-specific integrin $\alpha3$ subunit in mice caused massive proteinuria before 3 weeks and nephrotic syndrome by 6 weeks of their age [156]. Detachment of podocytes is substantiated by their presence in the urine in experimental and clinical studies of both diabetic and nondiabetic glomerular diseases. Many of these urinary podocytes are even viable and accompany micro to overt proteinuria and can be recognized as another important marker for glomerular disease [155, 157, 158].

(3) Foot Process Effacement. Foot process effacement (FPE) is characterized by retraction of the foot processes resulting in shortening of its length and increasing the width and the widening of foot processes are associated with the reduction in the podocytes number. The FPE usually replaces slit diaphragm by occluding junctions leading to sealing of the filtration slits. Reportedly, FPE is induced by reorganization of cytoskeletal proteins (e.g., α-actinin-4 and synaptopodin), dysregulation of slit diaphragm proteins, and interference with podocyte-GBM interaction which increasingly result from oxidative stress-induced injury in diabetic settings. It has been observed that deletion or mutation of any of the slit diaphragm-associated proteins such as nephrin, podocin, P-cadherin, CD2AP, and zonula occludens-1 (ZO-1) accelerates foot process effacement followed by proteinuria [137, 159]. Attenuated expression and/or increased loss of these slit proteins have also been observed in ROS-mediated diabetic and nondiabetic experimental models of glomerular abnormalities. Very recently, do Nascimento et al. [160] assessed mRNA levels of various podocyte proteins in urine collected from diabetic, prediabetic, and control patients and observed that mRNA levels of slit diaphragm proteins (e.g., nephrin and podocin) and podocyte cytoskeletal proteins (e.g., α-actinin-4 and synaptopodin) have been significantly increased in diabetic patients with normoalbuminuria, microalbuminuria, and macroalbuminuria. Increased urinary expression of these proteins in normoalbuminuric diabetic subjects suggests that podocyte damage may occur in early stage of diabetic injury. Similarly, nephrin expression has been inversely decreased with regard to ROS levels in mouse podocytes cultured in high glucose compared to normal glucose treatment group. Similar result was also found in OLETF diabetic rat models. Treatment with taurine and resveratrol (antioxidant agents) has restored nephrin mRNA levels and improved albuminuria, indicating the role of ROS in downregulation of nephrin in diabetes [161]. Furthermore, streptozotocin-induced diabetic spontaneously hypertensive rats showed decreased nephrin expression with consequent albuminuria which may result from reactive oxidants [162].

On the other hand, in nondiabetic in vivo and in vitro studies treated with puromycin aminonucleoside (PAN), loss of nephrin and podocin expression has been observed in line with increased foot process effacement and cytoskeletal actin reorganization of podocytes. Actin reorganization that is accompanied by loss of synaptopodin may induce FPE. These pathological modulations are found to be caused by an underlying mechanism of ROS generation and subsequent activation of p38-MAPK pathway. Triptolide has showed restoration of nephrin and podocin levels with remarkable improvement in cytoskeleton and foot processes by reducing ROS levels and p38-MAPK activation and ultimately decreased proteinuria [163]. In consistency with these findings, another recent study conducted by Lan et al. [164] demonstrated that slit diaphragm constituting proteins such as nephrin, podocin, and CD2AP and cytoskeletal synaptopodin are decreased in morphine treated mice with increased foot process retraction and cytoskeleton disruption. This can be attributed in part to morphine-induced oxidative stress which is likely to activate JNK, AKT, and p38 pathways. However, downregulation of nephrin, podocin, and CD2AP by activated AKT in morphine treated mice is a contradiction to the evidence that nephrin, podocin, and CD2AP themselves activate AKT via activation of PI3K to promote survival of podocytes [165]. It is pertinent to note that PI3K/AKT signaling can contribute to hypertrophy of mesangial cells upon activation by TGF-$\beta1$ [166], whereas podocytes may also undergo hypertrophic change in response to high glucose, intraglomerular pressure, and Ang II (Figure 3) [167]. Although ROS can activate PI3K/AKT signaling pathway by inducing AKT phosphorylation [54, 168], they can also be accountable for inactivation of AKT by its diminished phosphorylation [103, 169, 170]. For example, AGE-induced ROS generation as evident in diabetic milieu is likely to inhibit phosphorylation of AKT, leading to its deactivation which in turn promotes podocyte apoptosis [103]. In addition, ROS generated from mitochondrial dysfunction of aldosterone-treated podocytes (both in vitro and in vivo) are responsible for significant reduction of nephrin [141], which impairs nephrin-AKT interaction, resulting in podocyte death (Figure 3).

Moreover, diabetes is characterized not only by oxidative stress levels but also by other complications including insulin resistance, reduced adiponectin, and increased inflammatory mediators which are highly common in obese subjects. Thus, obese patients with diabetes are more susceptible to renal injury. This notion is supported by a recent study where the investigators using normoglycemic Zucker-fatty rats showed that some podocyte proteins such as nephrin, podocin, podocalyxin, and CD2AP are remarkably downregulated which can be attributed to increased oxidative and inflammatory mediators [171]. In conformation with this, Sharma et al. [172] demonstrated that obese patients with normoglycemia showed negative correlation of adiponectin with albuminuria. This indicates the importance of adiponectin in regulation of podocyte permeability by integration of SD-associated proteins. This is further supported by the findings that zona occludens-1 (ZO-1), an SD protein, can be translocated from cytoplasmic site to the plasma membrane via an AMPK-dependent pathway. Interestingly, ROS generating Nox4 can downregulate adiponectin and AMPK levels leading to impaired translocation of ZO-1 which cause increased permeability of slit diaphragm followed by excessive albuminuria. Similar observations were also found in adiponectin knock-out mice with or without diabetes suggesting that adiponectin-mediated regulation of SD permeability is critical to prevent albuminuria.

All the hyperglycemia-induced ROS-mediated pathological events discussed above are adequate to initiate protein leakage across structurally and functionally impaired glomerular barrier resulting in primary urine with excessive proteins. Though increased leakage of protein through glomerulus is the initiating point for microalbuminuria, other factors such as inability of renal tubule to increase protein reabsorption corresponding to increased protein levels in the tubular filtrate and decreased capacity of tubular reabsorption of proteins due to increased injury to the tubular cells can be held responsible for eventual increased urinary excretion of protein or albumin leading to microalbuminuria which, with progress of time, results in macroalbuminuria with advanced pathological changes in the kidney.

(4) Autophagy in Podocytes. Autophagy is an evolutionary conserved housekeeping process by which eukaryotic cells themselves degrade and recycle their cytoplasmic macromolecules and organelles in defense against cellular stress. This cellular self-degradation pathway is activated under environmental stress conditions and various pathological situations and is important for cell survival during these stressful conditions. Based on morphological and mechanistic characteristics, three forms of autophagy are recognized to date: macroautophagy, microautophagy, and chaperone-mediated autophagy (CMA) [138, 173]. Macroautophagy involves sequestration of any type of cellular contents including large organelles such as mitochondria and ribosomes within a double membrane bound vacuole called the autophagosome. In the second form of autophagy, microautophagy, cytosolic macromolecules and small organelles are directly engulfed by the lytic organelles through invagination of the lysosomal or vacuolar membrane. Chaperone-mediated autophagy is quite distinct from other types of autophagy and involves elimination of no organelles. This mechanism is selective for digestion of proteins that contain a certain amino acid sequence, namely, KFERQ (for lysine-phenylalanine-glutamate-arginine-glutamine). It has been noted that impaired CMA increases macroautophagy, implying an interaction between different forms of autophagy [173].

Podocytes are terminally differentiated cells with a limited proliferative capacity. Therefore, the fate of a podocyte depends on its ability to cope with the stress. Fortunately, podocytes exhibit a high level of autophagy even under nonstress conditions, suggesting that podocytes need to keep cellular homeostasis under basal conditions [174].

Evidently, autophagy plays an important renoprotective role by mainly maintaining homeostasis of podocytes in diabetic nephropathy. It has been manifested by podocyte-specific expression of autophagy related proteins such as Beclin-1, Atg5–Atg12, and LC3 (rat microtubule-associated protein 1 light chain 3) which results in increased basal level of autophagy in podocytes [175]. However, under certain diabetic conditions, including high glucose in vitro conditions, high basal levels of autophagy in podocytes became defective and defective autophagy facilitates podocyte injury. This evidence is supported by decreased expression of Beclin-1, Atg5–Atg12, and LC3 both in podocytes of STZ-induced diabetic mice and in cells cultured in high glucose [175]. In agreement with this observation, a very recent study showed insufficient autophagy in podocytes of diabetic patients and rodents with massive proteinuria which indicates autophagy to be implicated in the pathogenesis of diabetic nephropathy [176].

The mechanism underlying diabetes-induced impairment of podocyte autophagy is still ambiguous. However, in podocytes of diabetic mice and patients, mTORC1 (mammalian target of rapamycin complex 1) is highly activated and may be involved in the mechanisms of diabetes-induced autophagy inhibition in podocytes [177]. Interestingly, increased mTOR activity accompanied by human diabetic nephropathy induces early glomerular hypertrophy and hyperfiltration, whereas genetic deletion of mTORC1 in mouse podocytes results in proteinuria and progressive glomerulosclerosis, suggesting the requirement for tightly balanced mTOR activity in podocyte homeostasis [177]. Moreover, podocyte-specific activation of mTORC1 results in many features of DN, such as mesangial expansion, glomerular basement membrane (GBM) thickening, podocyte loss, and proteinuria in nondiabetic mice. Since mTORC1 attenuates autophagy, inhibition of mTORC1 can restore the autophagy of podocytes to basal levels resulting in the improvement of the features of diabetic nephropathy [178]. This has been supported by evidence that treatment of experimental models of type 1 and type 2 diabetic animals with the mTORC1 inhibitor, rapamycin, reduced the development of diabetic nephropathy [179].

Cell Cycle Abnormalities in Podocytes. The cell cycle involves five tightly controlled phases, that is, G_0 (resting) phase, G_1 phase, S phase, G_2 phase, and M (mitosis) phase. Proper cell cycle progression through all these phases can give rise to new cells which is very important for cellular homeostasis in tissue. Cell cycle entry begins with G_1 phase and ends within G_0 phase where newly divided cells remain quiescent and fulfill their physiological functions with the tissue. Mature podocytes are thought to be quiescent cells arrested in G_0 (resting) phase. The cell cycle has also some integrated checkpoints to ensure the fidelity of the cell division. For example, the first checkpoint, G_1/S, checks for the presence of damage DNA, and if any damaged DNA is found, it stalls for DNA repair. The G_2/M checkpoint will determine whether or not the cell proceeds to complete mitosis. Finally, metaphase or spindle checkpoints ensure proper chromosome alignment prior to cell division. In addition, normal cell cycle functions are regulated by three classes of proteins: cyclic proteins (cyclins), cyclin-dependent kinases (CDKs), and cyclin-dependent kinase inhibitors (CKIs). Podocytes express cyclin A, B1, and D1 as well as CDK inhibitors, such as p21, p27, and p57. Any abnormality in cell cycle components and/or checkpoints which is beyond the scope of automatic repair (e.g., DNA damage) may warrant for cell cycle arrest at distinct restriction points mediated by p53 and p27 cell cycle regulatory proteins [138, 180].

Mature podocytes reduce expression of Ki-67, a proliferation marker, cyclin A, and cyclin B1, while CKIs and cyclin D1 are intensively increased. Cyclins and CDKs can be modulated in human and experimental podocyte injury. For example, in the cellular type of human FSGS (focal segmental glomerulosclerosis), studies have found absent p27, p57, and cyclin D1 expression and increased cyclin E, cyclin A, cyclin B1, CDK2, and p21 [138]. In adriamycin-induced podocyte injury, the presence of CDK inhibitor p21 is protective for podocytes in this model of toxic podocytopathy. Conversely, in membranous nephropathy, podocytes upon immune-mediated injury increase DNA synthesis in S phase and upregulation of cyclin A and CDK2 and finally enter mitosis but are unable to divide resulting in multinucleated podocytes [180].

Podocyte hypertrophy is a characteristic of diabetic nephropathy. It occurs in different diabetic animal models due to increased expression of CKIs. For example, Zucker diabetic rats and db/db mice, both models of type 2 diabetes, or type 1 models, induced by streptozotocin administration, increase the expression of p27 and p21 resulting in podocyte's cell cycle arrest in response to injury induced DNA damage and this in turn causes glomerular hypertrophy and development of progressive renal failure [180, 181]. Interestingly, exposure of cultured mouse podocytes to cyclic mechanical stretch showed decrease in cyclins D1, A, and B1 and increase in CDK inhibitors p21 and p27, prompting the podocyte to adopt a hypertrophic phenotype [181]. Similarly, AGEs which are abundantly produced in hyperglycemic milieu can induce podocyte hypertrophy through upregulation of CDK inhibitor p27, which causes cell cycle arrest [57]. All these cell cycle related abnormalities are prominent during the early stages of diabetic nephropathy which may progress toward irreversible damage through changes of podocytes from their hypertrophic to increased apoptotic phenotypes.

6.2. Glomerular Hyperfiltration. Increased glomerular filtration rate (GFR) or hyperfiltration also marks the early sign of diabetic renal injury and may play a major role in the pathogenesis of diabetic nephropathy. Glomerular hyperfiltration occurs due to increased dilation of afferent arterioles leading to increased blood flow to the glomeruli. This afferent arteriolar dilation can be attributed to increased prostaglandin E2 synthesis, impaired responsiveness to vasoconstrictors (i.e., thromboxane and norepinephrine), elevated levels of atrial natriuretic peptide (ANP), and hyperglycemia-mediated inactivation of tubuloglomerular feedback (TGF) [182]. In diabetes, inactivated TGF results from increased glucose reabsorption along with Na^+ from the proximal tubule leading to decreased sodium delivery to macula densa (MD) cells. This phenomenon can further be interpreted by the fact that hyperglycemia usually increases glucose concentration in tubular filtrate and upregulates expression of both sodium glucose linked transporters-1 and -2 (SGLT1 and SGLT2) in the proximal tubule that causes increased cotransportation of glucose and Na^+ [182, 183]. However, role of TGF in hyperfiltration in diabetes has been debated since A1 adenosine-receptor (AA1R) null mice, previously shown to lack a functional TGF, still exhibit pronounced hyperfiltration when diabetes is induced [183, 184]. In addition, diabetic hyperfiltration may also result from increased pressure gradient across glomerular membrane which arises from increased capillary hydrostatic/colloidal pressure and reduced hydrostatic pressure in Bowman's capsule or proximal tubule. Interestingly, pressure in the proximal tubule is reduced due to increased reabsorption of Na^+ and Cl^- resulting from persistent hyperglycemia-mediated oxidative stress [183]. Additionally, prostaglandin E_2 (PGE_2) mediated reduction of hyperfiltration was explained by Kiritoshi et al. who showed increased PGE_2 synthesis in human mesangial cells (HMCs). They also found that prostaglandins synthesis in HMCs is increased due to ROS-mediated upregulation of cyclooxygenase-2 (COX-2) mRNA and increased activation of NF-κB. Prostaglandins in turn may modulate afferent arteriolar vasoconstriction after stimulation of TGF [185]. Moreover, high glomerular capillary pressure elicited from increased vasoconstriction of efferent arterioles also may contribute to hyperfiltration [186].

7. Progression of Renal Injury through Diverse Signaling Pathways

Though microalbuminuria may be initiating step for glomerular damage, progression of damage actually is achieved through activation of diverse pathological pathways. We have already discussed some of the signaling molecules that evoke some structural and functional damage to the filtration barrier to increase glomerular permeability. Now we will have a holistic view on some more signaling mediators in greater detail which are responsible for advanced pathological damage to the glomerulus if initial symptoms are not corrected. Of note, signaling mediators can be activated in any part of the glomerulus in response to high glucose, AGEs, and/or ROS. However, their activation in any glomerular cell type may affect surrounding cells as the whole glomerulus acts as a coordinated unit to regulate its functions.

7.1. Protein Kinase C (PKC). PKC is also an important signaling molecule playing central role in glomerular injury. In high glucose ambience, PKC is activated by diacylglycerol (DAG), a signaling molecule increasingly produced from an intermediate product of glycolytic pathway such as glyceraldehyde-3-phosphate (G3P) which is abundantly produced from high glucose flux into glycolytic pathway. Interestingly, under high glucose conditions, PKC can also be activated by higher concentrations of ROS, perhaps through tyrosine phosphorylation or DAG synthesis. Moreover, PKC-β2 can stimulate NADPH oxidase to produce more ROS resulting in vicious cycle of enhanced PKC activation (Figure 3) [187–189]. Activation of PKC (e.g., PKC-α) causes proteinuria by degradation of nephrin of slit diaphragm. Activated PKC

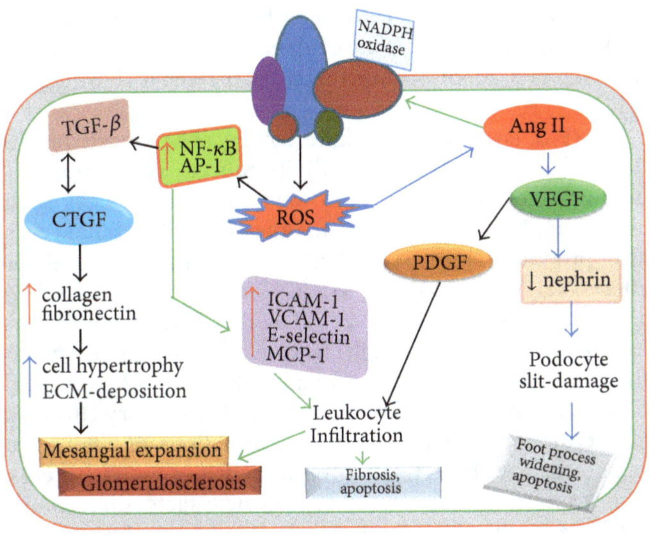

FIGURE 4: Major signaling pathways for induction of ECM accumulation following mesangial expansion, increased GBM, glomerulosclerosis, and fibrosis. This results in subsequent end-stage renal damage.

can also attenuate expression of P-cadherin mRNA and protein in experimental glomeruli and high glucose-stimulated podocytes, which suggests a potential role of P-cadherin loss in the development of excessive proteinuria [187, 190]. In addition, the activated PKC can promote endothelial dysfunction and increased production of endothelin-1, TGF-β, VEGF, and NF-κB leading to alteration in blood flow, capillary permeability, and extracellular matrix deposition.

7.2. Transcription Factors

Nuclear Factor-Kappa B (NF-κB). This is a redox-sensitive transcription factor that can be activated by a wide variety of stimuli including oxidative stress in various renal cells such as podocytes and endothelial, mesangial, and tubular cells [191]. ROS-mediated activation of NF-κB can interfere with the transcription of a wide range of proinflammatory and profibrotic genes coding for cytokines, adhesion molecules, and growth factors causing vascular dysfunction, atherosclerosis, and inflammation. Therefore, proinflammatory cytokines such as TNF-α, IL-1β, IL-2, IL-6, and IL-12, leukocyte adhesion molecules (e.g., E-selectin, VCAM-1, and ICAM-1), growth factors (TGF-β), and chemokines (MCP-1) are upregulated during persistent oxidative stress-induced NF-κB activation (Figure 4) [192]. In resting cells, NF-κB is continuously present in inactive state, when NF-κB remains bound to the inhibitory IκB proteins, preventing its translocation to nucleus. Activation of NF-κB requires the phosphorylation of IκB which causes ubiquitination of IκB implying its destruction by proteasome. IκB kinases (IKK) can phosphorylate IκB to facilitate ubiquitination and degradation of IκB followed by release of IκB-bound NF-κB, thereby translocating NF-κB to the nucleus to initiate gene transcription [191]. However, ROS have also been considered to phosphorylate IκB on its tyrosine residue instead of serine; the latter is usually seen in IKK-mediated phosphorylation, thus translocating NF-κB to the nucleus. Besides ROS-mediated activation, however, ROS have also been reported to inhibit NF-κB binding with DNA by oxidizing its Rel homology domain in nuclear region showing differential roles in cytoplasm and nucleus. These differences can be attributed to the study of different upstream pathways and cell-specific differences [193].

7.3. Activator Protein-1 (AP-1). AP-1 is another redox-regulated transcription factor involved in transcription of various inflammatory genes in response to activation by diverse stimuli. ROS can activate AP-1 through phosphorylation of upstream MAPKs such as ERK and p38 kinases as shown by a study [194]. In another study, it was shown that high glucose can lead to PKCβ1-mediated ROS generation through NADPH oxidase with subsequent RhoA activation in mesangial cells. This RhoA in turn activates downstream AP-1 through Rho kinase leading to activation of TGF-β1 [195]. In consistency with these observations, Weigert et al. [196] demonstrated that AP-1 activation is responsible for increased TGF-β1 expression through PKC- and p38-MAPK-dependent pathways.

7.4. Hypoxia Inducible Factor (HIF). HIF is a heterodimeric transcription factor that is composed of two subunits, an oxygen sensitive HIF-α subunit and a constitutively expressed HIF-β subunit. HIF-1α was the first isoform of HIF-α to be cloned. HIF-1α is activated in response to cellular hypoxia and induces transcription of various genes encoding erythropoietin, VEGF, glucose transporters, CTGF, and PAI-1, all of which are considered to aggravate extracellular matrix deposition in the glomerulus. Hypoxia, a common inducer of HIF-1α, can occur in the diabetic kidney resulting from increased consumption of oxygen by renal tubule and superoxide-mediated increased Na-K-2Cl cotransporter activity in the thick ascending limb (TAL) [197, 198]. In high glucose condition, HIF-1α has been upregulated in mesangial cells as evidenced in streptozotocin-induced diabetic mice and in vitro studies. Moreover, in addition to hypoxia, other factors such as angiotensin II, TGF-β1, PKC, and ROS which are found to be upregulated in diabetes can also activate HIF-1α, thereby exacerbating glomerular injury even in nonhypoxic condition [9]. For example, a study reported that Ang II increased HIF-1α protein levels in mesangial cells through stimulation of ROS generation which in turn activate PI3K/Akt pathway [199]. Since HIF-1α is capable of increasing transcription of profibrotic genes, it can greatly contribute to the renal fibrosis in diabetes with or without hypoxia leading to end-stage renal failure [200].

Other transcription factors including CREB (c-AMP-response-element-binding protein), NFAT (nuclear factor of activated T cells), and Sp1 (stimulating protein 1) are also activated in hyperglycemic milieu. These transcription factors can also regulate genes related to inflammation and ECM turnover [201]. Ang II-mediated podocyte injury can be induced by CREB which carries signal from calmodulin-dependent protein kinase II (CaMK II) to downstream Wnt/β-catenin signaling pathway to increase Wnt mRNA expression and β-catenin phosphorylation leading to inhibition of podocin and nephrin expression. Inhibition of CREB has improved podocyte injury by restoring podocin and nephrin levels confirming its role in renal injury [202].

7.5. Inflammatory Cytokines. Cytokines are small, nonstructural proteins with low molecular weights having autocrine, paracrine, and juxtacrine effects and very complex activities. They can act as regulators of host response to infection, immune response, trauma, and inflammation with their both pro- and anti-inflammatory role based on the type of cell, the time of action, and cellular environment. There are a lot of proinflammatory cytokines that can be activated in response to high glucose or oxidative stress. These include IL-1, IL-6, IL-18, and TNF-α which are mainly involved in the development and progression of diabetic nephropathy [203]. These cytokines are also transcribed by various transcription factors in inflammatory conditions.

IL-1β expression is increased in the glomeruli of streptozotocin-induced diabetic rat model which has been accompanied by augmentation in chemokines (MCP-1) and cell adhesion molecules (VCAM-1 and ICAM-1) expression. Macrophage infiltration can accompany MCP-1, VCAM-1, and ICAM-1 overexpression in different renal cells, including endothelial, mesangial, and tubular epithelial cells and also concomitantly overexpress α1-chain type IV collagen. This effects cause structural changes in renal cells by accumulating ECM proteins resulting in glomerulosclerosis in both type 1 and type 2 diabetic models [204, 205].

IL-6 has also been reported to be significantly high in type 2 diabetic patients with nephropathy (DN) in comparison to DM patients without DN. Analysis of kidney biopsies in patients with type 2 DN evidenced increased expression of IL-6 in cells infiltrating mesangium, interstitium, and tubules. Moreover, there is a positive relationship between mesangial expansion (glomerulopathy) and expression of IL-6 mRNA in both mesangial cells and podocytes, implying an important role of IL-6 in influencing extracellular matrix dynamics at mesangial and podocyte levels [206]. Recently, Choudhary and Ahlawat analyzed serum levels of IL-6 in type 2 diabetic patients to find a correlation between IL-6 and albuminuria. They have found significant positive correlation between IL-6 and albuminuria, suggesting contributory role of IL-6 in renal injury [207]. In conformation with this observation, another study also found positive correlation between IL-6 and UAE in type 1 DM patients [208]. These observations implicate IL-6 as having pathological role in diabetic renal injury progression toward renal failure.

IL-18 is potent inflammatory cytokine that is involved in different functions, such as induction of interferon-γ (IFN-γ) [209], production of proinflammatory cytokines (IL-1 and TNF-α) [210], overexpression of ICAM and VCAM molecules [210, 211], and increased apoptosis of endothelial cells via TNF-α and Fas (members of TNF family) [212]. IFN-γ further stimulates functional chemokine receptors expression in human mesangial cells [213]. Interestingly, similar to IL-6, IL-18 has also been reported to be enhanced in serum and urine samples of patients with diabetic nephropathy compared to controlled subjects, and higher IL-18 levels in turn increase UAE as evidenced by many clinical studies [214–216]. Therefore, it is evident that elevated IL-18 in diabetes is a predisposing threat to the renal dysfunction [216].

TNF-α is another cytokine having pronounced proinflammatory roles and mainly produced in monocytes, macrophages, and T cells. However, host renal cells such as mesangial, glomerular, endothelial, and tubular cells also produce TNF-α [217–220]. TNF-α mediates cellular effects via two receptors: (1) TNF-α receptor-1 (TNFR1) and (2) TNF-α receptor-2 (TNFR2). TNFR1 modulates immune response through IL-6 synthesis and apoptosis through apoptotic signal-regulating kinase-1 (ASK-1) and NF-κB, whereas TNFR2 mediates proinflammatory effects in glomerulonephritis [205]. Prominent actions of TNF-α on renal cells are the activation of second messenger systems, transcription factors, synthesis of growth factors, receptors, cytokines, cell adhesion molecules, and more importantly promotion of local ROS generation in diverse cells, including mesangial cells [206, 221]. TNF-α can also induce changes of intraglomerular blood flow and GFR resulting from hemodynamic imbalances between vasoconstrictors and vasodilators [222] and alters endothelial permeability. In addition, it can alter location of receptors involved in cell-cell adhesion and prevents the formation of F-actin stress fibers leading to modification of intercellular junctions followed by loss of endothelial permeability [223]. TNF-α can also induce cytotoxicity and apoptosis [224, 225]. Many experimental diabetic rat models showed increased TNF-α levels in renal cortex [226, 227], whereas clinical data of type 2 diabetic patients exhibited higher serum levels of TNF-α with significant microalbuminuria [214].

7.6. Other Cytokines/Growth Factors (GFs). Growth factors are activated by different effectors to induce secretion of matrix forming proteins to increase mesangial expansion as well as GBM thickness and express many cellular entities to promote cellular hypertrophy, apoptosis, and foot process effacement. Major GFs that play critical role in the pathogenesis of renal injury include TGF-β, VEGF, CTGF, and PDGF.

7.6.1. Transforming Growth Factor-β (TGF-β). TGF-β is a widely studied multifunctional cytokine that modulates cell proliferation, differentiation, apoptosis, adhesion, and migration of diverse cell types and induces the production of ECM proteins. TGF-β is expressed in many cell types including immature hematopoietic cells, activated T and B cells, macrophages, neutrophils, and dendritic cells which are sensitive to its effects [145]. It induces podocyte apoptosis via different downstream effectors including p38-MAPK, Smad, Bax, and caspase 3 (discussed above). Moreover, podocyte apoptosis can also be induced through TGF-β-mediated p21, a cyclin-dependent kinase (CDK) inhibitor [228]. This idea is supported by the findings that, like TGF-β, p21 has been reported to be increased in different experimental models of glomerular diseases such as membranous nephropathy (PHN model) [229], streptozotocin-induced diabetic nephropathy [230], and minimal change nephropathy. Wada et al. [228] reported that TGF-β increases p21 levels in cultured podocytes which coincides with their increased apoptosis. This is confirmed by the findings that TGF-β treatment of p21-null podocytes in culture decreased apoptosis, whereas wild type enhanced apoptotic response. However, transfection of p21 in p21-null podocytes has retained the apoptotic response to TGF-β, suggesting the implication of p21 as a downstream effector in TGF-β-induced apoptosis. Moreover, TGF-β can also induce apoptosis mesangial and glomerular endothelial cells. In addition, p21 and its another family member, p27, can also induce hypertrophy of mesangial cells as well as podocytes by inhibiting cell cycle progression [138, 230].

In addition to its apoptotic role, TGF-β can stimulate MCs to induce ECM deposition by producing types I, III, and IV collagen, laminin, and fibronectin and by inhibiting matrix degrading proteins called MMPs. Matrix expansion results in mesangial cell hypertrophy and apoptosis and decreases glomerular surface area for fluid filtration which leads to gradual diminution of GFR. In addition, TGF-β can also promote similar ECM-producing proteins in GBM, thereby increasing its thickness [231, 232]. Interestingly, high glucose, AGEs, and ROS push the disease forward to more complications by inducing TGF-β and other matrices and apoptosis influencing effector molecules. Increased mesangial expansion and GBM thickness ultimately cause more podocyte apoptosis advancing the disease toward renal failure.

7.6.2. Vascular Endothelial Growth Factor (VEGF). VEGF being expressed predominantly by podocytes and in some cases by mesangial cells in the kidney can induce angiogenesis and vascular permeability. VEGF elicits its action by interacting with its receptor located on the endothelium and mesangial cells [233, 234]. Many experimental diabetic rat models, such as type 1 (STZ-induced diabetic rats) and type 2 (e.g., Otsuka-Long-Evans-Tokushima-Fatty (OLETF) rats and Zucker Diabetic Fatty (ZDF-rats)) rats, demonstrated elevated expression of VEGF mRNA in the glomerulus [235–237]. In in vitro study, podocytes cultured in high glucose increases VEGF mRNA expression by increasing PKC-mediated ROS production, while antioxidant therapy reversed the expression implying an important role of ROS in the pathogenesis of podocyte injury in diabetic renal disease [238].

At initial stage, though VEGF increases filtration rate accompanied by microalbuminuria via enhanced neoangiogenesis, its subsequent reduction resulting from increased podocyte loss during progressive period of the disease eventually diminishes GFR [239]. This is supported by increased urinary excretion of VEGF and its high mRNA expression in the glomerulus during early stage of diabetic nephropathy in OLETF rats [235]. Interestingly, increased urinary VEGF levels showed a significant positive correlation with UAE and serum creatinine indicating its role in the pathogenesis of renal injury [235].

Though many studies exhibited the salutary effects of anti-VEGF agents to treat diabetic nephropathy, some other studies have shown potential complications associated with anti-VEGF treatment. Studies have found that administration of anti-VEGF neutralizing antibodies can significantly decrease hyperfiltration, albuminuria, and glomerular hypertrophy [240–242]. Furthermore, inhibition of VEGF binding with its receptor or impairment of VEGF receptor-mediated downstream signaling by sFlt-1 (soluble VEGF receptor-1) in podocytes has effectively improved diabetes-induced albuminuria, mesangial expansion, GBM thickening, podocyte foot process fusion, and TGF-β expression in diabetic mice [243]. In agreement with this study, Sung et al. [244] showed that inhibition of VEGF receptor phosphorylation through blocking the VEGF-tyrosine kinase activity ameliorated albuminuria, GBM thickening, and restored nephrin levels in diabetic mice. It is interesting to note that some collagen derivatives such as tumstatin (cleavage product of collagen IV) and endostatin (cleavage product of collagen XVIII) have been reported to prevent neovascularization in streptozotocin-induced diabetic mice by inhibiting some angiogenic factors including VEGF and suppressed glomerular hypertrophy, hyperfiltration, and albuminuria [245, 246]. Similarly, these peptides have decreased glomerular mesangial expansion, extracellular matrix accumulation, monocyte/macrophage deposition, TGF-β expression (inhibited only by endostatin), and type IV collagen expression which are potential pathological events induced in diabetic nephropathy. However, both peptides significantly increased nephrin expression in podocyte maintaining the integrity of slit-diaphragm leading to prevention of excess protein leakage [245, 246]. Recently, sulodexide, a compound made up of heparan and dermatan sulfate types of GAGs, has suppressed podocyte-specific VEGF synthesis through inhibition of high glucose-induced p38-MAPK in OLETE rats, a type 2 diabetic animal model, and it has elicited all aforementioned anti-VEGF agent-mediated renoprotective effects including decreased urinary albumin excretion and expression of profibrotic molecules [247]. Taken together, these results suggest that antiangiogenic therapy might be helpful in maintaining the glomerular barrier, resulting in the amelioration of albuminuria and other nephrotic syndromes.

In contrast to these renoprotective effects, many investigations found deleterious effects associated with anti-VEGF therapy for neoplastic diseases. These deleterious effects may include but are not limited to proteinuria, hypertension, and thrombotic microangiopathy [248, 249]. For instance, cancer patients treated with bevacizumab, a humanized monoclonal antibody against VEGF, experienced aggravated pathological events including proteinuria, hypertension, extensive foot process effacement, and thrombotic microangiopathy [250]. Administration of anti-VEGF agent, mutation, or gene deletion of podocyte-specific VEGF in murine models also exhibited similar adverse consequences. In addition, some studies have shown a beneficial role of VEGF which includes the prevention of progressive capillary rarefaction, promotion of capillary repair, improvement of renal injury, and prevention of functional and histologic abnormalities in diabetic nephropathy [250, 251]. In support of this evidence, Oltean et al.'s [251] transgenic podocyte-specific overexpression of VEGF-A165b in streptozotocin-induced diabetic mice demonstrated less glomerular hypertrophy, less mesangial expansion, and less GBM thickening. Similarly, systemic administration of VEGF-A165b in streptozotocin-induced diabetic mice improved proteinuria and GBM thickening but not mesangial expansion [251]. Based on these studies, it is obvious that VEGF expression should be optimum in renal cells, imbalance of which triggers injurious effects manifested by nephrotic syndromes and cardiovascular abnormalities.

7.6.3. Connective Tissue Growth Factor (CTGF). CTGF is an important downstream mediator of TGF-β1 signaling cascade and executes profibrotic as well as hypertrophic functions of TGF-β1 [252, 253]. Therefore, CTGF plays a pivotal role in TGF-β1-induced ECM production which causes mesangial expansion and increased GBM thickness leading to glomerulosclerosis and interstitial fibrosis, the progressive stage of renal injury [254, 255]. It also induces hypertrophy of mesangial cells through activation of $p21^{Cip1}$ and $p27^{kip1}$ and causes functional impairment as well as loss of podocytes resulting in diminished regulatory functions of the glomerulus [253, 256]. In addition, CTGF can activate proinflammatory signaling molecule NF-κB which in turn upregulates various chemokines (e.g., MCP-1 and ICAM-1) and cytokines (e.g., IL-6 and IL-4) leading to increased interstitial infiltration of immune cells such as monocytes/macrophages and/or T cells to worsen renal injury [257]. In diabetic condition, CTGF is upregulated in mesangial cells and podocytes to advance its fibrotic process which is aggravated by CTGF-mediated inhibition of matrix degradation through increased production of TIMPs (tissue inhibitor of metalloproteinases) [258].

7.6.4. Platelet-Derived Growth Factor (PDGF). PDGF is a cytokine that is involved in mediating and modulating many biological processes which occurred during renal injury. PDGF mediates its diverse effects, including proliferation, differentiation, extracellular matrix accumulation, tissue permeability, pro- as well as anti-inflammatory mediators, and migration of mesenchymal cells. It evokes its actions by interacting with its receptor, PDGFR, which can be expressed on mesenchymal, mesangial, and glomerular endothelial cells. PDGF is also important for physiological angiogenesis by the recruitment of perivascular cells, for example, pericytes, and it regulates vascular tone and platelet aggregation. PDGF binding with its receptor can trigger many signaling pathways, for example, Ras-MAPK, JAK/STAT, PLC-γ, and PI3K pathways, to induce transcription of genes involved in proliferation, migration, and survival. In renal injury, PDGF causes pronounced mesangial cell proliferation resulting in mesangioproliferative nephritis and renal interstitial fibrosis. PDGF-mediated stimulation of MC also promotes increased expression of many inflammatory mediators, including TGF-β1, PAI-1, IL-6, endothelin-1, and iNOS to increase extracellular matrix production, intraglomerular pressure, and vascular resistance, thus reducing renal blood flow as well as GFR [257, 259, 260].

7.6.5. Adhesion Molecules. Adhesion molecules such as ICAM-1 (intercellular adhesion molecule-1) and VCAM-1 (vascular cell adhesion molecule-1) play crucial role in infiltration of immune cells to endothelium, mesangium, and GBM. Invasion of immune cells (leukocytes) follows few steps: cell tethering, selectin-mediated rolling of cell on the endothelium, chemokine-dependent integrin activation and leukocyte adhesion, and finally transmigration of leukocytes across the endothelium. Interestingly, these processes can be advanced by the help of any adhesion molecules mentioned above to initiate immune response in local tissues [261].

ICAM-1 is a cell surface glycoprotein belonging to Ig superfamily and binds to β_2 integrins, such as lymphocyte function-associated antigen-1 (LFA-1) and macrophage-1 antigen (Mac-1), which are located on most leukocytes, thereby helping leukocytes to firmly attach to the endothelium. ICAM-1 is upregulated in response to certain kinds of stimuli, such as proinflammatory cytokines (e.g., TNF-α and IL-1), high glucose, AGEs, oxidative stress, shear stress, and protein kinase C activation [262, 263]. In addition, ICAM-1 expression is also upregulated in both type 1 [264] and type 2 [265] models of diabetic nephropathy accompanied by disease progression. In order to ascertain damaging role of ICAM-1 in type 2 diabetic nephropathy, Chow et al. [266] evaluated the development of renal injury in both ICAM-1 intact and deficient db/db mice with similar glucose level and obesity and found that ICAM-1 deficient db/db mice showed significantly attenuated glomerular hypertrophy and renal fibrosis accompanied by reduced glomerular and interstitial infiltration of macrophages. Similarly, Okada et al. [267] showed that ICAM-1 knock-out mice have been able to prevent the progression of albuminuria, glomerular infiltration of macrophages, glomerular hypertrophy, and interstitial fibrosis at 6 months after the induction of diabetes mellitus, whereas ICAM-$1^{+/+}$ demonstrated the opposite outcome. However, degree of albuminuria between ICAM-1-null mice and wild type mice was not different at 1 month after the injection of streptozotocin suggesting noninvolvement of ICAM-1 in increased albuminuria in the early stages of diabetic renal injury. Taken together, it is evident that OCAM-1-mediated inflammation observed in the diabetic kidney probably contributes to the progression of the disease rather than its onset.

VCAM-1, a member of Ig superfamily, is also a cell surface protein expressed on endothelial cells and some leukocytes such as macrophages and helps in their adhesion. It has been reported to be overexpressed on endothelial cells and infiltrating leukocytes in renal interstitium in diabetic animal models. In type 2 diabetes, serum level of VCAM-1 is likely to be increased and it positively correlates with albuminuria [262]. VCAM-1 expression is increased in response to several stimuli, including TNF-α, IFN-γ [268], high glucose, AGEs, oxidative stress, and Ang II [269].

7.7. Chemokines. Chemokines are small cytokines that are secreted by cells/leukocytes to induce recruitment of leukocytes to nearby host cells. They are induced and activated by primary proinflammatory mediators, for example, IL-1 and TNF-α. There are some common chemokines, such as MCP-1, MIP-1 α/β, and RANTES, which play crucial role in vascular and renal inflammation. They are briefly discussed below.

7.7.1. Monocyte Chemotactic Protein-1 (MCP-1). This is a potent chemokine belonging to CC chemokine family that is also recognized as chemokine (C-C motif) ligand 2 (CCL2). MCP-1 plays a key role in migration of monocytes, T cells, and macrophages to the diabetic kidney. In diabetic nephropathy, MCP-1 can be excessively produced by both inflammatory and renal resident cells which in turn induce progressive glomerular and tubule-interstitial injury by increasing macrophage infiltration. Its increased expression in type 2 diabetes is confirmed by its elevated urinary excretion accompanied with progressive tubulointerstitial damage [270]. It has been reported that MCP-1 is upregulated in response to high glucose concentrations, AGEs, oxidative stress, protein kinase C, and Ang II. Increased MCP-1 level in urine has been positively correlated with albumin excretion. However, diabetic MCP-1-null mice reduced macrophage infiltration and progression of diabetic renal injury [271, 272]. Based on these observations, it is evident that hyperglycemia-induced overexpression of MCP-1 eventually causes more advanced damage to the kidney.

In addition, macrophage inflammatory protein-1α (also known as CCL3) and CCL5/RANTES (regulated on activation, normal T cell expressed and secreted) are also upregulated in diabetic kidney. Increasing evidence shows that MIP-1α is overproduced and functionally activated to induce migration of T cells and macrophages to the kidney during diabetic and nondiabetic chronic kidney diseases [273, 274]. MIP-1α is increased in urine of patients with crescentic glomerulonephritis, whereas its cognate receptors, CCR1 and CCR5, are expressed In $CD3^{++}$ T cells and CD 68^{+} macrophages which infiltrate the glomeruli and interstitium. CCR5 acts as receptor for several ligands including MIP-1α, MIP-1β, and RANTES and its activation correlates with the recruitment of T cells and monocytes, whereas deletion of this receptor does not decrease but increases the degree of inflammatory cells' infiltration because of increased interaction of ligands with still intact CCR1 receptor. However, deletion of blockade of CCR1 significantly attenuates renal chemokine expression, T cell infiltration, and glomerular crescent formation in CCR5 knock-out mice. This suggests the functional importance of CCR1 receptor and its all ligands in ultimate renal injury [273].

7.8. Vasoactive Substances. These are circulating substances that regulate vascular tone and systemic as well as local blood pressure. Among many, angiotensin II and endothelin have been reported to be increased in response to high glucose, ROS, and AGEs in diabetic kidney and impair structural and functional integrity of the glomerulus.

7.8.1. Angiotensin II (Ang II). Ang II not only increases vasoconstriction of glomerular capillary followed by intraglomerular pressure but also elicits more progressive pathological change to the glomerulus and renal tubules. Increasing evidence of experimental and clinical studies has shown injurious effects of Ang II during progressive kidney injury that ranges from vascular and mesangial cell proliferation, hypertrophy, podocyte apoptosis, and increased synthesis of matrix forming proteins to eventual glomerular and tubular sclerosis by induction of profibrotic mediators, namely, TGF-β, and various cytokines and by stimulation of fibroblasts, chemokines, and oxidative stress. Ding et al. [275] showed direct apoptosis of podocytes in culture medium treated with Ang II through activation of TGF-β and its downstream proapoptotic molecules and the apoptotic effect is mediated through AT1R. Ang II also accelerates nephrin loss from podocytes and induces progressive proteinuria and glomerulosclerosis which are attenuated by ACE inhibitors [276]. Together, these observations suggest that Ang II plays a key role in podocyte apoptosis and its depletion followed by proteinuria and glomerulosclerosis.

An example of damage inflicted by Ang II is matrix protein synthesis in mesangial cells. Kagami et al. [277] has shown that in vitro cell culture of mesangial cells with Ang II induces ECM accumulation via TGF-β-dependent mechanism. Moreover, Ang II and high glucose concentration induced mesangial cell proliferation and ECM deposition through induction of activator protein-1 (AP-1) [278], suggesting an obvious role of Ang II in progression of renal damage toward renal failure. Interestingly, to make matter worse, Ang II can also induce ROS generation through activation of NADPH oxidase system and ROS in turn enhances profibrotic effects of Ang II and podocyte apoptosis, thereby aggravating the injury through ROS-dependent activation of a complex network of signaling pathways (Figure 4) [279–281]. Blockade of angiotensin II type I receptor (AT1R) or angiotensin converting enzyme inhibitor has shown promising improvement in chronic hyperglycemia-induced renal injury.

On the other hand, endothelin-1 is a potent vasoconstrictor that is highly produced in diabetic kidney. In addition to its vasoconstriction effect, endothelin-1 can induce proteinuria, proinflammatory mediators, ECM accumulation, and infiltration of macrophages in kidney of streptozotocin-induced diabetic rats [282]. It can also promote hypertrophy, proliferation, and ROS formation in diabetic milieu. Endothelin-1 mediates all of its effects through endothelin type A (ET_A) receptor, blockade of which reduces all these pathological events restoring normal function and structural integrity of kidney [282, 283]. In consistency with these observations, another study showed increased expression of proinflammatory cytokines (e.g., IL-6) and chemokines (MCP-1) in mesangial cells accompanied with increased collagen synthesis leading to ECM remodeling and renal fibrosis [284].

8. Advanced Renal Damage/ESRD

At the outset of diabetes, though renal injury is triggered by ROS-mediated loss of podocyte to a certain threshold level following microalbuminuria, major structural and functional changes occur in progressive stage which are induced by activation of diverse mediators and their signaling pathways. Major progressive pathological changes that have already been discussed include increased mesangial expansion, ECM deposition, hypertrophy and proliferation of mesangial cells, increased apoptosis of podocytes beyond threshold level, increased GBM thickening resulting from matrix forming protein deposition and expression of TIMPs, glomerular sclerosis that may have a nodular appearance (classic Kimmelstiel-Wilson nodules), inflammatory cell infiltration, and tubulointerstitial fibrosis (Figure 4). All these effects impair cross-talk among glomerular components which further exacerbates the functional and structural integrity of the whole glomerulus. This stage also induces severe renal tubular damage leading to even severe loss of nephron.

Moreover, denuded GBM which has already been left by increased podocytes depletion is no longer able to resist glomerular hydrostatic pressure allowing the GBM to be stretched to come in contact with the parietal cells of Bowman's capsule resulting in synechiae formation through capillary tuft adhesion to Bowman's capsule (adhesion of capillary basement membrane with Bowman's capsule). This tuft adhesion further degenerates the remaining podocytes located at the flanks of an adhesion leading to more podocyte loss that invokes excessive protein leakage that is termed "overt proteinuria" (macroalbuminuria) [285].

Progressively increased tubular protein load in tubular filtrate appears to keep the renal tubule under continuous challenge that results from its sustained exposure to diverse bioactive molecules including proteins. It is assumed that excessive proteins in the tubular infiltrate may elicit proinflammatory and profibrotic effects that directly contribute to chronic tubulointerstitial damage. This is initiated through the interaction of filtered proteins with proximal tubular cells, which excrete increased chemokines (e.g., MCP-1, RANTES, and complement component 3), profibrotic molecules (e.g., TGF-β), vasoactive substances (e.g., endothelin and Ang II), and cytokines (e.g., TNF-α), resulting in leukocytes infiltration, inflammation, myotransformation of interstitial fibroblasts, fibrosis, tubular atrophy, and apoptosis. Leukocyte such as macrophage migration to the tubulointerstitium can further promote production of TGF-β, endothelin, and Ang II exhibiting sustained profibrotic and proapoptotic effects. Moreover, imbalanced local production of endothelin, Ang II, and NO in tubules and peritubular capillary decreases peritubular capillary plasma flow and causes rarefaction of postglomerular capillaries, resulting in local hypoxia and tubular atrophy leading to increased nephron loss. Furthermore, loss of nephron can also be accelerated due to obstruction of urinary flow along the distal tubule by protein casts formed from protein overload leading to exacerbation of tubulointerstitial damage [286–289]. Together, these pathological events eventually lead to end-stage renal damage (ESRD).

As a result, at a point, kidney mass greatly reduces resulting in gradual decrease in glomerular blood flow and filtration rate. A limited number of nephrons also receive higher workload necessitating higher filtration pressure which can further weaken the attachment of podocytes to GBM. These are also complicated by increased mesangial expansion that reduces the filtration surface, thereby significantly reducing filtration rate and increasing intraglomerular pressure. Reduction of GFR can be used to represent severity of renal injury. For example, in the patient without kidney disease, GFR usually remains >90 mL/min/1.73 m^2. However, GFR reduces to the range between 59 and 30 mL/min/1.73 m^2 during moderate renal failure which further comes down to 15–29 mL/min/1.73 m^2 in patients with severe renal failure. Moreover, GFR having <15 mL/min/1.73 m^2 indicates end-stage renal damage requiring either dialysis or kidney transplantation [290]. The latter stage is achieved if the progressive signaling cascades are not intervened with pharmacological agents.

9. Conclusion

Chronic hyperglycemia is one of the most important risk factors for progressive renal damage. Patients having diabetes are more likely to develop microalbuminuria (proteinuria) that is used as a marker for abnormal renal function. High glucose plays pivotal role in causing abnormal renal function through stimulation of ROS generation. Increasing body of evidence shows that ROS is elevated in diabetic milieu both in vivo and in vitro. ROS are considered as important second messengers for different signaling pathways which maintain necessary biochemical interactions for the functions and survival of the tissues. However, accumulation of ROS resulting from their imbalanced generation and neutralization promotes diverse aberrant signaling pathways. Abnormal signaling in the kidney causes functional and structural changes of the glomerulus which is the center for renal damage. Though being generated from many sources, ROS originated from mitochondria and NADPH oxidase are thought to cause the onset of albuminuria followed by progression of renal damage through podocyte depletion.

It is assumed that all the components of glomerular filtration barrier remain under persistent strain in oxidative stress environment. But many studies have attributed initial renal damage to highly sensitive podocytes (visceral epithelial layer) that undergo apoptosis, foot process effacement, and detachment in high glucose-induced ROS environment. Accumulation of ROS in hyperglycemic ambience activates proapoptotic signaling pathways through upregulation and activation of p38-MAPK and caspase-3 which are downstream mediators of TGF-β. Increased TGF-β levels can also promote apoptosis through elevated production of SMAD7 (independent of p38-MAPK and caspase-3) and SMAD2/3 (via caspase-3 activation) (Figure 3) [135, 291]. Moreover, a recent study showed that increased TGF-β1 levels can stimulate expression of cytosolic cathepsin L (CatL) via nuclear translocation of dendrin from SD diaphragm of podocytes lacking CD2AP protein. Cytosolic CatL in turn causes reorganization of the actin cytoskeleton by proteolytically processing dynamin and synaptopodin. Alteration in the actin cytoskeleton renders podocytes hypersensitive to proapoptotic signals leading to their accelerated death [292]. Hyperglycemia can also facilitate podocyte detachment from GBM by downregulating $\alpha3\beta1$ integrin that helps podocyte attach to GBM. High glucose levels can also attenuate expression of some slit diaphragm proteins such as nephrin, podocin, P-cadherin, CD2AP, and ZO-1 through diverse mechanisms leading to foot process effacement followed by proteinuria.

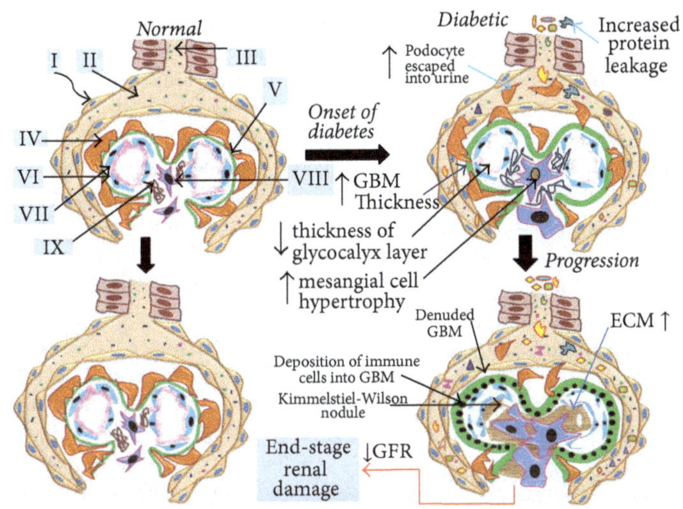

FIGURE 5: Comparison between normal and diabetic glomeruli with regard to pathological events which occurred during onset and progression of diabetes. I, parietal epithelial cells; II, Bowman's capsule; III, primary urine majorly containing water, urea, electrolytes, glucose, and so forth; IV, podocyte; V, glomerular basement membrane (GBM); VI, endothelial cells; VII, glycocalyx layer; VIII, mesangial cells; IX, extracellular matrix (ECM) proteins.

Increased albuminuria from the compromised functions of glomerular filtration barrier sets the platform for excessive activation of diverse signaling molecules. Among many, we have discussed transcription factors, inflammatory agents, growth factors, cytokines, chemokines, and vasoactive molecules in this paper in detail. Dysregulation of these abnormal signaling molecules advances the renal injury from progression of abnormal renal hemodynamics, increased glomerular basement membrane (GBM) thickness, mesangial expansion, extracellular matrix accumulation, interstitial fibrosis, and glomerulosclerosis to eventual end-stage renal damage. Lack of pharmacological intervention during progression of abnormal functional and histological change of the glomerulus may evoke irreversible end-stage renal damage which is marked by invasion of excess immune cells, classic Kimmelstiel-Wilson nodule and critically decreased glomerular filtration rate (<15 mL/min/1.73 m^2) (Figure 5). To understand the complex signaling pathways involved in renal damage, more studies are required to uncover hidden role of glucose, ROS, and ROS-generating components in causing pathological propagation.

Competing Interests

The authors declare that there are no competing interests.

References

[1] American Diabetes Association, "Diagnosis and classification of diabetes mellitus," *Diabetes Care*, vol. 33, no. 1, pp. S62–S69, 2010.

[2] Centers for Disease Control and Prevention, *National Diabetes Statistics Report: Estimates of Diabetes and Its Burden in the United States, 2014*, Department of Health and Human Services, Atlanta, Ga, USA, 2014.

[3] *Global Status Report on Noncommunicable Diseases 2014*, World Health Organization, Geneva, Switzerland, 2012.

[4] C. D. Mathers and D. Loncar, "Projections of global mortality and burden of disease from 2002 to 2030," *PLoS Medicine*, vol. 3, no. 11, article e442, 2006.

[5] Centers for Disease Control and Prevention (CDC), *National Chronic Kidney Disease Fact Sheet: General Information and National Estimates on Chronic Kidney Disease in the United States, 2014*, US Department of Health and Human Services, Atlanta, Ga, USA, 2014.

[6] B.-C. Liu, X. Song, X.-Y. Lu et al., "High glucose induces podocyte apoptosis by stimulating TRPC6 via elevation of reactive oxygen species," *Biochimica et Biophysica Acta*, vol. 1833, no. 6, pp. 1434–1442, 2013.

[7] P. Anil Kumar, G. I. Welsh, M. A. Saleem, and R. K. Menon, "Molecular and cellular events mediating glomerular podocyte dysfunction and depletion in diabetes mellitus," *Frontiers in Endocrinology*, vol. 5, 2014.

[8] K. K. Venkat, "Proteinuria and microalbuminuria in adults: significance, evaluation, and treatment," *Southern Medical Journal*, vol. 97, no. 10, pp. 969–979, 2004.

[9] G. Jarad and J. H. Miner, "Update on the glomerular filtration barrier," *Current Opinion in Nephrology and Hypertension*, vol. 18, no. 3, pp. 226–232, 2009.

[10] A. L. Sellers, N. Griggs, J. Marmorston, and H. C. Goodman, "Filtration and reabsorption of protein by the kidney," *The Journal of experimental medicine*, vol. 100, no. 1, pp. 1–10, 1954.

[11] G. C. Viberti, D. Mackintosh, R. W. Bilous, J. C. Pickup, and H. Keen, "Proteinuria in diabetes mellitus: role of spontaneous and experimental variation of glycemia," *Kidney International*, vol. 21, no. 5, pp. 714–720, 1982.

[12] A. I. Adler, R. J. Stevens, S. E. Manley, R. W. Bilous, C. A. Cull, and R. R. Holman, "Development and progression of nephropathy in type 2 diabetes: the United Kingdom prospective diabetes study (UKPDS 64)," *Kidney International*, vol. 63, no. 1, pp. 225–232, 2003.

[13] S. P. B. Ramirez, W. McClellan, F. K. Port, and S. I.-H. Hsu, "Risk factors for proteinuria in a large, multiracial, Southeast Asian population," *Journal of the American Society of Nephrology*, vol. 13, no. 7, pp. 1907–1917, 2002.

[14] C. M. Chan, "Hyperlipidaemia in chronic kidney disease," *Annals of the Academy of Medicine Singapore*, vol. 34, no. 1, pp. 31–35, 2005.

[15] American Diabetes Association, "Standards of medical care for patients with diabetes mellitus. (Posistion statement)," *Diabetes Care*, vol. 25, supplement 1, pp. S33–S49, 2002.

[16] A. S. A. Naderi and R. F. Reilly, "Primary care approach to proteinuria," *Journal of the American Board of Family Medicine*, vol. 21, no. 6, pp. 569–574, 2008.

[17] P. W. Mathieson, "The cellular basis of albuminuria," *Clinical Science*, vol. 107, no. 6, pp. 533–538, 2004.

[18] S. M. Bagshaw and R. Bellomo, "Early diagnosis of acute kidney injury," *Current Opinion in Critical Care*, vol. 13, no. 6, pp. 638–644, 2007.

[19] M. J. Karnovsky, "The ultrastructure of glomerular filtration," *Annual Review of Medicine*, vol. 30, pp. 213–224, 1979.

[20] A. Remuzzi and G. Remuzzi, "Glomerular perm-selective function," *Kidney International*, vol. 45, no. 2, pp. 398–402, 1994.

[21] M. P. Bohrer, C. Baylis, H. D. Humes, R. J. Glassock, C. R. Robertson, and B. M. Brenner, "Permselectivity of the glomerular capillary wall: *facilitated filtration of circulating polycations*," *Journal of Clinical Investigation*, vol. 61, no. 1, pp. 72–78, 1978.

[22] E. L. Bearer, L. Orci, and P. Sors, "Endothelial fenestral diaphragms: a quick-freeze, deep-etch study," *The Journal of Cell Biology*, vol. 100, no. 2, pp. 418–428, 1985.

[23] B. Haraldsson, J. Nyström, and W. M. Deen, "Properties of the glomerular barrier and mechanisms of proteinuria," *Physiological Reviews*, vol. 88, no. 2, pp. 451–487, 2008.

[24] B. J. Ballermann and R. V. Stan, "Resolved: capillary endothelium is a major contributor to the glomerular filtration barrier," *Journal of the American Society of Nephrology*, vol. 18, no. 9, pp. 2432–2438, 2007.

[25] S. Reitsma, D. W. Slaaf, H. Vink, M. A. M. J. Van Zandvoort, and M. G. A. Oude Egbrink, "The endothelial glycocalyx: composition, functions, and visualization," *European Journal of Physiology*, vol. 454, no. 3, pp. 345–359, 2007.

[26] S. Weinbaum, J. M. Tarbell, and E. R. Damiano, "The structure and function of the endothelial glycocalyx layer," *Annual Review of Biomedical Engineering*, vol. 9, pp. 121–167, 2007.

[27] M. J. C. Dane, B. M. Van Den Berg, M. C. Avramut et al., "Glomerular endothelial surface layer acts as a barrier against albumin filtration," *American Journal of Pathology*, vol. 182, no. 5, pp. 1532–1540, 2013.

[28] M. Jeansson and B. Haraldsson, "Morphological and functional evidence for an important role of the endothelial cell glycocalyx in the glomerular barrier," *American Journal of Physiology—Renal Physiology*, vol. 290, no. 1, pp. F111–F116, 2006.

[29] A. Singh, S. C. Satchell, C. R. Neal, E. A. McKenzie, J. E. Tooke, and P. W. Mathieson, "Glomerular endothelial glycocalyx constitutes a barrier to protein permeability," *Journal of the American Society of Nephrology*, vol. 18, no. 11, pp. 2885–2893, 2007.

[30] M. Jeansson and B. Haraldsson, "Glomerular size and charge selectivity in the mouse after exposure to glucosaminoglycan-degrading enzymes," *Journal of the American Society of Nephrology*, vol. 14, no. 7, pp. 1756–1765, 2003.

[31] E. Sawanobori, N. Terada, Y. Fujii, K. Higashida, S. Nakazawa, and S. Ohno, "Ultrastructural study of human glomerular capillary loops with igA nephropathy using quick-freezing and deep-etching method," *Histology and Histopathology*, vol. 23, no. 3, pp. 297–307, 2008.

[32] J. Patrakka and K. Tryggvason, "Molecular make-up of the glomerular filtration barrier," *Biochemical and Biophysical Research Communications*, vol. 396, no. 1, pp. 164–169, 2010.

[33] M. C. Menon, P. Y. Chuang, and C. J. He, "The glomerular filtration barrier: components and crosstalk," *International Journal of Nephrology*, vol. 2012, Article ID 749010, 9 pages, 2012.

[34] P. D. Yurchenco, "Basement membranes: cell scaffoldings and signaling platforms," *Cold Spring Harbor Perspectives in Biology*, vol. 3, no. 2, Article ID a004911, 2011.

[35] S. J. Harvey and J. H. Miner, "Revisiting the glomerular charge barrier in the molecular era," *Current Opinion in Nephrology and Hypertension*, vol. 17, no. 4, pp. 393–398, 2008.

[36] A. J. Groffen, M. A. Ruegg, H. Dijkman et al., "Agrin is a major heparan sulfate proteoglycan in the human glomerular basement membrane," *Journal of Histochemistry and Cytochemistry*, vol. 46, no. 1, pp. 19–27, 1998.

[37] J. A. Jefferson, S. J. Shankland, and R. H. Pichler, "Proteinuria in diabetic kidney disease: a mechanistic viewpoint," *Kidney International*, vol. 74, no. 1, pp. 22–36, 2008.

[38] S. J. Harvey, G. Jarad, J. Cunningham et al., "Disruption of glomerular basement membrane charge through podocyte-specific mutation of agrin does not alter glomerular permselectivity," *American Journal of Pathology*, vol. 171, no. 1, pp. 139–152, 2007.

[39] T. J. M. Wijnhoven, J. F. M. Lensen, R. G. P. Wismans et al., "*In vivo* degradation of heparan sulfates in the glomerular basement membrane does not result in proteinuria," *Journal of the American Society of Nephrology*, vol. 18, no. 3, pp. 823–832, 2007.

[40] T. J. M. Wijnhoven, J. F. M. Lensen, R. G. P. Wismans et al., "Removal of heparan sulfate from the glomerular basement membrane blocks protein passage," *Journal of the American Society of Nephrology*, vol. 18, no. 12, pp. 3119–3127, 2007.

[41] A. Greka and P. Mundel, "Cell biology and pathology of podocytes," *Annual Review of Physiology*, vol. 74, pp. 299–323, 2012.

[42] J.-L. R. Michaud and C. R. J. Kennedy, "The podocyte in health and disease: insights from the mouse," *Clinical Science*, vol. 112, no. 5-6, pp. 325–335, 2007.

[43] J. Wartiovaara, L. Öfverstedt, J. Khoshnoodi et al., "Nephrin strands contribute to a porous slit diaphragm scaffold as revealed by electron tomography," *The Journal of Clinical Investigation*, vol. 114, no. 10, pp. 1475–1483, 2004.

[44] M. Gekle, "Renal tubule albumin transport," *Annual Review of Physiology*, vol. 67, pp. 573–594, 2005.

[45] H. Pavenstädt, W. Kriz, and M. Kretzler, "Cell biology of the glomerular podocyte," *Physiological Reviews*, vol. 83, no. 1, pp. 253–307, 2003.

[46] M. M. Löwik, P. J. Groenen, E. N. Levtchenko, L. A. Monnens, and L. P. Van Den Heuvel, "Molecular genetic analysis of podocyte genes in focal segmental glomerulosclerosis—a review," *European Journal of Pediatrics*, vol. 168, no. 11, pp. 1291–1304, 2009.

[47] J. D. Stockand and S. C. Sansom, "Glomerular mesangial cells: electrophysiology and regulation of contraction," *Physiological Reviews*, vol. 78, no. 3, pp. 723–744, 1998.

[48] D. Schlöndorff and B. Banas, "The mesangial cell revisited: no cell is an island," *Journal of the American Society of Nephrology*, vol. 20, no. 6, pp. 1179–1187, 2009.

[49] P. Levéen, M. Pekny, S. Gebre-Medhin, B. Swolin, E. Larsson, and C. Betsholtz, "Mice deficient for PDGF B show renal, cardiovascular, and hematological abnormalities," *Genes and Development*, vol. 8, no. 16, pp. 1875–1887, 1994.

[50] J. Lee, N. Koo, and D. B. Min, "Reactive oxygen species, aging, and antioxidative nutraceuticals," *Comprehensive Reviews in Food Science and Food Safety*, vol. 3, no. 1, pp. 21–33, 2004.

[51] Y. Taniyama and K. K. Griendling, "Reactive oxygen species in the vasculature: molecular and cellular mechanisms," *Hypertension*, vol. 42, no. 6, pp. 1075–1081, 2003.

[52] J. S. Johansen, A. K. Harris, D. J. Rychly, and A. Ergul, "Oxidative stress and the use of antioxidants in diabetes: linking basic science to clinical pratice," *Cardiovascular Diabetology*, vol. 4, article no. 5, 2005.

[53] J. F. Turrens, "Mitochondrial formation of reactive oxygen species," *Journal of Physiology*, vol. 552, no. 2, pp. 335–344, 2003.

[54] Y. Gorin, K. Block, J. Hernandez et al., "Nox4 NAD(P)H oxidase mediates hypertrophy and fibronectin expression in the diabetic kidney," *Journal of Biological Chemistry*, vol. 280, no. 47, pp. 39616–39626, 2005.

[55] M. Satoh, S. Fujimoto, Y. Haruna et al., "NAD(P)H oxidase and uncoupled nitric oxide synthase are major sources of glomerular superoxide in rats with experimental diabetic nephropathy," *American Journal of Physiology: Renal Physiology*, vol. 288, no. 6, pp. F1144–F1152, 2005.

[56] H. Cheng, H. Wang, X. Fan, P. Paueksakon, and R. C. Harris, "Improvement of endothelial nitric oxide synthase activity retards the progression of diabetic nephropathy in db/db mice," *Kidney International*, vol. 82, no. 11, pp. 1176–1183, 2012.

[57] C. Rüster, T. Bondeva, S. Franke, M. Förster, and G. Wolf, "Advanced glycation end-products induce cell cycle arrest and hypertrophy in podocytes," *Nephrology Dialysis Transplantation*, vol. 23, no. 7, pp. 2179–2191, 2008.

[58] S. Munusamy and L. A. MacMillan-Crow, "Mitochondrial superoxide plays a crucial role in the development of mitochondrial dysfunction during high glucose exposure in rat renal proximal tubular cells," *Free Radical Biology and Medicine*, vol. 46, no. 8, pp. 1149–1157, 2009.

[59] K. Shahzad, F. Bock, W. Dong et al., "Nlrp3-inflammasome activation in non-myeloid-derived cells aggravates diabetic nephropathy," *Kidney International*, vol. 87, no. 1, pp. 74–84, 2015.

[60] V. Thallas-Bonke, J. C. Jha, S. P. Gray et al., "Nox-4 deletion reduces oxidative stress and injury by PKC-α-associated mechanisms in diabetic nephropathy," *Physiological Reports*, vol. 2, no. 11, Article ID e12192, 2014.

[61] K. Bedard and K.-H. Krause, "The NOX family of ROS-generating NADPH oxidases: physiology and pathophysiology," *Physiological Reviews*, vol. 87, no. 1, pp. 245–313, 2007.

[62] K. K. Griendling, C. A. Minieri, J. D. Ollerenshaw, and R. W. Alexander, "Angiotensin II stimulates NADH and NADPH oxidase activity in cultured vascular smooth muscle cells," *Circulation Research*, vol. 74, no. 6, pp. 1141–1148, 1994.

[63] T. Chabrashvili, A. Tojo, M. L. Onozato et al., "Expression and cellular localization of classic NADPH oxidase subunits in the spontaneously hypertensive rat kidney," *Hypertension*, vol. 39, no. 2 I, pp. 269–274, 2002.

[64] J.-M. Li and A. M. Shah, "Intracellular localization and preassembly of the NADPH oxidase complex in cultured endothelial cells," *Journal of Biological Chemistry*, vol. 277, no. 22, pp. 19952–19960, 2002.

[65] B. Lassègue, D. Sorescu, K. Szöcs et al., "Novel gp91^{phox} homologues in vascular smooth muscle cells: noxl mediates angiotensin II-induced superoxide formation and redox-sensitive signaling pathways," *Circulation Research*, vol. 88, pp. 888–894, 2001.

[66] P. L. Hordijk, "Regulation of NADPH oxidases: the role of Rac proteins," *Circulation Research*, vol. 98, no. 4, pp. 453–462, 2006.

[67] R. E. Clempus and K. K. Griendling, "Reactive oxygen species signaling in vascular smooth muscle cells," *Cardiovascular Research*, vol. 71, no. 2, pp. 216–225, 2006.

[68] M.-H. Paclet, S. Berthier, L. Kuhn, J. Garin, and F. Morel, "Regulation of phagocyte NADPH oxidase activity: identification of two cytochrome b_{558} activation states," *The FASEB Journal*, vol. 21, no. 4, pp. 1244–1255, 2007.

[69] C. Y. Han, T. Umemoto, M. Omer et al., "NADPH oxidase-derived reactive oxygen species increases expression of monocyte chemotactic factor genes in cultured adipocytes," *Journal of Biological Chemistry*, vol. 287, no. 13, pp. 10379–10393, 2012.

[70] M. Chopra, K. Kaul, J. Tarr, R. Choudhury, E. M. Kohner, and R. Chibber, "Oxidative stress in diabetic neuropathy: source of reactive oxygen species," *Endocrinology Studies*, vol. 2, no. 2, 2012.

[71] K. Sakai, K. Matsumoto, T. Nishikawa et al., "Mitochondrial reactive oxygen species reduce insulin secretion by pancreatic β-cells," *Biochemical and Biophysical Research Communications*, vol. 300, no. 1, pp. 216–222, 2003.

[72] T. Nishikawa, D. Edelstein, X. L. Du et al., "Normalizing mitochondrial superoxide production blocks three pathways of hyperglycaemic damage," *Nature*, vol. 404, no. 6779, pp. 787–790, 2000.

[73] S. R. Pieczenik and J. Neustadt, "Mitochondrial dysfunction and molecular pathways of disease," *Experimental and Molecular Pathology*, vol. 83, no. 1, pp. 84–92, 2007.

[74] G. Lenaz, "The mitochondrial production of reactive oxygen species: mechanisms and implications in human pathology," *IUBMB Life*, vol. 52, no. 3-5, pp. 159–164, 2001.

[75] Q. Chen, E. J. Vazquez, S. Moghaddas, C. L. Hoppel, and E. J. Lesnefsky, "Production of reactive oxygen species by mitochondria: central role of complex III," *Journal of Biological Chemistry*, vol. 278, no. 38, pp. 36027–36031, 2003.

[76] J. F. Turrens and A. Boveris, "Generation of superoxide anion by the NADH dehydrogenase of bovine heart mitochondria," *Biochemical Journal*, vol. 191, no. 2, pp. 421–427, 1980.

[77] K. Green, M. D. Brand, and M. P. Murphy, "Prevention of mitochondrial oxidative damage as a therapeutic strategy in diabetes," *Diabetes*, vol. 53, no. 1, pp. S110–S118, 2004.

[78] M. P. Murphy, "How mitochondria produce reactive oxygen species," *Biochemical Journal*, vol. 417, no. 1, pp. 1–13, 2009.

[79] M. Watabe and T. Nakaki, "Mitochondrial complex I inhibitor rotenone-elicited dopamine redistribution from vesicles to cytosol in human dopaminergic SH-SY5Y cells," *Journal of Pharmacology and Experimental Therapeutics*, vol. 323, no. 2, pp. 499–507, 2007.

[80] W. J. H. Koopman, S. Verkaart, H.-J. Visch et al., "Inhibition of complex I of the electron transport chain causes O_2^{-}•-mediated mitochondrial outgrowth," *American Journal of Physiology—Cell Physiology*, vol. 288, no. 6, pp. C1440–C1450, 2005.

[81] A. Anedda, E. Rial, and M. M. González-Barroso, "Metformin induces oxidative stress in white adipocytes and raises uncoupling protein 2 levels," *Journal of Endocrinology*, vol. 199, no. 1, pp. 33–40, 2008.

[82] R. Fato, C. Bergamini, M. Bortolus et al., "Differential effects of mitochondrial complex I inhibitors on production of reactive oxygen species," *Biochimica et Biophysica Acta (BBA)—Bioenergetics*, vol. 1787, no. 5, pp. 384–392, 2009.

[83] K. Sakai, K. Matsumoto, T. Nishikawa et al., "Mitochondrial reactive oxygen species reduce insulin secretion by pancreatic β-cells," *Biochemical and Biophysical Research Communications*, vol. 300, no. 1, pp. 216–222, 2003.

[84] A. Panov, S. Dikalov, N. Shalbuyeva, R. Hemendinger, J. T. Greenamyre, and J. Rosenfeld, "Species- and tissue-specific relationships between mitochondrial permeability transition and generation of ROS in brain and liver mitochondria of rats and mice," *American Journal of Physiology - Cell Physiology*, vol. 292, no. 2, pp. C708–C718, 2007.

[85] A. Panov, S. Dikalov, N. Shalbuyeva, G. Taylor, T. Sherer, and J. T. Greenamyre, "Rotenone model of Parkinson disease: multiple brain mitochondria dysfunctions after short term systemic rotenone intoxication," *The Journal of Biological Chemistry*, vol. 280, no. 51, pp. 42026–42035, 2005.

[86] M. A. Aon, S. Cortassa, E. Marbán, and B. O'Rourke, "Synchronized whole cell oscillations in mitochondrial metabolism triggered by a local release of reactive oxygen species in cardiac myocytes," *The Journal of Biological Chemistry*, vol. 278, no. 45, pp. 44735–44744, 2003.

[87] D. F. Stowe and A. K. S. Camara, "Mitochondrial reactive oxygen species production in excitable cells: modulators of mitochondrial and cell function," *Antioxidants & Redox Signaling*, vol. 11, no. 6, pp. 1373–1414, 2009.

[88] S. Dröse, "Differential effects of complex II on mitochondrial ROS production and their relation to cardioprotective pre- and postconditioning," *Biochimica et Biophysica Acta - Bioenergetics*, vol. 1827, no. 5, pp. 578–587, 2013.

[89] A. Anderson, A. Bowman, S. J. Boulton, P. Manning, and M. A. Birch-Machin, "A role for human mitochondrial complex II in the production of reactive oxygen species in human skin," *Redox Biology*, vol. 2, pp. 1016–1022, 2014.

[90] J. M. Forbes, M. T. Coughlan, and M. E. Cooper, "Oxidative stress as a major culprit in kidney disease in diabetes," *Diabetes*, vol. 57, no. 6, pp. 1446–1454, 2008.

[91] S. S. Korshunov, V. P. Skulachev, and A. A. Starkov, "High protonic potential actuates a mechanism of production of reactive oxygen species in mitochondria," *FEBS Letters*, vol. 416, no. 1, pp. 15–18, 1997.

[92] Y. Liu, G. Fiskum, and D. Schubert, "Generation of reactive oxygen species by the mitochondrial electron transport chain," *Journal of Neurochemistry*, vol. 80, no. 5, pp. 780–787, 2002.

[93] A. Boveris, N. Oshino, and B. Chance, "The cellular production of hydrogen peroxide," *Biochemical Journal*, vol. 128, no. 3, pp. 617–630, 1972.

[94] H. Raza, S. K. Prabu, A. John, and N. G. Avadhani, "Impaired mitochondrial respiratory functions and oxidative stress in streptozotocin-induced diabetic rats," *International Journal of Molecular Sciences*, vol. 12, no. 5, pp. 3133–3147, 2011.

[95] A. Stirban, T. Gawlowski, and M. Roden, "Vascular effects of advanced glycation endproducts: clinical effects and molecular mechanisms," *Molecular Metabolism*, vol. 3, no. 2, pp. 94–108, 2014.

[96] A. Goldin, J. A. Beckman, A. M. Schmidt, and M. A. Creager, "Advanced glycation end products: sparking the development of diabetic vascular injury," *Circulation*, vol. 114, no. 6, pp. 597–605, 2006.

[97] M. Koch, S. Chitayat, B. M. Dattilo et al., "Structural basis for ligand recognition and activation of RAGE," *Structure*, vol. 18, no. 10, pp. 1342–1352, 2010.

[98] D. Xu and J. M. Kyriakis, "Phosphatidylinositol 3′-kinase-dependent activation of renal mesangial cell Ki-Ras and ERK by advanced glycation end products," *Journal of Biological Chemistry*, vol. 278, no. 41, pp. 39349–39355, 2003.

[99] T. M. Wendt, N. Tanji, J. Guo et al., "RAGE drives the development of glomerulosclerosis and implicates podocyte activation in the pathogenesis of diabetic nephropathy," *American Journal of Pathology*, vol. 162, no. 4, pp. 1123–1137, 2003.

[100] A. L. Y. Tan, J. M. Forbes, and M. E. Cooper, "AGE, RAGE, and ROS in diabetic nephropathy," *Seminars in Nephrology*, vol. 27, no. 2, pp. 130–143, 2007.

[101] E. Linden, W. Cai, J. C. He et al., "Endothelial dysfunction in patients with chronic kidney disease results from advanced glycation end products (AGE)-mediated inhibition of endothelial nitric oxide synthase through RAGE activation," *Clinical Journal of the American Society of Nephrology*, vol. 3, no. 3, pp. 691–698, 2008.

[102] N. Lin, H. Zhang, and Q. Su, "Advanced glycation end-products induce injury to pancreatic beta cells through oxidative stress," *Diabetes and Metabolism*, vol. 38, no. 3, pp. 250–257, 2012.

[103] P. Y. Chuang, Q. Yu, W. Fang, J. Uribarri, and J. C. He, "Advanced glycation endproducts induce podocyte apoptosis by activation of the FOXO4 transcription factor," *Kidney International*, vol. 72, no. 8, pp. 965–976, 2007.

[104] M.-P. Wautier, O. Chappey, S. Corda, D. M. Stern, A. M. Schmidt, and J.-L. Wautier, "Activation of NADPH oxidase by AGE links oxidant stress to altered gene expression via RAGE," *American Journal of Physiology—Endocrinology and Metabolism*, vol. 280, no. 5, pp. E685–E694, 2001.

[105] W. K. Alderton, C. E. Cooper, and R. G. Knowles, "Nitric oxide synthases: structure, function and inhibition," *Biochemical Journal*, vol. 357, no. 3, pp. 593–615, 2001.

[106] M. E. Murphy and H. Sies, "Reversible conversion of nitroxyl anion to nitric oxide by superoxide dismutase," *Proceedings of the National Academy of Sciences of the United States of America*, vol. 88, no. 23, pp. 10860–10864, 1991.

[107] U. Förstermann and T. Münzel, "Endothelial nitric oxide synthase in vascular disease: from marvel to menace," *Circulation*, vol. 113, no. 13, pp. 1708–1714, 2006.

[108] C. F. B. Witteveen, J. Giovanelli, and S. Kaufman, "Reduction of quinonoid dihydrobiopterin to tetrahydrobiopterin by nitric oxide synthase," *Journal of Biological Chemistry*, vol. 271, no. 8, pp. 4143–4147, 1996.

[109] B. Thöny, G. Auerbach, and N. Blau, "Tetrahydrobiopterin biosynthesis, regeneration and functions," *Biochemical Journal*, vol. 347, no. 1, pp. 1–16, 2000.

[110] T. J. Guzik, S. Mussa, D. Gastaldi et al., "Mechanisms of increased vascular superoxide production in human diabetes mellitus: role of NAD(P)H oxidase and endothelial nitric oxide synthase," *Circulation*, vol. 105, no. 14, pp. 1656–1662, 2002.

[111] Y. Xia, L. J. Roman, B. S. S. Masters, and J. L. Zweier, "Inducible nitric-oxide synthase generates superoxide from the reductase domain," *The Journal of Biological Chemistry*, vol. 273, no. 35, pp. 22635–22639, 1998.

[112] S. Pou, W. S. Pou, D. S. Bredt, S. H. Snyder, and G. M. Resen, "Generation of superoxide by purified brain nitric oxide synthase," *The Journal of Biological Chemistry*, vol. 267, no. 34, pp. 24173–24176, 1992.

[113] G. M. Rosen, P. Tsai, J. Weaver et al., "The role of tetrahydrobiopterin in the regulation of neuronal nitric-oxide synthase-generated superoxide," *Journal of Biological Chemistry*, vol. 277, no. 43, pp. 40275–40280, 2002.

[114] M. Inoue, E. F. Sato, M. Nishikawa et al., "Mitochondrial generation of reactive oxygen species and its role in aerobic life," *Current Medicinal Chemistry*, vol. 10, no. 23, pp. 2495–2505, 2003.

[115] Y. B. Y. Sun, X. Qu, X. Zhang, G. Caruana, J. F. Bertram, and J. Li, "Glomerular endothelial cell injury and damage precedes that of podocytes in adriamycin-induced nephropathy," *PLOS ONE*, vol. 8, no. 1, Article ID e55027, 2013.

[116] K. Sison, V. Eremina, H. Baelde et al., "Glomerular structure and function require paracrine, not autocrine, VEGF-VEGFR-2 signaling," *Journal of the American Society of Nephrology*, vol. 21, no. 10, pp. 1691–1701, 2010.

[117] D. R. Abrahamson, B. G. Hudson, L. Stroganova, D.-B. Borza, and P. L. St John, "Cellular origins of type IV collagen networks in developing glomeruli," *Journal of the American Society of Nephrology*, vol. 20, no. 7, pp. 1471–1479, 2009.

[118] R. Moseley, R. J. Waddington, and G. Embery, "Degradation of glycosaminoglycans by reactive oxygen species derived from stimulated polymorphonuclear leukocytes," *Biochimica et Biophysica Acta*, vol. 1362, no. 2-3, pp. 221–231, 1997.

[119] C. B. S. Henry and B. R. Duling, "TNF-α increases entry of macromolecules into luminal endothelial cell glycocalyx," *American Journal of Physiology—Heart and Circulatory Physiology*, vol. 279, no. 6, pp. H2815–H2823, 2000.

[120] A. Singh, R. D. Ramnath, R. R. Foster et al., "Reactive oxygen species modulate the barrier function of the human glomerular endothelial glycocalyx," *PLOS ONE*, vol. 8, no. 2, Article ID e55852, 2013.

[121] A. Singh, V. Fridén, I. Dasgupta et al., "High glucose causes dysfunction of the human glomerular endothelial glycocalyx," *American Journal of Physiology: Renal Physiology*, vol. 300, no. 1, pp. F40–F48, 2011.

[122] R. F. Van Golen, T. M. Van Gulik, and M. Heger, "Mechanistic overview of reactive species-induced degradation of the endothelial glycocalyx during hepatic ischemia/reperfusion injury," *Free Radical Biology and Medicine*, vol. 52, no. 8, pp. 1382–1402, 2012.

[123] H. Kolárová, B. Ambruzová, L. S. vihálková et al., "Modulation of endothelial glycocalyx structure under inflammatory conditions," *Meidiators of Inflammation*, vol. 2014, Article ID 694312, 17 pages, 2014.

[124] E. A. Jaimes, P. Hua, R.-X. Tian, and L. Raij, "Human glomerular endothelium: interplay among glucose, free fatty acids, angiotensin II, and oxidative stress," *American Journal of Physiology: Renal Physiology*, vol. 298, no. 1, pp. F125–F132, 2010.

[125] S. Savard, P. Lavoie, C. Villeneuve, M. Agharazii, M. Lebel, and R. Larivire, "ENOS gene delivery prevents hypertension and reduces renal failure and injury in rats with reduced renal mass," *Nephrology Dialysis Transplantation*, vol. 27, no. 6, pp. 2182–2190, 2012.

[126] T. Nakagawa, K. Tanabe, B. P. Croker et al., "Endothelial dysfunction as a potential contributor in diabetic nephropathy," *Nature Reviews Nephrology*, vol. 7, no. 1, pp. 36–44, 2011.

[127] C. J. I. Raats, M. A. H. Bakker, J. Van Den Born, and J. H. M. Berden, "Hydroxyl radicals depolymerize glomerular heparan sulfate *in vitro* and in experimental nephrotic syndrome," *Journal of Biological Chemistry*, vol. 272, no. 42, pp. 26734–26741, 1997.

[128] C. J. I. Raats, J. Van Den Born, and J. H. M. Berden, "Glomerular heparan sulfate alterations: mechanisms and relevance for proteinuria," *Kidney International*, vol. 57, no. 2, pp. 385–400, 2000.

[129] N. Kashihara, Y. Watanabe, H. Makino, E. I. Wallner, and Y. S. Kanwar, "Selective decreased de novo synthesis of glomerular proteoglycans under the influence of reactive oxygen species," *Proceedings of the National Academy of Sciences of the United States of America*, vol. 89, no. 14, pp. 6309–6313, 1992.

[130] S. J. Klebanoff, M. G. Kinsella, and T. N. Wight, "Degradation of endothelial cell matrix heparan sulfate proteoglycan by elastase and the myeloperoxidase-H_2O_2-chloride system," *The American Journal of Pathology*, vol. 143, no. 3, pp. 907–917, 1993.

[131] J. H. Suh and J. H. Miner, "The glomerular basement membrane as a barrier to albumin," *Nature Reviews Nephrology*, vol. 9, no. 8, pp. 470–477, 2013.

[132] E. I. Mohamed, N. M. Fahmi, S. M. El Kholy, and S. M. Sallam, "Effects of reactive oxygen species on *in vitro* filtration of water and albumin across glomerular basement membrane," *International Journal of Biomedical Science*, vol. 2, no. 2, pp. 85–100, 2006.

[133] D. Kerjaschki, D. J. Sharkey, and M. G. Farquhar, "Identification and characterization of podocalyxin—the major sialoprotein of the renal glomerular epithelial cell," *Journal of Cell Biology*, vol. 98, no. 4, pp. 1591–1596, 1984.

[134] K. Matsui, S. Breiteneder-Geleff, A. Soleiman, H. Kowalski, and D. Kerjaschki, "Podoplanin, a novel 43-kDa membrane protein, controls the shape of podocytes," *Nephrology Dialysis Transplantation*, vol. 14, no. 1, pp. 9–11, 1999.

[135] T. W. Huang and J. C. Langlois, "Podoendin. A new cell surface protein of the podocyte and endothelium," *Journal of Experimental Medicine*, vol. 162, no. 1, pp. 245–267, 1985.

[136] K. Susztak, A. C. Raff, M. Schiffer, and E. P. Böttinger, "Glucose-induced reactive oxygen species cause apoptosis of podocytes and podocyte depletion at the onset of diabetic nephropathy," *Diabetes*, vol. 55, no. 1, pp. 225–233, 2006.

[137] S. J. Shankland, "The podocyte's response to injury: role in proteinuria and glomerulosclerosis," *Kidney International*, vol. 69, no. 12, pp. 2131–2147, 2006.

[138] H. Liapis, P. Romagnani, and H.-J. Anders, "New insights into the pathology of podocyte loss: mitotic catastrophe," *American Journal of Pathology*, vol. 183, no. 5, pp. 1364–1374, 2013.

[139] S. Greiber, T. Münzel, S. Kästner, B. Müller, P. Schollmeyer, and H. Pavenstädt, "NAD(P)H oxidase activity in cultured human podocytes: effects of adenosine triphosphate," *Kidney International*, vol. 53, no. 3, pp. 654–663, 1998.

[140] A. Whaley-Connell, J. Habibi, R. Nistala et al., "Attenuation of NADPH oxidase activation and glomerular filtration barrier remodeling with statin treatment," *Hypertension*, vol. 51, no. 2, pp. 474–480, 2008.

[141] C. Zhu, S. Huang, Y. Yuan et al., "Mitochondrial dysfunction mediates aldosterone-induced podocyte damage: a therapeutic target of PPARγ," *American Journal of Pathology*, vol. 178, no. 5, pp. 2020–2031, 2011.

[142] L. Gu, S. Hagiwara, Q. Fan et al., "Role of receptor for advanced glycation end-products and signalling events in advanced glycation end-product-induced monocyte chemoattractant protein-1 expression in differentiated mouse podocytes," *Nephrology Dialysis Transplantation*, vol. 21, no. 2, pp. 299–313, 2006.

[143] A. Piwkowska, D. Rogacka, M. Jankowski, M. H. Dominiczak, J. K. Stepiński, and S. Angielski, "Metformin induces suppression of NAD(P)H oxidase activity in podocytes," *Biochemical and Biophysical Research Communications*, vol. 393, no. 2, pp. 268–273, 2010.

[144] J. Toyonaga, K. Tsuruya, H. Ikeda et al., "Spironolactone inhibits hyperglycemia-induced podocyte injury by attenuating ROS production," *Nephrology Dialysis Transplantation*, vol. 26, no. 8, pp. 2475–2484, 2011.

[145] I. Loeffer and G. Wolf, "Transforming growth factor-β and the progression of renal disease," *Nephrology Dialysis Transplantation*, vol. 29, supplement 1, pp. i37–i45, 2014.

[146] M. Schiffer, M. Bitzer, I. S. D. Roberts et al., "Apoptosis in podocytes induced by TGF-β and Smad7," *Journal of Clinical Investigation*, vol. 108, no. 6, pp. 807–816, 2001.

[147] S. C. Lee, S. H. Han, J. J. Li et al., "Induction of heme oxygenase-1 protects against podocyte apoptosis under diabetic conditions," *Kidney International*, vol. 76, no. 8, pp. 838–848, 2009.

[148] M. C. Iglesias-De La Cruz, P. Ruiz-Torres, J. Alcamí et al., "Hydrogen peroxide increases extracellular matrix mRNA through TGF-β in human mesangial cells," *Kidney International*, vol. 59, no. 1, pp. 87–95, 2001.

[149] J. H. Oh, H. Ha, M. R. Yu, and H. B. Lee, "Sequential effects of high glucose on mesangial cell transforming growth factor-β1 and fibronectin synthesis," *Kidney International*, vol. 54, no. 6, pp. 1872–1878, 1998.

[150] H. B. Lee, M.-R. Yu, Y. Yang, Z. Jiang, and H. Ha, "Reactive oxygen species-regulated signaling pathways in diabetic nephropathy," *Journal of the American Society of Nephrology*, vol. 14, no. 8, S3, pp. S241–S245, 2003.

[151] C. D. Bondi, N. Manickam, D. Y. Lee et al., "NAD(P)H oxidase mediates TGF-β1-induced activation of kidney myofibroblasts," *Journal of the American Society of Nephrology*, vol. 21, no. 1, pp. 93–102, 2010.

[152] M. Jain, S. Rivera, E. A. Monclus et al., "Mitochondrial reactive oxygen species regulate transforming growth factor-β signaling," *The Journal of Biological Chemistry*, vol. 288, no. 2, pp. 770–777, 2013.

[153] G. Wolf, S. Chen, and F. N. Ziyadeh, "From the periphery of the glomerular capillary wall toward the center of disease: podocyte injury comes of age in diabetic nephropathy," *Diabetes*, vol. 54, no. 6, pp. 1626–1634, 2005.

[154] P. V. Kitsiou, A. K. Tzinia, W. G. Stetler-Stevenson et al., "Glucose-induced changes in integrins and matrix-related functions in cultured human glomerular epithelial cells," *American Journal of Physiology—Renal Physiology*, vol. 284, no. 4, pp. F671–F679, 2003.

[155] M. F. Bek, M. Bayer, B. Müller et al., "Expression and function of C/EBP homology protein (GADD153) in podocytes," *The American Journal of Pathology*, vol. 168, no. 1, pp. 20–32, 2006.

[156] N. Sachs, M. Kreft, M. A. Van Den Bergh Weerman et al., "Kidney failure in mice lacking the tetraspanin CD151," *The Journal of Cell Biology*, vol. 175, no. 1, pp. 33–39, 2006.

[157] A. T. Petermann, R. Krofft, M. Blonski et al., "Podocytes that detach in experimental membranous nephropathy are viable," *Kidney International*, vol. 64, no. 4, pp. 1222–1231, 2003.

[158] T. Nakamura, C. Ushiyama, S. Suzuki et al., "Urinary excretion of podocytes in patients with diabetic nephropathy," *Nephrology Dialysis Transplantation*, vol. 15, no. 9, pp. 1379–1383, 2000.

[159] J. J. Li, S. J. Kwak, D. S. Jung et al., "Podocyte biology in diabetic nephropathy," *Kidney International*, vol. 72, no. 106, pp. S36–S42, 2007.

[160] J. F. do Nascimento, L. H. Canani, F. Gerchman et al., "Messenger RNA levels of podocyte-associated proteins in subjects with different degrees of glucose tolerance with or without nephropathy," *BMC Nephrology*, vol. 14, article 214, 2013.

[161] J. H. Koh, E. S. Lee, M. Hyun et al., "Taurine alleviates the progression of diabetic nephropathy in type 2 diabetic rat model," *International Journal of Endocrinology*, vol. 2014, Article ID 397307, 11 pages, 2014.

[162] F. Bonnet, M. E. Cooper, H. Kawachi, T. J. Allen, G. Boner, and Z. Cao, "Irbesartan normalises the deficiency in glomerular nephrin expression in a model of diabetes and hypertension," *Diabetologia*, vol. 44, no. 7, pp. 874–877, 2001.

[163] C.-X. Zheng, Z.-H. Chen, C.-H. Zeng, W.-S. Qin, L.-S. Li, and Z.-H. Liu, "Triptolide protects podocytes from puromycin aminonucleoside induced injury *in vivo* and *in vitro*," *Kidney International*, vol. 74, no. 5, pp. 596–612, 2008.

[164] X. Lan, P. Rai, N. Chandel et al., "Morphine induces albuminuria by compromising podocyte integrity," *PLoS ONE*, vol. 8, no. 3, Article ID e55748, 2013.

[165] T. B. Huber, B. Hartleben, J. Kim et al., "Nephrin and CD2AP associate with phosphoinositide 3-OH kinase and stimulate AKT-dependent signaling," *Molecular and Cellular Biology*, vol. 23, no. 14, pp. 4917–4928, 2003.

[166] A. Lan and J. Du, "Potential role of Akt signaling in chronic kidney disease," *Nephrology Dialysis Transplantation*, vol. 30, no. 3, pp. 385–394, 2015.

[167] G. Manda, A.-I. Checherita, M. V. Comanescu, and M. E. Hinescu, "Redox signaling in diabetic nephropathy: hypertrophy versus death choices in mesangial cells and podocytes," *Mediators of Inflammation*, vol. 2015, Article ID 604208, 13 pages, 2015.

[168] H. E. Yoon, S. J. Kim, S. J. Kim, S. Chung, and S. J. Shin, "Tempol attenuates renal fibrosis in mice with unilateral ureteral obstruction: the role of PI3K-Akt-FoxO3a signaling," *Journal of Korean Medical Science*, vol. 29, no. 2, pp. 230–237, 2014.

[169] S.-X. Guo, Q. Fang, C.-G. You et al., "Effects of hydrogen-rich saline on early acute kidney injury in severely burned rats by suppressing oxidative stress induced apoptosis and inflammation," *Journal of Translational Medicine*, vol. 13, article 183, 2015.

[170] S. Turdi, Q. Li, F. L. Lopez, and J. Ren, "Catalase alleviates cardiomyocyte dysfunction in diabetes: role of Akt, Forkhead transcriptional factor and silent information regulator 2," *Life Sciences*, vol. 81, no. 11, pp. 895–905, 2007.

[171] J. F. Ndisang and S. Tiwari, "Mechanisms by which heme oxygenase rescue renal dysfunction in obesity," *Redox Biology*, vol. 2, pp. 1029–1037, 2014.

[172] K. Sharma, S. RamachandraRao, G. Qiu et al., "Adiponectin regulates albuminuria and podocyte function in mice," *The Journal of Clinical Investigation*, vol. 118, no. 5, pp. 1645–1656, 2008.

[173] A. Terman, B. Gustafsson, and U. T. Brunk, "Autophagy, organelles and ageing," *Journal of Pathology*, vol. 211, no. 2, pp. 134–143, 2007.

[174] L. Fang, Y. Zhou, H. Cao et al., "Autophagy attenuates diabetic glomerular damage through protection of hyperglycemia-induced podocyte injury," *PLOS ONE*, vol. 8, no. 4, Article ID e60546, 2013.

[175] A. Tagawa, M. Yasuda, S. Kume et al., "Impaired podocyte autophagy exacerbates proteinuria in diabetic nephropathy," *Diabetes*, vol. 65, no. 3, pp. 755–767, 2016.

[176] K. Yamahara, M. Yasuda, S. Kume, D. Koya, H. Maegawa, and T. Uzu, "The role of autophagy in the pathogenesis of diabetic nephropathy," *Journal of Diabetes Research*, vol. 2013, Article ID 193757, 9 pages, 2013.

[177] M. Gödel, B. Hartleben, N. Herbach et al., "Role of mTOR in podocyte function and diabetic nephropathy in humans and mice," *Journal of Clinical Investigation*, vol. 121, no. 6, pp. 2197–2209, 2011.

[178] Y. Ding and M. E. Choi, "Autophagy in diabetic nephropathy," *Journal of Endocrinology*, vol. 224, no. 1, pp. R15–R30, 2015.

[179] D. P. Cinà, T. Onay, A. Paltoo et al., "Inhibition of MTOR disrupts autophagic flux in podocytes," *Journal of the American Society of Nephrology*, vol. 23, no. 3, pp. 412–420, 2012.

[180] D. Thomasova and H.-J. Anders, "Cell cycle control in the kidney," *Nephrology Dialysis Transplantation*, vol. 30, no. 10, pp. 1622–1630, 2015.

[181] C. B. Marshall and S. J. Shankland, "Cell cycle and glomerular disease: a minireview," *Nephron - Experimental Nephrology*, vol. 102, no. 2, pp. e39–e48, 2006.

[182] V. Vallon, K. Richter, R. C. Blantz, S. Thomson, and H. Osswald, "Glomerular hyperfiltration in experimental diabetes mellitus: potential role of tubular reabsorption," *Journal of the American Society of Nephrology*, vol. 10, no. 12, pp. 2569–2576, 1999.

[183] P. Persson, P. Hansell, and F. Palm, "Tubular reabsorption and diabetes-induced glomerular hyperfiltration," *Acta Physiologica*, vol. 200, no. 1, pp. 3–10, 2010.

[184] R. Faulhaber-Walter, L. Chen, M. Oppermann et al., "Lack of A1 adenosine receptors augments diabetic hyperfiltration and glomerular injury," *Journal of the American Society of Nephrology*, vol. 19, no. 4, pp. 722–730, 2008.

[185] S. Kiritoshi, T. Nishikawa, K. Sonoda et al., "Reactive oxygen species from mitochondria induce cyclooxygenase-2 gene expression in human mesangial cells: potential role in diabetic nephropathy," *Diabetes*, vol. 52, no. 10, pp. 2570–2577, 2003.

[186] N. Bank, "Mechanisms of diabetic hyperfiltration," *Kidney International*, vol. 40, no. 4, pp. 792–807, 1991.

[187] B. Teng, M. Duong, I. Tossidou, X. Yu, and M. Schiffer, "Role of protein kinase C in podocytes and development of glomerular damage in diabetic nephropathy," *Frontiers in Endocrinology*, vol. 5, article 179, 2014.

[188] Y. Ohshiro, Y. Lee, and G. L. King, "Mechanism of diabetic nephropathy: role of protein kinase-C activation," *Advanced Studies in Medicine*, vol. 5, no. 1A, pp. S10–S19, 2005.

[189] H. Konishi, M. Tanaka, Y. Takemura et al., "Activation of protein kinase C by tyrosine phosphorylation in response to H_2O_2," *Proceedings of the National Academy of Sciences of the United States of America*, vol. 94, no. 21, pp. 11233–11237, 1997.

[190] Z.-G. Xu, D.-R. Ryu, T.-H. Yoo et al., "P-Cadherin is decreased in diabetic glomeruli and in glucose-stimulated podocytes in vivo and in vitro studies," *Nephrology Dialysis Transplantation*, vol. 20, no. 3, pp. 524–531, 2005.

[191] A. B. Sanz, M. D. Sanchez-Niño, A. M. Ramos et al., "NF-κB in renal inflammation," *Journal of the American Society of Nephrology*, vol. 21, no. 8, pp. 1254–1262, 2010.

[192] L. M. Pedruzzi, M. B. Stockler-Pinto, M. Leite Jr., and D. Mafra, "Nrf2-keap1 system versus NF-κB: the good and the evil in chronic kidney disease?" *Biochimie*, vol. 94, no. 12, pp. 2461–2466, 2012.

[193] M. J. Morgan and Z.-G. Liu, "Crosstalk of reactive oxygen species and NF-κB signaling," *Cell Research*, vol. 21, no. 1, pp. 103–115, 2011.

[194] M. Ding, X. Shi, Y. Lu et al., "Induction of activator protein-1 through reactive oxygen species by crystalline silica in JB6 cells," *The Journal of Biological Chemistry*, vol. 276, no. 12, pp. 9108–9114, 2001.

[195] Y. Zhang, F. Peng, B. Gao, A. J. Ingram, and J. C. Krepinsky, "High glucose-induced RhoA activation requires caveolae and PKCβ1-mediated ROS generation," *American Journal of Physiology - Renal Physiology*, vol. 302, no. 1, pp. 159–172, 2012.

[196] C. Weigert, U. Sauer, K. Brodbeck, A. Pfeiffer, H. U. Häring, and E. D. Schleicher, "AP-1 proteins mediate hyperglycemia-induced activation of the human TGF-β1 promoter in mesangial cells," *Journal of the American Society of Nephrology*, vol. 11, no. 11, pp. 2007–2016, 2000.

[197] V. Vallon and S. C. Thomson, "Renal function in diabetic disease models: the tubular system in the pathophysiology of the diabetic kidney," *Annual Review of Physiology*, vol. 74, pp. 351–375, 2012.

[198] T. Isoe, Y. Makino, K. Mizumoto et al., "High glucose activates HIF-1-mediated signal transduction in glomerular mesangial cells through a carbohydrate response element binding protein," *Kidney International*, vol. 78, no. 1, pp. 48–59, 2010.

[199] T.-H. Chen, J.-F. Wang, P. Chan, and H.-M. Lee, "Angiotensin II stimulates hypoxia-inducible factor 1α accumulation in glomerular mesangial cells," *Annals of the New York Academy of Sciences*, vol. 1042, pp. 286–293, 2005.

[200] V. H. Haase, "Hypoxia-inducible factor signaling in the development of kidney fibrosis," *Fibrogenesis & Tissue Repair*, vol. 5, supplement 1, article S16, 2012.

[201] J. Wada and H. Makino, "Inflammation and the pathogenesis of diabetic nephropathy," *Clinical Science*, vol. 124, no. 3, pp. 139–152, 2013.

[202] L. Jiang, L. Xu, Y. Song et al., "Calmodulin-dependent protein kinase II/cAMP response element-binding protein/Wnt/β-catenin signaling cascade regulates angiotensin II-induced podocyte injury and Albuminuria," *Journal of Biological Chemistry*, vol. 288, no. 32, pp. 23368–23379, 2013.

[203] P. M. García-García, M. A. Getino-Melián, V. Domínguez-Pimentel, and J. F. Navarro-González, "Inflammation in diabetic kidney disease," *World Journal of Diabetes*, vol. 5, no. 4, pp. 431–443, 2014.

[204] C. Sassy-Prigent, D. Heudes, C. Mandet et al., "Early glomerular macrophage recruitment in streptozotocin-induced diabetic rats," *Diabetes*, vol. 49, no. 3, pp. 466–475, 2000.

[205] A. K. H. Lim and G. H. Tesch, "Inflammation in diabetic nephropathy," *Mediators of Inflammation*, vol. 2012, Article ID 146154, 12 pages, 2012.

[206] J. F. Navarro-González and C. Mora-Fernández, "The role of inflammatory cytokines in diabetic nephropathy," *Journal of the American Society of Nephrology*, vol. 19, no. 3, pp. 433–442, 2008.

[207] N. Choudhary and R. S. Ahlawat, "Interleukin-6 and C-reactive protein in pathogenesis of diabetic nephropathy: new evidence linking inflammation, glycemic control, and microalbuminuria," *Iranian Journal of Kidney Diseases*, vol. 2, no. 2, pp. 72–79, 2008.

[208] S. Shelbaya, H. Amer, S. Seddik et al., "Study of the role of interleukin-6 and highly sensitive C-reactive protein in diabetic nephropathy in type 1 diabetic patients," *European Review for Medical and Pharmacological Sciences*, vol. 16, no. 2, pp. 176–182, 2012.

[209] H. Okamura, H. Tsutsui, T. Komatsu et al., "Cloning of a new cytokine that induces IFN-γ production by T cells," *Nature*, vol. 378, no. 6552, pp. 88–90, 1995.

[210] S.-M. Dai, H. Matsuno, H. Nakamura, K. Nishioka, and K. Yudoh, "Interleukin-18 enhances monocyte tumor necrosis factor α and interleukin-1β production induced by direct contact with T lymphocytes: implications in rheumatoid arthritis," *Arthritis and Rheumatism*, vol. 50, no. 2, pp. 432–443, 2004.

[211] R. J. L. Stuyt, M. G. Netea, T. B. H. Geijtenbeek, B. J. Kullberg, C. A. Dinarello, and J. W. M. Van Der Meer, "Selective regulation of intercellular adhesion molecule-1 expression by interleukin-18 and interleukin-12 on human monocytes," *Immunology*, vol. 110, no. 3, pp. 329–334, 2003.

[212] E. Mariño and J. E. Cardier, "Differential effect of IL-18 on endothelial cell apoptosis mediated by TNF-α and Fas (CD95)," *Cytokine*, vol. 22, no. 5, pp. 142–148, 2003.

[213] M. Schwarz, M. Wahl, K. Resch, and H. H. Radeke, "IFNγ induces functional chemokine receptor expression in human mesangial cells," *Clinical and Experimental Immunology*, vol. 128, no. 2, pp. 285–294, 2002.

[214] Y. Moriwaki, T. Yamamoto, Y. Shibutani et al., "Elevated levels of interleukin-18 and tumor necrosis factor-α in serum of patients with type 2 diabetes mellitus: relationship with diabetic nephropathy," *Metabolism: Clinical and Experimental*, vol. 52, no. 5, pp. 605–608, 2003.

[215] A. Nakamura, K. Shikata, M. Hiramatsu et al., "Serum interleukin-18 levels are associated with nephropathy and atherosclerosis in Japanese patients with type 2 diabetes," *Diabetes Care*, vol. 28, no. 12, pp. 2890–2895, 2005.

[216] S. Araki, M. Haneda, D. Koya et al., "Predictive impact of elevated serum level of IL-18 for early renal dysfunction in type 2 diabetes: an observational follow-up study," *Diabetologia*, vol. 50, no. 4, pp. 867–873, 2007.

[217] T. Nakamura, M. Fukui, I. Ebihara et al., "mRNA expression of growth factors in glomeruli from diabetic rats," *Diabetes*, vol. 42, no. 3, pp. 450–456, 1993.

[218] X. Dong, S. Swaminathan, L. A. Bachman, A. J. Croatt, K. A. Nath, and M. D. Griffin, "Resident dendritic cells are the predominant TNF-secreting cell in early renal ischemia-reperfusion injury," *Kidney International*, vol. 71, no. 7, pp. 619–628, 2007.

[219] A. M. Jevnikar, D. C. Brennan, G. G. Singer et al., "Stimulated kidney tubular epithelial cells express membrane associated and secreted TNFα," *Kidney International*, vol. 40, no. 2, pp. 203–211, 1991.

[220] T. J. Neale, B. M. Ruger, H. Macaulay et al., "Tumor necrosis factor-α is expressed by glomerular visceral epithelial cells in human membranous nephropathy," *The American Journal of Pathology*, vol. 146, no. 6, pp. 1444–1454, 1995.

[221] H. H. Radeke, B. Meier, N. Topley, J. Flöge, G. G. Habermehl, and K. Resch, "Interleukin 1-α and tumor necrosis factor-α induce oxygen radical production in mesangial cells," *Kidney International*, vol. 37, no. 2, pp. 767–775, 1990.

[222] L. Baud, J. Perez, G. Friedlander, and R. Ardaillou, "Tumor necrosis factor stimulates prostaglandin production and cyclic AMP levels in rat cultured mesangial cells," *FEBS Letters*, vol. 239, no. 1, pp. 50–54, 1988.

[223] B. Wójciak-Stothard, A. Entwistle, R. Garg, and A. J. Ridley, "Regulation of TNF-α-induced reorganization of the actin cytoskeleton and cell-cell junctions by Rho, Rac, and Cdc42 in human endothelial cells," *Journal of Cellular Physiology*, vol. 176, no. 1, pp. 150–165, 1998.

[224] S. M. Laster, J. G. Wood, and L. R. Gooding, "Tumor necrosis factor can induce both apoptic and necrotic forms of cell lysis," *Journal of Immunology*, vol. 141, no. 8, pp. 2629–2634, 1988.

[225] T. Bertani, M. Abbate, C. Zoja et al., "Tumor necrosis factor induces glomerular damage in the rabbit," *The American Journal of Pathology*, vol. 134, no. 2, pp. 419–430, 1989.

[226] J. F. Navarro, F. J. Milena, C. Mora et al., "Tumor necrosis factor-α gene expression in diabetic nephropathy: relationship with urinary albumin excretion and effect of angiotensin-converting enzyme inhibition," *Kidney International*, vol. 68, supplement 99, pp. S98–S102, 2005.

[227] J. F. Navarro, F. J. Milena, C. Mora, C. León, and J. García, "Renal pro-inflammatory cytokine gene expression in diabetic nephropathy: effect of angiotensin-converting enzyme inhibition and pentoxifylline administration," *American Journal of Nephrology*, vol. 26, no. 6, pp. 562–570, 2006.

[228] T. Wada, J. W. Pippen, Y. Terada, and S. J. Shankland, "The cyclin-dependent kinase inhibitor p21 is required for TGF-β1-induced podocyte apoptosis," *Kidney International*, vol. 68, no. 4, pp. 1618–1629, 2005.

[229] S. J. Shankland, J. Floege, S. E. Thomas et al., "Cyclin kinase inhibitors are increased during experimental membranous nephropathy: potential role in limiting glomerular epithelial cell proliferation *in vivo*," *Kidney International*, vol. 52, no. 2, pp. 404–413, 1997.

[230] C. J. Kuan, M. Al-Douahji, and S. J. Shankland, "The cyclin kinase inhibitor p21^{WAF1,CIP1} is increased in experimental diabetic nephropathy: potential role in glomerular hypertrophy," *Journal of the American Society of Nephrology*, vol. 9, no. 6, pp. 986–993, 1998.

[231] G. Gruden, P. C. Perin, and G. Camussi, "Insight on the pathogenesis of diabetic nephropathy from the study of podocyte and mesangial cell biology," *Current Diabetes Reviews*, vol. 1, no. 1, pp. 27–40, 2005.

[232] G. Wolf and F. N. Ziyadeh, "Cellular and molecular mechanisms of proteinuria in diabetic nephropathy," *Nephron—Physiology*, vol. 106, no. 2, pp. p26–p31, 2007.

[233] M. Khamaisi, B. F. Schrijvers, A. S. de Vriese, I. Raz, and A. Flyvbjerg, "The emerging role of VEGF in diabetic kidney disease," *Nephrology Dialysis Transplantation*, vol. 18, no. 8, pp. 1427–1430, 2003.

[234] K. Iijima, N. Yoshikawa, D. T. Connolly, and H. Nakamura, "Human mesangial cells and peripheral blood mononuclear cells produce vascular permeability factor," *Kidney International*, vol. 44, no. 5, pp. 959–966, 1993.

[235] D. R. Cha, Y. S. Kang, S. Y. Han et al., "Vascular endothelial growth factor is increased during early stage of diabetic nephropathy in type II diabetic rats," *Journal of Endocrinology*, vol. 183, no. 1, pp. 183–194, 2004.

[236] M. E. Cooper, D. Vranes, S. Youssef et al., "Increased renal expression of vascular endothelial growth factor (VEGF) and its receptor VEGFR-2 in experimental diabetes," *Diabetes*, vol. 48, no. 11, pp. 2229–2239, 1999.

[237] S. Hoshi, Y. Shu, F. Yoshida et al., "Podocyte injury promotes progressive nephropathy in zucker diabetic fatty rats," *Laboratory Investigation*, vol. 82, no. 1, pp. 25–35, 2002.

[238] E.-Y. Lee, C. H. Chung, J. H. Kim, H.-J. Joung, and S. Y. Hong, "Antioxidants ameliorate the expression of vascular endothelial growth factor mediated by protein kinase C in diabetic podocytes," *Nephrology Dialysis Transplantation*, vol. 21, no. 6, pp. 1496–1503, 2006.

[239] T. Eleftheriadis, G. Antoniadi, G. Pissas, V. Liakopoulos, and I. Stefanidis, "The renal endothelium in diabetic nephropathy," *Renal Failure*, vol. 35, no. 4, pp. 592–599, 2013.

[240] A. S. De Vriese, R. G. Tilton, M. Elger, C. C. Stephan, W. Kriz, and N. H. Lameire, "Antibodies against vascular endothelial growth factor improve early renal dysfunction in experimental diabetes," *Journal of the American Society of Nephrology*, vol. 12, no. 5, pp. 993–1000, 2001.

[241] B. F. Schrijvers, A. Flyvbjerg, R. G. Tilton, N. H. Lameire, and A. S. De Vriese, "A neutralizing VEGF antibody prevents glomerular hypertrophy in a model of obese type 2 diabetes, the Zucker diabetic fatty rat," *Nephrology Dialysis Transplantation*, vol. 21, no. 2, pp. 324–329, 2006.

[242] A. Flyvbjerg, F. Dagnæs-Hansen, A. S. De Vriese, B. F. Schrijvers, R. G. Tilton, and R. Rasch, "Amelioration of long-term renal changes in obese type 2 diabetic mice by a neutralizing vascular endothelial growth factor antibody," *Diabetes*, vol. 51, no. 10, pp. 3090–3094, 2002.

[243] C.-H. Ku, K. E. White, A. D. Cas et al., "Inducible overexpression of sFlt-1 in podocytes ameliorates glomerulopathy in diabetic mice," *Diabetes*, vol. 57, no. 10, pp. 2824–2833, 2008.

[244] S. H. Sung, F. N. Ziyadeh, A. Wang, P. E. Pyagay, Y. S. Kanwar, and S. Chen, "Blockade of vascular endothelial growth factor signaling ameliorates diabetic albuminuria in mice," *Journal of the American Society of Nephrology*, vol. 17, no. 11, pp. 3093–3104, 2006.

[245] Y. Yamamoto, Y. Maeshima, H. Kitayama et al., "Tumstatin peptide, an inhibitor of angiogenesis, prevents glomerular hypertrophy in the early stage of diabetic nephropathy," *Diabetes*, vol. 53, no. 7, pp. 1831–1840, 2004.

[246] K. Ichinose, Y. Maeshima, Y. Yamamoto et al., "Antiangiogenic endostatin peptide ameliorates renal alterations in the early of a type 1 diabetic nephropathy model," *Diabetes*, vol. 54, no. 10, pp. 2891–2903, 2005.

[247] J. J. Cha, Y. S. Kang, Y. Y. Hyun et al., "Sulodexide improves renal function through reduction of vascular endothelial growth factor in type 2 diabetic rats," *Life Sciences*, vol. 92, no. 23, pp. 1118–1124, 2013.

[248] V. Eremina, J. A. Jefferson, J. Kowalewska et al., "VEGF inhibition and renal thrombotic microangiopathy," *The New England Journal of Medicine*, vol. 358, no. 11, pp. 1129–1136, 2008.

[249] X. Zhu, S. Wu, W. L. Dahut, and C. R. Parikh, "Risks of proteinuria and hypertension with bevacizumab, an antibody against vascular endothelial growth factor: systematic review and meta-analysis," *American Journal of Kidney Diseases*, vol. 49, no. 2, pp. 186–193, 2007.

[250] A. Mima, W. Qi, and G. L. King, "Implications of treatment that target protective mechanisms against diabetic nephropathy," *Seminars in Nephrology*, vol. 32, no. 5, pp. 471–478, 2012.

[251] S. Oltean, Y. Qiu, J. K. Ferguson et al., "Vascular endothelial growth factor-A_{165}b is protective and restores endothelial glycocalyx in diabetic nephropathy," *Journal of the American Society of Nephrology*, vol. 26, no. 8, pp. 1889–1904, 2015.

[252] M. R. Duncan, K. S. Frazier, S. Abramson et al., "Connective tissue growth factor mediates transforming growth factor β-induced collagen synthesis: down-regulation by cAMP," *FASEB Journal*, vol. 13, no. 13, pp. 1774–1786, 1999.

[253] N. A. Wahab, B. S. Weston, T. Roberts, and R. M. Mason, "Connective tissue growth factor and regulation of the mesangial cell cycle: Role in cellular hypertrophy," *Journal of the American Society of Nephrology*, vol. 13, no. 10, pp. 2437–2445, 2002.

[254] S. E. Thomson, S. V. McLennan, P. D. Kirwan et al., "Renal connective tissue growth factor correlates with glomerular basement membrane thickness and prospective albuminuria in a non-human primate model of diabetes: possible predictive marker for incipient diabetic nephropathy," *Journal of Diabetes and Its Complications*, vol. 22, no. 4, pp. 284–294, 2008.

[255] L. R. James, C. Le, H. Doherty, H.-S. Kim, and N. Maeda, "Connective tissue growth factor (CTGF) expression modulates response to high glucose," *PLoS ONE*, vol. 8, no. 8, Article ID e70441, 2013.

[256] H. Yokoi, M. Mukoyama, K. Mori et al., "Overexpression of connective tissue growth factor in podocytes worsens diabetic nephropathy in mice," *Kidney International*, vol. 73, no. 4, pp. 446–455, 2008.

[257] E. Sánchez-López, S. Rayego, R. Rodrigues-Díez et al., "CTGF promotes inflammatory cell infiltration of the renal interstitium by activating NF-κB," *Journal of the American Society of Nephrology*, vol. 20, no. 7, pp. 1513–1526, 2009.

[258] S. V. McLennan, X. Y. Wang, V. Moreno, D. K. Yue, and S. M. Twigg, "Connective tissue growth factor mediates high glucose effects on matrix degradation through tissue inhibitor of matrix metalloproteinase type 1: implications for diabetic nephropathy," *Endocrinology*, vol. 145, no. 12, pp. 5646–5655, 2004.

[259] J. Floege, F. Eitner, and C. E. Alpers, "A new look at platelet-derived growth factor in renal disease," *Journal of the American Society of Nephrology*, vol. 19, no. 1, pp. 12–23, 2008.

[260] P. Boor, T. Ostendorf, and J. Floege, "PDGF and the progression of renal disease," *Nephrology Dialysis Transplantation*, vol. 29, supplement 1, pp. i45–i54, 2014.

[261] D. E. Staunton, S. D. Marlin, C. Stratowa, M. L. Dustin, and T. A. Springer, "Primary structure of ICAM-1 demonstrates interaction between members of the immunoglobulin and integrin supergene families," *Cell*, vol. 52, no. 6, pp. 925–933, 1988.

[262] K. Shikata and H. Makino, "Microinflammation in the pathogenesis of diabetic nephropathy," *Journal of Diabetes Investigation*, vol. 4, no. 2, pp. 142–149, 2013.

[263] C. W. Park, J. H. Kim, J. W. Lee et al., "High glucose-induced intercellular adhesion molecule-1 (ICAM-1) expression through an osmotic effect in rat mesangial cells is PKC-NF-kappa B-dependent," *Diabetologia*, vol. 43, no. 12, pp. 1544–1553, 2000.

[264] H. Sugimoto, K. Shikata, K. Hirata et al., "Increased expression of intercellular adhesion molecule-1 (ICAM-1) in diabetic rat glomeruli: glomerular hyperfiltration is a potential mechanism of ICAM-1 upregulation," *Diabetes*, vol. 46, no. 12, pp. 2075–2081, 1997.

[265] T. M. Coimbra, U. Janssen, H. J. Gröne et al., "Early events leading to renal injury in obese Zucker (fatty) rats with type II diabetes," *Kidney International*, vol. 57, no. 1, pp. 167–182, 2000.

[266] F. Y. Chow, D. J. Nikolic-Paterson, E. Ozols, R. C. Atkins, and G. H. Tesch, "Intercellular adhesion molecule-1 deficiency is protective against nephropathy in type 2 diabetic db/db mice," *Journal of the American Society of Nephrology*, vol. 16, no. 6, pp. 1711–1722, 2005.

[267] S. Okada, K. Shikata, M. Matsuda et al., "Intercellular adhesion molecule-1-deficient mice are resistant against renal injury after

induction of diabetes," *Diabetes*, vol. 52, no. 10, pp. 2586–2593, 2003.

[268] Y. Hosokawa, I. Hosokawa, K. Ozaki, H. Nakae, and T. Matsuo, "Cytokines differentially regulate ICAM-1 and VCAM-1 expression on human gingival fibroblasts," *Clinical and Experimental Immunology*, vol. 144, no. 3, pp. 494–502, 2006.

[269] E. Di Marco, S. P. Gray, and K. Jandeleit-Dahm, "Diabetes alters activation and repression of pro- and anti-inflammatory signaling pathways in the vasculature," *Frontiers in Endocrinology*, vol. 4, article 68, 2013.

[270] T. Wada, K. Furuichi, N. Sakai et al., "Up-regulation of monocyte chemoattractant protein-1 in tubulointerstitial lesions of human diabetic nephropathy," *Kidney International*, vol. 58, no. 4, pp. 1492–1499, 2000.

[271] B. Amann, R. Tinzmann, and B. Angelkort, "ACE inhibitors improve diabetic nephropathy through suppression of renal MCP-1," *Diabetes Care*, vol. 26, no. 8, pp. 2421–2425, 2003.

[272] F. Y. Chow, D. J. Nikolic-Paterson, E. Ozols, R. C. Atkins, B. J. Rollin, and G. H. Tesch, "Monocyte chemoattractant protein-1 promotes the development of diabetic renal injury in streptozotocin-treated mice," *Kidney International*, vol. 69, no. 1, pp. 73–80, 2006.

[273] A. C. K. Chung and H. Y. Lan, "Chemokines in renal injury," *Journal of the American Society of Nephrology*, vol. 22, no. 5, pp. 802–809, 2011.

[274] J. F. Ndisang, A. Jadhav, and M. Mishra, "The heme oxygenase system suppresses perirenal visceral adiposity, abates renal inflammation and ameliorates diabetic nephropathy in zucker diabetic fatty rats," *PLoS ONE*, vol. 9, no. 1, Article ID e87936, 2014.

[275] G. Ding, K. Reddy, A. A. Kapasi et al., "Angiotensin II induces apoptosis in rat glomerular epithelial cells," *American Journal of Physiology—Renal Physiology*, vol. 283, no. 1, pp. F173–F180, 2002.

[276] S. Blanco, J. Bonet, D. López, I. Casas, and R. Romero, "ACE inhibitors improve nephrin expression in Zucker rats with glomerulosclerosis," *Kidney International*, vol. 67, supplement 93, pp. S10–S14, 2005.

[277] S. Kagami, W. A. Border, D. E. Miller, and N. A. Noble, "Angiotensin II stimulates extracellular matrix protein synthesis through induction of transforming growth factor-β expression in rat glomerular mesangial cells," *The Journal of Clinical Investigation*, vol. 93, no. 6, pp. 2431–2437, 1994.

[278] J. D. Ahn, R. Morishita, Y. Kaneda et al., "Transcription factor decoy for AP-1 reduces mesangial cell proliferation and extracellular matrix production in vitro and in vivo," *Gene Therapy*, vol. 11, no. 11, pp. 916–923, 2004.

[279] A. Sachse and G. Wolf, "Angiotensin II-induced reactive oxygen species and the kidney," *Journal of the American Society of Nephrology*, vol. 18, no. 9, pp. 2439–2446, 2007.

[280] K. N. Campbell, L. Raij, and P. Mundel, "Role of angiotensin II in the development of nephropathy and podocytopathy of diabetes," *Current Diabetes Reviews*, vol. 7, no. 1, pp. 3–7, 2011.

[281] C. Cabello-Verrugio, M. J. Acuña, M. G. Morales, A. Becerra, F. Simon, and E. Brandan, "Fibrotic response induced by angiotensin-II requires NAD(P)H oxidase-induced reactive oxygen species (ROS) in skeletal muscle cells," *Biochemical and Biophysical Research Communications*, vol. 410, no. 3, pp. 665–670, 2011.

[282] J. M. Sasser, J. C. Sullivan, J. L. Hobbs et al., "Endothelin A receptor blockade reduces diabetic renal injury via an anti-inflammatory mechanism," *Journal of the American Society of Nephrology*, vol. 18, no. 1, pp. 143–154, 2007.

[283] C. Reichetzeder, O. Tsuprykov, and B. Hocher, "Endothelin receptor antagonists in clinical research—lessons learned from preclinical and clinical kidney studies," *Life Sciences*, vol. 118, no. 2, pp. 141–148, 2014.

[284] M. S. Simonson and F. Ismail-Beigi, "Endothelin-1 increases collagen accumulation in renal mesangial cells by stimulating a chemokine and cytokine autocrine signaling loop," *The Journal of Biological Chemistry*, vol. 286, no. 13, pp. 11003–11008, 2011.

[285] W. Kriz, N. Gretz, and K. V. Lemley, "Progression of glomerular diseases: is the podocyte the culprit?" *Kidney International*, vol. 54, no. 3, pp. 687–697, 1998.

[286] A. A. Eddy, "Molecular basis of renal fibrosis," *Pediatric Nephrology*, vol. 15, no. 3-4, pp. 290–301, 2000.

[287] A. A. Eddy, "Proteinuria and interstitial injury," *Nephrology Dialysis Transplantation*, vol. 19, no. 2, pp. 277–281, 2004.

[288] A. A. Eddy, "Interstitial nephritis induced by protein-overload proteinuria," *American Journal of Pathology*, vol. 135, no. 4, pp. 719–733, 1989.

[289] W. Kriz, H. Hosser, B. Hähnel, N. Gretz, and A. P. Provoost, "From segmental glomerulosclerosis to total nephron degeneration and interstitial fibrosis: a histopathological study in rat models and human gomerulopathies," *Nephrology Dialysis Transplantation*, vol. 13, no. 11, pp. 2781–2798, 1998.

[290] C. Thomas and L. Thomas, "Renal failure—measuring the glomerular filtration rate," *Deutsches Ärzteblatt International*, vol. 106, no. 51-52, pp. 849–854, 2009.

[291] R. Das, S. Xu, X. Quan et al., "Upregulation of mitochondrial Nox4 mediates TGF-β-induced apoptosis in cultured mouse podocytes," *American Journal of Physiology: Renal Physiology*, vol. 306, no. 2, pp. F155–F167, 2014.

[292] S. Yaddanapudi, M. M. Altintas, A. D. Kistler et al., "CD2AP in mouse and human podocytes controls a proteolytic program that regulates cytoskeletal structure and cellular survival," *The Journal of Clinical Investigation*, vol. 121, no. 10, pp. 3965–3980, 2011.

17

Administration of RAS Inhibitor before the Onset of Diabetic Nephropathy Counteracts the Adverse Effect of Chronic Hyperglycemia and Reduces the Augmentation of Urinary Albumin Excretion

Hidenori Hirukawa, Shinji Kamei, Tomohiko Kimura, Atsushi Obata, Kenji Kohara, Fuminori Tatsumi, Masashi Shimoda, Shuhei Nakanishi, Tomoatsu Mune, Kohei Kaku, and Hideaki Kaneto

Department of Diabetes, Endocrinology and Metabolism, Kawasaki Medical School, Japan

Correspondence should be addressed to Hidenori Hirukawa; hirukawa@med.kawasaki-m.ac.jp

Academic Editor: Kim Connelly

It is very important to explore how we can reduce urinary albumin excretion which is an independent risk factor for ischemic heart disease. In this study, we retrospectively evaluated the effects of RAS inhibitor therapy on diabetic nephropathy in Japanese subjects whose urinary albumin levels were within normal range. We enrolled 100 subjects with type 2 diabetes who did not take any renin-angiotensin system (RAS) inhibitor. We defined the subjects taking RAS inhibitor for more than 3 years as RAS inhibitor group. RAS inhibitor exerted protective effect on the progression of urinary albumin excretion in subjects with type 2 diabetes without diabetic nephropathy. In addition, RAS inhibitor exerted more protective effects on renal function especially in subjects with poor glycemic control. In conclusion, RAS inhibitor could protect renal function against the deleterious effect of chronic hyperglycemia in Japanese subjects with type 2 diabetes even before the onset of diabetic nephropathy.

1. Introduction

It is known that the augmentation of urinary albumin excretion (UAE) is associated with vascular endothelium disorder and is an independent risk factor for ischemic heart disease [1–5]. In addition, the increase of UAE leads to the ratio of cardiovascular disease-related mortality even before the onset of diabetic nephropathy [6, 7]. Therefore, it is very important to explore how we can reduce UAE. Hyperglycemia and subsequent activation of renin-angiotensin system (RAS) are associated with the development of diabetic nephropathy [8–12]. It was reported that RAS inhibitors suppressed the progression of overt diabetic nephropathy [13–16]. It remained unclear, however, whether RAS inhibitors exert such beneficial effects even before the onset of diabetic nephropathy. In this study, we retrospectively evaluated the effects of RAS inhibitor therapy on diabetic nephropathy in Japanese subjects whose urinary albumin levels were within normal range.

2. Methods

We enrolled the subjects with type 2 diabetes who visited Department of Diabetes, Endocrinology and Metabolism in Kawasaki Medical School and did not take any RAS inhibitor. We defined the subjects who started taking RAS inhibitor and continued for more than 3 years as RAS inhibitor group and the subjects who did not start any RAS inhibitor as control group. In RAS inhibitor group, 57 subjects had angiotensin II receptor blocker, 2

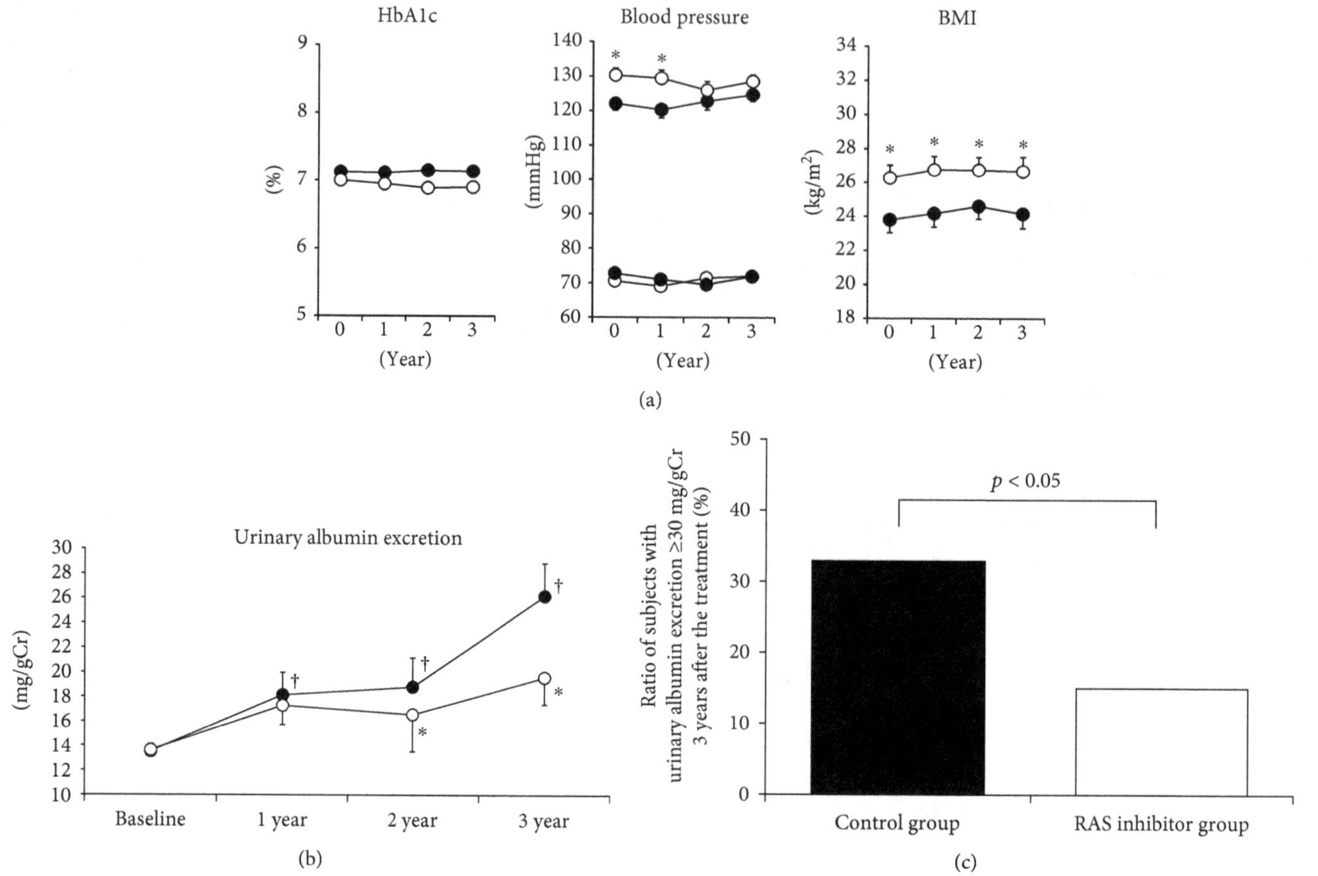

FIGURE 1: (a) Alteration of HbA1c, blood pressure, and BMI during 3-year observational period. Closed circle, control group; open circle, RAS inhibitor group. $^*p < 0.05$. (b) Alteration of urinary albumin excretion during 3-year observational period. Closed circle, control group; open circle, RAS inhibitor group. $^*p < 0.05$ vs. control group, $^\dagger p < 0.05$ vs. baseline value in control group. (c) Ratio of subjects with urinary albumin excretion ≥ 30 mg/gCr in subjects with and without RAS inhibitor treatment.

subjects had angiotensin-converting-enzyme inhibitor, and 1 subject had renin inhibitor. The study protocol was approved by our hospital ethics committee (no. 2419).

Clinical characteristics at baseline in RAS inhibitor group ($n = 60$, male/female = 35/25) and control group ($n = 100$, male/female = 60/40) were as follows: age, 60.0 ± 1.1 vs. 63.0 ± 1.4 years old (not significant (n.s.)); duration of diabetes, 11.3 ± 1.1 vs. 9.5 ± 1.1 years (n.s.); HbA1c, 7.09 ± 0.09% vs. 7.01 ± 0.13% (n.s.); Hb, 14.0 ± 0.2 g/dL vs. 13.6 ± 0.1 g/dL (n.s.); BMI, 23.8 ± 0.4 kg/m^2 vs. 26.3 ± 0.8 kg/m^2 ($p < 0.05$); LDL cholesterol, 103.2 ± 2.7 mg/dL vs. 104.4 ± 3.5 mg/dL (n.s.); HDL cholesterol, 54.0 ± 1.6 mg/dL vs. 55.1 ± 2.5 mg/dL (n.s.); triglyceride, 131.9 ± 9.3 mg/dL vs. 127.6 ± 10.8 mg/dL (n.s.); systolic blood pressure, 122.1 ± 1.8 mmHg vs. 130.3 ± 2.0 mmHg ($p < 0.05$); diastolic blood pressure, 70.6 ± 1.3 mmHg vs. 72.8 ± 1.6 mmHg (n.s.); urinary albumin excretion (UAE), 13.3 ± 0.6 mg/gCr vs. 13.6 ± 0.9 mg/gCr (n.s.); eGFR, 83.8 ± 2.3 mL/min/1.73m^2 vs. 79.4 ± 2.3 mL/min/1.73m^2; uric acid, 5.6 ± 0.2 mg/dL vs. 5.3 ± 0.1 mg/dL (n.s.); prevalence of diabetic retinopathy, 14.3% vs. 9.3% (n.s.); smoking status, 40.8% vs. 44.4% (n.s.); and family history of diabetes, 55.6% vs. 58.1% (n.s.). There was no difference in the ratio of antidiabetic drug use between the 2 groups. Similarly, there was no difference in the ratio of lipid-lowering drug use between the 2 groups: statin, 45.0% vs. 46.0% (RAS inhibitor group vs. control group) (n.s); fibrates, 8.3% vs. 6.0% (n.s.); and ezetimibe, 55.6% vs. 58.1% (n.s.).

An analysis of the relative odds of the occurrence of the outcome was performed with the use of a logistic regression model.

3. Results

There was no difference in HbA1c levels between RAS inhibitor group and control group through the 3-year observation period (Figure 1(a)). Systolic blood pressure in RAS inhibitor group was higher compared to that in control group at baseline and 1 year after starting RAS inhibitor ($p < 0.05$), but there was no difference between them 2 and 3 years after the treatment. There was no difference in diastolic blood pressure between the 2 groups. BMI in RAS inhibitor group was higher compared to that in control group through the observation period ($p < 0.05$).

Urinary albumin excretion (UAE) in control group was significantly increased compared to baseline (from 13.5 ± 0.5 mg/gCr to 26.2 ± 2.2 mg/gCr) ($p < 0.05$), whereas there was no significant difference in RAS inhibitor group between at

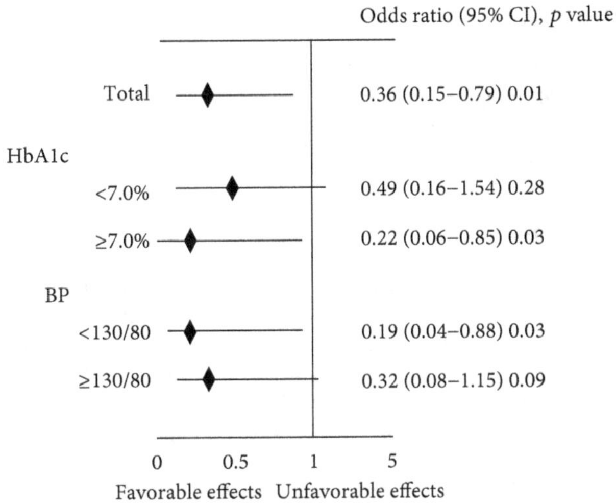

FIGURE 2: Odds ratio (95% CI) for favorable effect of RAS inhibitor on urinary albumin excretion. Comparison of odds ratio between the subjects with HbA1c < 7.0% and ≥7.0% and between the subjects with blood pressure < 130/80 mmHg and ≥130/80 mmHg.

baseline and 3 years after the treatment (13.6 ± 0.6 mg/gCr and 19.6 ± 2.7 mg/gCr) (Figure 1(b)). The alteration of UAE in RAS inhibitor group and control group was 2.5 ± 1.6 mg/gCr and 11.4 ± 2.2 mg/gCr, respectively. In addition, 2 and 3 years after the treatment, there was significant difference in UAE between the 2 groups ($p < 0.05$). UAE in 33% of control group increased up to ≥30 mg/gCr whereas only 15% of RAS inhibitor group increased up to ≥30 mg/gCr (Figure 1(c)). These data suggest that RAS inhibitor therapy exerts protective effect on the progression of UAE.

Next, we evaluated odds ratio about the progression of diabetic nephropathy. As shown in Figure 2, odds ratio (95% CI) for favorable effect of RAS inhibitor on UAE in all subjects was 0.36 (0.15–0.79), suggesting that RAS inhibitor exerted favorable effects. Odds ratio for favorable effect of RAS inhibitor on UAE in subjects with HbA1c < 7.0% and ≥7.0% was 0.49 (0.16–1.54) and 0.22 (0.06–0.85), respectively. These data suggest that RAS inhibitor exerted more beneficial effects in subjects with poor glycemic control. Odds ratio for favorable effect of RAS inhibitor on UAE in subjects with blood pressure < 130/80 mmHg and ≥130/80 mmHg was 0.19 (0.04–0.88) and 0.32 (0.08–1.15), respectively. These data suggest that blood pressure control is important for RAS inhibitor to exert beneficial effect.

Finally, to evaluate the possible association between the alteration of UAE and various clinical parameters, we performed univariate analysis. As shown in Table 1, the alteration of UAE was closely associated with annual mean HbA1c level through 3-year observational period in control group ($r = 0.406$, $p < 0.0005$), but such association was not observed in RAS inhibitor group ($r = 0.003$, p: n.s.). There was no association in both groups between the alteration of UAE and various other clinical parameters including age, duration of diabetes, eGFR at baseline, and annual mean of HbA1c levels, systolic and diastolic blood pressure, CRP, BMI, triglyceride, and LDL and HDL cholesterol.

TABLE 1: Association between the alteration of urinary albumin excretion and various clinical parameters: univariate analysis.

	Control group		RAS inhibitor group	
	r	p	r	p
HbA1c, annual mean	0.406	<0.0005	0.003	n.s.
Age, baseline	−0.083	n.s.	0.146	n.s.
Duration of diabetes, baseline	−0.002	n.s.	−0.104	n.s.
Systolic BP, annual mean	0.021	n.s.	0.250	n.s.
Diastolic BP, annual mean	0.041	n.s.	−0.004	n.s.
CRP, annual mean	0.199	n.s.	−0.090	n.s.
TG, annual mean	0.093	n.s.	0.069	n.s.
HDL-C, annual mean	−0.146	n.s.	−0.083	n.s.
LDL-C, annual mean	−0.031	n.s.	0.101	n.s.
BMI annual mean	0.035	n.s.	−0.033	n.s.
eGFR, baseline	0.202	n.s.	0.066	n.s.

Abbreviations: n.s., not significant; BP, blood pressure; TG, triglyceride; LDL-C, low-density lipoprotein cholesterol; HDL-C, high-density lipoprotein cholesterol; BMI, body mass index; RAS, renin-angiotensin system.

TABLE 2: Association between the alteration of urinary albumin excretion and various clinical parameters: multivariate analysis.

	Control group		RAS inhibitor group	
	β	p	β	p
HbA1c, annual mean	7.574	<0.005	−1.749	n.s.
Age, baseline	0.208	n.s.	0.171	n.s.
Systolic BP, annual mean	−0.021	n.s.	0.165	n.s.
Gender	0.533	n.s.	1.017	n.s.
eGFR, baseline	0.019	n.s.	0.142	n.s.

Abbreviations: n.s., not significant; BP, blood pressure; RAS, renin-angiotensin system.

Furthermore, to adjust the possible influence of blood pressure, eGFR, age, and gender on the alteration of UAE, we performed multivariate analysis using annual mean of HbA1c levels, systolic blood pressure, GFR and age at baseline, and gender as explanatory variables and the alteration of UAE as an objective variable. As shown in Table 2, annual mean of HbA1c levels was an independent determinant factor for the alteration of UAE in control group ($\beta = 7.574$, $p < 0.005$), but not in RAS inhibitor group ($\beta = -1.749$, p: n.s.). These data strengthened the idea that RAS inhibitor could protect renal function against the deleterious effect of chronic hyperglycemia in subjects with type 2 diabetes without diabetic nephropathy.

4. Discussion

It was known that RAS inhibitors suppressed the progression of overt diabetic nephropathy, but it remained unclear whether RAS inhibitors would bring out some favorable effects on renal function even before the onset of diabetic nephropathy. In this study, we showed that RAS inhibitor could exert protective effect on the progression of UAE and could counteract the adverse effect of hyperglycemia in subjects with type 2 diabetes even before the onset of diabetic nephropathy (Figure 1). RAS inhibitor exerted more protective effects on renal function in subjects with poor glycemic control (Figure 2). Therefore, it is likely that administration of RAS inhibitor reduces the adverse effect of hyperglycemia on the progression of UAE. In addition, these data suggest that it is more important to use RAS inhibitor when glycemic control is poor. Poor glycemic control was an independent determinant factor for the alteration of UAE in control group, but such findings were not observed in RAS inhibitor group (Table 2). These data suggest that deleterious effect of chronic hyperglycemia on renal function was reduced by the usage of RAS inhibitor in subjects with type 2 diabetes before the onset of diabetic nephropathy. In addition, RAS inhibitor exerted more protective effects on renal function in subjects with good control of blood pressure (Figure 2). These data suggest that it is very important to maintain good control of blood pressure so that RAS inhibitor could bring out more favorable effect on the progression of UAE and protection of renal function. Taken together, it is likely that RAS inhibitor exerts more beneficial effects in subjects with poor glycemic control and good control of blood pressure.

There are several limitations in this study. First, this is a retrospective study, but not a prospective study. Therefore, it would be necessary to perform a prospective study with a placebo control in order to strengthen our hypothesis. Second, the data in this study are influenced by lifestyle, diet, and other factors such as alternative medicine. Therefore, it would be necessary to perform some intervention to various factors including lifestyle so that we can demonstrate our hypothesis.

In conclusion, RAS inhibitor could protect renal function against the deleterious effect of chronic hyperglycemia in Japanese subjects with type 2 diabetes even before the onset of diabetic nephropathy.

Conflicts of Interest

Hideaki Kaneto has received honoraria for lectures and received scholarship grants from Sanofi, Novo Nordisk, Lilly, Boehringer Ingelheim, MSD, Takeda, Ono Pharma, Daiichi Sankyo, Sumitomo Dainippon Pharma, Mitsubishi Tanabe Pharma, Pfizer, Kissei Pharma, AstraZeneca, Astellas, Novartis, Kowa, Chugai, and Taisho Pharma. Kohei Kaku has been an advisor to, received honoraria for lectures from, and received scholarship grants from Novo Nordisk Pharma, Sanwa Kagaku Kenkyusho, Takeda, Taisho Pharmaceutical Co. Ltd, MSD, Kowa, Sumitomo Dainippon Pharma, Novartis, Mitsubishi Tanabe Pharma, AstraZeneca, Nippon Boehringer Ingelheim Co. Ltd, Chugai, Daiichi Sankyo, and Sanofi.

Funding

This work was supported by a Grant-in-Aid from the Japan Society for the Promotion of Science (no. 16K09770 to H. K.) and Research Project Grants from the Kawasaki Medical School (no. 28-021 to H. K.).

References

[1] H. Ibsen, M. H. Olsen, K. Wachtell et al., "Does albuminuria predict cardiovascular outcomes on treatment with losartan versus atenolol in patients with diabetes, hypertension, and left ventricular hypertrophy? The LIFE study," *Diabetes Care*, vol. 29, no. 3, pp. 595–600, 2006.

[2] P. Gæde, P. Vedel, N. Larsen, G. V. H. Jensen, H.-H. Parving, and O. Pedersen, "Multifactorial intervention and cardiovascular disease in patients with type 2 diabetes," *New England Journal of Medicine*, vol. 348, no. 5, pp. 383–393, 2003.

[3] M. Afkarian, M. C. Sachs, B. Kestenbaum et al., "Kidney disease and increased mortality risk in type 2 diabetes," *Journal of the American Society of Nephrology*, vol. 24, no. 2, pp. 302–308, 2013.

[4] H. B. Al-Saffar, H. Nassir, A. Mitchell, and S. Philipp, "Microalbuminuria in non-diabetic patients with unstable angina/non ST-segment elevation myocardial infarction," *BMC Research Notes*, vol. 8, no. 1, p. 371, 2015.

[5] H. Ota, N. Takehara, T. Aonuma et al., "Association between microalbuminuria predicting in-stent restenosis after myocardial infarction and cellular senescence of endothelial progenitor cells," *PLoS One*, vol. 10, no. 4, article e0123733, 2015.

[6] H. C. Gerstein, J. F. Mann, Q. Yi et al., "Albuminuria and risk of cardiovascular events, death, and heart failure in diabetic and nondiabetic individuals," *JAMA*, vol. 286, no. 4, pp. 421–426, 2001.

[7] F. Persson, M. Lindhardt, P. Rossing, and H.-H. Parving, "Prevention of microalbuminuria using early intervention with renin-angiotensin system inhibitors in patients with type 2 diabetes: a systematic review," *Journal of the Renin-Angiotensin-Aldosterone System*, vol. 17, no. 3, 2016.

[8] UK Prospective Diabetes Study (UKPDS) Group, "Intensive blood-glucose control with sulphonylureas or insulin compared with conventional treatment and risk of complications in patients with type 2 diabetes (UKPDS 33)," *The Lancet*, vol. 352, no. 9131, pp. 837–853, 1998.

[9] B. M. Brenner, M. E. Cooper, D. de Zeeuw et al., "Effects of losartan on renal and cardiovascular outcomes in patients with type 2 diabetes and nephropathy," *New England Journal of Medicine*, vol. 345, no. 12, pp. 861–869, 2001.

[10] E. J. Lewis, L. G. Hunsicker, W. R. Clarke et al., "Renoprotective effect of the angiotensin-receptor antagonist irbesartan in patients with nephropathy due to type 2 diabetes," *New England Journal of Medicine*, vol. 345, no. 12, pp. 851–860, 2001.

[11] S. Nakatani, E. Ishimura, T. Naganuma et al., "Poor glycemic control and decreased renal function are associated with increased intrarenal RAS activity in type 2 diabetes mellitus," *Diabetes Research and Clinical Practice*, vol. 105, no. 1, pp. 40–46, 2014.

[12] J. Gu, M. Yang, N. Qi et al., "Olmesartan prevents microalbuminuria in db/db diabetic mice through inhibition of angiotensin II/p38/SIRT1-induced podocyte apoptosis," *Kidney & Blood Pressure Research*, vol. 41, no. 6, pp. 848–864, 2016.

[13] Heart Outcomes Prevention Evaluation (HOPE) Study Investigators, "Effects of ramipril on cardiovascular and microvascular outcomes in people with diabetes mellitus: results of the HOPE study and MICRO-HOPE substudy," *The Lancet*, vol. 355, no. 9200, pp. 253–259, 2000.

[14] M. Haneda, R. Kikkawa, H. Sakai, R. Kawamori, and Candesartan in Diabetic Nephropathy Study Group, "Antiproteinuric effect of candesartan cilexetil in Japanese subjects with type 2 diabetes and nephropathy," *Diabetes Research and Clinical Practice*, vol. 66, no. 1, pp. 87–95, 2004.

[15] M. Urushihara and S. Kagami, "Role of the intrarenal renin-angiotensin system in the progression of renal disease," *Pediatric Nephrology*, vol. 32, no. 9, pp. 1471–1479, 2017.

[16] J. Paeng, J. Park, J. E. Um et al., "The locally activated renin-angiotensin system is involved in albumin permeability in glomerular endothelial cells under high glucose conditions," *Nephrology, Dialysis, Transplantation*, vol. 32, pp. 61–72, 2017.

Hyperglycemia Induced by Glucokinase Deficiency Accelerates Atherosclerosis Development and Impairs Lesion Regression in Combined Heterozygous Glucokinase and the Apolipoprotein E-Knockout Mice

Damilola D. Adingupu,[1] Suvi E. Heinonen,[1] Anne-Christine Andréasson,[1] Mikael Brusberg,[1] Andrea Ahnmark,[1] Margareta Behrendt,[1] Brendan Leighton,[2] and Ann-Cathrine Jönsson-Rylander[1]

[1] *CVMD iMED, AstraZeneca R&D, Gothenburg, Sweden*
[2] *The Research Network, Sandwich, UK*

Correspondence should be addressed to Ann-Cathrine Jönsson-Rylander; ann-cathrine.jonsson-rylander@astrazeneca.com

Academic Editor: Bernard Portha

Aim. Models combining diabetes and atherosclerosis are important in evaluating the cardiovascular (CV) effects and safety of antidiabetes drugs in the development of treatments targeting CV complications. Our aim was to evaluate if crossing the heterozygous glucokinase knockout mouse ($GK^{+/-}$) and hyperlipidemic mouse deficient in apolipoprotein E ($ApoE^{-/-}$) will generate a disease model exhibiting a diabetic and macrovascular phenotype. *Methods.* The effects of defective glucokinase on the glucose metabolism and on the progression and regression of atherosclerosis on high-fat diets were studied in both genders of $GK^{+/-}ApoE^{-/-}$ and $ApoE^{-/-}$ mice. Coronary vascular function of the female $GK^{+/-}ApoE^{-/-}$ and $ApoE^{-/-}$ mice was also investigated. *Results.* $GK^{+/-}ApoE^{-/-}$ mice show a stable hyperglycemia which was increased on Western diet. In oral glucose tolerance test, $GK^{+/-}ApoE^{-/-}$ mice showed significant glucose intolerance and impaired glucose-stimulated insulin secretion. Plasma lipids were comparable with $ApoE^{-/-}$ mice; nevertheless the $GK^{+/-}ApoE^{-/-}$ mice showed slightly increased atherosclerosis development. *Conclusions.* The $GK^{+/-}ApoE^{-/-}$ mice showed a stable and reproducible hyperglycemia, accelerated atherosclerotic lesion progression, and no lesion regression after lipid lowering. This novel model provides a promising tool for drug discovery, enabling the evaluation of compound effects against both diabetic and cardiovascular endpoints simultaneously in one animal model.

1. Introduction

Diabetes is rising globally, with the prevalence of type 2 diabetes (T2D) especially starting to reach epidemic proportions [1]. The metabolic abnormalities that characterize T2D have long been shown to induce molecular mechanisms that contribute to accelerated atherosclerosis progression [2]. Moreover, individuals with T2D have an increased risk of developing cardiovascular diseases and higher cardiovascular mortality rates compared with individuals without T2D [3]. Despite the advances in antidiabetic treatments, effective glycemic control is not always achieved in patients and cardiovascular benefits of treatments are not always demonstrated. To address the need for antidiabetic treatments that are effective against both underlying pathology in T2D and associated cardiovascular complications, studies testing novel drug candidates require a predictive and translational animal model which closely represents the disease pathology.

In the pancreas, glucokinase (GK) determines the rate of glucose-stimulated insulin secretion (GSIS), whereas in the liver the rates of glucose utilization and glycogen synthesis are regulated by the GK activity. Thus, GK plays a critical role in the regulation of blood glucose by acting as the glucose sensor in both pancreas and liver [4, 5]. In humans, heterozygous point mutations in the glucokinase (GK) gene result in reduced enzymatic activity and decreased insulin secretion, causing maturity onset diabetes of the young (MODY) with early-onset and persistent hyperglycemia [6]. Reduced GK activity has been suggested to contribute to impaired insulin secretion, as well as to the abnormalities in hepatic glucose balance in humans with T2D [7–10].

Animal models of GK depletion have been developed in the past, but with limited success. β-cell specific GK knockout is lethal; therefore, a nonleptin dependent global heterozygous depletion of glucokinase gene was generated at AstraZeneca [11]: a model that has proven responsive to standard-of-care antidiabetic agents like metformin, sitagliptin, exendin, glipizide, and GK activators [12]. This heterozygous glucokinase knockout ($GK^{+/-}$) mouse model has a global disruption of one allele for the GK gene, causing decreased GK activity in both pancreas and liver and leading to reduced insulin secretion and elevated blood glucose levels [11]. The $GK^{+/-}$ mice were recently shown to back-translate the effects of various standard-of-care antidiabetic agents with different mechanism of actions at clinically translatable free-drug exposure levels [13]. Additionally, these authors also showed that, due to the stability of its diabetic phenotype, the $GK^{+/-}$ mouse can be used for long-term safety studies of novel glucose-lowering agents [13]. These characteristics make the $GK^{+/-}$ mouse an attractive model to be used in drug development programs for new antidiabetic agents.

In order to develop a diabetic atherosclerotic mouse model with characteristics that closely resemble the human T2D driven cardiovascular disease, we cross-bred the above-mentioned mouse model ($GK^{+/-}$) into an apolipoprotein E ($ApoE^{-/-}$) deficient background, to derive a heterozygous glucokinase and apolipoprotein E-knockout mouse ($GK^{+/-}ApoE^{-/-}$). In this study, we describe the generation of the $GK^{+/-}ApoE^{-/-}$ mice and characterize their phenotypes, diabetic as well as lipid. In addition, the progression and regression of the atherosclerotic disease process were compared with nondiabetic $ApoE^{-/-}$ mice. The coronary vascular function of the female $GK^{+/-}ApoE^{-/-}$ mice was evaluated. The main goal was to accomplish a model that would be suitable for the evaluation of combined T2D and cardiovascular endpoints in drug development.

2. Materials and Methods

2.1. Animals. Animal care and experiments conform to the Directive 2010/63/EU of the European Parliament on the guidelines for the protection of animals used for scientific purposes and were approved by The Regional Animal Ethics Committee for Experimental Animals, University of Gothenburg. Studies are reported in accordance with the ARRIVE guidelines for reporting experiments involving animals [14].

Mice deficient in apolipoprotein E ($ApoE^{-/-}$) on the C57BL/6N background (AstraZeneca, Sweden) were crossed with C57BL/6J mice with a global deletion in one glucokinase allele ($GK^{+/-}$). Detailed description of the generation of the $GK^{+/-}$ was given in a previously published article [11]. $GK^{+/-}ApoE^{-/-}$ colony was maintained by backcrossing to $ApoE^{-/-}$ mice and thus the $GK^{+/-}ApoE^{-/-}$ mice gradually acquired a complete C57BL/6N genetic background. ApoE deficient ($ApoE^{-/-}$) littermates with functional GK were used as controls in all experiments.

Male mice were housed individually and female mice in groups of five in rooms with regulated temperature, humidity, and a 12 hours' light-dark cycle (lights off 19:00). They had free access to normal Chow diet (R3; Lactamin AB, Kimstad, Sweden) and water, unless stated otherwise in substudies. Body weights were monitored weekly during the studies. Mice were sacrificed during anesthesia with 5% isoflurane, following blood withdrawal from left ventricle.

2.2. Characterization of Diabetic Phenotype. The effect of high-fat Western diet (WD) (R638; Lactamin AB, Kimstad, Sweden) on the diabetic phenotype of the $GK^{+/-}ApoE^{-/-}$ mice was investigated in 10 male and 10 female $GK^{+/-}ApoE^{-/-}$ mice compared with the sex matched wild-type $ApoE^{-/-}$ mice ($n = 20$). Basal levels of blood glucose and insulin were measured in the mice which were fed normal Chow diet before starting the WD (Figure 1(a)). Blood glucose was measured after 4-hour fasting at 4, 8, and 14 and 21 weeks after starting WD, using a hand-held Accu-Chek glucose monitor glucometer (Accu-Chek, Roche Diagnostics, Mannheim, Germany) in the awake mice. At the same time points, a blood sample of ~20 μL was collected for insulin measurement.

Oral glucose tolerance and insulin sensitivity were examined by performing a tolerance test in the $GK^{+/-}ApoE^{-/-}$ mice and the $ApoE^{-/-}$ mice for comparison after 14 weeks on WD. Oral glucose tolerance tests (OGTT) were performed at 13:00 hour after 4-hour fasting by an oral administration of glucose (2 g/kg) and 15–20 μL blood was drawn from the tail vein at 0 (right before the dosing), 15, 30, 60, and 120 min for the measurement of glucose (2 μL, Accu-Chek, Roche Diagnostics, Mannheim, Germany) and insulin ($2 \times 5\,\mu$L, Ultra-Sensitive Mouse Insulin ELISA Kit, Crystal Chemical, Downers Grove, IL) levels. Area under the curve (AUC) values were calculated for glucose and insulin as total area under the curve and corrected for differences in baseline values.

Plasma insulin levels were measured with a radioimmunoassay (SRI-13K, Millipore Corporation, USA) on a 1470 Automatic Gamma Counter (PerkinElmer, USA). Whole blood insulin was measured with an ELISA kit (Ultra-Sensitive Mouse Insulin ELISA Kit; Crystal Chem, Downers Grove, IL).

2.3. Atherosclerosis Progression and Regression. To investigate atherosclerosis progression on different high-fat diets, $GK^{+/-}ApoE^{-/-}$ mice and $ApoE^{-/-}$ males and females (n = 10/gender/genotype) were switched from normal Chow diet to Lard diet (821424; 21% fat from pork lard, 0.15% cholesterol; Special Diets Services, Essex, UK) for 14 weeks, or Western

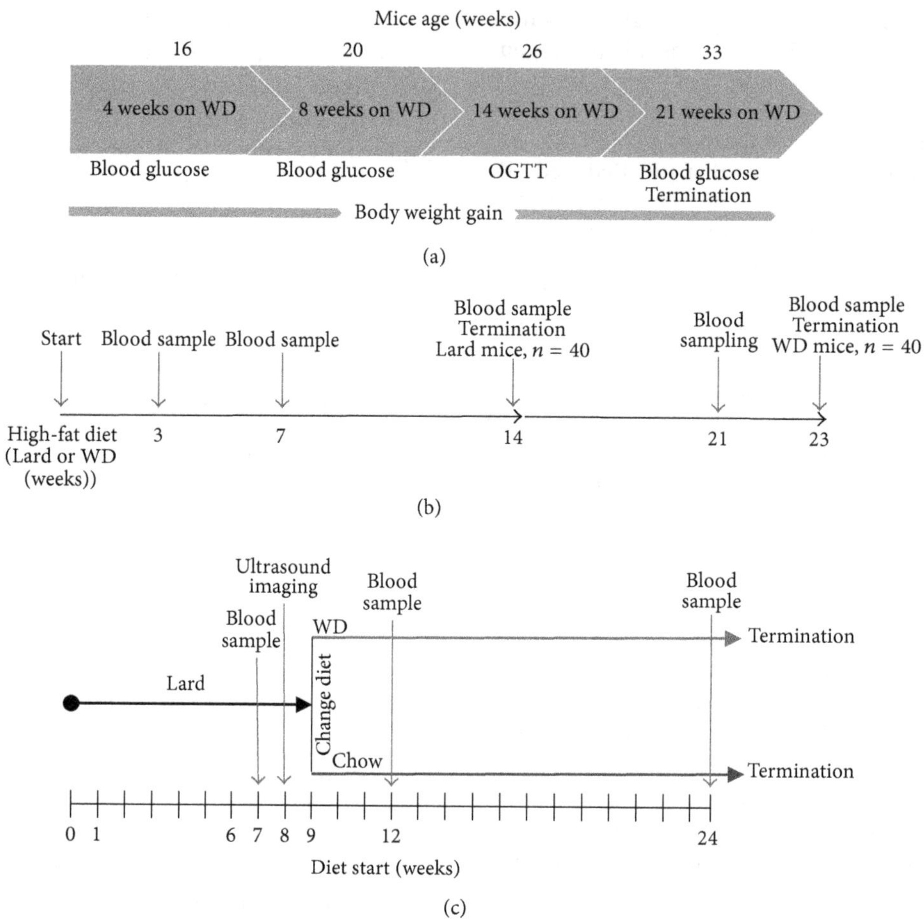

FIGURE 1: Study design for the characterization of the diabetic phenotype of the $GK^{+/-}ApoE^{-/-}$ and the $ApoE^{-/-}$ mice on Western diet (WD) (a), study design for the atheroprogression study (b), and atheroregression study (c).

diet (WD) (R638; 21% fat/cocoa butter, 0.15% cholesterol; Lantmännen, Kimstad, Sweden) for 23 weeks (Figure 1(b)). This aimed to accelerate the hyperlipidemia progress and pathological cardiovascular phenotype. Cholesterol was measured at 3 and 7 weeks after diet commenced and at termination (14 weeks in the Lard diet group and 23 weeks in the WD group).

In addition, to investigate atherosclerosis regression, 18-week-old $GK^{+/-}ApoE^{-/-}$ and $ApoE^{-/-}$ males and females ($n = 10$/gender/genotype) were first transferred from Chow to Lard diet (821424; 21% fat from pork lard, 0.15% cholesterol; Special Diets Services, Essex, UK) for 9 weeks to establish atherosclerotic lesions and then split into two groups (1) Chow diet and (2) WD for 14 weeks (Figure 1(c)). Animals were allocated to the different diet intervention groups by randomization based on plaque size in the brachiocephalic artery (BCA) measured by noninvasive ultrasound imaging.

2.4. Analyses of Plasma Lipid Levels. Blood samples during the study were drawn from the saphenous vein and by cardiac puncture at termination, placed into MiniCollect K3E EDTA tubes (Greiner Bio-One GmbH, Kremsmünster, Austria) on ice, and centrifuged (2800 rpm, 4°C, 10 min). Plasma was stored at −80°C until analysis. Plasma lipid concentrations were measured using enzymatic colorimetric methods (total cholesterol: kit number A11A01634, Horiba ABX, France; triglycerides: kit number 12146029, Roche Diagnostics GmbH, Germany; nonesterified fatty acids: NEFA-HR (2) assay, 434-91795 and 436-91995, Wako Chemicals GmbH, Germany).

2.5. Histological Analyses. Heart, BCA, and thoracic aorta were dissected out and fixed in 4% phosphate-buffered formaldehyde (number 02176, HistoLab Products, Gothenburg, Sweden). Thoracic aortas were cleaned from the adventitia and opened longitudinally and macroscopic lesions were quantified *en face* and photographed and images were imported into BioPix IQ 2.1.8 image analysis system (BioPix AB, Gothenburg, Sweden) which was used for quantification. Samples of aortic sinus, ascending aorta, and BCA were embedded in paraffin and serial 4 μm sections were cut (Histocenter, Gothenburg, Sweden). Sections were either stained with conventional stains (hematoxylin-eosin, Miller's elastin, or Picrosirius red; Histocenter, Gothenburg, Sweden) or immunostained for smooth muscle cells (α-actin, 1:100, clone 1A4, Dako, M0851) or macrophages (MAC-2,

1:10000, clone M3/38, CL8942AP, Cedarlane) using DAB (BC-BDB2004, Biocare) as the chromogen. Immunostaining was performed as single or dual stain using an automated stainer (Intellipath, Biocare). Slides were then scanned in an automated slide scanner (Mirax Scan, Zeiss) and images were analyzed with BioPix IQ 2.1.8 image analysis system (BioPix AB, Gothenburg, Sweden). Plaque area and area of positive staining were measured. Positive staining was related to plaque area. All histological procedures and analyses were performed in a blinded fashion.

2.6. Coronary Flow Velocity Reserve (CFVR) Measured Using Ultrasound Imaging. Transthoracic echocardiography was performed using noninvasive high-frequency ultrasound imaging in the atherosclerosis regression study on 18-week-old $GK^{+/-}ApoE^{-/-}$ and $ApoE^{-/-}$ female mice to characterize coronary vascular function. All mice were anesthetized with Isoba® vet isoflurane (Schering-Plough Ltd., England) in a closed chamber with 3% isoflurane in oxygen for 2 to 5 minutes until immobile and 1.0–1.5% isoflurane in oxygen during the examination. Each mouse was placed supine on a heated procedure board with isoflurane initially at 1.5% supplied by a nose cone connected to the anesthesia vaporizer. Chest hair was removed with chemical cream (Veet, Reckitt Benckiser, UK). Imaging was done with a high-resolution ultrasound scanner (Vevo 770, Visualsonics Inc., Toronto, Canada) using a 40 MHz mechanical transducer with a focal depth of 6 mm. Isoflurane was reduced to 1% to lower coronary flow to a baseline level and velocity profile in the left coronary artery was measured in a modified long-axis view, recorded with a pulsed-wave Doppler for 3 minutes to ensure stable signal was achieved, after which signals were collected and stored. Isoflurane level was then increased to 2.5% to increase the coronary flow, and velocity profile was monitored for up to 4 minutes during which time signals were stored for offline analysis of maximum hyperemic response. Isoflurane was reduced back to 1%, and mice were allowed to stabilize. Detailed protocol using isoflurane to induce hyperemia has been described elsewhere [15]. Plaque size and CFVR analysis were measured offline (Vevo770 software, Visualsonics Inc., Toronto, Canada) in a blinded fashion.

CFVR was calculated as the ratio of peak diastolic flow velocities at baseline obtained using 1% isoflurane and during hyperemia obtained using 2.5% isoflurane (CFVR = hyperemic coronary flow velocity/basal coronary flow velocity).

2.7. Statistical Analyses. To detect a 20% difference in blood glucose at $p < 0.05$ with 80% power, we would require group size of $n = 8$. However, since detecting differences in atherosclerosis requires bigger group sizes due to expected larger variation, group sizes were $n = 10$. Numerical values for each measurement are shown as mean ± SEM. Statistical significance was evaluated using 1-sided (blood glucose, plaque size, *en face* lesion area) or 2-sided (body weight, insulin, cholesterol, and triglyceride (TG)) Student's t-test. Significant statistical difference was considered at $p < 0.05$. For the OGTT, ANOVA of repeated measures and Tukey's correction for multiple comparisons were used. All statistical analyses were performed using GraphPad Prism version 6.01 (GraphPad Prism version 6.01 for Windows, GraphPad Software, La Jolla, California, USA).

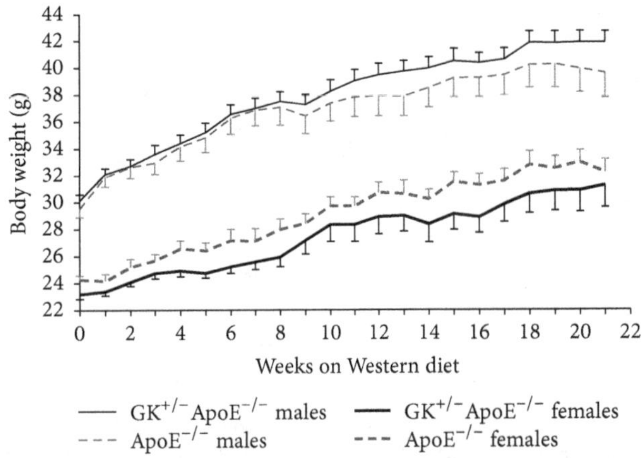

FIGURE 2: Body weight development of the $GK^{+/-}ApoE^{-/-}$ mice compared with the $ApoE^{-/-}$ mice on WD. $GK^{+/-}ApoE^{-/-}$ males have a higher body weight compared with the $ApoE^{-/-}$ males after 21 weeks on WD. $ApoE^{-/-}$ females have a higher body weight from baseline Chow diet and maintained the weight difference on WD compared with $GK^{+/-}ApoE^{-/-}$ female mice. Values are presented as means and standard error of mean (SEM).

3. Results

Body weight increased in both genotypes with age reflecting the growth of the animals. There were gender differences in the genotypes, where $GK^{+/-}ApoE^{-/-}$ males have a higher body weight compared with the $ApoE^{-/-}$ males after 21 weeks on WD. Conversely, $ApoE^{-/-}$ females have a higher body weight from baseline on Chow diet and maintained the weight difference on WD compared with $GK^{+/-}ApoE^{-/-}$ female mice (Figure 2).

3.1. Progression of Diabetes

3.1.1. Characterization of Diabetic Phenotype. On Chow diet, the $GK^{+/-}ApoE^{-/-}$ mice displayed significantly higher fasting blood glucose levels (15.2 ± 0.6 mmol/L in males and 12.2 ± 0.6 mmol/L in females), compared to the normoglycemic $ApoE^{-/-}$ controls (8.3 ± 0.3 mmol/L and 8.1 ± 0.4 mmol/L in males and females, resp.) (Figure 3). When challenged with WD, the glucose levels increased steadily to a 30% higher level in the $GK^{+/-}ApoE^{-/-}$ mice (19.8 ± 0.4 mmol/L, $p < 0.0001$, in males and 15.9 ± 0.6 mmol/L, $p = 0.0001$, in females). In $ApoE^{-/-}$ controls a significant 18% increase was seen in male mice (9.8 ± 0.6 mmol/L, $p < 0.05$), whereas in females the change was smaller and not statistically significant (15%, 9.3 ± 0.5 mmol/L, $p = 0.1266$).

In an oral glucose tolerance test performed after 14 weeks on WD (Figure 4), $GK^{+/-}ApoE^{-/-}$ mice showed significant glucose intolerance with 2.3-fold increased $AUC_{glucose}$ (Figure 4(b)) and impaired GSIS with $AUC_{insulin}$ reduced by

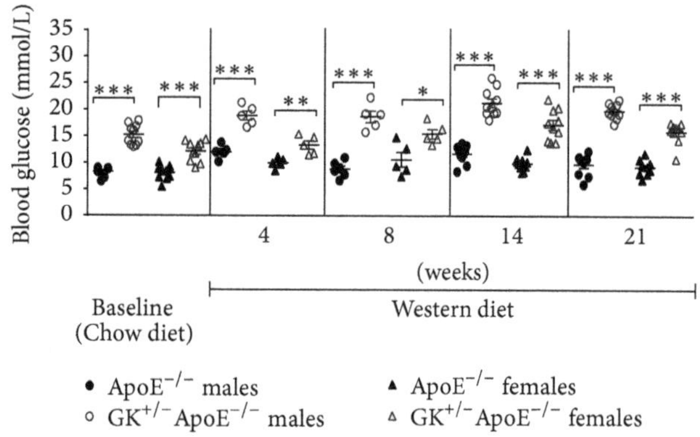

FIGURE 3: Fasting blood glucose is higher in $GK^{+/-}ApoE^{-/-}$ mice on normal Chow diet and WD at 4, 8, 14, and 21 weeks compared with $ApoE^{-/-}$ mice. Values are presented as individual data points and means. Statistical analysis was performed using t-test and a p value of less than 0.05 was considered significant. $^{*}p < 0.05$, $^{**}p < 0.005$, and $^{***}p < 0.0001$.

49% and 27% (in males and females, resp.) compared to $ApoE^{-/-}$ mice (Figure 4(d)). Defective GSIS was reflected also in basal insulin values, which in general tended to be lower in the $GK^{+/-}ApoE^{-/-}$ than $ApoE^{-/-}$ mice (Figure 4(c)).

3.1.2. Atheroprogression and Atheroregression Studies. In the atheroprogression and atheroregression studies, hyperglycemia was very stable and more profound in $GK^{+/-}ApoE^{-/-}$ mice compared to ApoE mice (data not presented).

3.2. Lipids

3.2.1. Atheroprogression Study. Reduction in the GK function did not affect total plasma cholesterol or triglyceride levels (Table 1). In general, cholesterol levels were higher on Lard diet compared with WD in both genotypes already after 3 weeks. $GK^{+/-}ApoE^{-/-}$ male mice have a trend for lower cholesterol from study start and show a declining tendency with time. The triglyceride levels were stable in $GK^{+/-}ApoE^{-/-}$ mice despite different diets, and there was a trend for lower values in $GK^{+/-}ApoE^{-/-}$ mice compared to $ApoE^{-/-}$ mice (Table 1).

3.2.2. Atheroregression Study. Priming with Lard diet for 9 weeks in the atherosclerosis regression study induced a 3-fold increase in total cholesterol and these levels remained the same after changing to WD with a similar cholesterol content (0.15%). On the contrary, after switching from Lard to Chow diet, the total cholesterol levels decreased significantly (43–55%) in all groups.

3.3. Atherosclerosis

3.3.1. Atheroprogression. On WD, in the BCA the female $GK^{+/-}ApoE^{-/-}$ had the largest plaques (230112 ± 20124) versus female $ApoE^{-/-}$ (188057 ± 15816) $p = 0.0587$ (Figure 5(a)). In the ascending aorta, there was a trend for $GK^{+/-}ApoE^{-/-}$ mice to have larger lesions with less variability compared with $ApoE^{-/-}$ (Figure 5(b)). However, statistically significant difference was seen only with female mice on Lard diet ($GK^{+/-}ApoE^{-/-}$ versus $ApoE^{-/-}$, 2602000 ± 403800 versus 1355000 ± 297600, $p = 0.0115$) (males on Lard: $GK^{+/-}ApoE^{-/-}$ versus $ApoE^{-/-}$ 4284000 ± 615660 versus 3201000 ± 465241, $p = 0.0858$).

On lard diet, there was also a trend in BCA for female $GK^{+/-}ApoE^{-/-}$ to have the largest plaque (228298 ± 22675) versus female $ApoE^{-/-}$ (190804 ± 16158), $p = 0.0974$. There were no statistically significant differences in plaque size in the brachiocephalic artery (WD 220188 ± 12279 versus 199578 ± 9759, Lard 264854 ± 28916 versus 286013 ± 23494) on either high-fat diets for the male group ($GK^{+/-}ApoE^{-/-}$ versus $ApoE^{-/-}$). Lesion was equally advanced in the brachiocephalic artery in the two strains illustrated in Figure 6.

3.3.2. Atheroregression. Despite lower plasma cholesterol levels in both males and females $GK^{+/-}ApoE^{-/-}$ and $ApoE^{-/-}$ mice after dietary change (Lard to Chow diet) compared with the Lard to WD (Figure 7(a)), plaque size in the brachiocephalic artery (Figure 7(b)) and in the aortic sinus (Figure 7(c)) remained comparable. In other vascular sites, there was also impaired lesion regression (*en face* lesion area in thoracic aorta, ascending aorta, and left coronary artery) (data not presented).

3.4. Coronary Flow Velocity Reserve (CFVR). Basal flow velocity and hyperemic flow velocity (cm/s) were not significantly different in either genotype. Furthermore, CFVR was not significantly different between $ApoE^{-/-}$ and $GK^{+/-}ApoE^{-/-}$ at 18 weeks of age (Table 2).

4. Discussion

The present study characterized heterozygous glucokinase knockout apolipoprotein E deficient mice ($GK^{+/-}ApoE^{-/-}$), a novel mouse model of diabetes and atherosclerosis. We demonstrate that this mouse model has very stable hyperglycemia, indications of increased atherosclerosis development on high-fat diet, and impaired lesion regression after lipid lowering. The atherosclerosis is stable on WD and the $GK^{+/-}ApoE^{-/-}$ knockout shows comparable coronary vascular function to the apolipoprotein E (ApoE) deficient mice at 18 weeks of age.

For a rodent model to be considered T2D model, fasting blood glucose levels of around 150–300 mg/dL^{-1} (8.3–16.7 mmol/L) are recommended [16]. Our model has glucose levels which exceed the minimum threshold and should therefore be considered as a diabetic model. There are other commonly used animal models of T2D (leptin-mutated ob/ob, leptin-receptor deficient db/db mice, and male missense mutated leptin-receptor Zucker Diabetic Fatty (ZDF) rats); however, they have a wide but unstable hyperglycemic range [12, 17]. In the fasted state, insulin levels were similar between the $GK^{+/-}ApoE^{-/-}$ knockout mice and the $ApoE^{-/-}$ mice despite higher glucose levels in the $GK^{+/-}ApoE^{-/-}$.

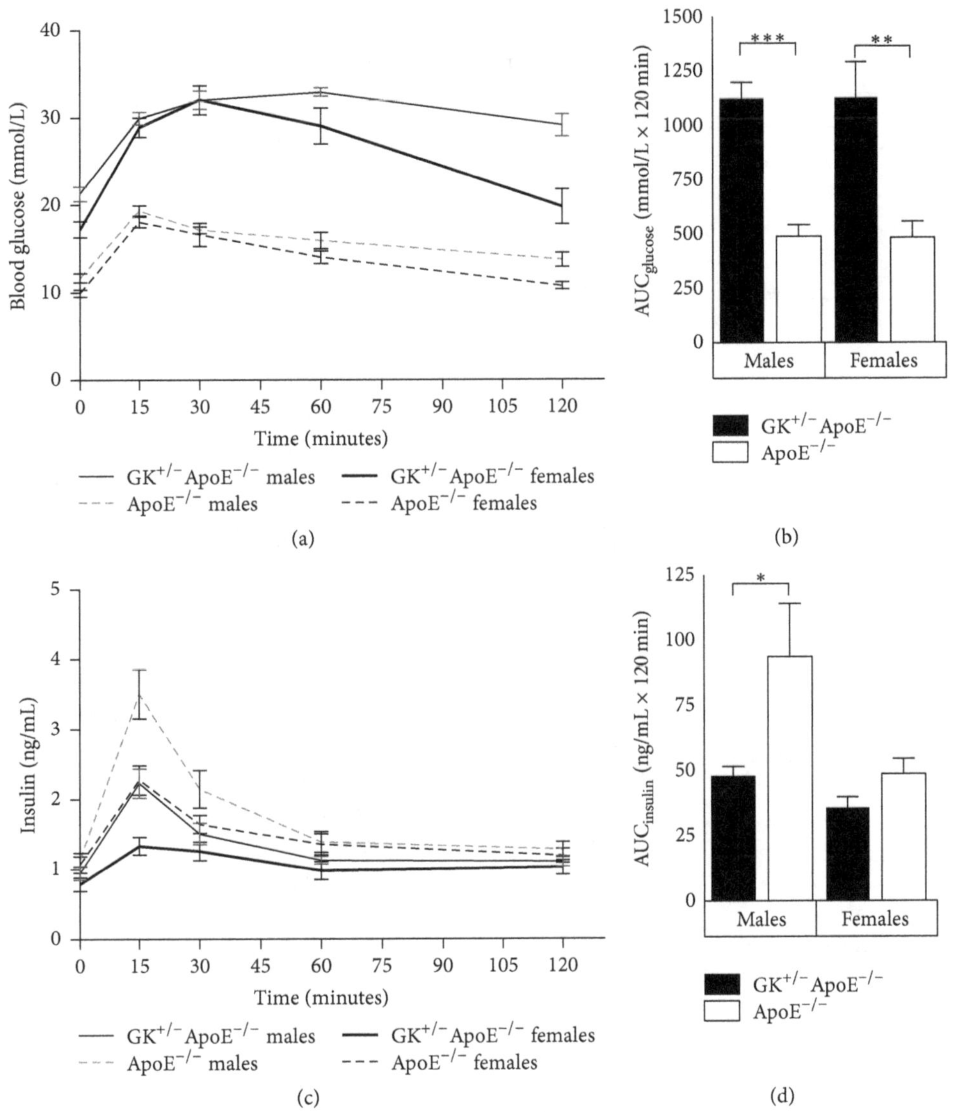

FIGURE 4: Oral Glucose tolerance test ((a) and (b)) and insulin ((c) and (d)) in the $GK^{+/-}ApoE^{-/-}$ mice compared with the $ApoE^{-/-}$ mice after 14 weeks on Western diet. Both male and female $GK^{+/-}ApoE^{-/-}$ mice display significantly impaired glucose-stimulated insulin secretion. Values are presented as means and standard error of mean (SEM). $^{*}p < 0.05$, $^{**}p < 0.005$, and $^{***}p < 0.0001$.

Higher glucose levels in the $GK^{+/-}ApoE^{-/-}$ would be expected to result in even higher insulin levels. This however was not the case, indicating that the hyperglycemia in the $GK^{+/-}ApoE^{-/-}$ knockout mice is predominantly due to inadequate compensatory insulin secretory response, possibly as a result of impaired β-cell function, an important determinant of type 2 diabetes [18, 19]. Insulin level measurement is an acceptable measure to indicate β-cell function in rodent models [20]; our findings are consistent with insulin response pattern in humans with advanced type 2 diabetes, where there is an insufficient insulin secretion to meet demand [19].

The $GK^{+/-}$ mouse model has been suggested to be a representative model of type 2 diabetes, which encompasses both the hepatic and the β-cell GK deficiencies found to occur in the disease [11]. On a high-fat diet, the $GK^{+/-}$ mouse has reduced islet GK activity and defects in glucose-stimulated insulin secretion [11, 21]; our current diabetic phenotype data on $GK^{+/-}ApoE^{-/-}$ knockout mice are comparable to those previously published on the $GK^{+/-}$ by above-mentioned authors. This indicates that the hepatic and the β-cell GK deficiencies in the parent $GK^{+/-}$ mice when cross-breed with the $ApoE^{-/-}$ were transferred to the offspring $GK^{+/-}ApoE^{-/-}$ knockout mice.

The $ApoE^{-/-}$ is a widely used mouse model of atherosclerosis [22]. Plasma lipid levels were comparable between the $GK^{+/-}ApoE^{-/-}$ and the $ApoE^{-/-}$ mice, but nevertheless the $GK^{+/-}ApoE^{-/-}$ mice showed slightly higher plaque burden in line with atherosclerotic progression in human T2D [23], as well as impaired lesion regression at different vascular sites. Even though the plaque burden is slightly higher in the $GK^{+/-}ApoE^{-/-}$ compared to the $ApoE^{-/-}$, both genotypes

TABLE 1: Lipid levels in $GK^{+/-}ApoE^{-/-}$ and $ApoE^{-/-}$ mice on Lard and Western diet measured in the atheroprogression study.

Diet	Gender	Time	Genotype	Cholesterol (mmol/L)	TG (mmol/L)	NEFA
Lard	Males	3 weeks	$ApoE^{-/-}$	38.86 ± 1.11	—	—
			$GK^{+/-}ApoE^{-/-}$	35.84 ± 1.91	—	—
		7 weeks	$ApoE^{-/-}$	38.20 ± 1.46	—	—
			$GK^{+/-}ApoE^{-/-}$	31.00 ± 1.52	—	—
		14 weeks	$ApoE^{-/-}$	38.32 ± 1.48	1.21 ± 0.11	0.49 ± 0.02
			$GK^{+/-}ApoE^{-/-}$	30.84 ± 1.81	0.86 ± 0.14	0.45 ± 0.02
	Females	3 weeks	$ApoE^{-/-}$	25.88 ± 1.00	—	—
			$GK^{+/-}ApoE^{-/-}$	22.78 ± 1.73	—	—
		7 weeks	$ApoE^{-/-}$	25.20 ± 0.97	—	—
			$GK^{+/-}ApoE^{-/-}$	23.40 ± 1.12	—	—
		14 weeks	$ApoE^{-/-}$	20.58 ± 0.62	0.52 ± 0.13	0.55 ± 0.04
			$GK^{+/-}ApoE^{-/-}$	20.11 ± 0.82	0.27 ± 0.06	0.50 ± 0.03
Western	Males	3 weeks	$ApoE^{-/-}$	20.84 ± 1.21	—	—
			$GK^{+/-}ApoE^{-/-}$	17.42 ± 2.47	—	—
		7 weeks	$ApoE^{-/-}$	22.40 ± 0.75	—	—
			$GK^{+/-}ApoE^{-/-}$	18.80 ± 2.82	—	—
		21 weeks	$ApoE^{-/-}$	31.65 ± 2.16	0.82 ± 0.09	0.39 ± 0.02
			$GK^{+/-}ApoE^{-/-}$	27.88 ± 2.78	0.81 ± 0.13	0.44 ± 0.02
	Females	3 weeks	$ApoE^{-/-}$	17.54 ± 1.04	—	—
			$GK^{+/-}ApoE^{-/-}$	20.62 ± 1.19	—	—
		7 weeks	$ApoE^{-/-}$	18.60 ± 0.51	—	—
			$GK^{+/-}ApoE^{-/-}$	18.40 ± 1.08	—	—
		21 weeks	$ApoE^{-/-}$	23.35 ± 1.57	0.36 ± 0.05	0.45 ± 0.03
			$GK^{+/-}ApoE^{-/-}$	20.57 ± 2.45	0.38 ± 0.06	0.43 ± 0.03

Lard diet induced higher cholesterol levels than Western diet. There is a trend for $ApoE^{-/-}$ mice to have higher cholesterol, triglycerides, and nonesterified fatty acids (NEFA) levels compared with $GK^{+/-}ApoE^{-/-}$. Data presented as mean ± SEM.

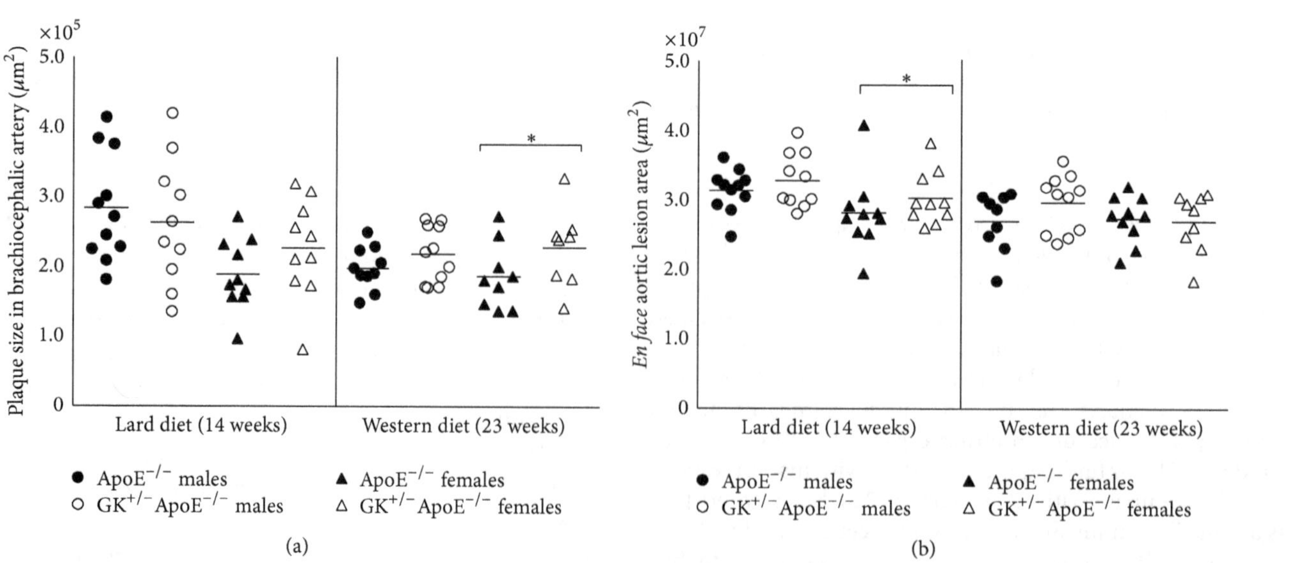

FIGURE 5: Histology evaluation of plaque size in the brachiocephalic artery (a) and *en face* lesion area in the thoracic aorta (b) measured in the atheroprogression study. There is a trend for $GK^{+/-}ApoE^{-/-}$ mice to have greater plaque compared with the $ApoE^{-/-}$, with female $GK^{+/-}ApoE^{-/-}$ having a more consistent pattern. Statistical analysis was performed using t-test and a p value of less than 0.05 was considered significant. $^{*}p < 0.05$.

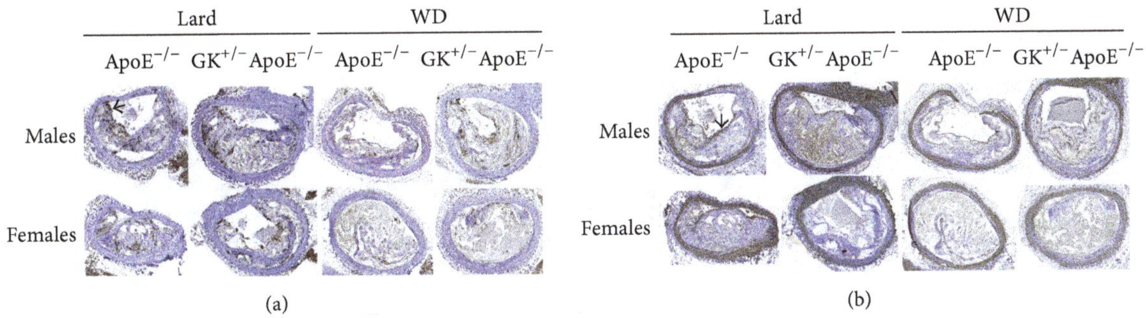

FIGURE 6: The atherosclerotic lesions of the brachiocephalic artery in both genotypes have become advanced and complicated after Lard and WD for 14 and 23 weeks, respectively. Large areas of the lesions consist of necrotic core and cholesterol clefts. (a) Only a few scattered macrophages (brown indicated by arrow on the figure) are detected by the macrophage antibody. (b) Smooth muscle cells (brown) are detected in the vessel wall by the alpha-actin antibody. A thin cap is sometimes seen in the lesions, indicated by arrow on the figure. Images in Figures 6(a) and 6(b) are consecutive sections from the same animal.

TABLE 2: Coronary flow velocity in female $ApoE^{-/-}$ and $GK^{+/-}ApoE^{-/-}$ mice at 18 weeks old.

	$ApoE^{-/-}$ ($n = 17$)	$GK^{+/-}ApoE^{-/-}$ ($n = 14$)
Basal flow velocity (cm/s)	35.1 ± 2.5	34.4 ± 2.7
Hyperemic flow velocity (cm/s)	59.1 ± 2.1	60.6 ± 2.3
CFVR	1.76 ± 0.18	1.86 ± 0.10

Data presented as mean ± SEM.

develop advanced and complicated lesions. There are only few detectable macrophages and thin protecting caps, if any. On the other hand, both genotypes have necrotic cores, cholesterol clefts, buried caps, and layered phenotype, hallmarks of complicated mice lesions [24]. Several clinical studies have shown in populations with atherosclerosis that dietary intervention may reduce the progression of the atherosclerotic plaque development [25, 26] and regression mediated by weight loss may even occur [27]. Furthermore, there are also data suggesting that coronary atherosclerosis may be regressed by diet and comprehensive lifestyle changes [28, 29]. For studies using animal models to investigate treatments targeting cardiovascular disease in diabetes, it is important that diabetic and atherosclerotic disease is stable.

This mouse model showed comparable coronary vascular function to the apolipoprotein E (ApoE) deficient mice at 18 weeks of age. Although there were no significant differences between the $GK^{+/-}ApoE^{-/-}$ and the $ApoE^{-/-}$ mice for coronary vascular function, values presented here for basal flow velocity and CFVR measured in both genotypes are higher and lower, respectively, when compared to published data for C57Bl/6J-lep^{ob} and age matched lean litter mates (+/?) of comparable age [30]. Furthermore, in a study by Hartley et al. [15], they showed that old $ApoE^{-/-}$ (2 years of age) mice have a higher baseline flow velocity and lower CFVR when compared to the $ApoE^{+/+}$ wild-type mice of similar age, which is in agreement with our findings [15]. Baseline coronary flow is based on cardiac metabolic demand (hemoglobin content, oxygen saturation, and baseline hemodynamics) [31, 32], and it is reasonable to assume that the high blood glucose and cholesterol in the $GK^{+/-}ApoE^{-/-}$ and the $ApoE^{-/-}$ mice will negatively influence their hemoglobin content, thereby increasing metabolic demand reflected by higher basal flow velocity. Correlation between CFVR and coronary atherosclerosis has been shown in mice [33]; furthermore, CFVR is reduced in atherosclerotic mice [32, 33]. In agreement, we observed low CFVR values in our mice model at 18 weeks of age and comparable plaque burden in the $GK^{+/-}ApoE^{-/-}$ and the $ApoE^{-/-}$ mice, supporting the lack of difference in the CFVR between the strains and emphasizing macrovascular burden to underlie the coronary vascular dysfunction. In man, CFVR is used to evaluate the severity of different cardiac pathologies and values ranging from 2.5 to 5.0 have been reported, with >3.0 used as the lower limit of normal [31]. Validation studies on the $GK^{+/-}ApoE^{-/-}$ are currently ongoing within our lab to characterize changes in coronary vascular function over time (mice from 6 weeks of age) using ultrasonography and to investigate effect of lipid lowering and standard-of-care treatments for diabetes.

The strength of the $GK^{+/-}ApoE^{-/-}$ mice lies in that it has stable hyperglycemia, and diabetes is not progressive. This makes it possible to use either young or old mice to carry out short or long studies without the disease phenotype changing with age. The ZDF rats and ob/ob or db/db mice have limited age window for treatments due to rapid disease progression and large variability, which requires large group sizes. These other rodent models of T2D (ZDF rats and ob/ob or db/db mice) are monogenic models of obesity which induces hyperglycemia, which weakens their translational value as obesity is seldom caused by a monogenic mutation [17, 20]. Diabetes induced by Streptozotocin (STZ) provides a non-physiological model, with variation dependent on STZ dose and sometimes severe adverse effect on rodents [34]. In the relatively long period of monitoring the $GK^{+/-}ApoE^{-/-}$ (up to 21 weeks), fasting blood glucose and cholesterol remained high and stable. This makes the $GK^{+/-}ApoE^{-/-}$ model suitable for investigations related to the combination of diabetes and atherosclerosis.

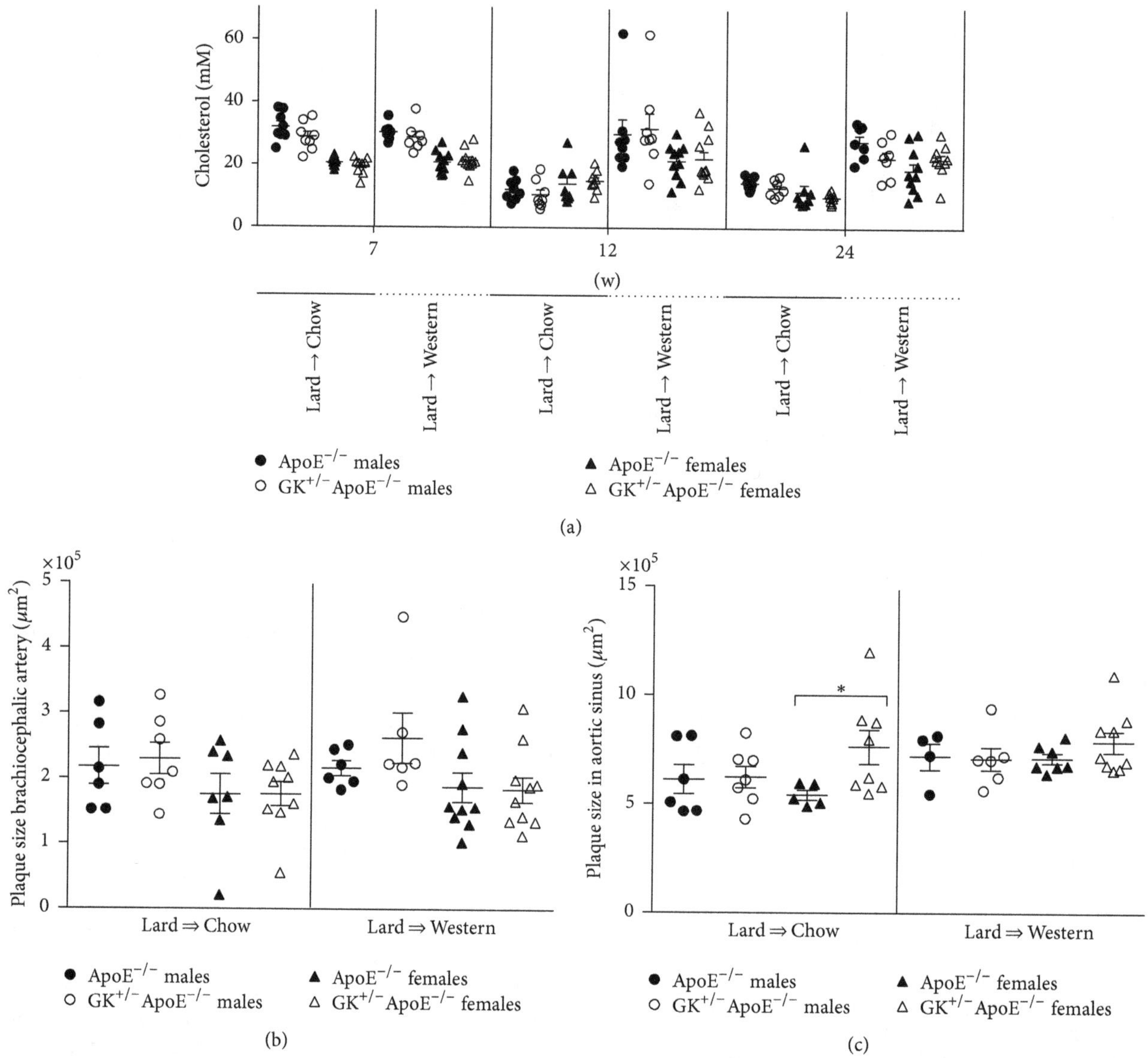

FIGURE 7: Nonfasting total plasma cholesterol measured after 7 weeks on Lard diet, 4 weeks after diet changed from Lard to WD or Lard to Chow, and 14 weeks after diet changed from Lard to WD or Lard to Chow (a). Plaque size in the brachiocephalic artery (b) and aortic sinus plaque size (c) measured after 14 weeks on Lard to WD or Lard to Chow diet in the atheroregression study. (a) Priming mice with Lard diet induced a 3-fold increase in total cholesterol and the levels remained the same after changing to WD, resulting in similar cholesterol levels at 7 weeks. Conversely, after switching from Lard to Chow diet, the total cholesterol levels decreased significantly in all groups. (b) Plaque sizes in the brachiocephalic artery in both diet groups were comparable, which indicates that the atherosclerosis did not regress on the Lard to Chow diet change. (c). Female $GK^{+/-}ApoE^{-/-}$ mice show equal amount of plaque in the aortic sinus in the Lard to Chow group compared to the Lard to WD despite lower plasma cholesterol levels in both $GK^{+/-}ApoE^{-/-}$ and $ApoE^{-/-}$ mice after dietary change (Lard to Chow diet). Statistical analysis was performed using t-test and a p value of less than 0.05 was considered significant. $^{*}p < 0.05$.

For decades, new diabetes drugs were approved primarily based on their glucose-lowering efficacy. However, after observations of increased cardiovascular risk with some medications, the regulatory agencies now demand studies showing that novel antidiabetic agents are at least neutral in their cardiovascular effects [35]. Although these new regulatory requirements as such apply only for clinical trials, they affect also preclinical research, as more accurate prediction of the cardiovascular effects is warranted. Secondly, instead of aiming just for cardiovascular neutrality, the future medical treatments will favor compounds that have beneficial cardiovascular effects in addition to their antidiabetic action (multifunctional compounds with hypolipidemic and antidiabetic action). Therefore, we need pharmacokinetic: pharmacodynamics (PK/PD) models, where both metabolic and cardiovascular endpoints can be studied in one and the same animal.

There are several positives in this novel animal model. The animal model has a stable hyperglycemic phenotype that is very reproducible from batch to batch, and there is little variation so that relatively small group sizes can be used. Diabetes does not cause increases in lipid levels, which is unlike most of the other used diabetes models. The etiology is rather relevant, since individuals with T2D exhibit high rates of hepatic glucose output and have reduced GK activity in liver and pancreas. These mice do not have any special health problems, so they are easy to breed and use in short- or long-term studies. The lipid profile is a negative against this model, since the ApoE$^{-/-}$ mice are a remnant model and thus do not resemble much the human lipoprotein profile and lack also all the other functions of ApoE. Reviewing the lipid levels shows that there is no exceptional difference in the GK$^{+/-}$ApoE$^{-/-}$ compared with the ApoE$^{-/-}$. Moreover, the diabetic GK$^{+/-}$ApoE$^{-/-}$ mice have a bit lower cholesterol and TG levels, which can be due to reduced GK activity in the liver and thus reduced lipogenesis. This is an important feature, since normally when diabetes is induced in mice, for example, with STZ or by crossing db/db mice with dyslipidemic strains, the lipid levels increase significantly and as a result supraphysiological lipid levels that easily overrun all other factors.

5. Conclusions

We conclude that, compared to normoglycemic ApoE$^{-/-}$ mice, the GK$^{+/-}$ApoE$^{-/-}$ mice showed a stable and reproducible hyperglycemia, which induced accelerated atherosclerotic lesion progression as well as impaired lesion regression after lipid lowering. Importantly, these effects were seen without increases in plasma lipid levels. This novel model provides a promising tool for drug discovery, enabling the evaluation of compound effects against both diabetic and cardiovascular endpoints simultaneously in one animal model.

Disclosure

Damilola D. Adingupu and Suvi E. Heinonen are joint first authors.

Competing Interests

The authors declare that they have no competing interests.

Authors' Contributions

Damilola D. Adingupu and Suvi E. Heinonen contributed equally to this work.

Acknowledgments

The authors thank Anna Tuneld and Gun-Britt Forsberg for excellent analytical support. We are also indebted to the animal facility at AstraZeneca in Alderly Park, UK, for the breeding of the mice and to the animal facility at AstraZeneca Mölndal, Sweden, for husbandry and help with blood sampling.

References

[1] G. Danaei, M. M. Finucane, Y. Lu et al., "National, regional, and global trends in fasting plasma glucose and diabetes prevalence since 1980: systematic analysis of health examination surveys and epidemiological studies with 370 country-years and 2.7 million participants," *The Lancet*, vol. 378, no. 9785, pp. 31–40, 2011.

[2] M. A. Creager, T. F. Lüscher, F. Cosentino, and J. A. Beckman, "Diabetes and vascular disease: pathophysiology, clinical consequences, and medical therapy—part I," *Circulation*, vol. 108, no. 12, pp. 1527–1532, 2003.

[3] T. F. Lüscher, M. A. Creager, J. A. Beckman, and F. Cosentino, "Diabetes and vascular disease: pathophysiology, clinical consequences, and medical therapy—part II," *Circulation*, vol. 108, no. 13, pp. 1655–1661, 2003.

[4] M. Coghlan and B. Leighton, "Glucokinase activators in diabetes management," *Expert Opinion on Investigational Drugs*, vol. 17, no. 2, pp. 145–167, 2008.

[5] F. M. Matschinsky, "Assessing the potential of glucokinase activators in diabetes therapy," *Nature Reviews Drug Discovery*, vol. 8, no. 5, pp. 399–416, 2009.

[6] K. K. Osbak, K. Colclough, C. Saint-Martin et al., "Update on mutations in glucokinase (GCK), which cause maturity-onset diabetes of the young, permanent neonatal diabetes, and hyperinsulinemic hypoglycemia," *Human Mutation*, vol. 30, no. 11, pp. 1512–1526, 2009.

[7] J. F. Caro, S. Triester, V. K. Patel, E. B. Tapscott, N. L. Frazier, and G. L. Dohm, "Liver glucokinase: decreased activity in patients with type II diabetes," *Hormone and Metabolic Research*, vol. 27, no. 1, pp. 19–22, 1995.

[8] A. Basu, R. Basu, P. Shah et al., "Effects of type 2 diabetes on the ability of insulin and glucose to regulate splanchnic and muscle glucose metabolism: evidence for a defect in hepatic glucokinase activity," *Diabetes*, vol. 49, no. 2, pp. 272–283, 2000.

[9] A. Basu, R. Basu, P. Shah et al., "Type 2 diabetes impairs splanchnic uptake of glucose but does not alter intestinal glucose absorption during enteral glucose feeding: additional evidence for a defect in hepatic glucokinase activity," *Diabetes*, vol. 50, no. 6, pp. 1351–1362, 2001.

[10] S. Del Guerra, R. Lupi, L. Marselli et al., "Functional and molecular defects of pancreatic islets in human type 2 diabetes," *Diabetes*, vol. 54, no. 3, pp. 727–735, 2005.

[11] T. Gorman, D. C. D. Hope, R. Brownlie et al., "Effect of high-fat diet on glucose homeostasis and gene expression in glucokinase knockout mice," *Diabetes, Obesity and Metabolism*, vol. 10, no. 10, pp. 885–897, 2008.

[12] D. J. Baker, A. M. Atkinson, G. P. Wilkinson, G. J. Coope, A. D. Charles, and B. Leighton, "Characterization of the heterozygous glucokinase knockout mouse as a translational disease model for glucose control in type 2 diabetes," *British Journal of Pharmacology*, vol. 171, no. 7, pp. 1629–1641, 2014.

[13] D. J. Baker, G. P. Wilkinson, A. M. Atkinson et al., "Chronic glucokinase activator treatment at clinically translatable exposures gives durable glucose lowering in two animal models of type 2 diabetes," *British Journal of Pharmacology*, vol. 171, no. 7, pp. 1642–1654, 2014.

[14] C. Kilkenny, W. Browne, I. C. Cuthill, M. Emerson, and D. G. Altman, "Animal research: reporting in vivo experiments: the ARRIVE guidelines," *British Journal of Pharmacology*, vol. 160, no. 7, pp. 1577–1579, 2010.

[15] C. J. Hartley, A. K. Reddy, S. Madala, L. H. Michael, M. L. Entman, and G. E. Taffet, "Effects of isoflurane on coronary blood flow velocity in young, old and ApoE$^{-/-}$ mice measured by doppler ultrasound," *Ultrasound in Medicine and Biology*, vol. 33, no. 4, pp. 512–521, 2007.

[16] E. H. Leiter, "Selecting the 'right' mouse model for metabolic syndrome and type 2 diabetes research," in *Type 2 Diabetes: Methods and Protocols*, C. Stocker, Ed., Humana Press, Totowa, NJ, USA, 2009.

[17] P. Lindstrom, "The physiology of obese-hyperglycemic mice [ob/ob mice]," *TheScientificWorldJournal*, vol. 7, pp. 666–685, 2007.

[18] American Diabetes Association, "Diagnosis and classification of diabetes mellitus," *Diabetes Care*, vol. 32, supplement 1, pp. S62–S67, 2009.

[19] M. E. Cerf, "Beta cell dysfunction and insulin resistance," *Frontiers in Endocrinology*, vol. 4, article 37, 2013.

[20] A. J. F. King, "The use of animal models in diabetes research," *British Journal of Pharmacology*, vol. 166, no. 3, pp. 877–894, 2012.

[21] Y. Terauchi, I. Takamoto, N. Kubota et al., "Glucokinase and IRS-2 are required for compensatory β cell hyperplasia in response to high-fat diet-induced insulin resistance," *The Journal of Clinical Investigation*, vol. 117, no. 1, pp. 246–257, 2007.

[22] A. A. Pendse, J. M. Arbones-Mainar, L. A. Johnson, M. K. Altenburg, and N. Maeda, "Apolipoprotein E knock-out and knock-in mice: atherosclerosis, metabolic syndrome, and beyond," *Journal of Lipid Research*, vol. 50, pp. S178–S182, 2009.

[23] C.-H. Yun, C. L. Schlett, I. S. Rogers et al., "Association between diabetes and different components of coronary atherosclerotic plaque burden as measured by coronary multidetector computed tomography," *Atherosclerosis*, vol. 205, no. 2, pp. 481–485, 2009.

[24] H. Williams, J. L. Johnson, K. G. S. Carson, and C. L. Jackson, "Characteristics of intact and ruptured atherosclerotic plaques in brachiocephalic arteries of apolipoprotein E knockout mice," *Arteriosclerosis, Thrombosis, and Vascular Biology*, vol. 22, no. 5, pp. 788–792, 2002.

[25] R. P. Wildman, L. L. Schott, S. Brockwell, L. H. Kuller, and K. Sutton-Tyrrell, "A dietary and exercise intervention slows menopause-associated progression of subclinical atherosclerosis as measured by intima-media thickness of the carotid arteries," *Journal of the American College of Cardiology*, vol. 44, no. 3, pp. 579–585, 2004.

[26] E. M. Hjerkinn, M. Abdelnoor, L. Breivik et al., "Effect of diet or very long chain ω-3 fatty acids on progression of atherosclerosis, evaluated by carotid plaques, intima-media thickness and by pulse wave propagation in elderly men with hypercholesterolaemia," *European Journal of Cardiovascular Prevention and Rehabilitation*, vol. 13, no. 3, pp. 325–333, 2006.

[27] I. Shai, J. D. Spence, D. Schwarzfuchs et al., "Dietary intervention to reverse carotid atherosclerosis," *Circulation*, vol. 121, no. 10, pp. 1200–1208, 2010.

[28] D. Ornish, S. E. Brown, J. H. Billings et al., "Can lifestyle changes reverse coronary heart disease?" *The Lancet*, vol. 336, no. 8708, pp. 129–133, 1990.

[29] G. F. Watts, B. Lewis, E. S. Lewis et al., "Effects on coronary artery disease of lipid-lowering diet, or diet plus cholestyramine, in the St Thomas' Atherosclerosis Regression Study (STARS)," *The Lancet*, vol. 339, no. 8793, pp. 563–569, 1992.

[30] H. U. Westergren, J. Grönros, S. E. Heinonen et al., "Impaired coronary and renal vascular function in spontaneously type 2 diabetic leptin-deficient mice," *PLoS ONE*, vol. 10, no. 6, Article ID e0130648, 2015.

[31] P. P. Dimitrow, M. Galderisi, and F. Rigo, "The non-invasive documentation of coronary microcirculation impairment: role of transthoracic echocardiography," *Cardiovascular Ultrasound*, vol. 3, article 18, 2005.

[32] J. Wikström, J. Grönros, and L.-M. Gan, "Adenosine induces dilation of epicardial coronary arteries in mice—relationship between coronary flow velocity reserve and coronary flow reserve *in vivo* using transthoracic echocardiography," *Ultrasound in Medicine and Biology*, vol. 34, no. 7, pp. 1053–1062, 2008.

[33] J. Wikström, J. Grönros, G. Bergström, and L.-M. Gan, "Functional and morphologic imaging of coronary atherosclerosis in living mice using high-resolution color Doppler echocardiography and ultrasound biomicroscopy," *Journal of the American College of Cardiology*, vol. 46, no. 4, pp. 720–727, 2005.

[34] M. L. Graham, J. L. Janecek, J. A. Kittredge, B. J. Hering, and H.-J. Schuurman, "The streptozotocin-induced diabetic nude mouse model: differences between animals from different sources," *Comparative Medicine*, vol. 61, no. 4, pp. 356–360, 2011.

[35] B. Hirshberg and A. Katz, "Cardiovascular outcome studies with novel antidiabetes agents: scientific and operational considerations," *Diabetes Care*, vol. 36, no. 2, pp. S253–S258, 2013.

19

Proteomic Analysis of Hippocampus and Cortex in Streptozotocin-Induced Diabetic Model Mice Showing Dementia

Kenji Matsuura,[1] Mieko Otani,[2] Masaoki Takano,[2] Keiichi Kadoyama,[3] and Shogo Matsuyama[4]

[1]*Faculty of Pharmacy, Osaka-Ohtani University, Tondabayashi 584-8540, Japan*
[2]*Department of Life Sciences Pharmacy, School of Pharmaceutical Sciences, Kobe Gakuin University, Kobe 650-8586, Japan*
[3]*Department of Pharmaceutical Health Care, Faculty of Pharmaceutical Sciences, Himeji Dokkyo University, Himeji 670-8524, Japan*
[4]*Biosignal Research Center, Kobe University, Kobe 657-8501, Japan*

Correspondence should be addressed to Shogo Matsuyama; shogo@platinum.kobe-u.ac.jp

Academic Editor: Hiroshi Okamoto

Aim. Diabetes with its associated hyperglycemia induces various type of peripheral damage and also impairs the central nervous system (CNS). This study is aimed at clarifying the precise mechanism of diabetes-induced dementia as an impairment of CNS. *Methods.* The proteomic analysis of the hippocampus and cortex in streptozotocin- (STZ-) treated mouse diabetic model showing dementia was performed using two-dimensional gel electrophoresis (2-DE) followed by mass spectrometry ($n = 3$ /group). *Results.* Significant changes in the expression of 32 proteins and 7 phosphoproteins were observed in the hippocampus and cortex. These identified proteins and phosphoproteins could be functionally classified as cytoskeletal protein, oxidoreductase, protein deubiquitination, energy metabolism, GTPase activation, heme binding, hydrolase, iron storage, neurotransmitter release, protease inhibitor, transcription, glycolysis, antiapoptosis, calcium ion binding, heme metabolic process, protein degradation, vesicular transport, and unknown in the hippocampus or cortex. Additionally, Western blotting validated the changes in translationally controlled tumor protein, ATP-specific succinyl-CoA synthetase beta subunit, and gamma-enolase isoform 1. *Conclusions.* These findings showed that STZ-induced diabetes changed the expression of proteins and phosphoproteins in the hippocampus and cortex. We propose that alterations in expression levels of these proteins play an important role in diabetes-induced dementia.

1. Introduction

Diabetes is a chronic and metabolic disease characterized by hyperglycemia resulting from defective insulin secretion and/or insulin resistance [1]. Diabetics are at a significantly elevated risk for nephropathy, peripheral neuropathy, and retinopathy. In the central nervous system (CNS), chronic hyperglycemia leads to the enhanced formation of advanced glycation end products (AGEs), which have potentially toxic effects on neurons, causing dementia [2]. Hyperglycemia also causes a significant increase in generation of reactive oxygen species (ROS), resulting in cerebral angiopathy and abnormalities of neurons and glia in the brain, and subsequent dementia [3]. The degree to which the neuronal abnormality is caused directly by hyperglycemia remains unclear [3]. Moreover, the development of diabetes-induced dementia is not only closely associated with hyperglycemia but also with the action of insulin [4].

Insulin and insulin receptors show abundant expression throughout the brain, especially in the hippocampus, which is involved in dementia [5]. Peripheral insulin crosses the blood-brain barrier (BBB) via an active transport mechanism to exert its effects within the CNS [6]. Insulin receptors in the brain are found at synapses on both neurons and astrocytes [7]. Insulin signaling acts as a neuromodulator that regulates the release and reuptake of neurotransmitters, such as acetylcholine and norepinephrine in rat locus coeruleus [8], and regulates neuronal and glial functions such as synaptogenesis and synaptic plasticity via energy homeostasis, gene expression, and cognition [9]. Interestingly, insulin administered by intranasal improved cognitive dysfunction and insulin signaling, reduced amyloid-β (Aβ) production and amyloid plaque burden, and increased neurogenesis in 4-month-old APP/PS1 mice showing early Alzheimer's disease (AD) pathologies [10]. Furthermore, intranasal insulin application improved cognitive performance in healthy subjects, aged subjects, AD patients, and experimental models of insulin resistance [11]. In the brain, insulin-degrading enzyme (IDE) is synthesized and secreted by neurons, oligodendrocytes, and microglia [12]. IDE degrades extracellular Aβ in microglial and neuronal cultures and insulin can prevent this degradation, thereby impairing the clearance of extracellular Aβ [13]. IDE mutant rats, which show reduced activity of the enzyme, lead to type 2 diabetes, resulting in the enhanced cerebral deposition of Aβ [14]. However, to clarify the precise mechanisms involved in the development of diabetes-induced dementia, further research will be required.

Streptozotocin (STZ), a glucosamine-nitrosourea compound, is a genotoxic methylating agent and preferentially destroys insulin-producing β cells of the pancreas through the generation of ROS and alkylation of DNA [15]. STZ is a chemical used for the generation of diabetes phenotypes in most strains of rodents [16]. A mouse model utilizing five doses of STZ at low dose (50–60 mg/kg/day) has been extensively used in studies of type 1 diabetes (T1D) due to the progressive destruction of pancreatic β cells induced [17]. Importantly, the STZ-induced diabetes of mouse resulted in spatial learning deficits and impaired hippocampal long-term potentiation (LTP), which is thought to affect the cellular mechanisms of learning and memory [18]. Accordingly, STZ-treated mice have been used extensively to examine the physiological and pathophysiological consequences of diabetes-induced dementia.

In the present study, changes in the expression of hippocampal and cortical proteins and phosphoproteins in STZ-treated mice were examined using two-dimensional gel electrophoresis followed by staining with SYPRO Ruby and Pro-Q Diamond, respectively, and subsequent mass spectrometry to elucidate the molecular mechanisms involved in diabetes-induced dementia.

2. Materials and Methods

2.1. Reagents. Streptozotocin (STZ), urea, thiourea, sodium dodecyl sulfate (SDS), 3-((3-cholamidopropyl) dimethylammonio)-1-propanesulfonate (CHAPS), 2-mercaptoethanol (2-ME), dithiothreitol (DTT), bromophenol blue, iodoacetamide, RNase A, and DNase I were purchased from Wako Pure Chemical Industries, Ltd. (Osaka, Japan). Source information for all other assay reagents and materials is stated in the Materials and Methods section described below.

2.2. Animals. C57BL/6 mice (Japan SLC, Inc., Shizuoka, Japan) were maintained in a standard 12 h light/dark environment (lights on at 7:00 A.M.). Food and water were available to mice ad libitum. All experimental procedures were performed in accordance with the National Institutes of Health Guidelines on the Care and Use of Animals and confirmed by the Himeji Dokkyo University Animal Experiment Committee. All efforts were made to minimize animal use and suffering.

2.3. Generation of Diabetic Model Mice. The diabetic model was set up by intraperitoneal injection of STZ 50 mg/kg once a day for 5 consecutive days [19]. Ten weeks after injection, the mice were tested for sufficient levels of hyperglycemia. Blood glucose level was assessed using blood glucometer (Terumo Co. Tokyo, Japan) by tail vein puncture blood sampling. A serum glucose level higher than 400 mg/dl was considered diabetic [20].

2.4. Protein Extraction. Protein extraction was performed as previously described [21]. Both the STZ- and vehicle-treated mice were killed under anesthesia with pentobarbital sodium. The hippocampi and cortices were isolated from three mice in each group, and mixed separately for the two groups. Two-DE analysis was repeated in triplicate. In brief, mouse hippocampal samples were homogenized in lysis buffer [7 M urea, 2 M thiourea, 5% CHAPS, 2% immobilized pH gradient (IPG) buffer (GE Healthcare UK Ltd., Buckinghamshire, UK), 50 mM 2-ME, 2.5 μg/ml DNase I, and 2.5 μg/ml RNase A]. Solubilized extracts were centrifuged at 15,000 ×g for 30 min, and the supernatant was used for further analysis.

2.5. Two-DE. Two-DE analysis was carried out as previously described [21, 22]. In brief, one-dimensional isoelectric focusing (IEF) gel electrophoresis was performed using IPG gel strips (pH 4–7; 7 cm; GE Healthcare, WI). Approximately 1000 μg of protein from each group was incubated with the IPG strips and run at 50 V for 6 h, at 100 V for 6 h, and finally at 2000 V for 6 h. After IEF gel electrophoresis, the IPG strips were equilibrated for 15 min in equilibration buffer [50 mM Tris-HCl, pH 8.8, 6 M urea, 1% SDS, 30% (v/v) glycerol, and 1% (w/v) DTT] and then for 15 min in equilibration buffer containing 2.5% (w/v) iodoacetamide instead of DTT. For the second dimension, the equilibrated IPG strips were transferred onto 15% SDS-PAGE gels at 5 mA/gel for 7 h.

2.6. Protein or Phosphoprotein Staining and Image Acquisition. Protein or phosphoprotein gel staining and image acquisition were carried out as previously described [21, 22]. Briefly, the gels were fixed three times in 200 ml immobilization solution [10% acetic acid and 50% methanol] for 30 min and washed five times with 200 ml of water for 15 min. Under the dark, the gels were stained with Pro-Q Diamond phosphoprotein gel stain (Life Technologies, Carlsbad, CA) for 120 min at room temperature with gentle agitation and then washed three times with destaining solution [50 mM sodium acetate, pH 4.0 and 20% (v/v) acetonitrile] for 30 min. Image acquisition was performed on Fluorophorestar 3000 image capture system (Anatech, Tokyo, Japan) with a 520 nm excitation and 575 nm emission filter for Pro-Q Diamond detection.

Next, gels were washed with washing solution [10% methanol and 7% acetic acid] for 30 min. The gels were incubated in SYPRO Ruby stain (Life Technologies) for 90 min in the dark. The gels were washed with destaining solution [10%

methanol and 7% acetic acid] for 30 min and rinsed with MilliQ H_2O. Image acquisition was carried out using a Fluorophorestar 3000 image capture system with a 470 nm excitation and 618 nm emission filter for SYPRO Ruby detection.

2.7. Image Analysis. Image analysis was performed as previously described [21, 22]. Image analysis and the quantification of gel spots were performed with Prodigy SameSpots software (Nonlinear Dynamics, Newcastle upon Tyne, UK). From the menu of SameSpots normalization options, we chose to normalize the intensity of each spot to the total intensity of all matched spots within each gel and to identify differentially expressed spots by comparing spot intensity differences between samples from STZ-treated mice and control mice using ANOVA.

2.8. Trypsin Digestion. In-gel digestion was performed using a method described [21]. Protein spots were cut from the gels, and the gel pieces were washed three times for 15 min each with 200 μl of 50 mM ammonium bicarbonate with 50% (v/v) acetonitrile and then dried under vacuum. The gel piece was rehydrated in 5 μl of sequencing-grade modified trypsin (10 ng/μl, Promega, Madison, WI) in 10 mM ammonium bicarbonate for 30 min at 4°C, and digestion was carried out for 18 h at 37°C. Peptides were extracted with 5 μl of extracting solution [50% (v/v) acetonitrile and 0.3% (v/v) trifluoroacetic acid] for 10 min by sonication.

2.9. Mass Spectrometry Analysis and Protein Identification. Mass spectrometry analysis was performed in accordance with the procedure described in our previous report [21]. In brief, mass spectra were obtained using a MALDI-TOF MS/MS analyzer (ABI PLUS 4800, Applied Biosystems, Foster City, CA). One μl of each sample was mixed with 1 μl matrix solution [1 μg/μl α-cyano-4-hydroxycinnamic acid (CHCA, Wako Pure Chemical Industries Ltd.) in 50% (v/v) acetonitrile and 0.3% (v/v) trifluoroacetic acid]. Analyte and matrix were spotted onto a stainless steel MALDI target plate and dried under ambient conditions. The peptides were analyzed using a MALDI-TOF MS/MS analyzer, and the authors searched the database with the Mascot search engine (http://www.matrixscience.com; Matrix Science, Boston, MA) using a Mascot MS/MS ion search through NCBInr databases. Proteins were considered as identified by MALDI-TOF MS if they had Mascot scores of 60 or higher ($P < 0.05$).

2.10. Western Blotting. The isolated hippocampus and cortex samples were homogenized in buffer containing 20 mM Tris-HCl, pH 7.0, 6 M urea, 150 mM NaCl, 2 mM EDTA, and 1% Triton X-100. The homogenates were subjected to 8% SDS-polyacrylamide gel electrophoresis and analyzed by Western blot using rabbit anti-TCTP (diluted 1 : 1000, Abcam, Cambridge, MA), rabbit anti-SUCLA2 (diluted 1 : 1000, Abcam), rabbit anti-NSE (diluted 1 : 1000, Abcam), and rabbit anti-GAPDH (diluted 1 : 10,000, AbFrontier, Seoul, Korea) antibodies at 4°C overnight. The membranes were incubated with the indicated secondary antibody (diluted 1 : 5000, GE Healthcare, Madison, WI). All values were corrected with reference to the value for GAPDH, used as an internal standard. Immunoreactivity was detected by using an Amersham ECL Prime Western blotting detection kit (GE Healthcare). Western blot images were quantified using the Multi Gauge version 2.2 software (Fuji Photofilm, Tokyo, Japan).

2.11. Statistical Analysis. Respective densitometric quantifications are shown as mean ± SEM. All data were tested by one-way ANOVA followed by Dunnett's multiple-comparisons tests to evaluate the differences between groups. $P < 0.05$ was considered statistically significant.

3. Results

The expression changes of proteins and phosphoproteins in the hippocampus and cortex of STZ-treated and untreated control mice were quantified and identified on 2-DE gels using Prodigy SameSpot software and MALDI-TOF MS/MS. Image analysis showed approximately 400 protein spots and 200 phosphoprotein spots on each SYPRO Ruby-stained 2-DE gel (Figure 1) and each Pro-Q Diamond-stained 2-DE gel (Figure 2), respectively. We detected 16 (5 up- and 11 downregulated) hippocampal proteins (Table 1), 16 (7 up- and 9 downregulated) cortical proteins (Table 2), 3 (1 up- and 2 downregulated) hippocampal phosphoproteins (Table 3), and 4 (2 up- and 2 downregulated) cortical phosphoproteins (Table 3). These proteins and phosphoproteins were categorized into functional groups as shown in Tables 1–3 using the PANTHER (http://www.pantherdb.org/) database.

3.1. Identification of Altered Proteins and Phosphoproteins in the Hippocampus of STZ-Treated Mice. The 5 proteins with increased expression levels were identified as type II peroxiredoxin 1, ATP-specific succinyl-CoA synthetase beta subunit, rho GDP-dissociation inhibitor 1, heme-binding protein, and phosphatidylethanolamine-binding protein 1, and the 11 proteins with decreased expression levels were identified as profilin-2, tubulin beta-5 chain, alpha-internexin, ketimine reductase mu-crystallin, L-lactate dehydrogenase B chain isoform 1, ubiquitin carboxy-terminal hydrolase L1, isoform CRA_a, proteasome subunit alpha type-3, N(G),N(G)-dimethylarginine dimethylaminohydrolase 1, ferritin heavy chain, translationally controlled tumor protein, and prohibitin (Table 1).

The phosphoprotein with increased expression level was identified as dihydropyrimidinase-related protein 2, and 2 phosphoproteins with decreased expression level were identified as proteasome subunit alpha type-3 and beta-soluble NSF attachment protein (Table 2).

3.2. Identification of Proteins and Phosphoproteins with Altered Expression in the Cortex of STZ-Treated Mice. The 7 proteins with increased expression levels were identified as alpha-tubulin, partial, tubulin alpha-1C chain, put. Beta-actin (aa 27–375), gamma-actin, alpha-internexin, beta-synuclein, and unnamed protein product, and the 9 proteins with decreased expression levels were identified as tubulin beta-5 chain, NADH dehydrogenase (ubiquinone) Fe-S protein 1, atp5b protein, partial, gamma-enolase isoform 1, calretinin,

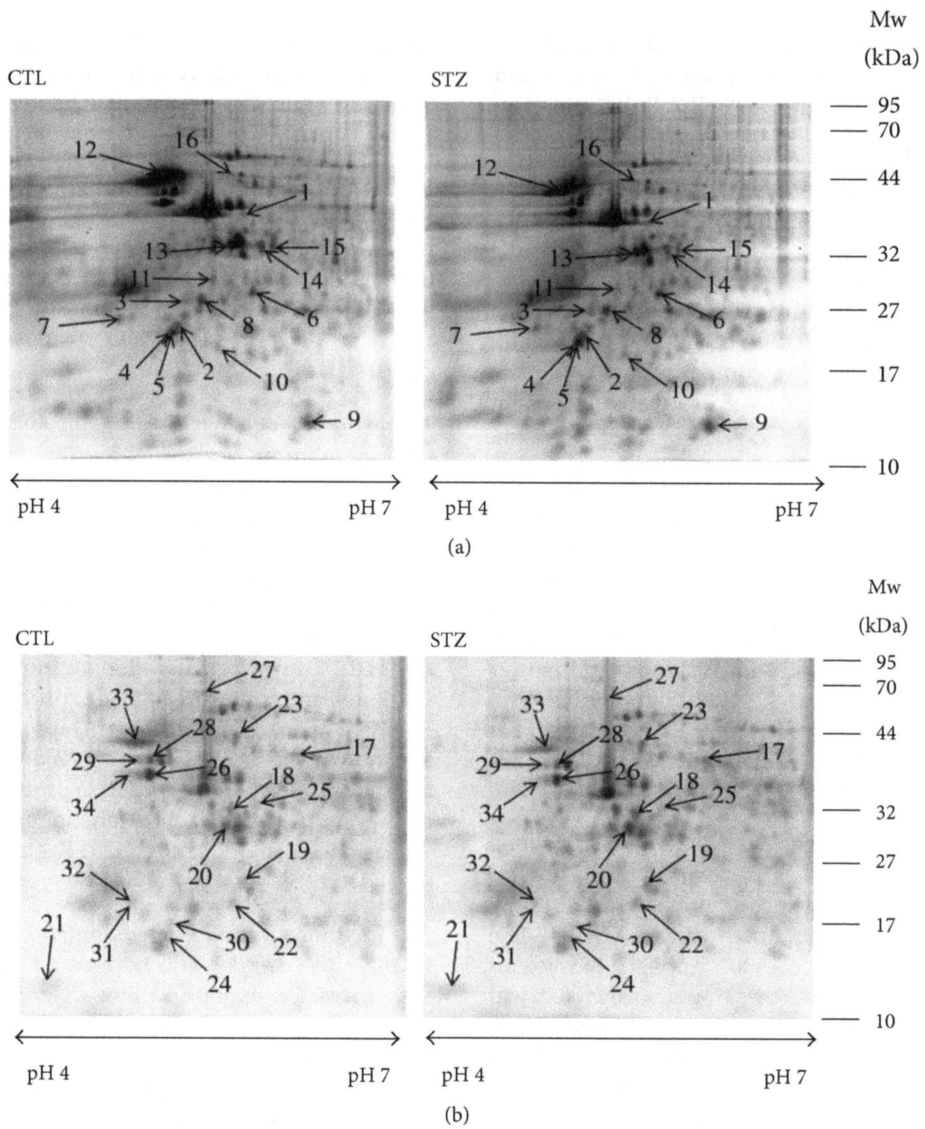

Figure 1: Two-DE images of hippocampal (a) and cortical (b) proteins in STZ-treated (STZ) and control (CTL) mice. IPG strips (pH 4–7) were used for the first dimension, and 15% polyacrylamide gels were used for the second dimension. Isoelectric points (PIs) and experimental masses are shown on the *x*- and *y*-axes. The differentially expressed proteins are identified by numbers that correspond to spot numbers in Tables 1 and 3. Experiments were repeated three times independently with similar results. Typical gel images are shown.

heme-binding protein, phosphatidylethanolamine-binding protein 1, COP9 signalosome complex subunit 4, and ubiquitin C-terminal hydrolase L3 (Table 3).

The 2 phosphoproteins with increased expression levels were identified as dihydropyrimidinase-related protein 2 and enolase 1B, retrotransposed, and the 2 phosphoproteins with decreased expression levels were identified as gamma-actin and proteasome subunit alpha type-3 (Table 2).

3.3. Western Blot Analysis of the Altered Proteins in the Hippocampus and Cortex of STZ-Treated Mice. Western blot analysis was performed to validate the identity of translationally controlled tumor protein and ATP-specific succinyl-CoA synthetase beta subunit as differentially expressed hippocampal proteins and the identity of gamma-enolase isoform 1 as differentially expressed cortical protein. The protein level of translationally controlled tumor protein was significantly decreased about 0.8-fold in the hippocampus of STZ-treated mice compared with untreated control ($P = 0.049$) (Figure 3(a)). The protein level of hippocampal ATP-specific succinyl-CoA synthetase beta subunit tended to increase ($P = 0.29$) (Figure 3(b)) and that of cortical gamma-enolase isoform 1 tended to decrease ($P = 0.057$) (Figure 3(c)).

4. Discussion

In this study, we used 2-DE coupled with MS to investigate changes in the expression of proteins and phosphoproteins in the hippocampus and cortex of STZ-treated mice, that

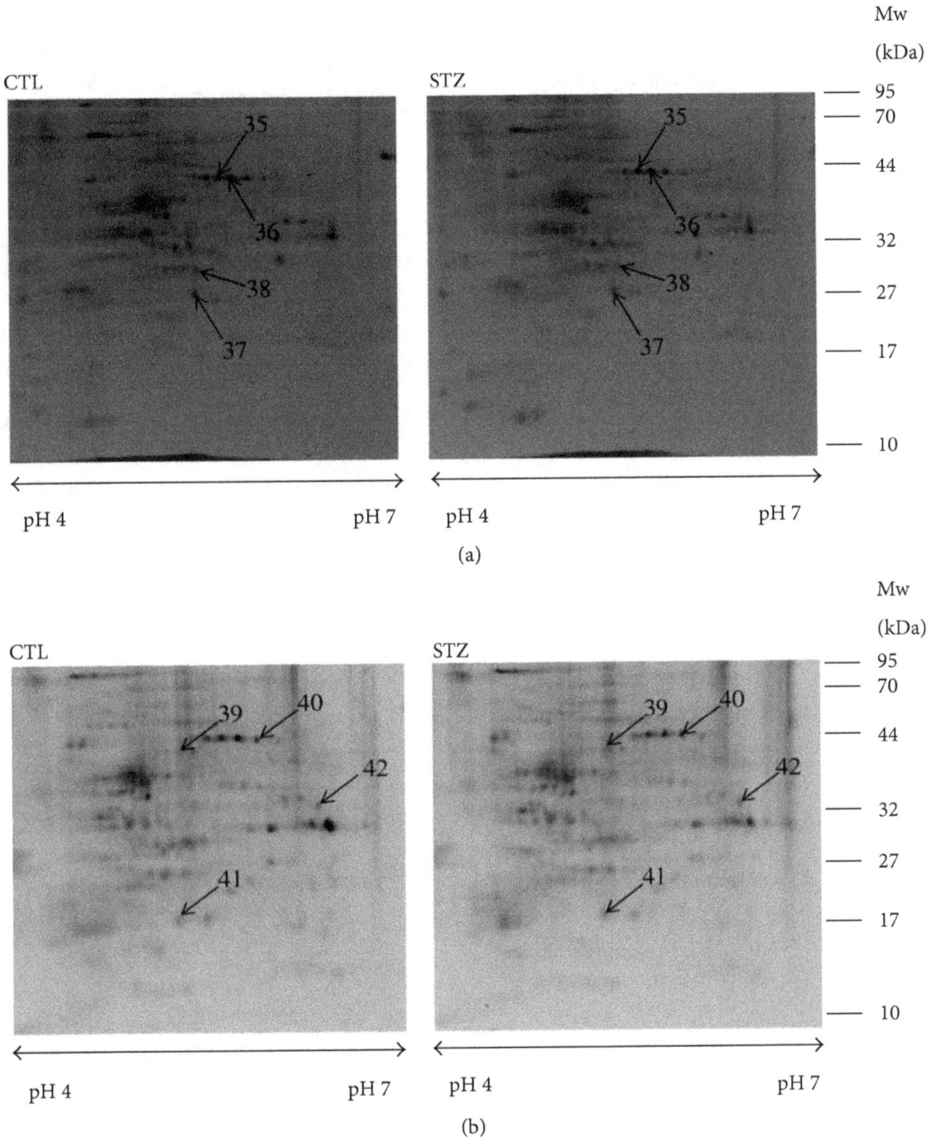

Figure 2: Two-DE images of hippocampal (a) and cortical (b) phosphoproteins in STZ-treated (STZ) and control (CTL) mice. IPG strips (pH 4–7) were used for the first dimension, and 15% polyacrylamide gels were used for the second dimension. Isoelectric points (PIs) and experimental masses are shown on the x- and y-axes. The differentially expressed phosphoproteins are identified by numbers that correspond to spot numbers in Table 2. Experiments were repeated three times independently with similar results. Typical gel images are shown.

is, diabetic model mice showing dementia, and revealed that the expression of 32 proteins and 7 phosphoproteins changed significantly.

4.1. Cellular Cytoskeleton. Micorotubules are composed of α- and β-tubulin heterodimers and are present throughout neuronal dendrites and axons. Microtubule dynamics regulate axonal outgrowth, dendritic spine morphology, and synaptic plasticity [23]. Treatment with paclitaxel, a microtubule dynamics inhibitor, leads to LTP deficits in the cortico-amygdala pathway in mouse brain slices [24]. Actin exists in both monomeric (G-actin) and polymerized (F-actin) forms and presents in dendritic spines. Actin dynamics are essential in synaptic function and memory formation [25]. Indeed, cytochalasin D, an inhibitor of F-actin polymerization, blocks the late phase of LTP but not the early phase [26]. Thus, changes in the expression of tubulin and actin might affect synaptic plasticity, being involved with diabetes-induced dementia.

4.2. Oxidoreductase. Peroxiredoxins (Prxs) are antioxidant enzymes that contain one or two cysteine (Cys) residues in their active site [27]. There are six isoforms divided into three groups: the 2-Cys Prxs (Prx 1, 2, 3, and 4), the atypical 2-Cys Prx (Prx 5), and the 1-Cys Prx (Prx 6) [27]. In neurons, intracellular Prxs, which are induced by various oxidative stimuli, protect against oxidative radical damage by ROS [28]. Type II Prx 1, also known as Prx 2, is predominantly

TABLE 1: Identified proteins in the hippocampus and their functional categories.

Spot no.	Accession no.	Identified protein	Observed Mw (kDa)/pI	Theoretical Mw (Da)/pI	Score	SC	Fold change (STZ/CTL)	ANOVA P value
Cytoskeletal protein								
9	gi|9506971	Profilin-2	12/6.2	15,364/6.55	145	28	0.8	0.048
12	gi|7106439	Tubulin beta-5 chain	43/5.0	50,095/4.78	295	14	0.8	0.012
16	gi|508538	Alpha-internexin	43/5.6	56,007/5.16	232	14	0.7	0.013
Oxidoreductase								
5	gi|3603241	Type II peroxiredoxin 1	21/5.1	21,949/5.20	136	9	1.1	0.032
13	gi|7710012	Ketimine reductase mu-crystallin	32/5.6	33,673/5.44	208	14	0.8	0.002
15	gi|6678674	L-Lactate dehydrogenase B chain isoform 1	32/5.9	36,834/5.70	233	14	0.7	0.041
Protein deubiquitination								
8	gi|148705825	Ubiquitin carboxy-terminal hydrolase L1, isoform CRA_a	26/5.3	24,977/5.05	221	21	0.9	0.018
11	gi|261824000	Proteasome subunit alpha type-3	28/5.4	28,615/5.29	201	17	0.8	0.043
Energy metabolism								
1	gi|3766201	ATP-specific succinyl-CoA synthetase beta subunit	37/5.7	46,557/5.65	170	8	1.8	0.014
GTPase activation								
3	gi|31982030	Rho GDP-dissociation inhibitor 1	26/5.2	23,450/5.12	114	15	1.2	0.038
Heme binding								
2	gi|3724328	Heme-binding protein	22/5.1	21,165/5.18	95	14	1.3	0.023
Hydrolase								
14	gi|38371755	N(G),N(G)-dimethylarginine dimethylaminohydrolase 1	31/5.8	31/5.8 31,760/5.64	125	8	0.7	0.011
Iron storage								
10	gi|6753912	Ferritin heavy chain	18/5.5	21,224/5.53	237	26	0.8	0.039
Neurotransmitter release								
7	gi|6678437	Translationally controlled tumor protein	24/4.7	19,564/4.76	98	5	0.9	0.015
Protease inhibitor								
4	gi|84794552	Phosphatidylethanolamine-binding protein 1	21/5.1	20,988/5.19	168	25	1.1	0.032
Transcription								
6	gi|6679299	Prohibitin	27/5.7	29,859/5.57	270	20	0.9	0.038

Spot numbers correspond to the 2-DE gel in Figure 1(a). Accession numbers were obtained from the National Center for Biotechnology Information (NCBI) database. Score and sequence coverage (SC) were obtained by Mascot database searching (http://www.matrixscience.com). P values were obtained by ANOVA, $P < 0.05$.

expressed in the brain [29]. The protein level of Prx 2 is increased in aging and AD brains, suggesting that Prx 2 is involved in the elevated neuronal antioxidant response under oxidative stress [30]. The proteomic analysis of the hippocampus in AD patients shows that the expression of Prx 2 increases compared with age-matched controls [31]. Prx 2-deficient mice show remarkably increased susceptibility to oxidative stress-induced tissue damage [32]. Therefore, the increased expression of Prx 2 might decrease oxidative damage, improving abnormalities of neurons and glia in the brain and subsequent dementia.

4.3. Neurotransmitter Release. Translationally controlled tumor protein (TCTP) is a multifunctional protein that is involved in immune responses, cell proliferation, cancer progression, and apoptosis [33]. TCTP, also known as histamine-releasing factor (HRF), induces the secretion of histamine that is widely distributed in the brain [34].

TABLE 2: Identified proteins in the cortex and their functional categories.

Spot no.	Accession no.	Identified protein	Observed Mw (kDa)/pI	Theoretical Mw (Da)/pI	Score	SC	Fold change (STZ/CTL)	ANOVA *P* value
Cytoskeletal protein								
17	gi|3642627	Alpha-tubulin, partial	40/6.1	11,058/4.85	70	15	1.4	0.016
18	gi|6678469	Tubulin alpha-1C chain	31/5.6	50,562/4.96	187	10	1.4	0.015
19	gi|49868	Put. beta-actin (aa 27–375)	25/5.7	39,446/5.78	126	8	1.3	0.035
22	gi|809561	Gamma-actin	22/5.6	41,335/5.56	221	10	1.3	0.037
23	gi|148539957	Alpha-internexin	44/5.6	55,520/5.35	567	19	1.2	0.045
33	gi|7106439	Tubulin beta-5 chain	41/4.9	50,095/4.78	426	12	0.7	0.031
Energy metabolism								
27	gi|13879366	NADH dehydrogenase (ubiquinone) Fe-S protein 1	59/5.4	80,724/5.51	264	10	0.9	0.002
28	gi|23272966	Atp5b protein, partial	39/5.0	56,632/5.24	535	22	0.8	0.007
29	gi|23272966	Atp5b protein, partial	39/4.9	56,632/5.24	470	19	0.8	0.008
Glycolysis								
26	gi|7305027	Gamma-enolase isoform 1	36/5.0	47,609/4.99	449	14	0.9	0.044
34	gi|7305027	Gamma-enolase isoform 1	36/4.8	47,609/4.99	249	11	0.6	0.004
Antiapoptosis								
21	gi|15809030	Beta-synuclein	16/4.2	14,043/4.38	122	29	1.3	0.024
Calcium ion binding								
31	gi|34098931	Calretinin	22/4.8	31,467/4.94	199	15	0.8	0.008
Heme metabolic process								
30	gi|4886904	Heme-binding protein	20/5.2	21,153/5.18	170	26	0.8	0.004
Protease inhibitor								
24	gi|84794552	Phosphatidylethanolamine-binding protein 1	19/5.1	20,988/5.19	203	32	0.9	0.007
Protein degradation								
25	gi|6753490	COP9 signalosome complex subunit 4	31/5.8	46,541/5.57	62	4	0.9	0.035
Protein deubiquitination								
32	gi|7578956	Ubiquitin C-terminal hydrolase L3	22/4.8	26,333/5.08	113	9	0.8	0.008
Unknown								
20	gi|74212109	Unnamed protein product	29/5.5	50,076/4.75	246	10	1.3	0.041

Spot numbers correspond to the 2-DE gel in Figure 1(b). Accession numbers were obtained from the National Center for Biotechnology Information (NCBI) database. Score and sequence coverage (SC) were obtained by Mascot database searching (http://www.matrixscience.com). *P* values were obtained by ANOVA, $P < 0.05$.

Histamine-expressing neurons project to wide areas of the brain, including regions especially important for cognitive functions such as the frontal cortex and hippocampus [35]. Histamine and TCTP are significantly reduced in AD brain compared to age-matched control, suggesting that decreased histamine levels impair cognitive function in AD [35]. Thus, the decreased expression of TCTP might decrease the histamine release and be one of the main causes of dementia.

4.4. Protein Deubiquitination. In humans, four ubiquitin carboxy-terminal hydrolase (UCH) proteins (UCH-L1, UCH-L3, UCH37/UCH-L5, and BAP1) have been identified, but only UCH-L1 and L3 have been studied in detail [36]. UCH-L1 is a neuronal deubiquitinase that cleaves peptide adducts from the C-terminus of ubiquitin [37]. UCH-L1 is predominantly expressed in the brain [37]. The proteomic analysis of the hippocampus in AβPPswe/PS1dE9 mice

Table 3: Identified phosphoproteins in the hippocampus and cortex, and their functional categories.

Spot no.	Accession no.	Identified protein	Observed Mw (kDa)/pI	Theoretical Mw (Da)/pI	Score	SC	Fold change (STZ/CTL)	ANOVA *P* value
Hippocampus								
Neuronal development								
35	gi|40254595	Dihydropyrimidinase-related protein 2	44/5.6	62,638/5.95	85	4	1.2	0.04
36	gi|40254595	Dihydropyrimidinase-related protein 2	44/5.8	62,638/5.95	144	6	1.1	0.015
Protein degradation								
37	gi|261824000	Proteasome subunit alpha type-3	28/5.3	28,615/5.29	88	9	0.9	0.037
Vesicular transport								
38	gi|29789104	Beta-soluble NSF attachment protein	30/5.3	33,878/5.32	177	16	0.8	0.04
Cortex								
Cytoskeletal protein								
42	gi|809561	Gamma-actin	43/5.3	41,335/5.56	254	13	0.7	0.039
Neuronal development								
39	gi|40254595	Dihydropyrimidinase-related protein 2	45/5.9	62,638/5.95	490	17	1.3	0.026
Protein degradation								
41	gi|261824000	Proteasome subunit alpha type-3	21/5.3	28,615/5.29	142	14	0.8	0.043
Unknown								
40	gi|70794816	Enolase 1B, retrotransposed	32/6.5	47,453/6.37	163	9	1.1	0.018

Spot numbers correspond to the 2-DE gel in Figure 2. Accession numbers were obtained from the National Center for Biotechnology Information. (NCBI) database. Score and sequence coverage (SC) were obtained by Mascot database searching (http://www.matrixscience.com). *P* values were obtained by ANOVA, $P < 0.05$.

shows that the expression of UCH-L1 decreases compared with age-matched wild-type mice [38]. UCH-L1 is downregulated in the brain of patients with Parkinson's disease and AD [39]. The administration of UCH-L1 protein fused to the transduction domain of HIV transactivator (TAT) protein into APP/PS1 model mice of AD provided a protective effect against amyloid-induced neurodegeneration in synaptic function and contextual memory [40]. UCH-L3 is universally expressed in all tissues [41]. UCH-L3-deficient mice exhibit significant impairment in learning and memory using Morris water maze and 8-arm radial maze task [42]. Indeed, our findings showed that UCH-L1 and L3 were downregulated in diabetes-induced dementia. Thus, the decreased expressions of UCH-L1 and L3 could contribute to neurodegeneration, resulting in dementia.

4.5. Antiapoptosis. The human synuclein family has 3 members, α-synuclein, β-synuclein, and γ-synuclein [43]. α-Synuclein and β-synuclein are predominantly localized at presynaptic nerve terminals in the CNS [44]. In contrast, γ-synuclein is abundant in the peripheral nervous system [45]. β-Synuclein protects neurons against apoptosis induced by staurosporine and 6-hydroxydopamine, which is linked to the suppression of p53 transcriptional activity [46]. Thus, the increased expression of β-synuclein could protect against neuronal apoptosis in diabetes-induced dementia.

4.6. Calcium Ion Binding. Calretinin is an EF-hand calcium-binding protein involved in calcium signaling [47]. Calretinin is expressed in hilar mossy cells and in widely distributed subsets of GABAergic interneurons in the normal mouse hippocampus [48]. Calretinin maintains appropriate calcium ion concentration in cells and participates in the modulation of neuronal activity and synaptic plasticity [49]. Knockout mice lacking calretinin show no alteration in basal synaptic transmission but impaired LTP in the dentate gyrus [48]. These findings indicate that the decreased expression of calretinin might be involved in diabetes-induced dementia.

4.7. Neuronal Development. Dihydropyrimidinase-related protein 2/collapsin response mediator protein 2 (DPYL2/CRMP2) binds to tubulin heterodimers to promote microtubule formation and stability, resulting in axonal growth and neuronal polarity [50]. Cyclin-dependent kinase 5 (Cdk5) and glycogen syntheses kinase 3β (GSK-3β) regulate DPYL2

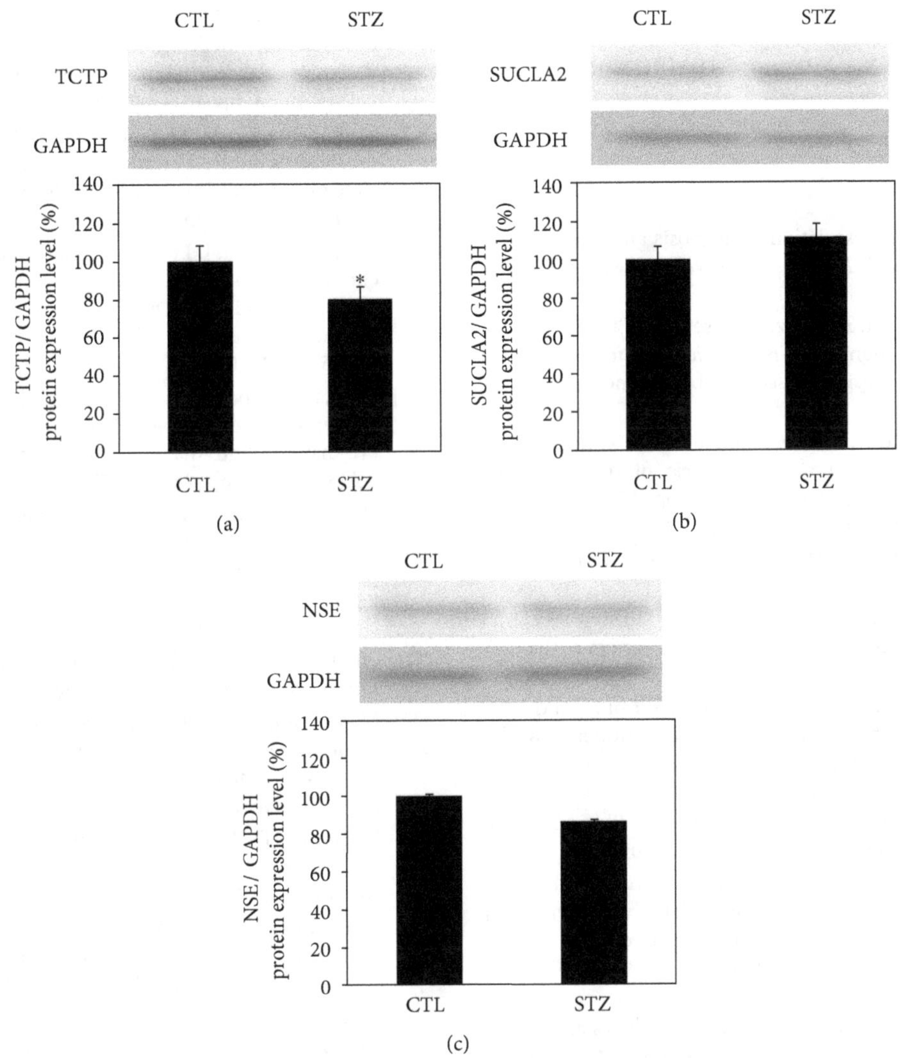

FIGURE 3: Representative images of Western blotting evaluating the expression of translationally controlled tumor protein (TCTP) (a), ATP-specific succinyl-CoA synthetase beta subunit (SUCLA2) (b) in the hippocampus, and gamma-enolase isoform 1 (NSE) (c) in the cortex from STZ-treated (STZ) and control (CTL) mice. The protein expression levels are normalized to glyceraldehyde 3-phosphate dehydrogenase (GAPDH) expression and indicated as the ratio relative to that in CTL. Data are presented as mean ± SEM of four independent experiments. Representative bands are shown above each graph. $^{*}P < 0.05$ versus control.

activity [51]. The phosphorylation of DPYL2 by GSK-3β can inactivate DPYL2 function [52]. DPYL2 is phosphorylated at Ser522 by Cdk5 and subsequently at Ser518, Thr514, and Thr509 by GSK-3β in brain tissue from human AD patients and in some mouse models of AD [53]. Aβ_{25-35}-induced impairment of cognitive function and LTP was not observed in DPYL2 phosphorylation-deficient knock-in mice, in which Ser522 of DPYL2 was replaced with alanine [54], suggesting that the phosphorylation of DPYL2 at Ser522 was associated with Aβ_{25-35}-induced cognitive memory deficit and impairment of LTP. Indeed, our findings showed that phosphorylated DPYL2 was increased in the hippocampus and cortex of STZ-treated mice. Taken together, it is suggested that phosphorylated DPYL2 plays an important role in diabetes-induced dementia. Interestingly, DPYL2 was identified from two phosphoprotein spots on 2-DE gels stained with Pro-Q Diamond staining in the hippocampus. The shift in the position of these phosphoprotein spots may imply translational modifications such as phosphorylation, acetylation, and degradation.

5. Conclusion

In conclusion, we found 32 proteins and 7 phosphoproteins with significantly altered levels in the hippocampus and cortex of STZ-treated mice. We propose that the identified proteins and phosphoproteins might play important roles in the molecular mechanisms involved in diabetes-induced dementia.

Conflicts of Interest

The authors declare no conflict of interest.

Acknowledgments

The authors thank Y. Kitamura (BMRC) for animal maintenance.

References

[1] American Diabetes Association, "Diagnosis and classification of diabetes mellitus," *Diabetes Care*, vol. 34, Supplement 1, pp. S62–S69, 2010.

[2] J. S. Roriz-Filho, T. M. Sá-Roriz, I. Rosset et al., "(Pre) diabetes, brain aging, and cognition," *Biochimica et Biophysica Acta (BBA) - Molecular Basis of Disease*, vol. 1792, no. 5, pp. 432–443, 2009.

[3] R. Mastrocola, F. Restivo, I. Vercellinatto et al., "Oxidative and nitrosative stress in brain mitochondria of diabetic rats," *Journal of Endocrinology*, vol. 187, no. 1, pp. 37–44, 2005.

[4] E. Candeias, A. I. Duarte, C. Carvalho et al., "The impairment of insulin signaling in Alzheimer's disease," *IUBMB Life*, vol. 64, no. 12, pp. 951–957, 2012.

[5] J. Havrankova, J. Roth, and M. Brownstein, "Insulin receptors are widely distributed in the central nervous system of the rat," *Nature*, vol. 272, no. 5656, pp. 827–829, 1978.

[6] C. L. Adam, P. A. Findlay, R. P. Aitken, J. S. Milne, and J. M. Wallace, "In vivo changes in central and peripheral insulin sensitivity in a large animal model of obesity," *Endocrinology*, vol. 153, no. 7, pp. 3147–3157, 2012.

[7] Z. Laron, "Insulin and the brain," *Archives of Physiology and Biochemistry*, vol. 115, no. 2, pp. 112–116, 2009.

[8] M. A. Reger, G. S. Watson, P. S. Green et al., "Intranasal insulin administration dose-dependently modulates verbal memory and plasma amyloid-beta in memory-impaired older adults," *Journal of Alzheimer's Disease*, vol. 13, no. 3, pp. 323–331, 2008.

[9] S. M. de la Monte, "Relationships between diabetes and cognitive impairment," *Endocrinology and Metabolism Clinics of North America*, vol. 43, no. 1, pp. 245–267, 2014.

[10] Y.-F. Mao, Z. Guo, T. Zheng et al., "Intranasal insulin alleviates cognitive deficits and amyloid pathology in young adult APPswe/PS1dE9 mice," *Aging Cell*, vol. 15, no. 5, pp. 893–902, 2016.

[11] J. T. Dou, M. Chen, F. Dufour, D. L. Alkon, and W. Q. Zhao, "Insulin receptor signaling in long-term memory consolidation following spatial learning," *Learning & Memory*, vol. 12, no. 6, pp. 646–655, 2005.

[12] H. G. Bernstein, U. Lendeckel, A. Bukowska et al., "Regional and cellular distribution patterns of insulin-degrading enzyme in the adult human brain and pituitary," *Journal of Chemical Neuroanatomy*, vol. 35, no. 2, pp. 216–224, 2008.

[13] K. Vekrellis, Z. Ye, W. Q. Qiu et al., "Neurons regulate extracellular levels of amyloid beta-protein via proteolysis by insulin-degrading enzyme," *Journal of Neuroscience*, vol. 20, no. 5, pp. 1657–1665, 2000.

[14] W. Farris, S. Mansourian, M. A. Leissring et al., "Partial loss-of-function mutations in insulin-degrading enzyme that induce diabetes also impair degradation of amyloid beta-protein," *American Journal of Pathology*, vol. 164, no. 4, pp. 1425–1434, 2004.

[15] T. Szkudelski, "The mechanism of alloxan and streptozotocin action in B cells of the rat pancreas," *Physiological Research*, vol. 50, no. 6, pp. 537–546, 2001.

[16] M. C. Deeds, J. M. Anderson, A. S. Armstrong et al., "Single dose streptozotocin-induced diabetes: considerations for study design in islet transplantation models," *Laboratory Animals*, vol. 45, no. 3, pp. 131–140, 2011.

[17] M. Radenkovic, M. Stojanovic, and M. Prostran, "Experimental diabetes induced by alloxan and streptozotocin: the current state of the art," *Journal of Pharmacological and Toxicological Methods*, vol. 78, pp. 13–31, 2016.

[18] Y. Wang, L. Wu, J. Li et al., "Synergistic exacerbation of mitochondrial and synaptic dysfunction and resultant learning and memory deficit in a mouse model of diabetic Alzheimer's disease," *Journal of Alzheimer's Disease*, vol. 43, no. 2, pp. 451–463, 2015.

[19] J. J. Ramos-Rodriguez, O. Ortiz, M. Jimenez-Palomares et al., "Differential central pathology and cognitive impairment in pre-diabetic and diabetic mice," *Psychoneuroendocrinology*, vol. 38, no. 11, pp. 2462–2475, 2013.

[20] H. S. Fox, "Androgen treatment prevents diabetes in nonobese diabetic mice," *The Journal of Experimental Medicine*, vol. 175, no. 5, pp. 1409–1412, 1992.

[21] K. Matsuura, M. Otani, M. Takano, K. Kadoyama, and S. Matsuyama, "The influence of chronic nicotine treatment on proteins expressed in the mouse hippocampus and cortex," *European Journal of Pharmacology*, vol. 780, pp. 16–25, 2016.

[22] M. Takano, T. Yamashita, K. Nagano et al., "Proteomic analysis of the hippocampus in Alzheimer's disease model mice by using two-dimensional fluorescence difference in gel electrophoresis," *Neuroscience Letters*, vol. 534, pp. 85–89, 2013.

[23] P. Penzes, D. P. Srivastava, and K. M. Woolfrey, "Not just actin? A role for dynamic microtubules in dendritic spines," *Neuron*, vol. 61, no. 1, pp. 3–5, 2009.

[24] G. P. Shumyatsky, G. Malleret, R. M. Shin et al., "Stathmin, a gene enriched in the amygdala, controls both learned and innate fear," *Cell*, vol. 123, no. 4, pp. 697–709, 2005.

[25] P. Hotulainen and C. C. Hoogenraad, "Actin in dendritic spines: connecting dynamics to function," *Journal of Cell Biology*, vol. 189, no. 4, pp. 619–629, 2010.

[26] T. Krucker, G. R. Siggins, and S. Halpain, "Dynamic actin filaments are required for stable long-term potentiation (LTP) in area CA1 of the hippocampus," *Proceedings of the National Academy of Sciences*, vol. 97, no. 12, pp. 6856–6861, 2000.

[27] S. G. Rhee, S. W. Kang, T. S. Chang, W. Jeong, and K. Kim, "Peroxiredoxin, a novel family of peroxidases," *IUBMB Life*, vol. 52, no. 1, pp. 35–41, 2001.

[28] C. Espinosa-Diez, V. Miguel, D. Mennerich et al., "Antioxidant responses and cellular adjustments to oxidative stress," *Redox Biology*, vol. 6, pp. 183–197, 2015.

[29] T. A. Sarafian, M. Anthony Verity, H. V. Vinters et al., "Differential expression of peroxiredoxin subtypes in human brain cell types," *Journal of Neuroscience Research*, vol. 56, no. 2, pp. 206–212, 1999.

[30] A. Patenaude, M. R. V. Murthy, and M. -E. Mirault, "Emerging roles of thioredoxin cycle enzymes in the central nervous system," *Cellular and Molecular Life Sciences*, vol. 62, no. 10, pp. 1063–1080, 2005.

[31] R. Sultana, D. Boyd-Kimball, J. Cai et al., "Proteomics analysis of the Alzheimer's disease hippocampal proteome," *Journal of Alzheimers Disease*, vol. 11, no. 2, pp. 153–164, 2007.

[32] T. H. Lee, S. U. Kim, S. L. Yu et al., "Peroxiredoxin II is essential for sustaining life span of erythrocytes in mice," *Blood*, vol. 101, no. >12, pp. 5033–5038, 2003.

[33] M. Gnanasekar, S. Thirugnanam, G. Zheng, A. Chen, and K. Ramaswamy, "Gene silencing of translationally controlled tumor protein (TCTP) by siRNA inhibits cell growth and induces apoptosis of human prostate cancer cells," *International Journal of Oncology*, vol. 34, no. 5, pp. 1241–1246, 2009.

[34] S. M. Macdonald, "Potential role of histamine releasing factor (HRF) as a therapeutic target for treating asthma and allergy," *Journal of Asthma and Allergy*, vol. 5, pp. 51–59, 2012.

[35] A. Zlomuzica, D. Dere, S. Binder, M. A. De Souza Silva, J. P. Huston, and E. Dere, "Neuronal histamine and cognitive symptoms in Alzheimer's disease," *Neuropharmacology*, vol. 106, pp. 135–145, 2016.

[36] Z. M. Eletr and K. D. Wilkinson, "Regulation of proteolysis by human deubiquitinating enzymes," *Biochimica et Biophysica Acta (BBA) - Molecular Cell Research*, vol. 1843, no. 1, pp. 114–128, 2014.

[37] C. N. Larsen, B. A. Krantz, and K. D. Wilkinson, "Substrate specificity of deubiquitinating enzymes: ubiquitin C-terminal hydrolases," *Biochemistry*, vol. 37, no. 10, pp. 3358–3368, 1998.

[38] Y. Fu, D. Zhao, B. Pan et al., "Proteomic analysis of protein expression throughout disease progression in a mouse model of Alzheimer's disease," *Journal of Alzheimer's Disease*, vol. 47, no. 4, pp. 915–926, 2015.

[39] J. Choi, A. I. Levey, S. T. Weintraub et al., "Oxidative modifications and down-regulation of ubiquitin carboxyl-terminal hydrolase L1 associated with idiopathic Parkinson's and Alzheimer's diseases," *Journal of Biological Chemistry*, vol. 279, no. 13, pp. 13256–13264, 2004.

[40] B. Gong, Z. Cao, P. Zheng et al., "Ubiquitin hydrolase Uch-L1 rescues beta-amyloid-induced decreases in synaptic function and contextual memory," *Cell*, vol. 126, no. 4, pp. 775–788, 2006.

[41] L. J. Kurihara, E. Semenova, J. M. Levorse, and S. M. Tilghman, "Expression and functional analysis of Uch-L3 during mouse development," *Molecular and Cellular Biology*, vol. 20, no. 7, pp. 2498–2504, 2000.

[42] M. A. Wood, M. P. Kaplan, C. M. Brensinger, W. Guo, and T. Abel, "Ubiquitin C-terminal hydrolase L3 (Uchl3) is involved in working memory," *Hippocampus*, vol. 15, no. 5, pp. 610–621, 2005.

[43] Y. H. Sung and D. Eliezer, "Residual structure, backbone dynamics, and interactions within the synuclein family," *Journal of Molecular Biology*, vol. 372, no. 3, pp. 689–707, 2007.

[44] R. Jakes, M. G. Spillantini, and M. Goedert, "Identification of two distinct synucleins from human brain," *FEBS Letters*, vol. 345, no. 1, pp. 27–32, 1994.

[45] A. N. Akopian and J. N. Wood, "Peripheral nervous system-specific genes identified by subtractive cDNA cloning," *Journal of Biological Chemistry*, vol. 270, no. 36, pp. 21264–21270, 1995.

[46] C. A. da Costa, E. Masliah, and F. Checler, "Beta-synuclein displays an antiapoptotic p53-dependent phenotype and protects neurons from 6 hydroxydopamine-induced caspase 3 activation: cross-talk with alpha-synuclein and implication for Parkinson's disease," *Journal of Biological Chemistry*, vol. 278, no. 39, pp. 37330–37335, 2003.

[47] J. H. Rogers, "Calretinin: a gene for a novel calcium-binding protein expressed principally in neurons," *Journal of Cell Biology*, vol. 105, no. 3, pp. 1343–1353, 1987.

[48] S. Schurmans, S. N. Schiffmann, H. Gurden et al., "Impaired long-term potentiation induction in dentate gyrus of calretinin-deficient mice," *Proceedings of the National Academy of Sciences*, vol. 94, no. 19, pp. 10415–10420, 1997.

[49] K. Rycerz, A. Krawczyk, J. Jaworska-Adamu, and I. Krawczyk-Marc, "Effects of monosodium glutamate treatment on calretinin-immunoreactive neurons in hippocampus of postnatal rats," *Folia Histochemica et Cytobiologica*, vol. 52, no. 4, pp. 281–288, 2014.

[50] N. Arimura, C. Menager, Y. Kawano et al., "Phosphorylation by rho kinase regulates CRMP-2 activity in growth cones," *Molecular and Cellular Biology*, vol. 25, no. 22, pp. 9973–9984, 2005.

[51] Y. Uchida, T. Ohshima, Y. Sasaki et al., "Semaphorin3A signalling is mediated via sequential Cdk5 and GSK3beta phosphorylation of CRMP2: implication of common phosphorylating mechanism underlying axon guidance and Alzheimer's disease," *Genes to Cells*, vol. 10, no. 2, pp. 165–179, 2005.

[52] T. Yoshimura, Y. Kawano, N. Arimura, S. Kawabata, A. Kikuchi, and K. Kaibuchi, "GSK-3β regulates phosphorylation of CRMP-2 and neuronal polarity," *Cell*, vol. 120, no. 1, pp. 137–149, 2005.

[53] A. R. Cole, W. Noble, L. van Aalten et al., "Collapsin response mediator protein-2 hyperphosphorylation is an early event in Alzheimer's disease progression," *Journal of Neurochemistry*, vol. 103, no. 3, pp. 1132–1144, 2007.

[54] T. Isono, N. Yamashita, M. Obara et al., "Amyloid-β_{25-35} induces impairment of cognitive function and long-term potentiation through phosphorylation of collapsin response mediator protein 2," *Neuroscience Research*, vol. 77, no. 3, pp. 180–185, 2013.

Permissions

All chapters in this book were first published in JDR, by Hindawi Publishing Corporation; hereby published with permission under the Creative Commons Attribution License or equivalent. Every chapter published in this book has been scrutinized by our experts. Their significance has been extensively debated. The topics covered herein carry significant findings which will fuel the growth of the discipline. They may even be implemented as practical applications or may be referred to as a beginning point for another development.

The contributors of this book come from diverse backgrounds, making this book a truly international effort. This book will bring forth new frontiers with its revolutionizing research information and detailed analysis of the nascent developments around the world.

We would like to thank all the contributing authors for lending their expertise to make the book truly unique. They have played a crucial role in the development of this book. Without their invaluable contributions this book wouldn't have been possible. They have made vital efforts to compile up to date information on the varied aspects of this subject to make this book a valuable addition to the collection of many professionals and students.

This book was conceptualized with the vision of imparting up-to-date information and advanced data in this field. To ensure the same, a matchless editorial board was set up. Every individual on the board went through rigorous rounds of assessment to prove their worth. After which they invested a large part of their time researching and compiling the most relevant data for our readers.

The editorial board has been involved in producing this book since its inception. They have spent rigorous hours researching and exploring the diverse topics which have resulted in the successful publishing of this book. They have passed on their knowledge of decades through this book. To expedite this challenging task, the publisher supported the team at every step. A small team of assistant editors was also appointed to further simplify the editing procedure and attain best results for the readers.

Apart from the editorial board, the designing team has also invested a significant amount of their time in understanding the subject and creating the most relevant covers. They scrutinized every image to scout for the most suitable representation of the subject and create an appropriate cover for the book.

The publishing team has been an ardent support to the editorial, designing and production team. Their endless efforts to recruit the best for this project, has resulted in the accomplishment of this book. They are a veteran in the field of academics and their pool of knowledge is as vast as their experience in printing. Their expertise and guidance has proved useful at every step. Their uncompromising quality standards have made this book an exceptional effort. Their encouragement from time to time has been an inspiration for everyone.

The publisher and the editorial board hope that this book will prove to be a valuable piece of knowledge for researchers, students, practitioners and scholars across the globe.

List of Contributors

Kirtikar Shukla, Pabitra Bikash Pal, Himangshu Sonowal, Satish K. Srivastava and Kota V. Ramana
Department of Biochemistry and Molecular Biology, University of Texas Medical Branch, Galveston, TX 77555, USA

Erick O. Hernández-Ochoa, Quinton Banks and Martin F. Schneider
Department of Biochemistry and Molecular Biology, University of Maryland School of Medicine, Baltimore, MD 21201, USA

Cristina Mega
Agrarian School of Viseu (ESAV), Polytechnic Institute of Viseu (IPV), 3500-606 Viseu, Portugal
Centre for the Study of Education, Technologies and Health (CI&DETS), Polytechnic Institute of Viseu (IPV), 3500-606 Viseu, Portugal
Institute of Pharmacology and Experimental Therapeutics and Institute for Biomedical Imaging and Life Sciences (IBILI), Faculty of Medicine, University of Coimbra, 3000-548 Coimbra, Portugal

Edite Teixeira-de-Lemos
Agrarian School of Viseu (ESAV), Polytechnic Institute of Viseu (IPV), 3500-606 Viseu, Portugal
Centre for the Study of Education, Technologies and Health (CI&DETS), Polytechnic Institute of Viseu (IPV), 3500-606 Viseu, Portugal

Rosa Fernandes and Flávio Reis
Institute of Pharmacology and Experimental Therapeutics and Institute for Biomedical Imaging and Life Sciences (IBILI), Faculty of Medicine, University of Coimbra, 3000-548 Coimbra, Portugal
CNC.IBILI Research Consortium, University of Coimbra, 3004-504 Coimbra, Portugal

Kei Takahashi, Hidetaka Nakamura, Hiroshi Sato, Kazuo Takada and Tomiko Tsuji
Department of Health and Nutrition, Faculty of Health and Human Life, Nagoya Bunri University, 365, Maeda, Inazawa-Cho, Inazawa City, Aichi, Japan

Hideto Matsuda
Department of Food and Nutrition, College of Nagoya Bunri University, 2-1, Sasazuka-Cho, Nishi-Ku, Nagoya, Aichi, Japan

Lixia Ji and Zhihong Yang
Department of Pharmacology, School of Pharmacy, Qingdao University, Qingdao, China

Lixia Cheng
Department of Endocrinology, People's Hospital of Weifang, Weifang, China

Guangwei Song, Da Lin, Licheng Bao, Qi Jiang, Yinan Zhang, Haihua Zheng and Qianying Gao
The Second Affiliated Hospital and Yuying Children's Hospital of Wenzhou Medical University, Wenzhou 325027, China
The Second School of Medicine, Wenzhou Medical University, Wenzhou 325027, China

Rie Oka
Department of Internal Medicine, Hokuriku Central Hospital, Kanazawa University Hospital, Kanazawa, Japan
Department of Cardiovascular and Internal Medicine, Kanazawa University Graduate School of Medicine, Kanazawa, Japan

Mitsuhiro Kometani, Masakazu Yamagishi and Takashi Yoneda
Department of Cardiovascular and Internal Medicine, Kanazawa University Graduate School of Medicine, Kanazawa, Japan

Kyoko Shibata and Kenichi Yoshimura
Department of Biostatistics, Innovative Clinical Research Center (iCREK), Kanazawa University Hospital, Kanazawa, Japan

Masaru Sakurai
Department of Social and Environmental Medicine, Kanazawa Medical University, Kanazawa, Japan

Kenneth N. Grisé, Matthew W. McDonald, Adwitia Dey, Mao Jiang and C.W. James Melling
Exercise Biochemistry Laboratory, School of Kinesiology, Faculty of Health Sciences, Western University, London, ON, Canada N6A 3K7

T. Dylan Olver
Neurovascular Research Laboratory, School of Kinesiology, Faculty of Health Sciences, Western University, London, ON, Canada N6A 3K7

James C. Lacefield
Department of Electrical and Computer Engineering, Department of Medical Biophysics and Robarts Research Institute, Western University, London, ON, Canada N6A 3K7

J. Kevin Shoemaker
Neurovascular Research Laboratory, School of Kinesiology, Faculty of Health Sciences, Western University, London, ON, Canada N6A 3K7
Department of Physiology and Pharmacology, Western University, London, ON, Canada N6A 3K7
Lawson Health Research Institute, London, ON, Canada N6C 2R5

Earl G. Noble
Exercise Biochemistry Laboratory, School of Kinesiology, Faculty of Health Sciences, Western University, London, ON, Canada N6A 3K7
Lawson Health Research Institute, London, ON, Canada N6C 2R5

Joshua A. David, William J. Rifkin, Piul S. Rabbani and Daniel J. Ceradini
Hansjörg Wyss Department of Plastic and Reconstructive Surgery, New York University School of Medicine, 430 East 29th Street, New York, NY 10016, USA

Anna Weiser, Pieter Giesbertz, Hannelore Daniel and Britta Spanier
Nutrition Physiology, Technische Universität München, Gregor-Mendel-Str. 2, 85350 Freising, Germany

Yang Wu, Yan Leng, Qingtao Meng, Rui Xue, Bo Zhao, Liying Zhan and Zhongyuan Xia
Department of Anesthesiology, Renmin Hospital of Wuhan University, Wuhan, Hubei Province 430060, China

Rina Su, Jie Yan and Huixia Yang
Department of Obstetrics and Gynecology, Peking University First Hospital, No. 8, Xishiku Street, XichengDistrict, Beijing 100034, China

Yoshiichi Takagi, Taichi Sugimoto, Masaya Kobayashi, Mitsuyuki Shirai and Fumitoshi Asai
Laboratory of Veterinary Pharmacology, School of Veterinary Medicine, Azabu University, Kanagawa, Japan

Xiangqun Deng
Department of Endocrinology, Wuhan Third Hospital, Wuhan University, Wuhan 430062, China

Min Xu, Moyu Shen and Jinluo Cheng
Department of Endocrinology, Changzhou No. 2 People's Hospital, Nanjing Medical University, Changzhou 213003, China

Fernanda Vacante, Pamela Senesi and Alice Frigerio
Metabolism Research Center, IRCCS Policlinico San Donato, San Donato Milanese, Milan, Italy

Livio Luzi
Metabolism Research Center, IRCCS Policlinico San Donato, San Donato Milanese, Milan, Italy
Department of Biomedical Sciences for Health, Università degli Studi di Milano, Milan, Italy

Anna Montesano and Ileana Terruzzi
Department of Biomedical Sciences for Health, Università degli Studi di Milano, Milan, Italy

Selim Fakhruddin, Wael Alanazi and Keith E. Jackson
Department of Basic Pharmaceutical Sciences, School of Pharmacy, University of Louisiana at Monroe (ULM), Pharmacy Building, 1800 Bienville Dr., Monroe, LA 71201, USA

Hidenori Hirukawa, Shinji Kamei, Tomohiko Kimura, Atsushi Obata, Kenji Kohara, Fuminori Tatsumi, Masashi Shimoda, Shuhei Nakanishi, Tomoatsu Mune, Kohei Kaku and Hideaki Kaneto
Department of Diabetes, Endocrinology and Metabolism, Kawasaki Medical School, Japan

Damilola D. Adingupu, Suvi E. Heinonen, Anne-Christine Andréasson, Mikael Brusberg, Andrea Ahnmark, Margareta Behrendt and Ann-Cathrine Jönsson-Rylander
CVMD iMED, AstraZeneca R&D, Gothenburg, Sweden

Brendan Leighton
The Research Network, Sandwich, UK

Kenji Matsuura
Faculty of Pharmacy, Osaka-Ohtani University, Tondabayashi 584-8540, Japan

Mieko Otani and Masaoki Takano
Department of Life Sciences Pharmacy, School of Pharmaceutical Sciences, Kobe Gakuin University, Kobe 650-8586, Japan

Keiichi Kadoyama
Department of Pharmaceutical Health Care, Faculty of Pharmaceutical Sciences, Himeji Dokkyo University, Himeji 670-8524, Japan

Shogo Matsuyama
Biosignal Research Center, Kobe University, Kobe 657-8501, Japan

Index

P

R

S

T

U

V

W

Z

www.ingramcontent.com/pod-product-compliance
Lightning Source LLC
LaVergne TN
LVHW060558210926
848485LV00005B/1339